Freed, recd.
2/3/81
complimentary copy

Virgil H. Freed

# ENVIRONMENTAL HEALTH CHEMISTRY

## The Chemistry of Environmental Agents as Potential Human Hazards

# ENVIRONMENTAL HEALTH CHEMISTRY

## The Chemistry of Environmental Agents as Potential Human Hazards

Edited by
James D. McKinney

ANN ARBOR SCIENCE
PUBLISHERS INC / THE BUTTERWORTH GROUP

230 Collingwood, P.O. Box 1425, Ann Arbor, Michigan 48106

Library of Congress Catalog Card Number 80-65510
ISBN 0-250-40352-8

Manufactured in the United States of America

# PREFACE

Society has only recently acknowledged that health problems can be derived from trace substances in our environment and that there is a need to prevent uncontrolled release of even small quantities of such substances into our environment. Environmental chemical agents can include elements and both natural and synthetic organic and inorganic compounds. However, the majority of chemicals in the biotic environment recognized to be hazardous are low- to medium-molecular-weight lipophilic organic compounds. The major reason for this is the rapidly rising research effort concerning synthetic organics, while that concerning inorganics has leveled off or possibly even diminished. The organic compounds are emphasized as a central theme and focus throughout this book, but the book is not limited to the organics, and this emphasis on organics does not reflect a lesser importance of inorganics as potential environmental human health hazards. On the contrary, it suggests the need for enhanced research effort in this area, particularly to enhance our understanding of the effects of toxic trace metals and their relevant species in the environment.

Although the "zero discharge philosophy" for controlling environmental agents represents an idealistic goal which could provide big payoffs in preventive medicine, *it seems impracticable on the basis of best available technology and perhaps even on the basis of best achievable technology*. Therefore, research in environmental health sciences must develop a knowledge base which recognizes that toxic trace substances are in the environment and are potential human health hazards.

It is clear that chemistry as a basic physical science has a very important role to play in the accomplishment of our mission in this area. The major divisions of environmental health sciences which are necessary to define a human health hazard are epidemiology, toxicology and chemistry. If one or more of these areas is lacking or incomplete in studies of environmental agents, then the health hazard potential cannot fully be assessed. Chemistry is essential in these relationships to provide timely and effective solutions to environmental health problems.

The interrelationships of the major divisions of environmental health sciences and the obvious areas of overlap are depicted in the drawing shown in Chapter 1. Environmental health chemistry is presented as a new subdiscipline that emphasizes the chemistry needed to establish these relationships and permit assessment of the potential human health hazards associated with chemical contamination of our environment. Although environmental analysis is recognized as a part of the overall environmental chemistry effort, it is identified separately because of its basic importance to environmental health research. Specifically, environmental health chemistry deals with the human exposure problem by developing, among other things, an understanding of the mechanisms, modes of action and body burdens of hazardous chemicals with an aim to prevent or reverse undesired biological effects in human populations.

Except Chapter 24, the material in this book came from the symposium program "Environmental Health Chemistry: The Chemistry of Environmental Agents as Potential Human Hazards," at the 178th National American Chemical Society Meeting, Washington, DC, September 1979. The book is organized to introduce the reader to environmental health chemistry and the role of the chemist in environmental health research (Section 1). This is followed by logical presentation of the more important, interactive and unifying chemistry aspects of solving potential health problems associated with exposure to environmental chemicals. This includes the identification of problems and methods in environmental analysis (Sections 1 and 2), biomechanism elucidation and toxicity prediction (Section 3), and toxicological testing aspects of the problem (Section 4). With regard to the toxicological testing of chemicals, the establishment of a National Toxicology Program (Chapter 25) is exemplary of the environmental health chemistry concept, since the chemistry aspects are essential in interrelating the various biological and toxicological aspects and providing for definitive and credible testing results.

It is hoped that this book will stimulate further interest, growth and development in the area. Ultimately, environmental health chemistry will be recognized in the environmental health sciences as a subdiscipline that facilitates and strengthens our ability to prevent and control environmentally related diseases.

One can conclude from the symposium and the book that we have many sophisticated methods and techniques for conducting effective and timely research in environmental health chemistry but that much still remains to be done. We have only begun to reap the benefits from merging specialties in this field of research endeavor.

James D. McKinney

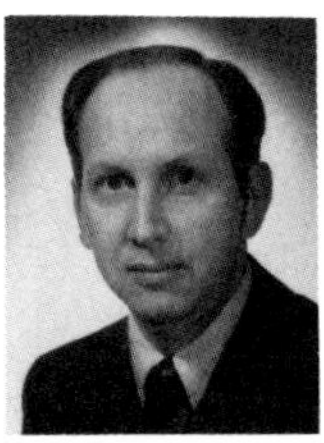

**James D. McKinney** is Chief of the Laboratory of Environmental Chemistry at the National Institute of Environmental Health Sciences (NIEHS), USPHS-DHHS, Research Triangle Park, North Carolina. He received his PhD in Organic Chemistry from the University of Georgia in 1968. Until 1969 he was a Commissioned Officer in the United States Public Health Service at the National Communicable Disease Center in Atlanta. Since joining NIEHS, he has been involved in diverse studies of the biologically significant chemistry of a variety of halogenated hydrocarbons including the chlorinated hydrocarbon pesticides of the polycyclodiene and DDT type, and the halogenated benzenes, naphthalenes, biphenyls, dibenzo-*p*-dioxins and dibenzofurans.

Dr. McKinney's work covers a range of approaches encompassing development of analytical chemical techniques, organic synthesis and metabolite identification and biomechanism elucidation using the tools of the bioorganic chemist. His work assessing the importance of structure-activity relationships in the toxicity of these compounds is widely accepted.

He has also organized and developed a nationally recognized program in environmental chemistry at NIEHS which utilizes intradisciplinary strategies in biology and chemistry aimed at solving environmental health problems. In recognition of these accomplishments, he received the NIH Directors Award in 1979. He has authored or co-authored numerous scientific publications in these areas, including 15 book chapters. Dr. McKinney has been an invited lecturer both nationally and internationally, served on numerous committees, as scientific consultant, as scientific journal editorial board member and reviewer and member of professional societies.

to

Dorothy, Peggy and Kristen

for their deep affection and unceasing inspiration

# CONTENTS

## Section 1
## Environmental Health Chemistry Perspectives



## Section 2
## Environmental Analysis

## Section 3
## Structure-Activity and Toxicity Prediction

**Section 4**
**Chemistry Aspects of Toxicological Testing**

# SECTION 1

# ENVIRONMENTAL HEALTH CHEMISTRY PERSPECTIVES

# CHAPTER 1

# ENVIRONMENTAL HEALTH CHEMISTRY–DEFINITIONS AND INTERRELATIONSHIPS: A CASE IN POINT

**James D. McKinney**

Laboratory of Environmental Chemistry
National Institutes of Environmental Health Sciences
Research Triangle Park, North Carolina

## INTRODUCTION

The mission of environmental health science is to perform and promote research to develop the knowledge base needed for preventive programs for environmentally related diseases in the broad environment and in the workplace. This includes basic research focused on the interaction between man and potentially toxic or harmful agents in his environment. It concentrates on recognizing, identifying and investigating environmental factors that may have deleterious effects on population groups, not just on individuals; on quantifying those effects; and on understanding the mechanisms of action of toxic agents in biological systems. In addition, this knowledge base permits assessment of the impact of environmental factors on human health, to aid those agencies charged with devising and instituting control or therapeutic measures. If the mission is to be accomplished, the knowledge base generated must be broad and complete enough to be immediately applicable to real environmental health problems. Once the hazard potential of toxic agents has been assessed for human populations, action by regulatory agencies can begin.

It is clear that chemistry as a basic physical science has a very important role to play in the accomplishment of this mission. In fact, research in environmental chemistry, particularly research on fate and distribution and predictive models, could provide big payoffs in preventive medicine. Diseases related to chemical environmental agents can be eliminated or substantially reduced if exposure to the causative chemicals can be prevented or minimized.

## ENVIRONMENTAL HEALTH CHEMISTRY

Environmental health chemistry deals with the exposure problem by developing an understanding of the mechanisms, modes of action and body burdens of hazardous chemicals with an aim to prevent or reverse undesired biological effects in human populations. It focuses on the chemistry needed to assess the potential human hazards associated with chemical contamination of the environment.

In the broad sense, environmental chemistry involves studies of the chemistry of foreign compounds and their mixtures present in the environment which result in deleterious effects on living organisms. Such environmental chemical agents can include elements and both natural and synthetic organic and inorganic compounds. However, the majority of chemicals in the biotic environment recognized to be hazardous are low- to medium-molecular weight lipophilic organic compounds. Environmental chemistry deals with the fate and distribution aspects of environmental pollution and the chemistry of ecosystems.

The major divisions of the environmental health sciences which are necessary to define a hazard are epidemiology, toxicology and chemistry. Because analysis is such an important part of environmental chemistry, it will be considered separately here. One or more of these areas is often lacking in studies of environmental agents; therefore, hazard potential cannot be assessed fully. Chemistry is essential in these relationships to provide timely and effective solutions to environmental health problems.

A schematic representation (Figure 1) can be drawn, depicting the interrelationships of the major divisions of environmental health science and the obvious areas of overlap. Epidemiology depends on the ability to identify and measure body burdens of environmental chemicals, and rests on the development of validated methods for deriving chemical data for correlation with biological effects data.

Analytical, organic, inorganic and physical chemistry are all important in the fate-and-distribution and structure-activity studies which make up environmental chemistry. It is of paramount importance to determine the

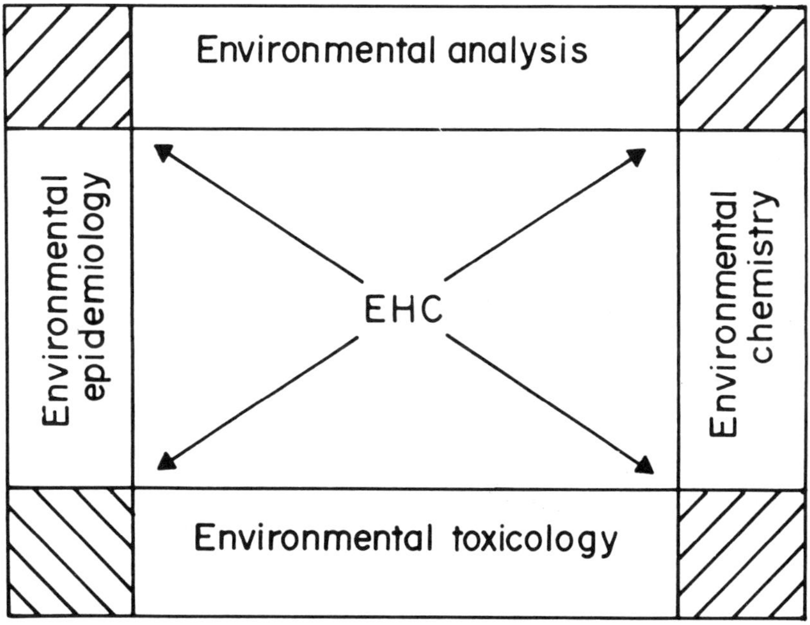


**Figure 1.** Interrelationships for major environmental health sciences.

exact nature and amounts of chemicals which reach man, whether they are the result of biological (e.g., microorganisms in soil and plants) or nonbiological (e.g., hydrolysis in the aquatic environment and photodegradation by sunlight) transformation processes. In such studies, a great deal is learned about the "chemical appearances" (e.g., stability and reactivity) of environmental chemicals, which is of value in structure-activity work and toxicity prediction.

Structure-activity work, in turn, is important to toxicology. Such work is of fundamental importance to understanding the mechanisms and modes of action of chemicals in biological systems. Prior knowledge of the structural requirements which elicit biological activity can be very useful in providing direction for further biological studies of related compounds, new compound design, synthesis for commercial uses and hazard prediction of associated contaminants of old and new products as they are discovered.

The relationship of environmental toxicology and environmental epidemiology is important in providing for the extrapolation of laboratory animal data to man. This interface has required relatively little chemistry input thus far. However, mathematical chemical approaches to toxicity prediction are becoming an increasingly active and important area of research. Considered all together, these activities embody environmental health chemistry.

## THE POLYCHLORINATED BIPHENYL PROBLEM

The history of polychlorinated biphenyls (PCB) use is a remarkable case in point of the continuing controversy of toxic substances in our environment and the public health [1,2]. The intent here is not to review the area of PCB research, but to trace the development of our attack on the PCB problem and the timing and sequence of events and involvement of various scientific disciplines (see Table I for summary). PCB are a complex mixture of chlorobiphenyl compounds with varying degrees and positions of chlorine substitution on the biphenyl nucleus. Of the 209 possible isomers and homologs, most are tetra- to hexa-substituted. However, many of these isomers do not occur at significant levels in commercial PCB mixtures such as the Aroclors®. The mixtures, of course, have been used extensively throughout the world as insulating and dielectric fluids.

The discovery of PCB as an environmental contaminant in 1966 in fish in the Baltic Sea set off the concentrated effort to examine the potential health effects of these compounds. PCB were first manufactured in the United States in 1929, and it was presumed that they were used primarily in closed systems. The complex nature of these mixtures, coupled with the fact that they have a complex fate and distribution in the environment which leads to

**Table I. Some History and Attack on the PCB Problem**

| |
|---|
| First manufactured in the U.S. in 1929 |
| Discovery in fish in Baltic Sea in 1966 |
| Identified as causative agent in "Yusho" disease in 1969 |
| Diverse toxicological studies focusing primarily on unused mixtures themselves |
| Synthesis and isolation of individual isomers and homologs of the PCB found in commercial mixtures |
| Diverse toxicological studies focusing on individual isomers and homologs |
| Discovery of qualitative and quantitative differences in biological activity and behavior for some of the individual isomers and homologs |
| Continued development and use of analytical and synthetic methods to support environmental studies |
| Recognition of associated contaminants in used mixtures and their complicating role in biological studies |
| Limited toxicological studies focusing on products of use conditions or transformation in the environment |
| Initiation of epidemiological studies investigating potential PCB exposure |

unrecognizable residue patterns, delayed their initial detection in the environment and has complicated attempts to control and regulate their continued use.

However, three years after being found in fish from the Baltic, they were identified as the causative agent in an outbreak of a disease in Japan now called "Yusho" or "oil" disease [2]. It is now known that this PCB problem derived from leakage of a heat-exchange fluid into rice oil is a much more complex problem, and not a simple PCB-exposure case. Chemical characterization[3] of this oil has shown that it contains several classes of chlorinated aromatic hydrocarbons, some in significantly increased concentrations (e.g., the chlorinated dibenzofurans) over that found in the original PCB mixture and other new ones (largely biphenyl dimers and trimers) in high concentrations.

The available evidence suggests that these changes are primarily the result of chemical transformations occurring under use conditions. Furthermore, it also appears that the products of use found in this heat exchange fluid are not the same as those found in a transformer fluid [4] where the original formulation as well as use conditions are different. The products of use of such commercial PCB mixtures are just now being realized for their potential as environmental contaminants derived from PCB. This, of course, has further complicated the regulatory problem.

Nevertheless, a great deal has been learned about the human health effects of PCB and related compounds from the "Yusho" disease. However, the studies that followed immediately afterwards were diverse toxicological studies with experimental animals, which focused primarily on the unused mixtures themselves with little understanding of the composition of those complex mixtures. Difficulty in interpreting and reproducing the data obtained from such studies led to increased efforts to chemically analyze and characterize the mixtures. This, in turn, led to the realization that to understand the toxicological findings, it would be necessary to study to some extent the individual components or at least individual classes of halogenated hydrocarbons normally found in the commercial mixtures. There was little concern at the time for the problem of other or similar compounds being formed under use conditions.

After some individual isomers and homologs of the PCB and associated contaminants, particularly the chlorinated dibenzofurans, became available from direct synthesis and were tested toxicologically, it was apparent that there were both qualitative and quantitative differences in the toxicopathology [1]. The differences were not only associated with the degree of chlorination but also with the position(s) of chlorination. This became especially clear in studies of symmetrical hexachlorobiphenyl (HCB) isomers in which the degree of chlorination remained constant and only the positional pattern was varied (as, for example, in 2,2′,3,3′,6,6′-HCB and 3,3′,4,4′,5,5′-HCB). Along with these types of studies came the discovery that certain non-*ortho*-substituted PCB (e.g., 3,3′,4,4′,5,5′-HCB) exhibited unusual toxicological properties presumably because of their ability to assume coplanar conformations and behave much like the planar chlorinated dibenzo-*p*-dioxins and dibenzofurans that are known to be highly toxic.

Such stereoelectronic properties of these compounds were also linked to lipophilicity and increased tissue levels. An underlying factor in the apparent symmetry requirement for high lipophilicity and toxicity for certain non-*ortho* PCB appears to be net polarizability of the molecule [5]. This property is thought to confer a noncovalent high-affinity binding to a specific bioreceptor. Diverse structure-activity studies of individual isomers and homologs have been much more illuminating with respect to mechanisms and mode of action of PCB. Structure-activity work is becoming increasingly important for understanding and predicting toxicity in environmental health chemistry.

In addition, metabolic pathways have been elucidated, some of which could have carcinogenic or mutagenic endpoints. The results of pharmacokinetic studies using labeled compounds were usually consistent with the toxicological data, and had predictive value. Again, studies of the symmetrical hexachlorobiphenyl isomers were particularly valuable in this regard. For example, 2,2′,3,3′,6,6′-HCB was the least toxic [6] and most rapidly metabolized [7] isomer studied. The nature of the metabolites strongly supports the intermediacy of an arene oxide as the predominant mechanism of PCB metabolism. Metabolism by direct insertion of a hydroxyl group is of importance only in the absence of vicinal (adjacent) unsubstituted carbon atoms, and is facilitated by the presence of unchlorinated *meta* positions. Oxidative metabolism can occur both with and without dechlorination (Figure 2).

Such studies have also helped delineate the role of covalent and noncovalent binding of PCB and their metabolites in affording toxic effects such as carcinogenesis. Formation of an arene oxide appears to be fundamental to the covalent binding process [8]. Non-*ortho* substitution with a high degree of *meta-para* substitution appears to be important for high affinity noncovalent binding [9]. There is an increasing body of evidence [10] that the PCB residues stored in the fat of humans in the general population are largely the *ortho*-substituted type, with high chlorine content, which are not eliminated or otherwise readily dealt with by any of these mechanisms. These isomers include the 2,2′,3,3′,5,5′- and 2,2′,4,4′,5,5′-HCB, which are neither rapidly metabolized nor particularly toxic on a short-term basis. It is the PCB which cannot be measured that may be of greater biological consequence. This suggest that measurement of such fatty stores of PCB is only an indirect measure of exposure to PCB and the potential for health effects. The exact

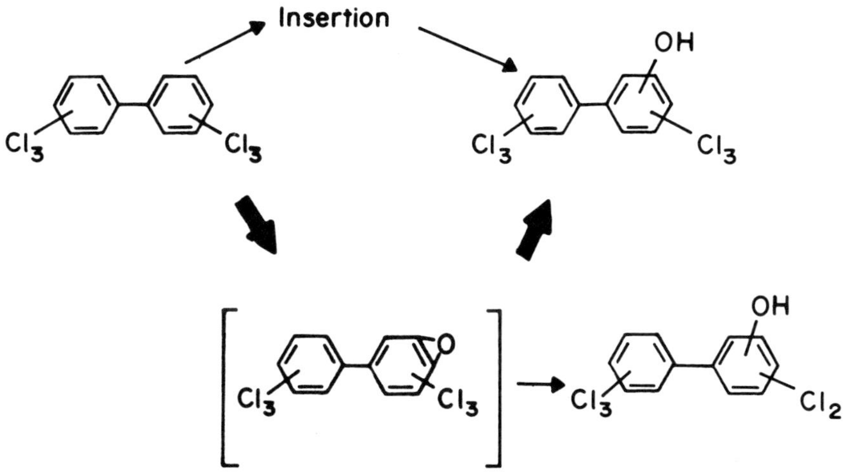


**Figure 2.** Major oxidative pathways for PCB.

nature, amount and effects of "bound" PCB residue in humans are not known at this time.

Analysis of PCB in environmental, including biological, samples continues and is still largely done using gas chromatography with electron capture detection (EC/GC). This method, although it can be reproducible, cannot provide absolute quantitation of PCB and is not definitive alone for specific isomers and homologs. More recent methods which rely on radioimmunoassay [11] and isotopic dilution techniques [12] offer some promise in this area. The radioisotope dilution assay overcomes the uncertainties in the estimation of total PCB by direct gas chromatography and eliminates the need for extreme measures to avoid handling losses. The radioimmunoassay method is able to provide information relative to the Aroclor product number, as well as to determine the concentration in the sample. All of these methods, however, depend on extractable (nonbound) residues for measurement.

The problem of PCB analysis illustrates the requirements of both sensitivity and specificity needed for analysis of environmental samples. Figure 3 illustrates the specific problem of analyzing for PCB in human milk by EC/GC. Although several peaks (particularly the ones numbered) appear to coincide with the standard, the pattern seen in milk is clearly different from the

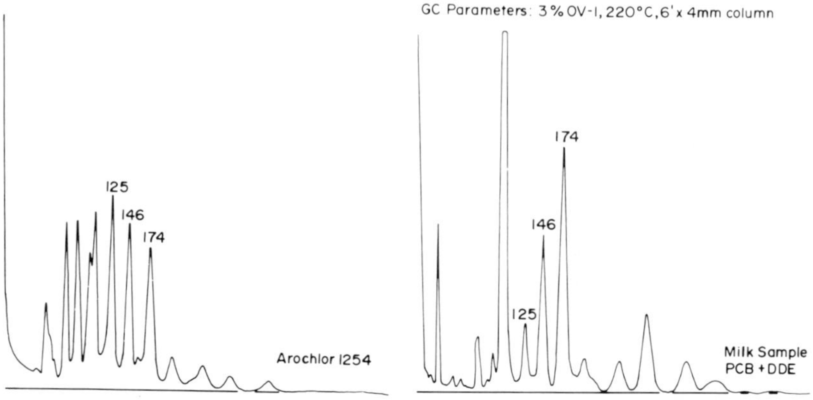


**Figure 3.** Comparison of gas chromatograms of PCB contained in standard mixture and human milk.

pattern from the standard. These peaks really cannot be compared, because each one likely contains more than one compound with varying responses to the detector. Therefore, there is no true standard for quantitation. The concentration is estimated assuming that some of these peaks are the same in both the milk and a commercial Aroclor standard mixture which seems to fit. The peak off scale is DDE, a ubiquitous metabolite and contaminant of DDT.

In developing analytical techniques, there are two very general questions that must be addressed [13]. The first is "What are appropriate levels of concern for toxic substances?" The second is "What are the restrictions to be placed on the methodology by the requirement that the screening procedures detect any unknown member of a broad class of toxic substances?" The first question can generally be answered as requiring nanogram ($10^{-9}$ g) detectability of quantities of toxic compounds in the presence of much larger quantities of biomolecules. A notable exception to this is the chlorinated dibenzo-*p*-dioxins which have required picogram ($10^{-12}$ g) detectability. The answer to the second question is much more difficult, but generally the requirement for screening imposes rather severe restrictions on sample cleanup procedures. The problems and approaches in this important and very difficult area of environmental analysis are just now being realized and fully appreciated.

Nevertheless, the problem of PCB and public health has come back to the analytical chemist to provide definitive analytical data for epidemiological purposes and to identify the more toxic components (including those formed during use and from environmental transformation) in the environment which reach the public. Table II classifies major compounds associated with the PCB problem that require different chemical and biological considerations in hazard assessment. Representative structures for these compounds are shown in Figure 4. Of course, such programs engage other chemists, such as the synthetic organic chemist who must synthesize compounds to be used as analytical standards and test compounds in animal experiments and develop model chemical reactions to simulate environmental transformation and use conditions.

Recent studies have sought to identify levels of these compounds in human milk, and a study is in progress that will attempt to correlate health effects in the developing infant with levels of PCB and related compounds measured in mother's milk. This study [14] has required the development of a method that will allow determination of total organic chlorine residues in body fluids and tissues, including both bound and unbound materials. Epidemiological studies of this type present many new and difficult problems. There are many unique chemistry problems in assessing chemical-derived disease problems such as this. Even if only the biphenyls associated with the PCB problem are considered, the toxicological picture is still not simple. The biphenyl problem can be possibly classified into two types (Figure 5): the non-*ortho* planar type and the *ortho* nonplanar type. In doing so, some common but yet some different pathways can be seen which might be operating in animals. Some processes are thought to be detoxifying and others are not.

**Table II. Classification and Occurrence of Compounds Associated with the PCB Problem**

| Compounds | In Commercial Mixtures | Product of Use or Transformation |
|---|---|---|
| PCB and Related Derivatives | | |
| *Non-ortho*-substituted with high *meta-para* substitution (Type I) | X | |
| *Ortho*-substituted | | |
| *Vicinal unsubstituted* carbon atoms absent (Type II) | X | |
| *Vicinal unsubstituted* carbon atoms present (Type III) | X | |
| Biphenyl dimers and trimers | | X[a] |
| Oxygenated Chlorinated Aromatic Compounds | | |
| Chlorinated dibenzofurans | X | X[a] |
| Chlorinated diphenylethers | | X[a] |
| Hydroxychlorinated biphenyls and related oxygen-containing compounds | | X[b] |

[a]This is based on preliminary data [4] from analysis of the used fluids as well as from analysis of model chemical reactions under simulated use conditions.
[b]Biological transformation.

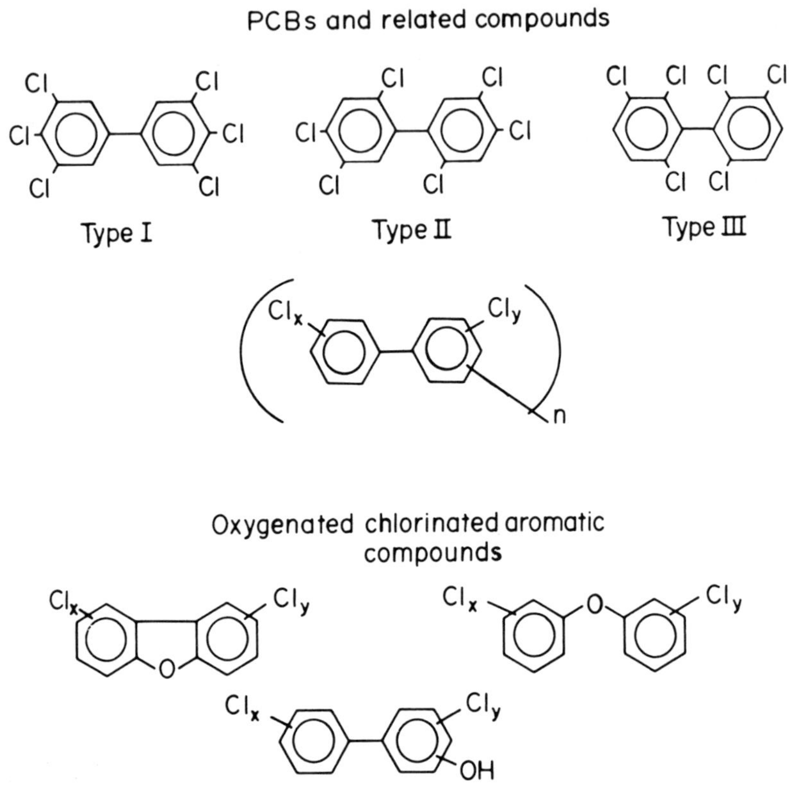


**Figure 4.** Structures of compounds associated with the PCB problem.

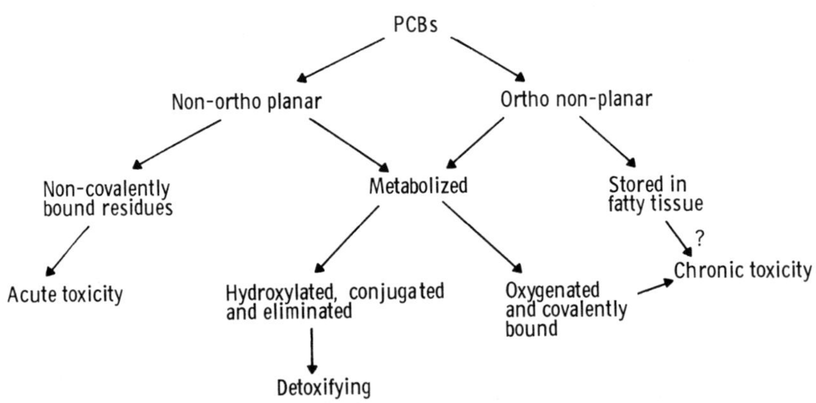


**Figure 5.** Fate of PCB in animals.

A great deal of research has been done on the PCB problem that is not particularly informative with respect to assessing the hazard potential of PCB. The lack of involvement of chemistry in the early stages of the toxicological work has been most alarming. If this work had been done in an interactive way using the environmental health chemistry approach described here, we would be better informed today about the PCB problem, in particular about the toxicological implications to humans of the compound classes presented in Table II. However, the current trend in toxicological testing is toward early and continued chemistry involvement, which is proving quite useful in meeting rapidly changing safety standards.

## CONCLUSIONS

In general, more attention should be paid to classification of environmental agents and subsequent study of the classes, much as we classify organic compounds according to similarities in structure and physicochemical properties. Furthermore, the sequence of investigative phases in toxicity evaluation and hazard assessment needs to be the most efficient and quickest possible. This includes the proper sequencing of the various chemistry aspects, including analytical methods development; identification and characterization of residues and components; synthesis of standards; and sturcture-activity work. In addition, the order of the various biological aspects is also important, which includes pharmacokinetic and metabolism studies; diverse toxicological studies which assess both short- and long-term effects; and epidemiological studies which can rely on pattern recognition established in the previous work. Thus, chemistry plays an underlying role in tying together these environmental health sciences. It is primarily these necessary interrelationships which define the area of environmental health chemistry. These relationships are described in greater detail in Chapter 2.

## REFERENCES

1. "General Summary and Conclusions of DHEW Subcommittee on Health Effects of PCBs and PBBs" *Environ. Health Persp.* 24:191-198 (1978).
2. *Proceedings of National Conference on PCBs,* U.S. EPA, Publication EPA-560/6-75-004 (1976).
3. McKinney, J. D., Laboratory of Environmental Chemistry, National Institute of Environmental Health Sciences. Unpublished observations (1978).

4. Albro, P. W., C. Parker and J. Corbett. "General Approach to the Fractionation and Class Determination of Complex Mixtures of Chlorinated Aromatic Hydrocarbons," *J. Chromatog.* (in press).
5. McKinney, J. D., P. Singh, L. Levy, and M. Walker. High Toxicity and Cocarcinogenic Potential of Certain Halogenated Aromatic Hydrocarbons," in *Safe Handling of Chemical Carcinogens, Mutagens and Teratogens and Highly Toxic Substances,* D. Walters, (Ann Arbor, MI: Ann Arbor Science Publishers, Inc., 1980).
6. McKinney, J. D., K. Chae, B. N. Gupta, J. A. Moore and J. A. Goldstein. "Toxicological Assessment of Hexachlorobiphenyl Isomers and 2,3,7,8-Tetrachlorodibenzofuran in Chicks. I. Relationship of Chemical Parameters," *Toxicol. Appl. Pharmacol.* 36:65-80 (1976).
7. Kato, S., J. D. McKinney and H. B. Matthews. "Metabolism of Symmetrical Hexachlorobiphenyl Isomers in the Rat," *Toxicol. Appl. Pharmacol.* 53:389-398 (1980).
8. Morales, N. M., and H. B. Matthews. "*In Vivo* Binding of 2,3,6,2′,3′,6′-Hexachlorobiphenyl and 2,4,5,2′,4′,5′-Hexachlorobiphenyl to Mouse Liver Macromolecules," *Chem.-Biol. Interact.* 27:99-110 (1979).
9. Poland, A., and E. Glover "Chlorinated Biphenyl Induction of Aryl Hydrocarbon Hydroxylase Activity: A Study of the Structure-Activity Relationship," *Mol. Pharmacol.* 13:924-937 (1977).
10. Nakamura, A., and T. Kashimoto. "Studies on a Calculation Method for Polychlorinated Biphenyl (PCB) Isomers," *Food Hygienic Soc. Japan* 18 (3):1-12 (1977).
11. Luster, M., P. Albro, G. Clark, K. Chae, S. Chaudhary, L. Lawson, J. Corbett and J. McKinney. "Production and Characterization of Antisera Specific for Chlorinated Biphenyl Species: Initiation of a Radioimmunoassay for Aroclors®," *Toxicol. Appl. Pharmacol.* 50:147-155 (1979).
12. Kohli, K. K., P. W. Albro and J. McKinney. "Radioisotope Dilution Assay (RIDA) for the Estimation of Polychlorinated Biphenyls (PCBs)," *J. Anal. Toxicol.* 3:125-128 (1979).
13. Dougherty, R. C., and E. A. Hett. "Negative Chemical Ionization Mass Spectrometry: Applications in Environmental Analytical Chemistry," in *Pentachlorophenol*, K. Ranga Rao, Ed. (New York: Plenum Publishing Corporation, (1978), pp. 339-350.
14. Fawkes, J., D. B. Walters, and J. D. McKinney. "Neutron Activation Analysis of Organically Bound Chlorine. Precautions to Minimize Extraneous Halide Contamination in Collection, Storage and Analysis of Human Milk and Formula," paper presented at the National Institute of Environmental Health Sciences Science Seminar, June 1, 1979; abstract published in *Environ. Health Persp.* 33:347 (1979).

# CHAPTER 2

# ENVIRONMENTAL AND TOXICOLOGICAL CHEMISTRY AT THE UNIVERSITY OF AMSTERDAM: FIVE YEARS OF PHILOSOPHY AND PRACTICE OF ENVIRONMENTAL HEALTH CHEMISTRY

**O. Hutzinger**

Laboratory of Environmental and Toxicological Chemistry
University of Amsterdam
Amsterdam, The Netherlands

## INTRODUCTION

In technologically advanced countries, increasing use of potentially toxic chemicals poses the threat of exposure and subsequent effects for humans and other organisms in the environment. Chemical and toxicological aspects of these problems have been studied for some time by industrial and government laboratories and, in academic institutions, in departments dealing with specific topics such as pesticide chemistry, wastewater technology, air chemistry, industrial hygiene and analytical chemistry. In the last few years a tendency toward integrated approaches is noticeable, and interdepartmental and multidisciplinary "environmental institutes" at universities are now common, some of them indeed having long and successful traditions.

The training of students in a new interdisciplinary field such as environmental chemistry is a challenge both on an undergraduate and graduate level [1,2], and four possible ways of training graduate environmental chemists have been proposed [1]:

1. The environmental chemist should take a traditional graduate degree in chemistry, and any necessary aspects of environmental science should be gained as job experience.
2. The environmental chemist should take a graduate chemistry degree within a program that provides courses, seminars and research relating to the chemistry of the environment. No emphasis should be placed on disciplines other than chemistry.
3. The environmental chemist should take a graduate chemistry degree within an interdisciplinary program that provides course and research opportunities relating to disciplines other than chemistry.
4. Training should be gained within a multidisciplinary program of environmental science. Balanced emphasis should be placed on all disciplines, and expertise in chemistry should be gained by specialization in this area.

Relatively few environmental chemistry laboratories in the strict sense of the word operate in universities, and little information is available on their programs, philosophies and success, although attention is being given to the subject [3].

Environmental Health research and training at U.S. universities has recently been assessed [4]. In 157 college and university programs, the number of people completing graduate studies in environmental health specialities at the master's, doctoral and postdoctoral levels have doubled in the period from 1967 to 1976. The environmental health specialty areas surveyed are:

| | |
|---|---|
| Air Pollution | Cancer Research |
| Water Pollution | Epidemiology |
| Soil Pollution | Environmental Physiology |
| Solid Wastes | Occupational Health |
| Pesticides | Ergonomics |
| Food | Accidental Injury |
| Radiation Protection | Multidisciplinary Training |
| Toxicology | |

Of the students completing doctoral programs, 76% were in water pollution, toxicology, radiation protection, air pollution and cancer research; 61% of those completing postdoctoral programs were in cancer research and toxicology.

In this chapter, the concept of "environmental health chemistry" as practiced at the Laboratory of Environmental and Toxicological Chemistry in the University of Amsterdam will be outlined.

The laboratory is multidisciplinary, with emphasis on chemistry; it is wholly within the faculty of chemistry and it developed alongside the classical disciplines such as organic, inorganic, analytical, physical and biochemistry. After five years of operation an attempt will now be made to assess the advantages and shortcomings of such an arrangement for environmental health chemistry. A short description of the Dutch University system can be found in Karasek and Hutzinger [5].

## PHILOSOPHY OF ENVIRONMENTAL HEALTH CHEMISTRY

### Chemicals and Health

We live in a chemical environment. The air we breathe, the food we eat and the soil on which plants grow are composed of chemicals. Chemicals are involved in the growth, life and decay of organisms. Many chemicals that occur in the environment are necessary and useful for life, or at least insignificant in the concentrations commonly available. Some chemical compounds of both natural and synthetic origin, however, have deleterious effects on life processes.

For the sake of philosophical argument we may, then, distinguish three types of chemicals as far as health is concerned:

1. chemicals which are, in varying concentrations, necessary for certain life processes (e.g., vitamins, essential elements and amino acids)
2. chemicals which have no noticeable effect on life (they are neither harmful nor necessary for life, e.g., argon, cellulose and granite) or which can be substituted easily by other chemicals (e.g., certain amino acids and carbohydrates).
3. chemicals which have an undesirable effect on some or all forms of life [they are toxic; e.g., mercury, lead and 2,3,7,8-tetrachlorodibenzo-*p*-dioxin (TCDD)].

This classification is useful as a first approximation, but is an oversimplification, particularly with respect to dose-response relationships. Many essential chemicals are toxic at high concentrations (e.g., copper, selenium, vitamin D and tryptophane). Figure 1 places these relationships in proper perspective.

Only compounds which show negative (toxic) effects are of interest in the "health-oriented" subject of environmental health chemistry and, depending on the chosen scope, only effects on humans (toxic effects on humans) or effects on all organisms in the environment (ecotoxicology) are of prime importance.

In recent years the greatest concern about health effects of chemicals is undoubtedly their possible carcinogenic potential. A large percentage of human cancers are said to be caused by environmental influences, largely chemicals [6]; with cancer being the second leading cause of death in all developed countries (Table I) the concern is understandable. Work on the source, environmental behavior, metabolism and mechanism of action of (potentially) carcinogenic compounds has therefore become one of the main topics in environmental health chemistry.

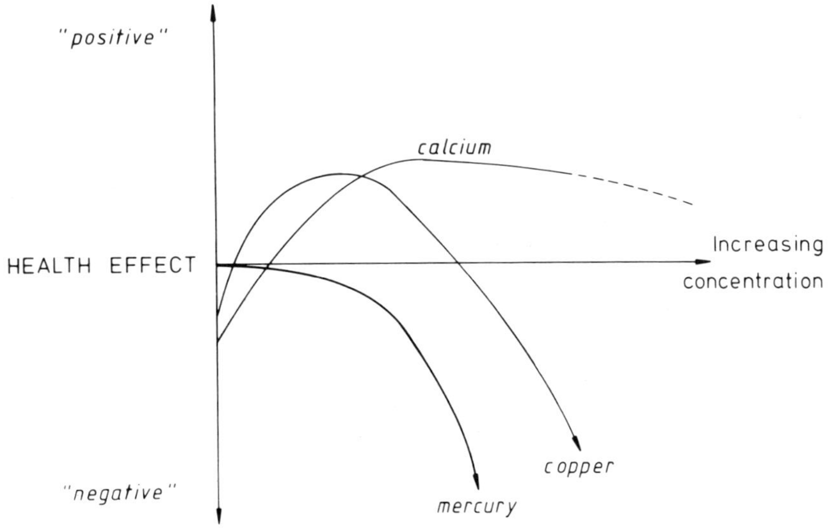


**Figure 1.** Schematic of the relationship between amount (dose) of several chemical species and effect on organisms. Mercury is toxic at all concentrations above a certain threshold value; copper is essential for this hypothetical organism but becomes toxic at higher concentrations, whereas calcium has no negative effects over a much wider concentration range.

**Table I. Major Causes of Death in the United States in 1975 [7]**

| Cause of Death | Number |
|---|---|
| Disease of the Heart and Circulatory System | 980,000 |
| Cancer | 370,000 |
| Infective and Parasitic Diseases | 72,000 |
| Diabetes | 36,000 |
| Respiratory Diseases | 26,000 |
| Birth Injury | 15,000 |
| Gastrointestinal Diseases | 14,000 |
| All Other Diseases | 210,000 |

## Environmental Health Chemistry: The Background

Humans (as an example of an organism) are constantly exposed to a multitude of chemicals. They enter the human body normally by three routes: oral (eating, drinking), by inhalation (via the lungs by breathing) and dermal (via the skin). The most important sources of chemicals to enter the human body are depicted in Figure 2. More than 95% of "foreign" or potentially hazardous chemicals are taken up from food (the average intake of food is about 2-3 lb/person/day). Drinking water contains only small quantities of chemicals. In some instances, however, hazardous products are present. The average daily intake is 1-2 qt/person.

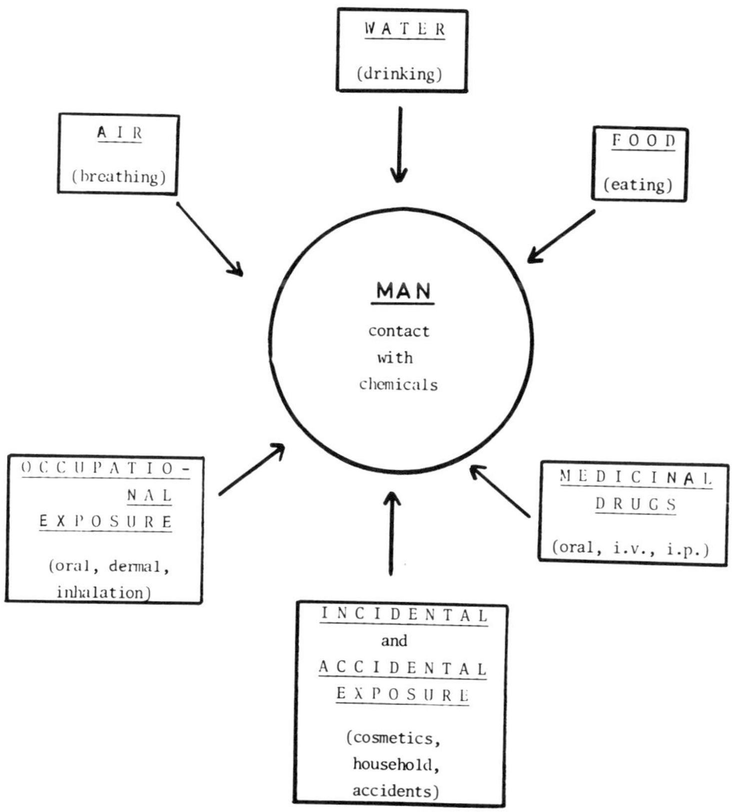


**Figure 2.** Routes of exposure and origin of chemicals to enter the human body.

Occupational exposure involves inhalation of vapors and dusts and, often, exposure to chemicals through the skin (e.g., cleaning fluids and solvents). The concentration of chemicals in air is low, even in heavily polluted areas. Uptake by the lung, however, is very efficient, and the lung itself is a very sensitive organ. The lungs of an average person move 20 $m^3$ air/day.

The intake of medicinal drugs is strictly controlled; however, many active drugs are extremely potent compounds with a potential for toxicity and side effects. Accidental and incidental exposure refers to (household) accidents, poisonings, contact with chemicals through cosmetics and exposures such as babies with chemically treated (flameproofed) sleepwear.

Strictly speaking, environmental exposure is only from air, water and, to a large extent, food. Direct contact by medicinal drugs is the subject of pharmacology, and exposure to chemicals at the workplace is dealt within the occupational health sciences. In the latter case, however, the compounds of concern are often identical (e.g., chlorinated compounds, asbestos, polycyclic hydrocarbons and heavy metals) to those of environmental concern, and an overlap of interest is inevitable. Poison centers have dealt with most of the problems of accidental exposure but, similarly, chemicals and mechanisms of exposure are often involved which are important also in the occupational and environmental areas (pesticides).

The relation of environmental exposure to other types of exposure as far as concentration, route and freedom of intake is concerned is shown in Table II. Whereas the toxicological concern in environmental health chemistry is the same as in pharmacology and occupational health, the distinguishing feature is the necessary involvement of the environment. In environmental health chemistry, three factors are involved: (1) the health of an organism (humans), (2) toxic (potentially) chemical compounds, and (3) the environment (Figure 3). The contact (exposure) of the organisms with the chemical has to be via the environment. It is therefore essential to understand the forces, processes and cycles which are characteristic for and operate in our environment.

**Table II. Comparison of Different Exposures to Chemicals**

| Agent | Concentration of Intake | Route of Intake | Freedom of Intake |
|---|---|---|---|
| Drugs | High | Direct | High |
| Chemicals at the workplace | Medium | Shortpath | Medium |
| Environmental Chemicals (via food, water or air) | Low | Often Very Indirect | Low |

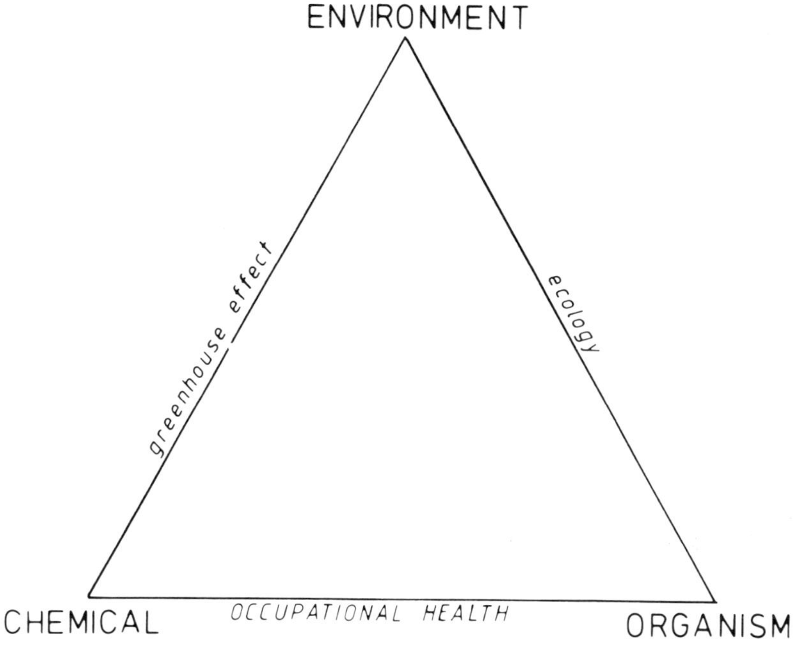


**Figure 3.** The essential features of environmental health chemistry. The organism that is affected, the environment that is the medium of exposure and the chemical compound that causes the toxic effect. Examples of effects or areas of study where one of the three factors is missing are outlined also.

## Environmental Health Chemistry: The Subject

Studies on the behavior and fate of chemicals in the environment and organisms, and the chemical mechanisms of toxic action are the most important topics in environmental health chemistry.

In the relationship:

$$\text{Chemical Compound} \longrightarrow \text{Biological Effect}$$

a number of factors are important: (1) from the point of view of response by the organisms, the "classical" parameters such as type of organism, species, sex, age, route of exposure etc.; and (2) on a molecular and mechanistic level, the amount and chemical identities of toxicant which becomes available at the "receptor site" for toxic action (e.g., nervous system, liver and DNA). This depends on the type of chemical (an intrinsic structure property of the molecule), on the dose (exposure concentration) and on the behavior (fate) of the compound in the organism in question, thus the pharmacokinetic properties—uptake, distribution, metabolism and excretion (Figure 4):

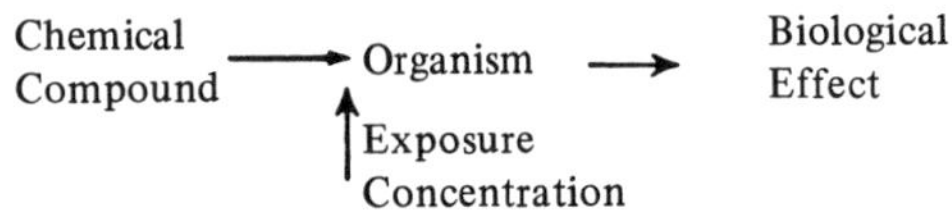


The exposure concentration (dose) for the target organism is easy to assess for medicinal drugs (a certain quantity is swallowed or injected) and even for occupational exposure where a relatively straightforward exposure, for instance, through inhalation of relatively steady concentrations of harmful vapors, can be monitored.

With environmental contaminants, the situation is more complicated because the environment is "between" the point of release and point of contact, i.e., these two events are separated in time and space.

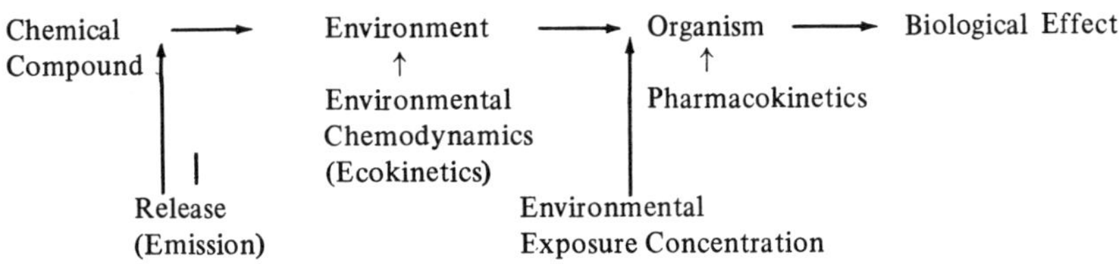


The type of compound and the environmental exposure concentration (the "what and how much" of a chemical compound that is available for contact with the organism) depends largely on what happened to the compound in the environment before contact with the organism.

It has been suggested to consider the environment as a complex super-organism in which chemicals behave—in analogy with pharmacokinetics—according to the principles of "ecokinetics" or "environmental chemodynamics" [8-13] (Figure 5). A compound may enter the environment in specific amounts and be transported and/or transformed to other structures by biological or (photo)chemical action. The compound or its transformation product(s), depending on their distribution and fate in air, water, soil or sediment, may become available for different organisms in various environmental subcompartments at different concentrations depending on their environmental behavior. Very volatile compounds, for example, will not be available to fish in high concentrations, and the same is true for compounds that are biodegraded rapidly. Compounds that adsorb strongly to sediment or have very low solubility in water, again, will not be found in high concentrations in water, but may become available at low concentrations over prolonged periods of time from the "reservoir" sediment.

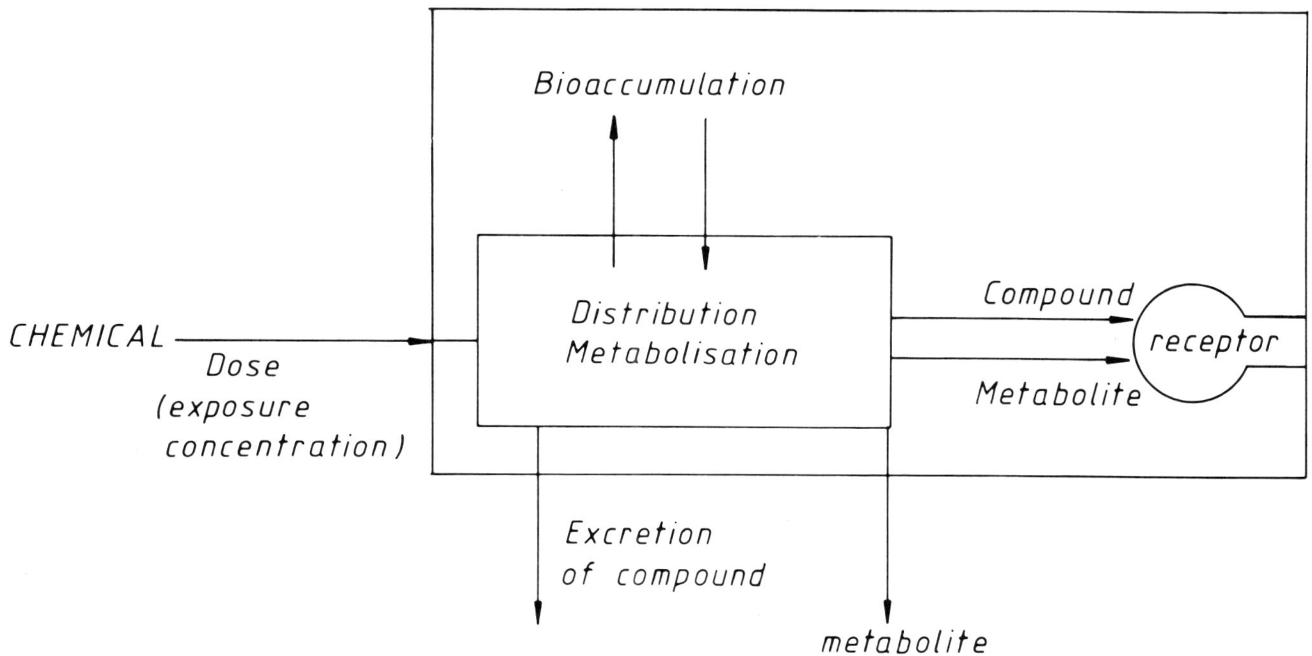


**Figure 4.** Schematic representation of pharmacokinetic properties of a chemical compound. The rectangle represents "an organism."

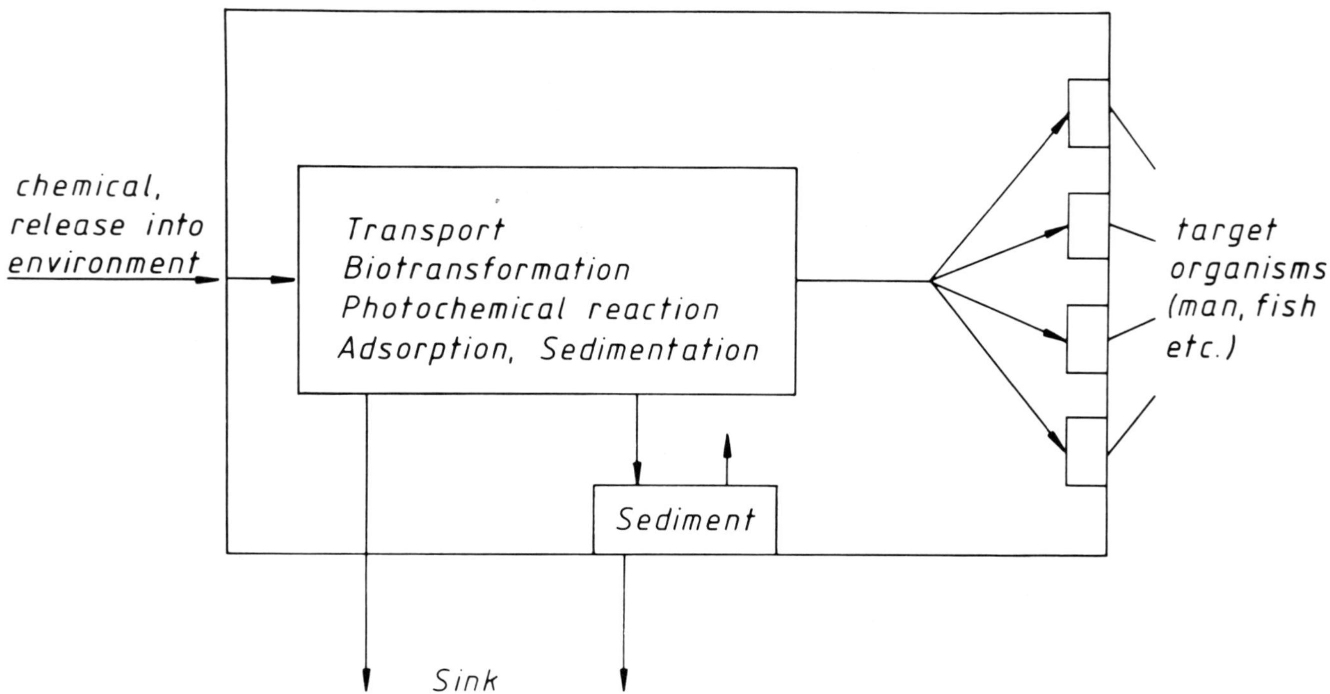


**Figure 5.** Schematic representation of ecokinetic properties of a chemical. The outer rectangle represents "the environment."

The amount of compound (toxicant) that becomes available to the organism (the dose) in a particular environmental subcompartment thus depends on the rate of release into the environment, the rate of disappearance in sinks and factors such as dispersion behavior, transport and bioaccumulation.

The two main mechanisms of removal of a compound from the environment are (1) biodegradation, which is actual disappearance of the compound from the environment, and which ideally is conversion to carbon dioxide, water and mineral elements, or at least to some other harmless substances, and (2) sedimentation and irreversible adsorption. These mechanisms remove the compound from circulation and thus effectively from the environment. A complicating factor arises through formation of metabolites or other transformation products which are pollutants in their own right (e.g., DDT → DDE).

The most important tasks of environmental health chemistry can now be summarized in schematic form and compared to related disciplines (Figure 6).

## Environmental Fate of Chemicals

Several groups of widely used chemicals such as medicinal drugs, pesticides and chemicals added to food and feed have been subject to government regulations for some time, and tests for acute and chronic toxicity have been common practice for these products.

For the types of compounds mentioned above, only human toxicity data are required, except for pesticides, where tests on environmental fate and effects on species in the environment are also required.

The Toxic Substances Control Act (TSCA) in the United States, and related laws in other countries [12] require extensive testing of large quantities of chemicals not only in the traditional toxicological disciplines but also as far as environmental fate is concerned. In this respect, these laws designed to minimize the risk from toxic chemicals have stimulated work and development of philosophies in environmental health chemistry tremendously. In environmental fate testing one considers what the environment does to the chemical (pollutant), rather than what effects the chemical (pollutant) has on components in the environment (Figure 7).

Chemicals in the environment are subjected to a complex interplay of forces which determine the occurrence, chemical species and concentration of substances, this concentration in an environmental subcompartment, often called the environmental pollutant concentration or environmental exposure concentration (available dose) can be used in combination with toxicity tests to assess the overall risk to different organisms, including humans.

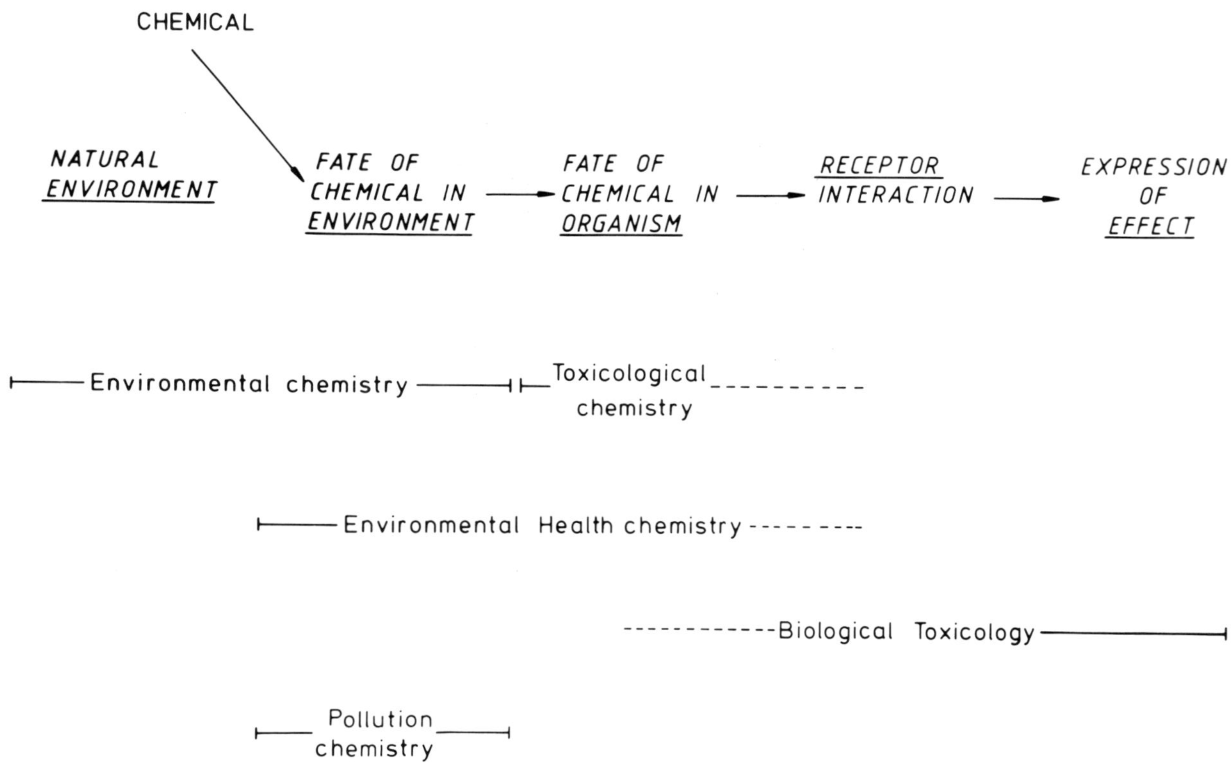


**Figure 6.** The subject of environmental health chemistry compared with related disciplines.

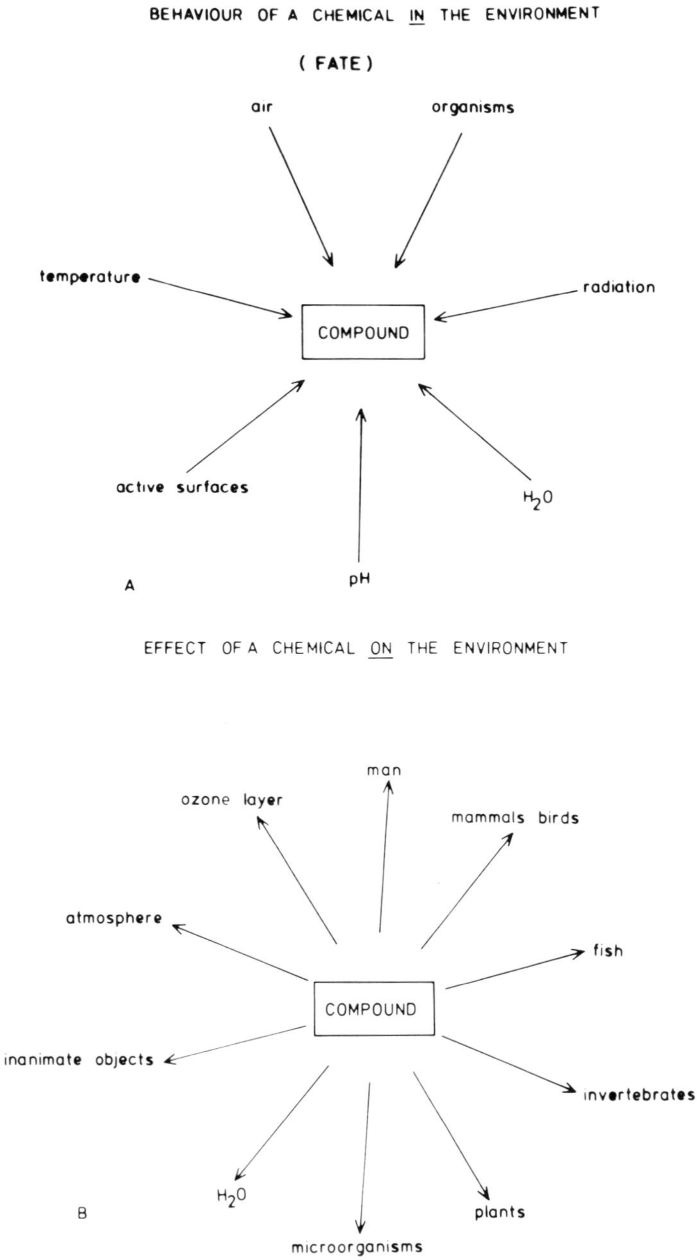


**Figure 7.** Representation of (A) fate of chemical in the environment (effect of environmental forces on the chemical); and (B) effect of the chemical on components in the environment.

The physical distribution can take place within the main environmental compartments or across the soil/water, sediment/water, water/air and air/soil interface. Transport of chemicals usually follows natural movements and cycles.

Transformations (structural change, reactions) of chemicals in the environment occur under the influence of:

- various chemical species (acids, bases, nucleophiles, radicals)
- the ultraviolet (UV) component of the sun's radiation (wavelengths equal to 300 nm or greater)
- action of enzymes (mainly microbial metabolism)

Conceptually it is convenient to describe transport and transformation as processes which occur separately, although in reality they happen concurrently (Table III).

**Table III. Transport and Transformation of Chemicals in the Environment**

**Chemical Compound**

| **Transport** | **Transformation** |
|---|---|
| air<br>water<br>soil<br>biota (food web) | air<br>water<br>soil |
| Transport between compartments while structure of chemical compounds remains unchanged<br>Important physicochemical properties for transport are:<br>Solubility in water<br>Partition Coefficient<br>Adsorptivity<br>Volatility | Change of the chemical compound's structure:<br>Chemical reactions<br>Photochemical reactions<br>Enzymatic reactions<br>(Microorganisms) |

## ENVIRONMENTAL FATE TESTING

Testing for environmental fate, like testing for other properties of chemicals, such as toxicity, is usually done in a so-called tier-system in which one proceeds from simple to more complex tests. The simple laboratory tests are generally relatively easy to set up in a university laboratory, and because of their value in teaching students the concept of environmental fate, the most important principles will be described. Often a difference is made between molecular properties (e.g., water solubility) and rate constants (e.g., hydrolysis of an ester at a specific pH). The outline in Table IV lists the most important physical constants and rates to be measured and tests to be done, as well as their relation to environmental fate.

**Table IV. Laboratory Tests for Environmental Fate and Their Importance for Environmental Processes**

| Measurement in Laboratory | Related to Environmental Behavior |
|---|---|
| *Physicochemical Parameters* (chemical mobility testing) | |
| Adsorptivity | Association with particulate matter in air, soil and sediment |
| Solubility in water | Mobility in aquatic environment, degree of adsorption and leaching |
| Vaporization behavior | Atmospheric mobility, rate of vaporization |
| Partition coefficient | Potential for bioaccumulation, adsorption by organic matter |
| *Chemical Reactivity* (chemical persistence testing) | Persistence in the environment |
| Hydrolysis | |
| Oxidation | |
| Photoreactivity | |
| *Biological Tests* | |
| Biodegradation | Persistence in the environment |
| Bioaccumulation | Bioaccumulation potential, food-web effects |

## Adsorption [14-17]

Adsorption (sorption) of chemicals from water to biotic and abiotic solids is probably the most important process which affects transport, degradation and bioavailability. Sorption, which reduces the concentration of a chemical in water, occurs by a number of mechanisms, depending on the nature of the chemical and adsorbent. For ions or insoluble organic chemicals, ion exchange and hydrophobic bonding, respectively, are most important. Sorption of chemicals by sediment and biota has been extensively studied and the following observations can be made [15].

1. Sorption of highly insoluble organics by sediments and microorganisms is rapid (that is, substantially complete in less than a few hours).
2. Sorption of highly insoluble organics by sediments and microorganisms is rapidly reversible.
3. Sediment sorption is strongest with the finer particle size fractions in the case of both cation and hydrophobic organics.
4. Unless cation exchange is involved, the most insoluble compounds are usually the most strongly sorbed or most highly accumulated.
5. Organic cations are likely to be strongly sorbed.

Measurements of adsorptive properties of a compound can be described by adsorption isotherms which give the relation between concentration of the chemical in the aqueous phase ($C_w$) and the concentration on the adsorbent ($C_s$) at equilibrium expressed in grams per liter and grams per gram.

The Freundlich adsorption isotherm is an empirical equation which gives the most general description of a variety of relationships:

$$C_s = K.C^n \text{ or } \log C_s = \log K + n \log C_w$$

K (or log K) and n are the important parameters of adsorption strength and shape of the curve. By the double-log plots of the measured equilibrium concentrations, the actual values of n and log K can be determined: n being the slope and log K the intercept of the line (Figure 8). For lipophilic compounds, n approaches unity, i.e., the amount adsorbed is then proportional to the water concentration. The adsorptive properties of lipophilics depend strongly on the organic content of the adsorbent [18,19] (Figure 9).

Leaching (desorption) tests are usually performed to study the behavior of chemicals (often pesticides) in soils, and are frequently accomplished by soil thin layer chromatography (TLC) or soil column techniques. In soil TLC, in analogy to conventional chromatography, compounds are chromatographed on TLC plates made from soil with water as the eluent. Soil column techniques have the advantages of being applicable to volatile compounds and being performed under more natural conditions (intact soil cores, long irrigation times).

Although lipophilic compounds strongly adsorb on microorganisms, biosorption is not an important environmental fate because the proportion of bacteria to other materials (clays, detritus, humic substances) in natural waters is usually very low (e.g., in an oligotrophic lake $10^{-7}$ - $10^{-6}$ and even in an eutrophic lake only $10^{-5}$). Even if biosorption is not an important fate from a quantitative viewpoint, it is significant because biosorption is often the first step to biomagnification, and should therefore be measured.

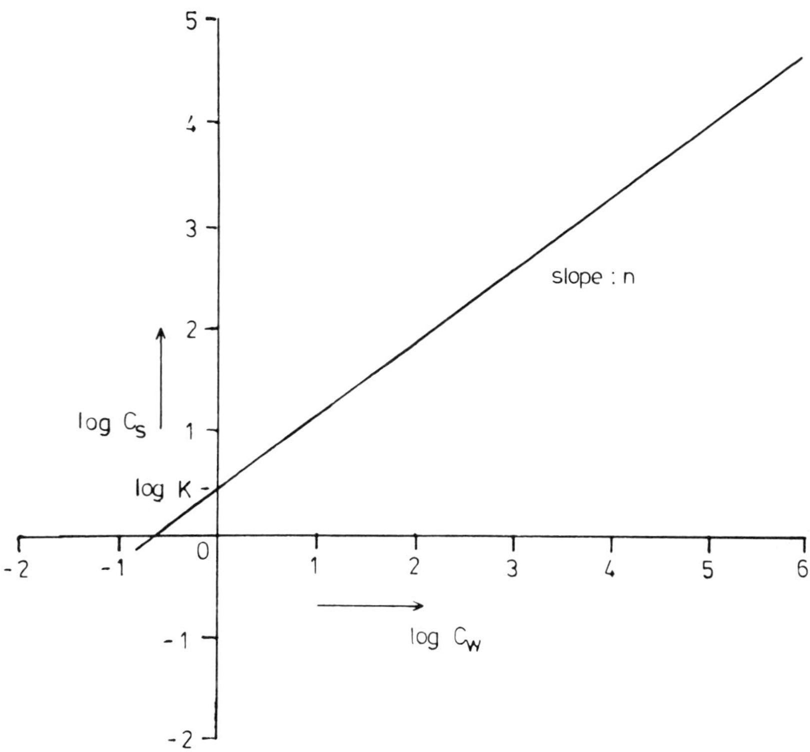


**Figure 8.** Typical Freundlich adsorption isotherm $C_s$ = concentration on the adsorbent; $C_w$ = concentration in the water; $0 < n \leqslant 1$. $C_s = K C_w^n$ or $\log C_s = n \log C_w + \log K$.

## Water Solubility [14,16,20-23]

The degree of water solubility often determines the ultimate fate of a substance in the environment. Water-soluble substances are generally more widely distributed than insoluble materials, and are more readily available for possible biodegradation by microorganisms. Many chemicals of environmental concern have a hydrophobic character and solubilities in the parts-per-billion range. This makes their exact determination difficult because it is often impossible to distinguish between true solutions in water and suspensions, micellar aggregates or colloidal systems. For these compounds, long-term equilibration or the loaded-column method are probably the most reliable experimental methods for the determination of aqueous solubility.

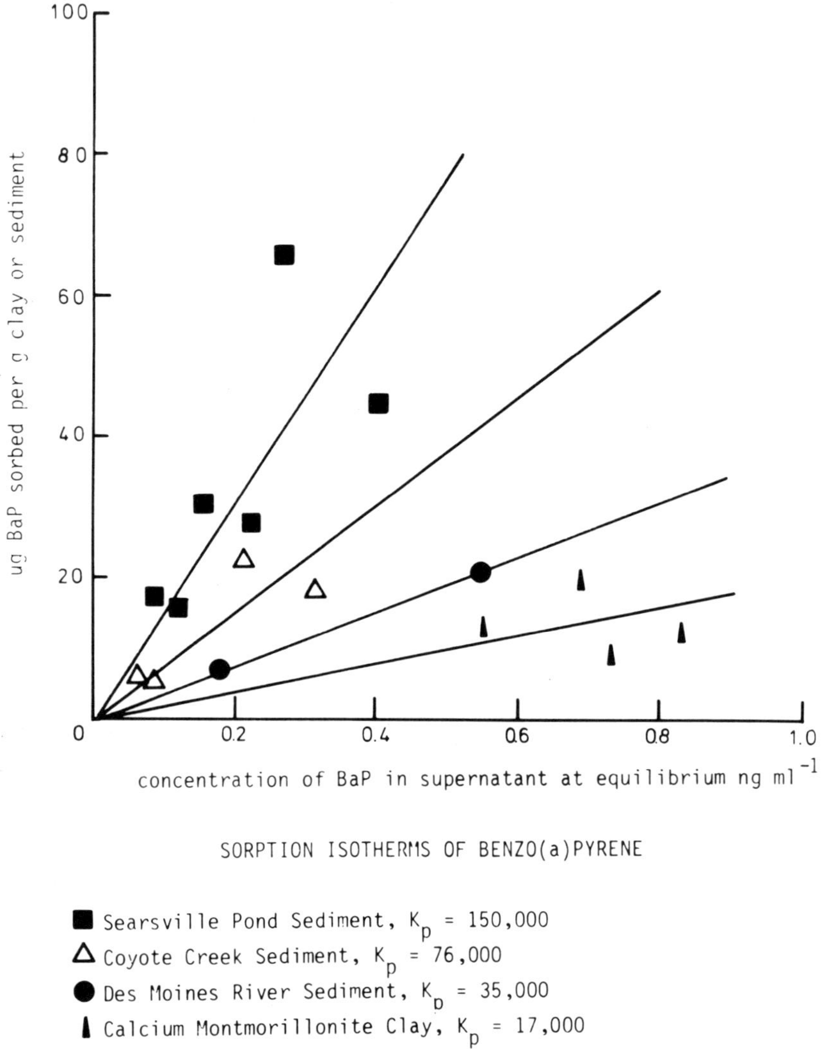


**Figure 9.** Sorption isotherms of benzo[a] pyrene [45].

## Volatilization [14,16,24]

Air-water transport is well studied for gases and volatile organic chemicals. The realization that air transport is important for lipophilic compounds of relatively low vapor pressure has stimulated research on the evaporation rates of these substances from water bodies. Good agreement has been found between measured half-lives of volatilization for about 20 chemicals with half-lives calculated by the method of Mackay and Leinonen [25]:

$$-\frac{d[S]}{dt} = \frac{k_{iL}([S] - Pi/Hi)}{L}$$

where L = depth of a completely mixed layer of water
Hi = Henry's law constant
Pi = partial pressure of the chemical
$k_{iL}$ = the mass transfer coefficient

An alternative approach, which is the basis for an experimental procedure, is based on the observation of Tsivoglou that the volatilization rates from water of several low-molecular-weight substances is constant over a wide range of turbulence conditions. For compounds A and B then, the ratio:

$$k_v^A/k_v^B = \text{constant}$$

If A is chosen as the substrate and B is oxygen, the law of microscopic reversibility requires that the rate of volatilization of substrate A from the water be equal to the rate of dissolution of oxygen in water. The ratio of substrate volatilization rate to the oxygen reaeration constant can be measured in the laboratory, and the volatilization rate of the substrate for the real water body for which the oxygen reaeration rate is known can thus be calculated. Experimentally, the substrate solution is purged with nitrogen to remove most dissolved oxygen. The concentration of substrate and oxygen is measured at the beginning of the experiment (t = 0) and successively at regular intervals while the solution is being stirred in a beaker which is open to the atmosphere.

The substrate concentration vs time data are fitted to an exponential decay curve:

$$[S_t] = [S_o]\, e^{-k_v^S t}$$

which is the integrated form of the first-order rate expression:

$$-\frac{d[S]}{dt} = k_v^S[S]$$

The oxygen concentration data are fitted to:

$$[O_2]_t = [O_2]_{sat} - ([O_2]_{sat} - [O_2]_o)\, e^{-k_v^s t}$$

which is the integrated form of:

$$\frac{d[O_2]}{dt} = k_v^o\left([O_2]_{sat} - [O_2]_t\right)$$

## Octanol-Water Partition Coefficient [16-19,23,26-31]

The octanol-water partition coefficient is the ratio of concentration of a chemical at equilibrium in octanol and water phases. It has been shown to be related to solubility, bioaccumulation, sediment sorption and even toxicity. Partition coefficients can be measured or calculated, and methods for estimating log P by reverse phase TLC and HPLC methods have recently been developed. Octanol-water partition coefficients have been particularly useful as a predictive tool for estimating bioaccumulation potential of chemicals (Figure 10). The bioaccumulation potential of a compound predicted by the octanol-water partition coefficient is generally considered as an "upper limit value." A number of mechanisms may reduce the bioaccumulation factor in a real organism. The most important ones are:

1. Effective metabolic conversion can significantly reduce bioaccumulated material.
2. Very lipophilic compounds ("superlipophilics" log P $>7$) for which a log P can still be calculated, may not pass biological membranes any more for reasons of lipophilicity, solubility or size.

The octanol-water partition coefficient has also recently been shown to correlate with strength of adsorption on sediments. For ten chemicals with log P from 2.1 to 6.3 it was found that (1) the adsorption isotherm as linear and (2) the adsorption coefficient per gram organic carbon ($K_{oc}$) was directly related to the *n*-octanol-water partition coefficient.

## Hydrolytic Reactions [14,16,32]

Many of the chemicals that enter the environment are esters of carboxylic and phosphoric acids, carbamates and related compounds which can be expected to hydrolyze at pH values available in the environment. The pH of water in the atmosphere is slightly acidic from dissolved $CO_2$. The pH of surface water is usually 5-9. A survey of 1300 U.S. cities has revealed 60 cities with drinking water of pH greater than 9, and 3 with

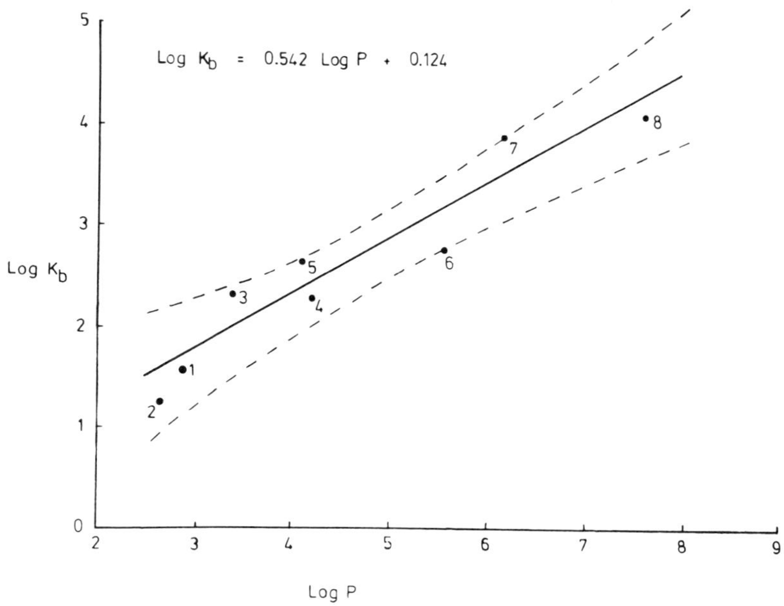


**Figure 10.** Linear regression between logarithms of partition coefficient and bioconcentration of chemicals in trout muscle [27]. (1) 1,1,2,2-tetrachloroethylene; (2) carbon tetrachloride; (3) *p*-dichlorobenzene; (4) diphenyl oxide; (5) diphenyl; (6) 2-biphenyl phenyl ether; (7) hexachlorobenzene; (8) 2,2′,4,4′-tetrachlorodiphenyl oxide.

pH greater than 10.5. Water in soil generally has a pH of 4–10. Under environmental conditions, carboxylic esters can hydrolyze under alkaline conditions, by acid catalysis and reaction with water itself. The overall rate expression for hydrolysis of the substrate (ester E) is:

$$-\frac{dE}{dt} = k_{obs.}[E] = k_{H^+}[E][H^+] + k_{OH^-}[E][OH^-]\, k_{H_2O}[E]$$

Because most natural waters have considerable buffering capacity and pollutant concentrations are low, the effective concentration of acid or base does not change during the reaction.

Pseudo-first-order kinetics are observed, and the observed first-order rate constant is given by:

$$k_{obs.} = k_{H^+}[H^+] + k_{OH^-}[OH^-] + k_{H_2O}$$

The pH thus effects the overall rate; at high or low pH one of the first two terms is usually dominant, while at pH 7 the last term can often be most important. The detailed relationship of pH and rate depends on the specific values of $k_{H^+}$, $k_{OH^-}$ and $k_{H_2O}$. At fixed pH the overall rate process is first-order, and the half-life of the substrate is independent of its concentration and is:

$$t_{1/2} = \ln 2/k_{obs}$$

## Photochemical Transformations [14-16,32,33]

Environmental photochemistry studies reactions that are initiated by electronic excitation of compounds which occur in the environment. The source of radiation is either the sun or an artificial source designed to simulate the sun's wavelength distribution as observed at ground level. Although the basic laws of photochemistry apply to environmental photochemistry, significant differences exist (Table V).

The cutoff for the solar spectrum in the troposphere is about 290 nm, and absorption of photons of only this or longer wavelength can result in photochemical reactions either by direct transformation or photosensitized reactions. In higher atmospheric layers low-wavelength radiation is available (~200 nm). Physical properties of molecules, such as the molar extinction coefficients and the nature of the excited species, and chemical properties, such as the strength of different bonds in the molecule, are responsible for their photoreactivity and thus stability against solar radiation. Table VI shows the correlation between the energy of radiation of different wavelength and bond strength of a number of bonds characteristics of compounds that occur in the environment. The choice of the proper phase for laboratory investigations depends on the physical properties of the compound in question.

Chemicals with low vapor pressure are likely to be found adsorbed on particles in the atmosphere, whereas very volatile compounds will be in the vapor phase and thus more available for radiation. Such compounds, if stable in the troposphere, may diffuse into the stratosphere and thus be exposed to radiation of higher energy (lower wavelength) there. Water-soluble compounds may occur in true solution, whereas lipophilic compounds are likely to be adsorbed on particles or found in the organic microlayer of water surfaces. Laboratory modeling has to take into account all of these facts.

Kinetics and mechanisms of direct photolysis of compounds can usually be understood and evaluated with our present understanding; however, details of sensitized photolyses are largely undefined.

Table V. Comparison of "Classical" and Environmental Photochemistry

| Parameter | Traditional Photochemistry | Environmental Photochemistry | Comment |
|---|---|---|---|
| Wavelength | Any, mostly $> 150$ nm often 254 nm | $> 290$ nm, except for simulation of stratospheric conditions | Experimental simulation of the tropospheric spectrum of the sun |
| Phase | Any, mostly inert organic solvent | Aqueous solution, vapor phase, adsorbed species | Imitation of the true natural state of pollutants |
| Substrate Concentration | $> 10^{-3}$ $M$ | $< 10^{-4}$ $M$ | Identification of trace amounts of products |
| Reactants, Gases, Mixtures | Usually $N_2$, one or two reactants, sometimes sensitizers and quenchers | Contaminant gases ($NO_X$, $SO_X$), mixtures, natural sensitizers and quenchers | Complex mixtures and reactions, which may influence each other |

**Table VI. Important Bond Strengths and Energy of Radiation at Different Wavelengths**

| | H | Cl | Br | I | OH |
|---|---|---|---|---|---|
| H - | 435 | 431 | 364 | 297 | 498 |
| $H_3C$ - | 435 | 352 | 293 | 235 | 385 |
| $H_5C_6$ - | 469 | 360 | 335 | 272 | 469 |
| $H_2C = CH$ - | 452 | 373 | | | |

| 605 | 390 | 302 | 243 | 201 | Energy (kJ/mol) |
|---|---|---|---|---|---|
| 200 | 300 | 400 | 500 | 600 | Wavelength (nm) |

++++++++++++ = Solar radiation

It was shown that in natural water samples disappearance of substrate obeys a first-order rate law of the form:

$$-\frac{d[S]}{dt} = k\, I\, \phi\, [S]$$

where I = the intensity of incident light
$\phi$ = the quantum yield
[S] = pollutant concentration.

The simplest and most direct method of using laboratory experiments for estimating environmental photolysis rates is to expose an aqueous solution of the chemical to outdoor sunlight and measure its rate of disappearance. However, sunlight intensity varies with the time of day, season, latitude and weather conditions (Figure 11). Another method for estimating environmental photolysis rates consists of calculating rate constants from extinction coefficients and quantum yields which are measured in the laboratory. The sunlight intensity with respect to time of day, season and latitude are available from the literature, and photolysis rates can thus be estimated for different locations.

## Biodegradations [14,15,34]

In the course of time microorganisms have evolved catabolic enzyme systems for the metabolism of naturally occurring compounds, and are thus the principal agents responsible for recycling organic matter in nature. Many manmade chemical products fit into this cycle of carbon, and microorganisms are responsible for the degradation of wastes and many of the

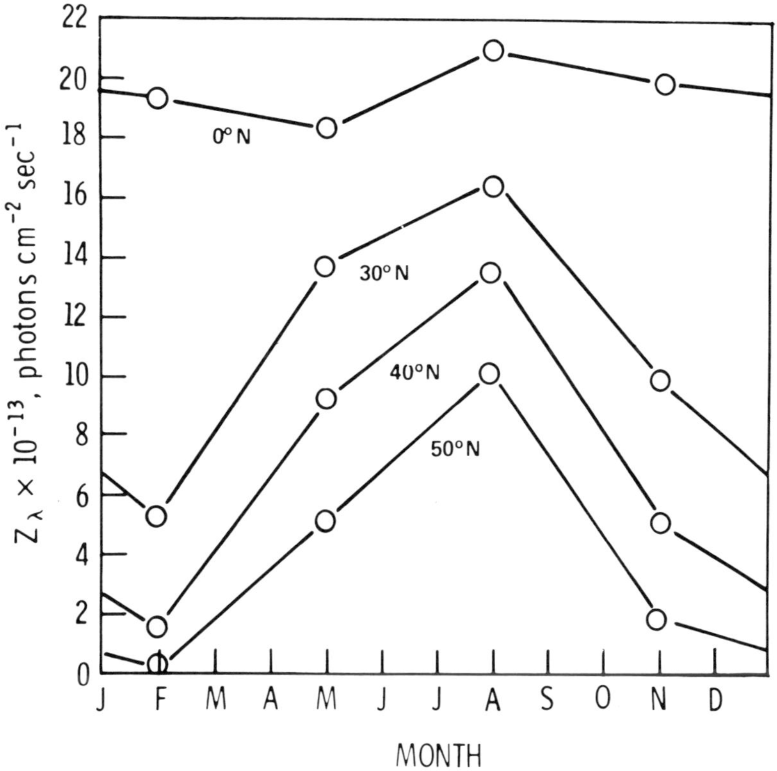


**Figure 11.** Dependence of short-wavelength solar UV irradiance upon season and latitude [32].

chemical products which enter the soil and water environments. Microorganisms either use these manmade chemicals as sources of carbon and energy, or degrade them by cooxidation or cometabolic mechanisms. Organic compounds that are not readily degraded are often referred to as persistent or recalcitrant. Persistence of a compound may have different causes but is often related to a structure for which degradative enzymes are not available or inducible in natural microbial populations. Because persistence is one of the least desirable properties for a compound in the environment, interest has been shown for years to identify such chemicals by laboratory tests.

Microorganisms used in biodegradation studies involve pure cultures from enrichment procedures or culture collections and mixed populations, either from natural sources or by cultural enrichment. Techniques involve measuring of biological oxygen demand, microbial growth, substrate disappearance, $^{14}CO_2$ evolution or identification and measurement of metabolites. To allow evaluation of biodegradation in an overall hazard assessment of chemical products, "biodegradation categories" have been proposed (Table VII). Only in a few examples have the structural features of a molecule been correlated with persistence.

**Table VII. Persistence Categories of Chemicals [35]**

| Class | Persistence in Unadapted Soil | Example |
|---|---|---|
| 1. Easily Degradable | 1–3 weeks | Acetic Acid |
| 2. Degradable | 1–3 months | Benzoic Acid |
| 3. Difficult to Degrade | 3 months–1 year | ε-Caprolactam |
| 4. Very Difficult to Degrade | 1–2 year | Chlorobenzene |
| 5. Refractory | 2 years | Hexachlorobenzene |

It is known, for instance that branching of hydrocarbons hinders the β-oxidative degradation.

$$R\text{-}CH_2\text{-}CH_2CH_3 \rightarrow R\text{-}CH_2\text{-}CH_2\text{-}CH_2\text{-}OH \rightarrow R\text{-}CH_2\text{-}CH_2COOH \rightarrow R\text{-}\underset{\displaystyle OH}{\underset{|}{CH}}\text{-}CH_2\text{-}COOH$$

Increasing chlorine content of aromatic rings generally retards microbiological degradation (Figure 12) and some highly chlorinated biphenyls for instance are considered essentially nondegradable [37,38]. Efforts to describe microbial degradation rates of chemicals have usually used modifications of Monod kinetics, and it appears that this provides a reasonable approximation to the rate of microbial degradation in aquatic systems:

$$-\frac{d[S]}{dt} = \frac{k\,[S]\,[M]}{k_s + [S]}$$

where $[M]$ = the concentration of active organisms
$k, k_S$ = constants

## Bioaccumulation [39,40]

In the most general definition, bioaccumulation denotes the presence of a chemical substance in an organism in higher concentrations than in the direct environment or in its food. Bioaccumulation becomes important when

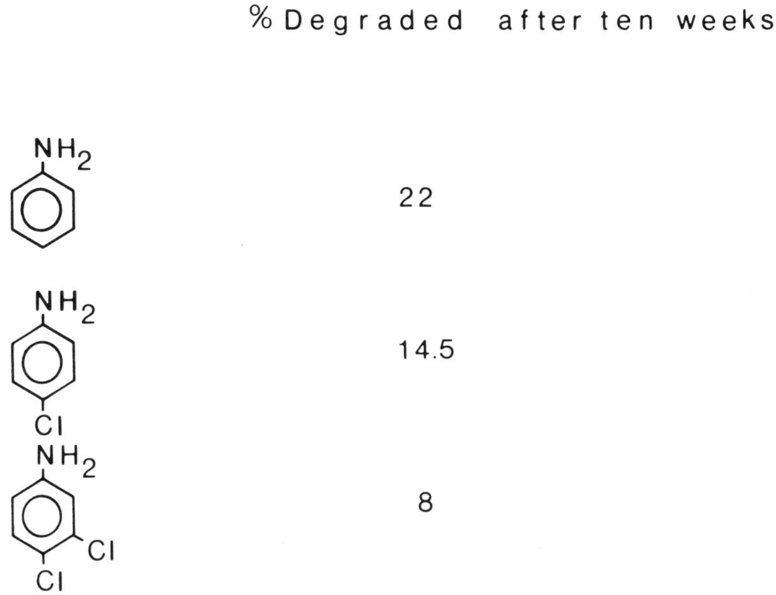


**Figure 12.** Influence of aromatic chlorine substitution on the ability of soil microorganisms to degrade a series of anilines [36].

potentially harmful substances are involved and when the ratio organism/environment gets higher than about 100-1000.

Although different mechanisms for bioaccumulation are known, the most important with respect to the many new organic compounds to be tested for bioaccumulation potential is the partitioning of lipophilic compounds into the fatty phase of organisms, particularly fish and other aquatic species. The route of accumulation for most chemicals in aquatic species is predominantly via exchange with water. Because aquatic organisms live in a relatively oxygen-poor environment (~10 mg/kg as opposed to ~200 g/kg in air), their exchange with the ambient environment and thus with potentially accumulative and hazardous chemicals is much more effective than in air-breathing organisms.

Bioaccumulation tests are therefore carried out similarly to aquatic toxicity tests, by exposing the organism (fish) through water and not through food as in mammals. The large quantity of water which daily passes the gills combined with the high extraction efficiency for lipophilic compounds and the ease of passage through lipoid membranes allows a partition equilibrium to establish relatively quickly. Experiments have shown that the accumulation process in fish can be described by a first-order model for reversible distribution over two compartments.

$$C_w \underset{k_2}{\overset{k_1}{\rightleftharpoons}} C_f$$

where $C_w$ = concentration in water
$C_f$ = concentration in fish

whereby the rate of transport into the fish depends on the concentration in the water, and the depuration dependent on the concentration in the fish (Figure 13).

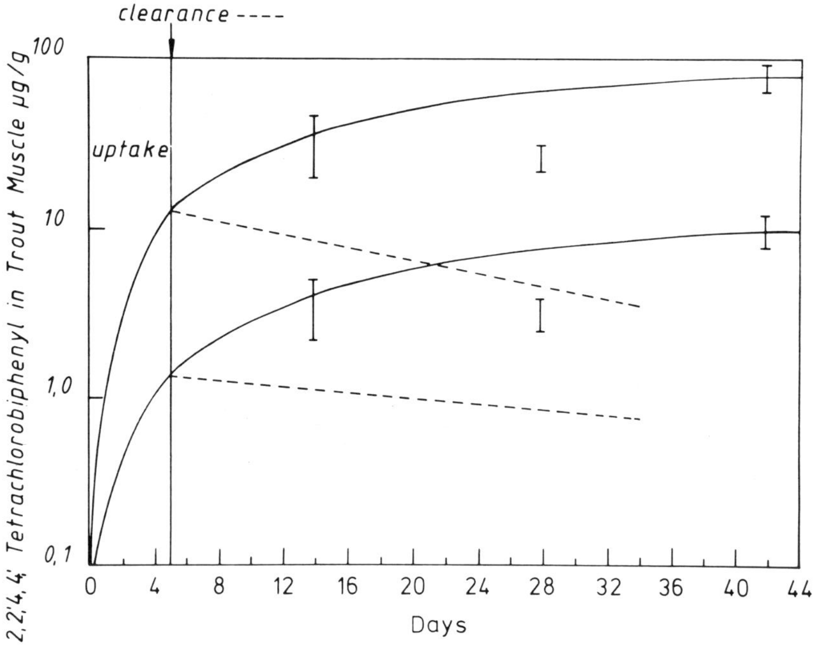


**Figure 13.** Concentrations of 2,2′,4,4′-tetrachlorobiphenyl in trout muscle in 42-day exposure (solid line). Depuration after transfer to clean water (broken line) [39].

$$\frac{dC_f}{dt} = k_1 C_w - k_2 C_f$$

where $k_1$ = first-order rate constant for uptake
$k_2$ = first-order rate constant for depuration

At equilibrium

$$\frac{dC_f}{dt} = 0$$

where $k_1 C_w = k_2 C_f$

or

$$\frac{C_f}{C_w} = \frac{k_1}{k_2} = K_b$$

$K_b$, the relation between the concentration in the fish and in water is the bioaccumulation factor (bioconcentration factor).

When contaminated fish are transferred to clean water, a process of elimination (depuration) begins, and the elimination half-life can be calculated when the concentration in the fish is periodically measured:

$$C_w = 0 \quad \frac{dC_f}{dt} = - k_2 C_f$$

$$ln_{C_{f_1}} - ln\ C_{f_2} = k_2(t_2 - t_1)$$

where $C_{f_1}$ and $C_{f_2}$ are the concentrations in the fish at times $t_1$ and $t_2$

$$t_{1/2} = \frac{ln_2}{k_2}$$

## Integrated Approaches: Microecosystems [41-44]

The natural environment consists of a large number of ecosystems of great diversity. No two ecosystems are exactly alike. Nevertheless, attempts have been made to set up specific, limited ecosystems in the laboratory (microecosystems, microcosms, model ecosystems) to study a variety of the phenomena that occur in natural ecosystems. The study of the fate of chemicals in such model ecosystems is appealing because these systems, in their basic functions, behave like pieces of real environment. The fate parameters that can most easily be obtained from such model ecosystem studies are, for instance for the commonly used "Metcalf system," biodegradability index and ecological magnification values. Data on sorption to soil or sediment can usually also be generated. Classification of model ecosystems can be according to the "source" of the system, i.e., whether a physical section of a natural ecosystem is being used or, on the other extreme, the most artificial where all components are assembled by the scientist to meet specific needs. Other classifications are according to the main "medium." The two main types are aquatic laboratory microecosystems designed, for instance, to simulate a pond or lake environment, and terrestrial systems where, as an example, the fate of a pesticide on cropland may be studied. One major advantage of the laboratory model ecosystem approach in a university setting is the instructive value for students.

## Integrated Systems: The Environmental Rates Approach [14,15,44,45]

According to the environmental rates approach, the overall disappearance of a chemical from an environmental compartment is controlled by transformation and transport processes that can be studied separately in the laboratory. There is a minimum of properties and rate processes which must be determined (or estimated) to make a prediction of fate possible. Two examples will be given. The first is a case study using laboratory data to predict the environmental concentration of the insecticide chlorpyrifos in a pond in Missouri.

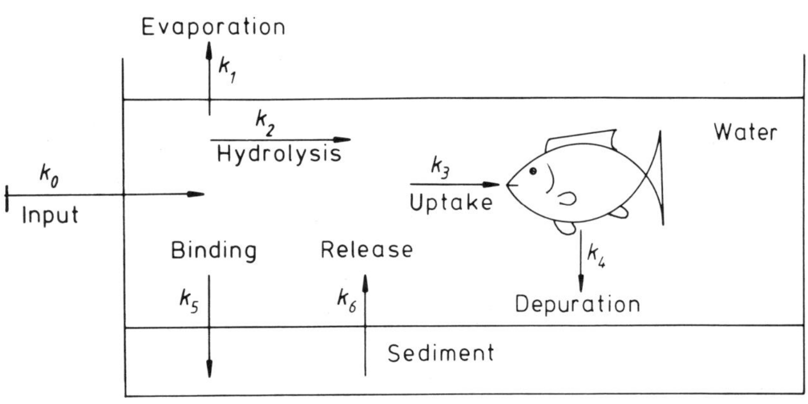


MATERIAL BALANCE EQUATION

$$V\frac{dC_W}{dt} = k_0 - k_1AC_W - k_2VC_W - k_3FC_W + k_4FC_f - k_5SC_W + k_6SC_S$$

**Figure 14.** Key properties and material balance equation for predicting the fate of chlorpyrifos in a pond [44]. V = Volume of water (ml); A = surface area ($cm^2$); F = fish mass (g); S = sediment mass (g); $C_W$ = concentration of chemical in water; k = rate constant, $C_F$ = concentrations of chemical in fish, $C_s$ = concentration of chemical in sediment.

Figure 14 shows the pond model, the key properties and the material balance equation for predicting the fate of chlorpyrifos in the pond. The predicted and experimentally found concentrations in fish and water (Table VIII) show good agreement.

**Table VIII. Predicting the Fate of Chlorpyrifos in a Pond: Seven-Day[a] Concentrations of Chlorpyrifos [44]**

| Water[b] μg/l | | Fish μg/g | |
|---|---|---|---|
| Predicted | Found | Predicted | Found |
| 1.0 | 1.0 | 0.8 | 1.0 |

| Compartment | % of Total 2 days | % of Total 25 days |
|---|---|---|
| Water | 48 | 0.8 |
| Soil | 25 | 0.5 |
| Fish | 0.8 | <0.1 |
| Air | 3.8 | 11.4 |
| Metabolized | 2.9 | 11.0 |
| Hydrolyzed | 25 | 76.0 |

[a]Similarly agreement at days 2, 4 and 28.
[b]5.75 μg/l at t = 0.

The second example describes a nine-compartment computer model which was developed by Stanford Research Institute and the U.S. Environmental Protection Agency (EPA). The model was designed to explore the impact of water body heterogenicity on the transport and transformation mechanisms investigated in laboratory studies [14] (Figure 15).

The model assumes a number of physical dimensions (Figure 16) and water quality parameters (number of bacteria, sediment loading, oxygen reaeration rate, photolysis activity index) for a pond, a river and a lake system. Further details are available in Branson [44].

As an example, the calculated distribution of benzo[a]pyrene is shown after an input concentration of 1 ng/ml in a two-compartment pond system (Figure 17) and in a nine-compartment oligotrophic lake (Figure 18) [45].

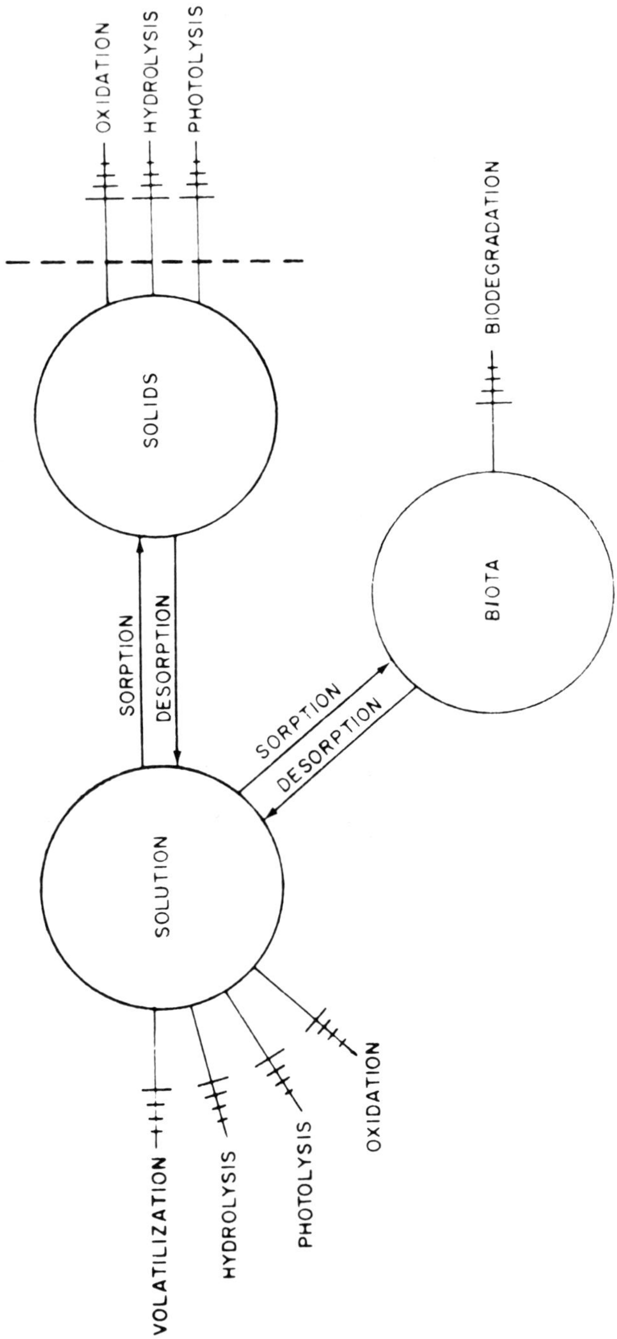


**Figure 15.** Schematic representation of transport and transformation routes simulated [14].

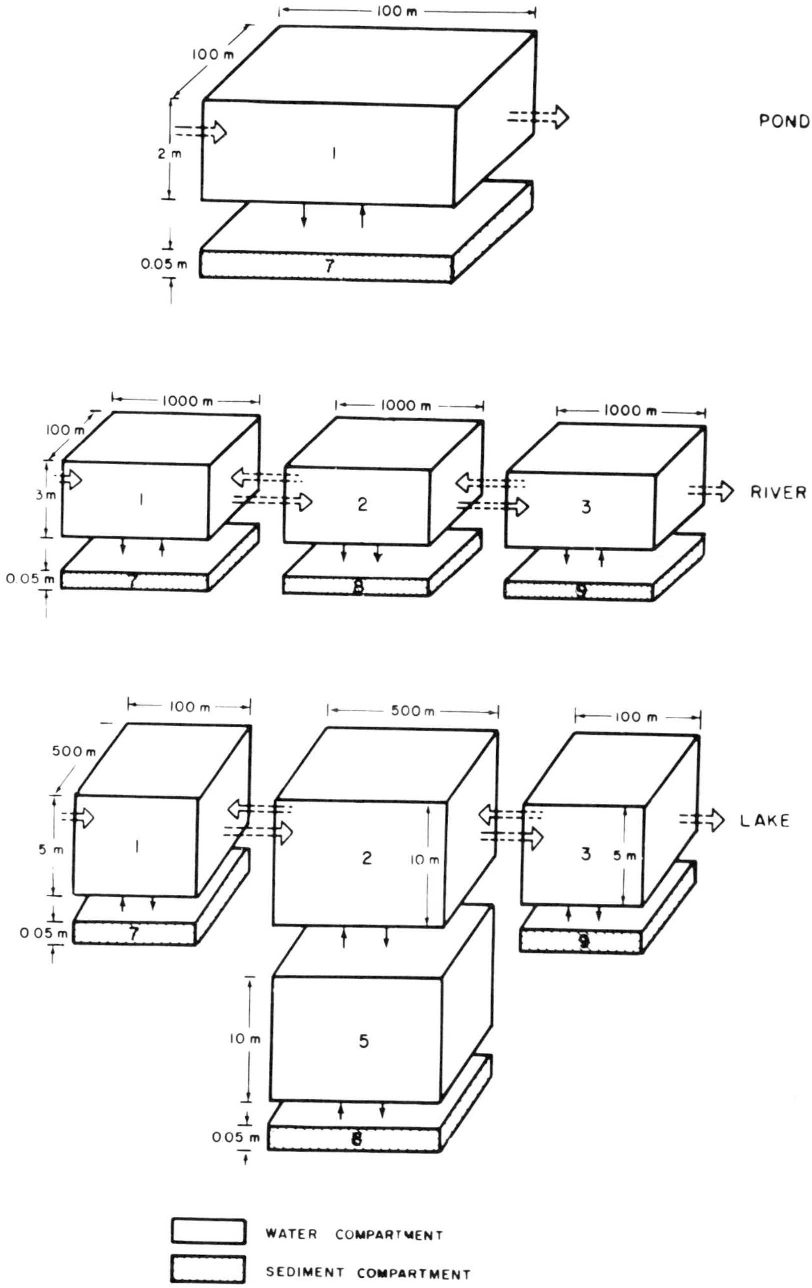


**Figure 16.** Physical configurations of the pond, river and lake simulations [14].

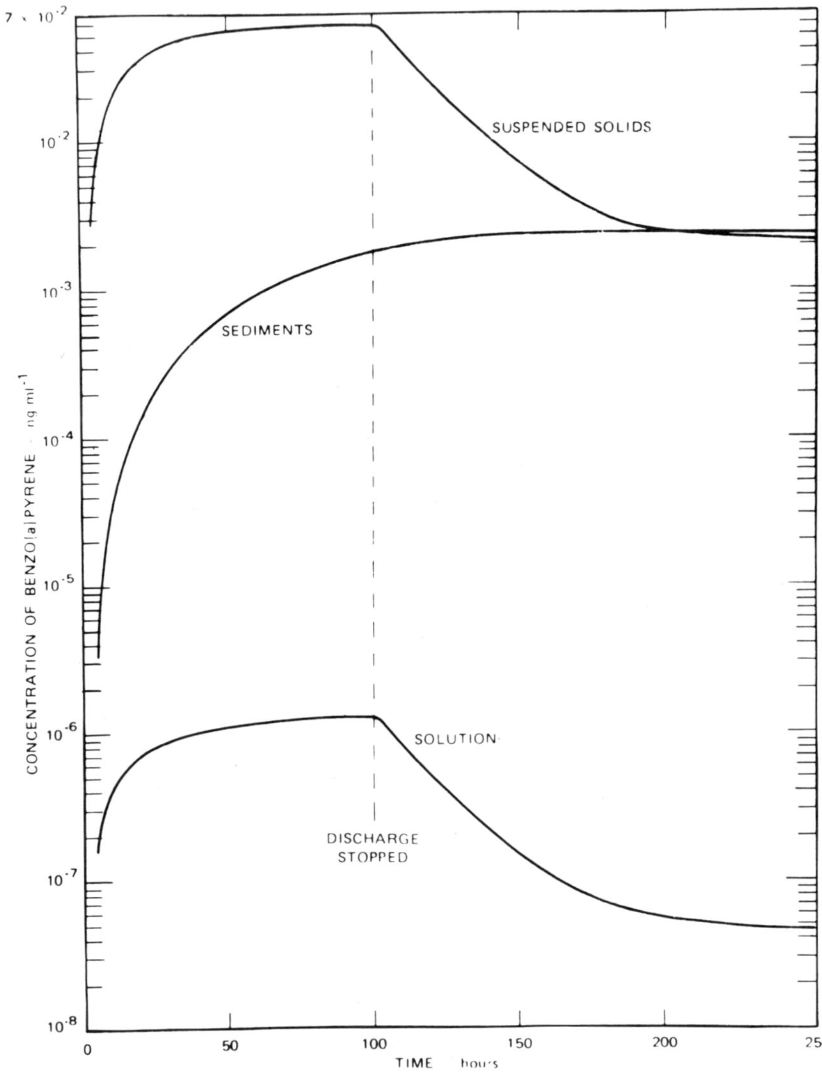


**Figure 17.** Persistence of benzo[a]pyrene in a two-compartment pond system (computer simulation) [45].

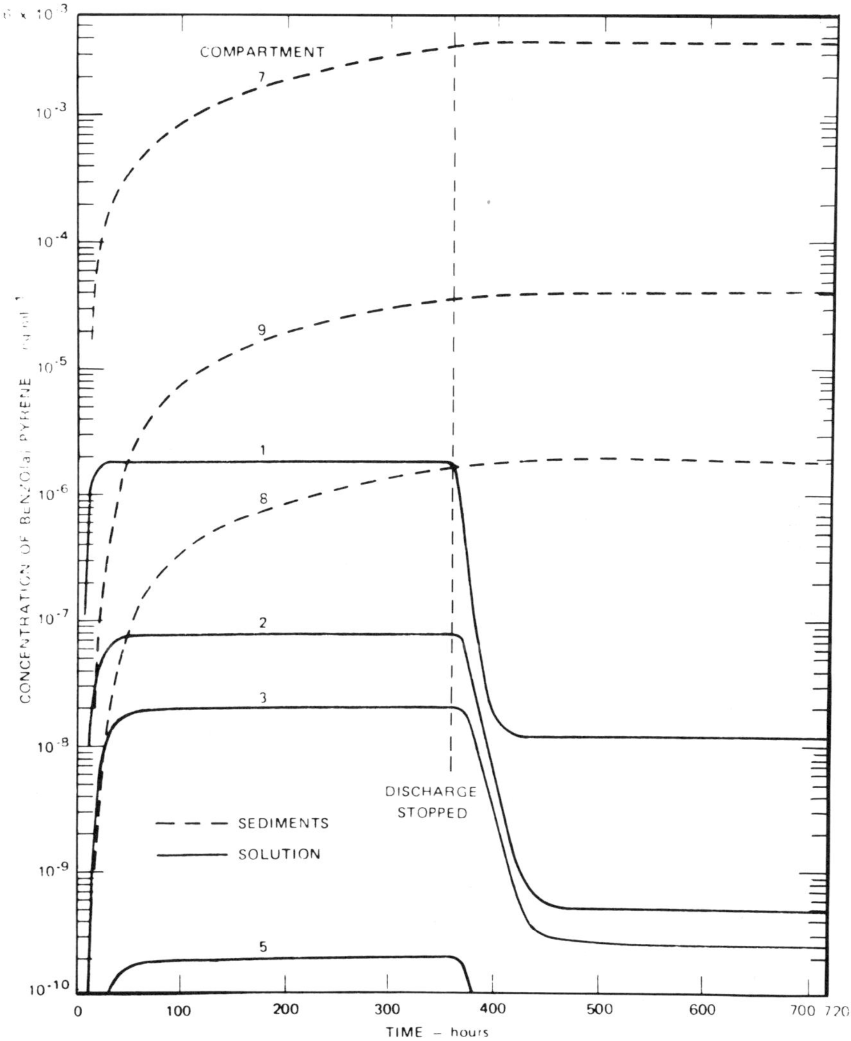


**Figure 18.** Persistence of benzo[a]pyrene in an oligotrophic lake (computer simulation) [45].

## PRACTICE OF ENVIRONMENTAL HEALTH CHEMISTRY

The Laboratory of Environmental and Toxicological Chemistry of the University of Amsterdam offers a complete program of teaching and research, beginning with a formal lecture course suitable for the last year two years of undergraduate study and up to a PhD program.

### Teaching

A formal lecture course, "General Environmental Chemistry," for undergraduates requires prior knowledge of most branches of chemistry, e.g., organic, inorganic physical and analytical chemistry. Most aspects of pollution are dealt with, as are chemical aspects of natural environment and toxicological problems with emphasis on the compounds involved. Although a number of books on pollution chemistry and environmental chemistry are now available [46-54], lecture notes [55] are the main basis for this course. The table of contents (Table IX) reflects the diversity of topics.

This series of lectures has been given yearly since 1974, and the material proved to be too much for one lecture period (about 30 hours). These lectures are given by one person rather than a team of experts. On this undergraduate level, familiarization with a number of topics outside chemistry (e.g., ecology and meteorology) is not too difficult for the lecturer, and the advantage is a uniform chemical-oriented approach without overlap or gaps.

"Advanced Topics in Environmental Chemistry" is a graduate course intended to provide up-to-date and in-depth knowledge on subjects of current interest. This series strongly relies on invited experts from outside the department and requires student participation. This course was offered for the first time in the fall of 1978, and most lectures were given by researchers from Dutch and other near-by European institutes, as well as by visitors and "resident foreigners" on sabbatical leave. Each of the following topics were scheduled for two hours but usually lasted a whole afternoon including discussion. The topics were:

- The Fate of Oil at Sea
- Transport and Transformations of Major Atmospheric Pollutants
- Chemistry and Fate of Polynuclear Aromatic Hydrocarbons in the Environment
- Heavy Metals in the Environment
- Atmospheric Distribution Models
- The Fate of Compounds in the Oceans
- Photochemical Fate of Organic Compounds in the Environment

**Table IX. Table of Contents, Lecture Notes for "General Environmental Chemistry," Given at the University of Amsterdam**

The Natural Chemical Environment–Ecochemistry
- Energy and Radiation
- The Atmosphere
- The Hydrosphere
- The Lithosphere
- The Biosphere
- Organic Compounds of Interest in the Ecosphere

General Pollution Chemistry
- Air Pollution
- Water Pollution (including waste water)
- Waste Disposal

Environmental Chemicals–Physical Factors in the Environment
- Transport
- Adsorption and Sedimentation Phenomena
- Accumulation

Environmental Chemicals–Structural Change in the Environment
- Persistence
- Chemical Reactions
- Photochemical Reactions
- Biochemical Reactions (metabolism, microorganisms, plants, animals)
- Discussion of Common Reaction Types

Environmental Chemicals–Toxic and Other Effects
- Effects of Chemicals on and in the Environment
- Effects on Humans–Toxicity

Environmental Chemicals–Analysis and Monitoring

Chemicals from Agriculture and Food Processing
- Pesticides (insecticides, nonlethal insect-control agents, fungicides, herbicides, other pesticides)
- Other Agricultural Chemicals
- Food and Feed Additives
- Natural Toxicants

Industrial Chemicals
- Inorganic Compounds
- Heavy Metals
- Radioactive Isotopes
- Organic Compounds and Materials (oil, polycyclic hydrocarbons, surfactants, synthetic polymers, halogenated compounds, other industrial compounds)

- The Fate of Persistent Halogenated Compounds in the Environment
- The Fate of Pesticides in Soil
- Sorption and Bioaccumulation in the Aquatic Environment
- Environmental Fate, Toxicity and Assessment of Risk

Reading material was taken from the recent literature. A new advanced text may provide background reading in the future [56].

A laboratory session is still in the preparatory phase. It is designed to give students practical experience in environmental fate studies. Laboratory models for bioaccumulation, biodegradation, photodegradation, physicochemical behavior (solubility, adsorption) and mammalian metabolism and pharmacokinetic studies as required by the new toxic substances laws are the subjects of this practical study. Several books deal with laboratory experiments in pollution studies; however, the levels of these general experiments are much too low for an advanced undergraduate course. A recent book handles more advanced experiments [57], but these are designed more for general pollution studies rather than environmental fate studies as envisaged in this laboratory session.

### Research

The general research theme of the Laboratory of Environmental and Toxicological Chemistry (LETC) is the behavior and fate of persistent lipophilic (mainly haloaromatic) compounds in the environment and organisms, with special emphasis on the relation between chemical structure and environmental properties. Table X shows an overall outline as an example of a research setup in environmental health chemistry. This, of course, represents an idealized situation. In the LETC, for instance, expertise in physical fate is largely, and for toxic effects is completely, missing. A well-rounded, properly functioning environmental health chemistry laboratory should strive, however, to have expertise in all "vertical" areas. Only then is proper hazard assessment of specific compounds ("horizontal" areas) possible.

## CONCLUSIONS

The advantages of operating an environmental health chemistry laboratory in a chemistry faculty (department) lie in the close association with fellow chemists. The standards of the chemical work are controlled by chemists, and the ready availability of colleagues for consultation, use of instrumentation and cooperation is a definite asset. Furthermore, the student population is

**Table X. Example of Research Outline in Environmental Health Chemistry**

| | Physical Fate Adsorption Solubility Volatility | Biodegradation (Microorganisms) | (Photo)-Chemical Degradation | Bioaccumulation Pharmacokinetics | Animal Metabolism | Toxic Effects |
|---|---|---|---|---|---|---|
| Theoretical, Structure Properties | Mathematical Models and Predictive Parameters | | | | | |
| Laboratory Model | Develop Test Methods for Toxic Substances Laws | | | | | |
| Environmental Data | Comparative Data from Real Environment | | | | | |
| Specific Compounds, for example, | | | | | | |
| Chloroaromatic compounds | → | → | → | → | → | |
| Flame retardants | → | → | → | → | → | |
| Chlorodibenzo-*p*-dioxins | → | → | → | → | → | |

reasonably homogeneous, with all of them having had adequate basic chemical training before.

The difficulties are entirely associated with the interdisciplinary nature of the program. Little financial support or even understanding and appreciation by the department can be expected for nonchemical parts of the program (biology, toxicology). Cooperation with colleagues from other disciplines (outside chemistry) becomes exceedingly difficult, particularly in the European university system, where different institutes are self-contained units and other faculties (departments) are often far removed physically. (The buildings of most European universities are scattered throughout cities and not located "on campus").

Another problem is funding from outside the university (grants). Agencies support either fundamental (pure) scientific effort (which according to popular definition, environmental health chemistry cannot be) or problem-oriented (problem-solving) research. Fundamental research in environmental health chemistry (i.e., research which is fundamental for the program such as for instance, studies on the relationship between chemical structure on the one hand and environmental behavior or toxicity on the other), fall neither in the pure or problem-oriented science package. Funds from health-oriented (medical) granting agencies, furthermore, are on the whole unavailable for chemists working in chemistry departments.

## ACKNOWLEDGMENTS

My sincere thanks are due to my colleagues and students for countless discussions about the concept of Environmental Health Chemistry. Drs. W.A. Bruggeman, Dr. A. A. M. Roof and Dr. M. Th. M. Tulp have been particularly helpful. Thanks are also due to Dr. G. L. Baughman, Dr. R. J. Moolenaar and Dr. R. G. Zepp for permission to use figures from their own papers or papers from their laboratories.

## REFERENCES

1. Natusch, D. F. S. "Conflicts in the Training of Graduate Environmental Chemists," *Am. Lab.* (July 1974) pp. 25-29.
2. Hutzinger, O., University of Amsterdam. "Report, Laboratory of Environmental Chemistry," Unpublished (1975).
3. Freed, V. H. "The Chemist and His Role in the Study of Transport and Fate of Toxic Substances," paper presented at the Division of Environmental Chemistry, American Chemical Society meeting, Miami, September 1978 (Abstracts pp. 52-53).

4. Moeller, W., B. Pahl and B. Hammond. "Trends in University Environmental Health Research and Training," *Am. J. Public Health* 69:125-129 (1979).
5. Karasek, F. W., and O. Hutzinger. "Environmental Chemistry in the Netherlands," *Res. Devel.* 26(9):40-46 (1975).
6. Higginson, J., and C. S. Muri. "Epidemiology of Cancer," in *Cancer Medicine, Vol. 3* J. F. Holland and E. Frei, Eds. (Philadelphia: Lea and Febiger, 1973), p. 241.
7. "Major Causes of Death in the U.S.," *Chem. Eng. News* (December 5, 1975) p. 36.
8. Blau, G. E., W. B. Neely and D. R. Branson. "Ecokinetics: A Study of the Fate and Distribution of Chemicals in Laboratory Ecosystems," *Am. Inst. Chem. Eng. J.* 21(5):854-861 (1975).
9. Haque, R., and V. H. Freed. "Behavior of Pesticides in the Environment: Environmental Chemodynamics," in *Residue Reviews,* F. A. Gunther, Ed. (New York: Springer-Verlag, 1974), p. 89.
10. Freed, V. H., C. T. Chiou and R. Haque. "Chemodynamics: Transport and Behaviour of Chemicals in the Environment–A Problem in Environmental Health," *Environ. Health Persp.* 20:55-70 (1977).
11. Hutzinger, O., M. Th. M. Tulp and V. Zitko. "Chemicals with Pollution Potential," in *Aquatic Pollutants, Transformation and Biological Effects,* O. Hutzinger, I. H. van Lelyveld and B. C. J. Zoeteman, Eds. (Oxford: Pergamon Press, 1978), p. 13.
12. Haque, R., and N. Ash. "Factors Affecting the Behavior of Chemicals in the Environment," in *Survival in Toxic Environments* (New York: Academic Press, Inc., 1974), p. 357.
13. Hutzinger, O., and A. A. M. Roof. "Hydrocarbons and Halogenated Hydrocarbons in the Aquatic Environment: Some Thoughts on the Philosophy and Practice of Environmental Chemistry," in *Proceedings of the International Symposium on Hydrocarbons and Halogenated Hydrocarbons,* B. K. Afghan and D. Mackay, Eds. (New York: Plenum Publishing Corporation, 1979).
14. "Environmental Pathways of Selected Chemicals in Freshwater Systems, Part I: Background and Experimental Procedures," U.S. EPA, Publication, EPA-600/7-77-113 (1977).
15. Baughman, G. L., and R. R. Lassiter. "Prediction of Environmental Pollutant Concentration," in *Estimating the Hazard of Chemical Substances to Aquatic Life,* J. Cairns, Jr., K. L. Dickson and A. W. Maki, Eds., Special Technical Publication 657 (Philadelphia: American Society for Testing and Materials, 1978), p. 35.
16. Stern, A. M., and C. P. Walker, "Hazard Assessment of Toxic Substances: Environmental Fate Testing of Organic Chemicals and Ecological Effects Testing," in *Estimating the Hazard of Chemical Substances to Aquatic Life,* J. Cairns, Jr., K. L. Dickson and A. W. Maki, Eds., Special Technical Publication 657 (Philadelphia: American Society for Testing and Materials, 1978), p. 81.
17. Haque, R. "Role of Adsorption in Studying the Dynamics of Pesticides in a Soil Environment," in *Environmental Dynamics of Pesticides,* R. Haque and V. H. Freed, Eds. (New York: Plenum Publishing Corporation, 1975), p. 97.

18. Pierce, R. H., C. E. Olney and G. T. Felbeck. "p,p′-DDT Adsorption to Suspended Particulate Matter in Sea Water," *Geochim. Cosmochim. Acta.* 38:1061-1073 (1974).
19. Karickhoff, S. W., D. S. Brown and T. A. Scott. "Sorption of Hydrophobic Pollutants on Natural Sediments," *Water Res.* 13:241-248 (1979).
20. Weil, L., G. Duré and K. E. Quentin. "Wasserlöslichkeit von Insektiziden, chlorierten Kohlenwasserstoffen und polychlorierten Biphenylen im Hinblick auf eine Gewässerbelastung mit diesen Stoffen," *Wasser-Abwasserforsch.* 7:169-175 (1974).
21. Veith, G. D., and V. M. Comstock. "Apparatus for Continuously Saturating Water with Hydrophobic Organic Chemicals," *J. Fish. Res. Board Can.* 32:1849-1851 (1975).
22. May, W. E., S. P. Wasik and D. H. Freeman. "Determination of the Aqueous Solubility of Polynuclear Aromatic Hydrocarbons by a Coupled Column Liquid Chromatographic Technique," *Anal. Chem.* 50:175-179 (1978).
23. Tulp, M. Th. M., and O. Hutzinger. "Some Thoughts on Aqueous Solubilities and Partition Coefficients of PCB, and the Mathematical Correlation Between Bioaccumulation and Physico-Chemical Properties," *Chemosphere* 7:849-860 (1978).
24. Mackay, D. "Volatilization of Pollutants from Water," in *Aquatic Pollutants: Transformation and Biological Effects,* O. Hutzinger, I. H. van Lelyveld and B. C. J. Zoeteman, Eds. (Oxford: Pergamon Press, 1978), p. 175.
25. Mackay, D., and P. J. Leinonen. "Rate of Evaporation of Low-Solubility Contaminants from Water Bodies to Atmosphere," *Environ. Sci. Technol.* 9(13):1178-1180 (1975).
26. Leo, A., C. Hansch and D. Elkins. "Partition Coefficients and Their Uses," *Chem. Rev.* 71:525-616 (1971).
27. Neely, W. B., D. R. Branson and G. E. Blau. "Partition Coefficient to Measure Bioconcentration Potential of Organic Chemicals in Fish," *Environ. Sci. Technol.* 8:1113-1115 (1974).
28. Rekker, R. F. *The Hydrophobic Fragmental Constant* (Amsterdam: Elsevier, 1977).
29. Veith, G. D., N. M. Austin and R. T. Morris. "A Rapid Method for Estimating log P for Organic Chemicals," *Water Res.* 13:43-47 (1979).
30. Tomlinson, E. "Chromatographic Hydrophobic Parameters in Correlation Analysis of Structure-Activity Relationships," *J. Chromatog.* 113:1-45 (1975).
31. Renberg, L., and G. Sundström. "Prediction of Bioconcentration Potential of Organic Compounds Using Partition Coefficients Derived from Reversed Phase Thin Layer Chromatography," *Chemosphere.* 8:449-459 (1979).
32. Wolfe, N. L., R. G. Zepp, G. L. Baughman, R. G. Fincher and J. A. Gordon. "Chemical and Photochemical Transformation of Selected Pesticides in Aquatic Systems," U.S. EPA, Publication EPA-600/3-76-067 (1976).
33. Zepp, R. G., and G. L. Baughman. "Prediction of Photochemical Transformation of Pollutants in the Aquatic Environment," in *Aquatic*

*Pollutants: Transformation and Biological Effects,* O. Hutzinger, I. H. van Lelyveld and B. C. J. Zoeteman, Eds. (Oxford: Pergamon Press, 1978), p. 237.

34. Paris, D. F., D. L. Lewis and N. L. Wolfe. "Rates and Degradation of Malathion by Bacteria Isolated from Aquatic Systems," *Environ. Sci. Technol.* 9(2):135-138 (1975).
35. Abrams, E. T., D. Derkics, C. V. Fong, D. K. Guinan and K. M. Slimak. "Identification of Organic Compounds in Effluents from Industrial Sources," U.S. EPA, Publication EPA-560/3-75-002 (1975).
36. Süsz, A., G. Fuchsbichler and C. Eben, "Abbau von Anilin, 4-Chloranilin und 3,4-Dichloranilin in verschiedenen Boden," *Z. Pflanzenernaehr. Bodenkd.* 141:57-66 (1978).
37. Zell, M., H. J. Neu and K. Ballschmiter. "Single Component Analysis of Polychlorinated Biphenyl (PCB) and Chlorinated Pesticide Residues in Marine Fish Samples," *Z. Anal. Chem.* 292:97-107 (1978).
38. Tulp, M. Th. M., R. Schnitz and O. Hutzinger. "The Bacterial Metabolism of 4,4′-Dichlorobiphenyl and Its Suppression by Alternative Carbon Sources," *Chemosphere* 1:103-108 (1978).
39. Branson, D. R., G. E. Blau, H. C. Alexander and W. B. Neely. "Bioconcentration of 2,2′,4,4′-Tetrachlorobiphenyl in Rainbow Trout as Measured by an Accelerated Test," *Trans. Am. Fish Soc.* 104:785-792 (1975).
40. Hamelink, J. L., and A. Spacie. "Fish and Chemicals: The Process of Accumulation," *Ann. Rev. Pharmacol. Toxicol.* 17:167-177 (1977).
41. Metcalf, R. L., G. K. Sangha and I. P. Kappor. "Model Ecosystem for the Evaluation of Pesticide Biodegradability and Ecological Magnification," *Environ. Sci. Technol.* 5:709-713 (1971).
42. Draggan, S., and J. M. Giddings. "Testing Toxic Substances for Protection of the Environment," *Sci. Total Environ.* 9:63-74 (1978).
43. Gile, J. D., and J. W. Gillet. "Fate of $^{14}C$-Dieldrin in a Simulated Terrestrial Ecosystem," *Arch. Environ. Contam. Toxicol.* 8:107-124 (1979).
44. Branson, D. R. "Predicting the Fate of Chemicals in the Aquatic Environment from Laboratory Data," (Philadelphia: American Society for Testing and Materials, Special Technical Publication 657, 1978), p. 55.
45. "Environmental Pathways of Selected Chemicals in Freshwater Systems. Part II: Laboratory Studies," U.S. EPA, Publication EPA-600/7-78-074 (1978).
46. Scientific American. *The Biosphere* (San Francisco: W. H. Freeman and Co., 1970).
47. Manahan, S. E. *Environmental Chemistry* (Boston: Willard Grant Press, 1974).
48. Higgins, I. J., and R. G. Burns. *The Chemistry and Microbiology of Pollution* (London: Academic Press, 1975).
49. Stoker, H. S., and S. L. Seager. *Environmental Chemistry: Air and Water Pollution* (Glenview, IL: Scott, Foresman and Company, 1976).
50. Moore, J. W., and E. M. Moore. *Environmental Chemistry* (New York: Academic Press, Inc., 1976).

51. Hodges, L. *Environmental Pollution* (New York: Holt Rinehart and Winston, 1977).
52. Bockris, J. O. M. *Environmental Chemistry* (New York: Plenum Publishing Corporation, 1977).
53. Baily, R. A., H. M. Clarke, J. P. Ferris, S. Kranse and R. L. Strong. *Chemistry of the Environment* (New York: Academic Press, Inc., 1978).
54. Horne, R. A. *The Chemistry of Our Environment* (New York: John Wiley & Sons, Inc., 1978).
55. Hutzinger, O. "Environmental Chemistry," lecture notes, University of Amsterdam (1977).
56. Hutzinger, O., Ed. *Handbook of Environmental Chemistry, Vol. 1-3* (Heidelberg: Springer-Verlag, 1980).
57. Connell, D. W., and P. D. Vowles. *Experiments in Environmental Chemistry* (Oxford: Pergamon Press, 1980).

# CHAPTER 3

# PHYSICOCHEMICAL FACTORS IN ROUTES AND RATES OF HUMAN EXPOSURE TO CHEMICALS

**V. H. Freed and C. T. Chiou**

Department of Agricultural Chemistry
Oregon State University
Corvallis, Oregon

## INTRODUCTION

The processes of life are carried on in an essentially chemical world. Chemical reactions are the basis of food use and the growth of cells and organisms. Regulation of growth is mediated by chemicals such as hormones; response to external agents, whether physical, biological, or chemical, results in a change in the chemistry of the organism. Xenobiotics, therefore, play an important role in the health and welfare of an organism [1-3]. Depending on the level and extent of exposure, such agents can significantly influence the organism's well-being.

With the escape or release of a chemical into the environment, there is a finite probability of human exposure because the dynamics of the chemical and the system into which it is introduced results in its movement [4]. Although many would wish for a zero exposure to xenobiotics, this is virtually unattainable as long as chemicals are manufactured and used [1,4-6]. Indeed, even if no chemical were manufactured and used by man, the naturally occuring products and elements would continue to provide exposure.

Many years ago, Paracelsus observed that "the dose makes the poison" [7]. The validity of this observation has been confirmed in toxicological experiments many times over. With any chemical, the intensity of effect and the time required to produce that effect is related to the amount of the chemical to which the organism is exposed [3,7]. It doesn't matter whether or not there is a threshold below which no observable effect is noted; once the dosage is increased, the response becomes shortened and augmented.

It is important, then, to know the level of exposure that humans may receive, to assess the likelihood of adverse effect, its nature and probable seriousness. The concentration or level of the chemical providing the exposure may be measured directly in the various environmental media, but the dynamics would require a continuous monitoring of this level to provide an integrated dose figure. Obviously, with the great number of chemicals in use today, continuous monitoring of all of them to determine the exposure level of the population is a formidable undertaking. Therefore, a fundamental means of estimating routes and rates of exposure would be of great value.

In only a relatively few instances have accurate measurements of human exposure to xenobiotics been made [2,4,8,9]. The principal examples of such measurement involves certain air pollutants such as sulfur dioxide, food additives and residues, and a few occupational exposures. Even these are fraught with uncertainty because of the unpredictability of human behavior [10-12].

## EXPOSURE

There are a number of ways in which man may be exposed to chemicals. The primary routes of exposure to environmental chemicals are dermal, respiratory and oral. These are inadvertent routes, whereas injections (intravenous, subcutaneous or intraperitoneal) are advertent or intended routes of exposure [7].

In the case of the environmental chemical, the predominant route of exposure will vary as to the nature of the activity, whether the compound is undergoing transport or is resident in a particular compartment of the environment, e.g., water or food, and on the physicochemical properties of the materials. Thus, with a compound of high vapor pressure, the probability of respiratory exposure is much greater than dermal or oral exposure unless the material is spilled on the skin. On the other hand, a compound of low vapor pressure and poor solubility might more frequently be encountered on oral ingestion.

The route of exposure is important, both as to the amount absorbed and the rapidity of the response. This is caused by the nature of the barrier, i.e., skin, intestinal mucosa, alveolar cells and the blood supply to the particular barrier or organ. There is also the matter of the chemistry of the absorbing organ as to whether it is preferential in taking up lipid-soluble materials or whether hydophilic substances pass with more ease across the barrier [8]. In general, the toxicity and rapidity of reaction decreases as the exposure occurs through intravenous, respiratory, oral or dermal routes.

Similarly, there is considerable difference in the determined LD50 (the dosage producing a 50% toxicity in a sample population) as indicated in Table I for toxaphene, an organochlorine insecticide. This difference in toxicity based on routes of exposure is probably caused partly by the speed with which the concentration of the chemical builds up in the susceptible organ or sites. Thus, one would expect for most substances that the skin, because of its *corneum stratum*, would provide a barrier that would reduce the rate of entry. Indeed, one finds a difference in dermal penetration depending on the portion of the body exposed. This is illustrated by the penetration of parathion on skin of different regions of the body (Table II).

With many environmental chemicals, exposure accrues through several routes, although one may be the predominant exposure route. However,

**Table I. Toxicity of Toxaphene to Rats**

| Route of Administration | LD50 (mg/kg) | Carrier |
|---|---|---|
| Intravenous | 13 | Peanut Oil |
| Oral | 90 | Peanut Oil |
| Dermal | 930 | Xylene |
| Inhalation LC50, (40% dust) | 3.4 mg/l | |

**Table II. Dermal Absorption of an Organophosphate**

| Body Area | Relative Absorption (%) |
|---|---|
| Hands | 12 |
| Forearm | 8 |
| Upperarm | 28 |
| Feet | 13 |
| Cheek | 46 |
| Forehead | 36 |
| Scrotum | 100 |

in an instance such as Love Canal, exposure is probably dermal, oral and respiratory. Thus, once the barrier seal of the dump was broken by construction, migration of the chemical was possible. Consequently, many of these substances would evaporate, even though of relatively low vapor pressure, to afford respiratory exposure. Some would be transported, adsorbed on dust particles affording dermal exposure and others getting into water, possibly resulting in oral exposure.

Regardless of route of exposure, the matter of fundamental importance is the amount or dose of the chemical received [7,13]. If one takes a group of animals and exposes them through oral, dermal or inhalation routes to a predetermined amount of the chemical, and likewise takes a similar group exposed to incrementally larger amounts of chemical, the number of animals responding to the exposure in any given group increases as the amount of chemical increases. This is the basic dose-response relationship. The dose below which there is no observable effect is often called the threshold or no-observable-effect level. For many toxic responses, there does appear to be a threshold below which no discernible adverse effect occurs. However, for carcinogenic responses, it is believed by many that the exposure to any level of chemical carries with it the potential for initiating cancer. Toxicologists are not in full agreement on the "no-threshold" concept, feeling that the variation in potency (toxicity) and nature of reactions is bound to vary across the array of chemicals; therefore, for some chemicals there indeed would be no threshold, whereas for others such a threshold may exist.

On the other hand, even if no threshold exists for carcinogenic action of the chemical, there is a dose-response effect. In this instance, as dosage increases, so does the yield of tumors; simultaneously there is a general shortening of the period between exposure and appearance of the tumor.

There is almost no chemical without toxicity to one or more species of organisms when administered in a sufficiently large dose by the right means. Considerable variations in the toxicity is observed among chemicals, leading to the conclusion that the particular kinds and arrangements of atoms determine an intrinsic property of toxicity. However, whether a particular chemical in the environment produces a toxic effect or hazard depends on a variety of factors, not the least of which are the physicochemical properties of the compound. The likelihood of adverse effect or hazard, therefore, may be said to be comprised of at least four factors:

1. the intrinsic toxicity;
2. the selectivity among species, which is a function of the species, route of exposure and properties of the compound;
3. the persistence of the chemical; and
4. the mobility of the chemical

The intrinsic toxicity would appear to be a property that depends on the kinds and number of atoms and their particular arrangement. Although many efforts have been made to relate structure and activity to chemical composition and arrangement, knowledge in this area is as yet imprecise, and rarely permits extrapolation from one class of compounds to another. The other factors involved in the potential for adverse effect of an environmental chemical can be shown to be related at least, in part, to the physicochemical properties of the compound as well as the processes in the environment. Take, for example, the matter of persistence in relation to hazard from a chemical. Tetraethylpyrophosphate was one of the early organophosphates developed for use as an insecticide. The material is highly toxic on either respiratory or dermal exposure, with an LD50 of a few milligrams per kilogram of body weight. A great deal of this material was used, but the number of poisoning cases was relatively low. The reason for the low number of poisoning cases was deduced to be the rapid hydrolysis of the compound in the environment, thus markedly lowering the hazard. Similarly, it is found that certain compounds will be highly toxic to one class of organisms and relatively low to another due to differences in physical properties. DDT, for example, is highly toxic to susceptible insects because it partitions favorably into the insect body (fat), but in contrast has a relatively low toxicity to mammals since their system does not afford so ready passage through the skin or intestinal mucosa.

It is thus apparent that physicochemical factors play an important role, both in whether or not exposure will occur and whether or not the chemical will find access to the organism. It has been concluded from a number of studies that the partition coefficient between lipids and water as indicated by the octanol-water partition coefficient is a factor in dermal adsorption [8]. There are upper and lower bounds to the partition coefficient favorable for absorption, and these have been defined for a number of different substances [12,14,15]. The utility of the partition coefficient as an indicator of ease of internal exposure, that is passage into the organism, was first propounded by Overton and Meyer in the nineteenth century. Though not the full answer in every situation, it has nonetheless proven a fairly good predictive tool, not only for dermal absorption, but for uptake of a variety of chemicals in a number of different species [16,17].

It is also intuitively obvious that the vapor pressure is a property of the compound that relates to exposure. Although it has long been appreciated that the low-boiling, high-vapor-pressure compounds, e.g., chloroform, vinyl chloride, ethylene dibromide and sulfur dioxide, when released would result in respiratory exposure; an appreciation of the extent of respiratory exposure accruing from low-vapor-pressure compounds spread over large areas has only been recently recognized. This has become increasingly apparent in cases of pesticide use or industrial waste disposal on soil surfaces. Thus, compounds with vapor pressure on the order of $10^{-5}$-$10^{-7}$ torr at 25°C will show substantial evaporative losses from a surface in a matter of a few days. The process, of course, depends in part, on water providing competitive adsorption to prevent the organic molecule from becoming "fixed" or adsorbed on colloidal particles. An approach [18] to understanding the quantitative aspects of this factor in exposure involves the modified Langmuir or Knudsen diffusion equation. For evaporative loss of a pure chemical, the expression is:

$$Q^{\circ}_i = \beta_i P_i \sqrt{\frac{M_i}{2\pi RT}}$$

where $Q^{\circ}_i$ = amount of chemical vaporizing per unit area per unit time
$P_i$ = vapor pressure
$\beta_i$ = air turbulence
$M_i$ = molecular weight
$R$ = gas constant
$T$ = temperature, °K

Table III shows the relatively good agreement between the calculated rate loss and that determined experimentally.

Similarly, the rate of loss from an aqueous system may be analyzed as follows [19]:

$$Q_i = \beta_i \alpha_i P_i \sqrt{\frac{M_i}{2\pi RT}}$$

where $\alpha_i$ = the relative solute depletion near the water surface compared to that in the bulk-water phase ($\leqslant 1$), and is a function of the chemical's Henry's law coefficient ($H_i$) and the subwater mixing efficiency
$P_i$ = the partial pressure corresponding to the bulk phase solute concentration.

In general, $\alpha_i = 1$ for poorly volatile solutes, i.e., low $H_i$, in all conditions. For highly volatile solutes (high $H_i$), $\alpha_i$ is less than 1 in an unmixed or poorly mixed solution, and is a function of $H_i$ for given system conditions. The relation between $\alpha_i$ and $H_i$ has been established under certain system conditions [19] to assess the evaporative losses of various solutes from water.

It is apparent from the foregoing examples that the properties of the chemical are indeed important as factors in human exposure to environmental chemicals. The physical properties and chemical reactivity are involved in the route and rate of exposure that is likely to be received. These factors also interact with the environmental processes in a predictable manner to either increase or decrease the probability of exposure [4,20]. Thus, the movement, distribution and persistence of the chemical, all of which relate to the possibility of exposure whether in an occupational or environmental setting, are a function of chemical properties and environmental processes [4,9,21].

Table III. Evaporation Rates of Chemicals

| Compound | P (mm Hg) | Evaporative Loss ($g/cm^2$-hr) Experimental | Calculated[a] |
|---|---|---|---|
| Dichlofenthion (20°C) | $5.6 \times 10^{-4}$ | $7.8 \times 10^{-7}$ | $2.3 \times 10^{-6}$ |
| Fenitrothion (20°C) | $2.2 \times 10^{-4}$ | $2.7 \times 10^{-7}$ | $8.7 \times 10^{-7}$ |
| Malathion (20°C) | $3.4 \times 10^{-4}$ | $5.8 \times 10^{-7}$ | $1.5 \times 10^{-6}$ |
| Parathion (20°C) | $3.8 \times 10^{-5}$ | $1.7 \times 10^{-7}$ | $1.5 \times 10^{-7}$ |
| Ronnel (20°C) | $5.5 \times 10^{-5}$ | $9.2 \times 10^{-8}$ | $2.3 \times 10^{-7}$ |
| Methyl Dursban (20°C) | $3.4 \times 10^{-5}$ | $3.8 \times 10^{-8}$ | $1.5 \times 10^{-7}$ |
| Dicapthon (20°C) | $3.6 \times 10^{-6}$ | $\sim 1.5 \times 10^{-8}$ | $\sim 1.5 \times 10^{-8}$ |
| 1,2-Dichlorobenzene (23.2°C) | 1.30 | $4.25 \times 10^{-3}$ | $3.71 \times 10^{-3}$ |
| *m*-Xylene (23.5°C) | 8.00 | $1.80 \times 10^{-2}$ | $1.96 \times 10^{-2}$ |
| 1,2-Dibromoethane (24°C) | 13.5 | $4.46 \times 10^{-2}$ | $4.37 \times 10^{-2}$ |
| Water (23.7°C; 30% relative humidity[b] | 22.0 | $1.81 \times 10^{-2}$ | $1.54 \times 10^{-2}$ |

[a] $Q_{cal} = \beta P(M/2\pi RT)^{1/2}$, where $\beta$ is the average evaporation constant and has a value of $\beta = 1.98 \times 10^{-5}$ (±9% SD); P is the vapor pressure at temperature T (°K).

[b] At 30% relative humidity, the effective vapor pressure of liquid water was calculated to be equal to 70% of the saturated value.

## PHYSICOCHEMICAL CONSIDERATIONS

If a chemical were essentially immobile and inert after release into the environment, human exposure would be a negligible problem. The chemicals, however, are neither immobile nor unreactive, and, as a consequence of their movement, result in exposure. Whether the movement or transport is through diffusion in air or water, or passive transport by these agents, varying amounts are carried from point of release to humans and other biota. The quantity, routes and rates of chemical transport are a function of the amount released, the intensity of environmental conditions and processes, and the property of the chemical itself. Thus, temperature, velocity of air movement, water, light and various biological factors play a role in transport and exposure. So also do the chemical and physical properties of the compound play a role. Thus, a substantial proportion of a highly volatile compound will be transported and afford an exposure as a vapor [9,21,22]. In contrast, compounds of low volatility are more likely to be transported in solution, adsorbed on particles, or accumulate as a residue in a food matrix.

Given that the physical and chemical properties are important to potential for transport and exposure, the environmental chemist is concerned with identifying these physicochemical properties and establishing the quantitative relationship to exposure. A number of such properties have been investigated through the years. A variety of physical and chemical properties have been studied in relation to transport, exposure and effect on the organism [7,23, 24]. These investigations have addressed such problems as vapor pressure, ionization, parachors, molecular volumes and some of the very sophisticated studies on geometry of molecules and electron distribution [14,15, 24,25].

Water solubility has been a property of concern, particularly as it relates to a transport. Very early, it was found that, at least with nonionizable compounds, water solubility shows an inverse correlation to adsorption. More recently, the octanol-water partition coefficient has been demonstrated to be related not only to biouptake and bioaccumulation, but also to adsorption, which appears to be a key phenomenon in environmental behavior. Table IV presents a listing of some physicochemical properties that have been found to be related to the transport and exposure.

**Table IV. Relationship Between Some Physical Properties of a Chemical, and Transport and Exposure**

| Physicochemical Property | Related to |
|---|---|
| Solubility in Water | Adsorption, route of absorption, mobility in environment |
| Latent Heat of Solution | Adsorption, leaching, vaporization from surfaces |
| Partition Coefficient | Bioaccumulation potential, sorption by organic matter |
| Hydrolysis | Persistence in environment or biota |
| Ionization | Route and mechanism of absorption or uptake, persistence, interaction with other molecular species |
| Vapor Pressure | Atmospheric mobility, persistence |

## Adsorption

When a chemical is released or escapes into the environment, it encounters many different types of solid surfaces. Interaction with these surfaces is important to the ultimate fate of the chemical, its transport and the exposure that is likely to be received. Although the nature of the surface is important, so also has been found the properties of the chemical in determining the the degree of interaction [26]. While nonionic compounds may interact through various forces (such as van der Waals), the ionic forms may interact through ion exchange. The overall reaction, however, may be written as:

$$[\text{Chemical}] + [\text{Surface}] \rightleftharpoons [\text{Chemical} \cdot \text{Surface}] + [\text{Surface*}] + [\text{Chemical*}]$$

Under specified conditions, this reaction attains an apparent equilibrium for which an equilibrium constant may be derived.

The energy involved in the adsorption now modifies the mobility of the chemical, both with water and air [26,27]. Thus, once adsorbed, the rate of evaporation may be reduced materially [27] or its rate of leaching, if it is in soil, can be modified [26,28,29]. Similarly, the bioavailability of the compound once adsorbed, is usually reduced. This, of course, is a well known phenomenon employed for years by physicians in treating human poisoning [7].

In dealing with the adsorption of nonionic compounds by soils, a number of investigators have observed the close correlation between adsorption and organic matter. Although the adsorption can also be correlated to the amount of clay, type of clay and other factors, the highest correlation coefficient is usually found with the organic content of the soil [26,29].

Once adsorbed, the mobility of the material will be reduced substantially. This may reduce its rate of evaporation from a plant or soil surface, or its mobility with water percolating through the soil. Such a relationship has been demonstrated by a number of investigators [21,22,27]. The relationship developed by Lambert et al. [28], although not as sophisticated as some of the others, is especially useful in assessing the concentration profile of the chemical moving with water as a function of the depth of penetration through soil, $\Delta x$.

$$C_i = \frac{Q_i}{\sigma\sqrt{2\pi}} \exp \frac{-(\Delta x)^2}{2\sigma^2}$$

Based on the soil-water equilibrium studies, it became interesting to speculate on the possibility that the nonionic compounds were, in fact, partitioning into the organic matter not unlike the phenomenon observed in the octanol-water partitioning. This speculation is augmented by the recent work of Chiou et al. [30], where soil-water equilibrium data are reported to be consistent with the hypothesis of solute partitioning in the soil organic matter. Assuming a partition concept, the reported correlations of the partitioning between soil organics with the octanol-water partition are presumably the result of similar equilibrium processes. The relation between the two is shown in Figure 1. In this case, the partitioning

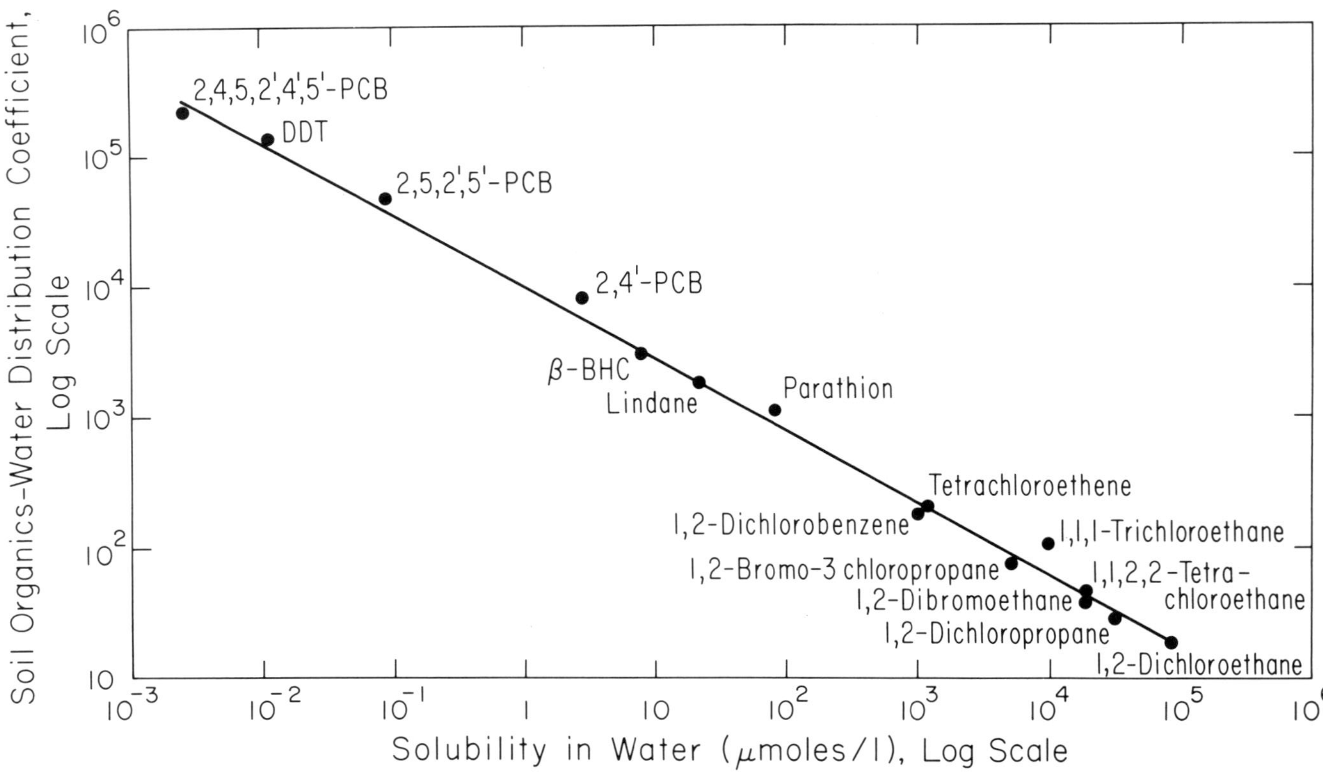


**Figure 1.** Relationship between water solubility and partitioning into soil organic matter.

between organic matter in soil and water is plotted against solubility which, as will be shown, is also related to the partition coefficient. The correlation coefficient where n equals 15 compounds is equal to 0.988. This would appear to provide another application of the partitioning phenomenon as a physicochemical factor in evaluating exposure and transport from chemicals.

## VAPOR BEHAVIOR

The potential for exposure from gases and high-vapor-pressure compounds has long been recognized. With many compounds of low vapor pressure, e.g., $10^{-5}$ and less, it was not until more sensitive methods of analysis existed that this could be established. These compounds also afforded respiratory exposure. With such compounds, losses as vapors can be appreciable when the surface area is large. For example, the work of Spencer et al. [21] and others [22,27] have shown appreciable quantities of DDT, a compound with a vapor pressure of about $1.9 \times 10^{-7}$ torr (at 20°C), to show substantial evaporative losses from soil shortly after application. Similarly, many industrial compounds and waste disposed on soil or in water may be lost to the atmosphere, thus resulting in respiratory exposure [1,6,17].

The quantitative relationship between the amount of chemical lost per unit area and vapor pressure was discussed in an earlier section.

When the chemical is present in a solid matrix such as soil or water, there is a modification of the behavior. The sorption on soil may substantially reduce the rate of evaporation, largely by reducing the apparent vapor pressure. Such is the case of trifuralin, reported by Spencer et al. [21]. When the surface of the soil dried and sorption occurred, the rate of vapor loss was reduced.

In water, evaporative losses are strongly influenced by Henry's constants as indicated in the previous discussion of vapor behavior.

## SOLUTION BEHAVIOR

Chemicals may reach water through direct injection as in disposal of waste through runoff from the surface or percolation through the soil profile [4,9, 17,20]. Contamination of water by chemicals is a significant factor, because subsequent use of such water for drinking results in oral ingestion.

Water chemistry and dynamics significantly influence the distribution and behavior of the chemical. Solubility, however, is an imporant factor, especially as it relates to biological availability and accumulation. Adsorption on particulate matter or partitioning to films of oil and proteins may contribute to significantly increasing the amount of chemical in water, allowing concentrations in excess of its solubility. Conversely, high salt concentrations may reduce the amount of material.

## PARTITIONING AND BIOACCUMULATION

The distribution of a chemical between phases or partitioning is recognized as an important and almost determinative factor in transport, behavior and exposure. Thus, adsorption is a partitioning between a solid phase and either gas or liquid that occurs in soil and in water; other examples of partitioning are between immiscible liquid phases and between gas or liquid phases and biota. This partitioning is significant in terms of behavior of the chemical, its uptake and bioaccumulation. One of the widely known examples of the role of partitioning in influencing uptake or exposure is that involving herbicides. It has been found that a soil-applied herbicide shows decreasing activity from sandy soil to clay to an organic soil [26,29]. The reason is the increasing adsorbtivity of the soil with greater partitioning into the solid phase with a subsequent reduction of bioavailability. Similar results have been noted in fish toxicology where the concentration (TLM96) in clear filtered water is much less than the TLM96 in muddy water [9,12,20,23].

As indicated earlier, partition or distribution coefficients have long been of interest to those concerned with biological activity of the chemicals. Starting in the nineteenth century, attempts were made to correlate biological activity to distribution coefficients between two liquid phases. Hansch et al. [14,25] greatly extended this concept and successfully applied it to a larger number of compounds. Partition or distribution coefficients have been found to play a role in many other instances, particularly some of those relating to exposure and uptake [8,15,16,18]. Thus, mobility in soil with subsequent movement to water has been shown to be related to the distribution coefficient between soil organic matter and the water phase [4,28]. A good correlation exists between the octanol-water partition coefficient and the organic carbon-water partition coefficient. In like manner, the octanol-water partition coefficient has been related in numerous studies to uptake by fish and in some instances, dermal uptake by mammals [8,12,15].

There appears to be a good correlation between water solubility of nonionic compounds and their partition coefficient as shown in Table V.

Table V. Solubilities and Partition Coefficients of Various Compounds

| Compound | Solubility in Water (ppm) | Log ($n$-Octanol/$H_2O$ Partition Coefficient) |
|---|---|---|
| Benzene | 820 (22°C)[a] | 2.13[b] |
| Toluene | 470 (16°)[a] | 2.69[b] |
| Fluorobenzene | 1540 (30°)[a] | 2.27[b] |
| Chlorobenzene | 448 (30°)[a] | 2.84[b] |
| Bromobenzene | 446 (30°)[a] | 2.99[b] |
| Iodobenzene | 340 (30°)[a] | 3.25[c] |
| *p*-Dichlorobenzene | 79 (25°)[a] | 3.38[d] |
| Naphthalene | 30[a] | 3.37[e] |
| Diphenyl Ether | 21 (25°)[d] | 4.20[d] |
| Tetrachloroethylene | 400 (25°)[d] | 2.60[d] |
| Chloroform | 7950 (25°)[d] | 1.97[f] |
| Carbon Tetrachloride | 800[a] | 2.64[g] |
| *p,p'*-DDT | 0.0031[h]-0.0034[i] | 6.19[j] |
| *p,p'*-DDE | 0.040 (20°) | 5.69[j] |
| Benzoic Acid | 2700 (18°)[a] | 1.87[b] |
| Salicylic Acid | 1800 (20°)[a] | 2.26[f] |
| Phenylacetic Acid | 16600 (20°)[a] | 1.41[b] |
| Phenoxyacetic Acid | 12000 (10°)[a] | 1.26[b] |
| 2,4-D | 890 (25°)[d] | 2.81[b] |
| 2,4,5,2',5'-PCB | 0.010 (24°) | 6.11 |
| 2,4,5,2',4',5'-PCB | 0.00095 (24°) | 6.72 |
| 4,4'-PCB | 0.062 (20°) | 5.58 |
| Phosalone | 2.12 (20°) | 4.30 |
| Methyl Chlorpyrifos | 4.76 (20°) | 4.31 |

[a] From Reference 31.
[b] From Reference 32.
[c] From Reference 33.
[d] From Reference 34.
[e] From Reference 35.
[f] From Reference 36.
[g] From Reference 37.
[h] From Reference 38.
[i] From Reference 39.
[j] From Reference 40.

## CONCLUSIONS

Many thousands of compounds, both synthetic and natural, exist in the environment. Chemical considerations would clearly indicate the high probability of exposure to many of these substances. It is desirable, almost crucial, to know the routes and rates of these exposures. Because of the interaction of the properties of the chemical with components and processes of the environment, it is clear that a number of physicochemical factors are involved. Investigation of these physicochemical factors permits us to begin the assessment of probable routes and rates by which the exposure will occur and to devise strategies to minimize the level of exposure. Advantage can also be taken of reactivity of many of the compounds as well as physical properties in both evaluating the exposure and methods of reducing it.

## REFERENCES

1. "Environmental Measurements of Chemicals for Assessment of Human Exposure," *Human Health and the Environment–Some Research Needs, Number 2* Report of the 2nd Task Force for Research Planning in Environmental Health Sciences, U.S. DHEW, NIEHS, (1977) pp. 217–242.
2. Kraybill, H. F. "Conceptual Approaches to the Assessment of Non-Occupational Environmental Cancer," in *Environmèntal Cancer,* H. F. Kraybill and M. A. Mehlman, Eds. (Washington: Hemisphere Publishing Corporation, 1977), pp. 27–62.
3. VanDuuren, V. L. "Chemical Structure, Reactivity and Carcinogenicity of Halo Hydrocarbons," *Environ. Health Persp.* 21:7–16 (1977).
4. Freed, V. H., C. T. Chiou and R. Haque. "Chemodynamics: Transport and Behavior of Chemicals in the Environment–A Problem in Environmental Health," *Environ. Health Persp.* 20:55–70 (1977).
5. Davies, J. E., and W. F. Edmundson. *Epidemiology of DDT* Mount Kisco, NY: Futura Publishing Company, 1972), pp. 1–157.
6. "Transport and Alteration of Pollutants, Waste Disposal, and Natural Sources of Toxicants," in *Human Health and the Environment–Some Research Needs, Number 2,* Report of the 2nd Task Force for Research Planning in Environmental Health Sciences, U.S. DHEW, NIEHS (1977) pp. 183–216.
7. Hayes, W. J., Jr. *Toxicology of Pesticides* (Baltimore: Williams and Wilkins Co., 1975).
8. Dugard, T. H. "Skin Permeability Theory in Relation to Measurement of Percutaneous Absorption in Toxicology," in *Dermatotoxicology and Pharmacology,* F. N. Marzulli and H. I. Maibach, Eds. (Washington, DC: Hemisphere Publishing Corporation, 1977), pp. 525–550.
9. Maltoni, C. "Recent Findings on the Carcinogenicity of Chlorinated Olefins," *Environ. Health Persp.* 21:1–6 (1977).

10. Davies, J. E. et al. "International Dynamics of Pesticide Poisonings," in *Environmental Dynamics of Pesticides,* R. Haque and V. H. Freed, Eds. (New York: Plenum Publishing Corporation, 1975), pp. 275-284.
11. Hoben, H. J., S. A. Ching and L. J. Casarett. "A Study of Inhalation of Pentachlorophenol by Rats, III, Inhalation Toxicity Study," *Bull. Environ. Contam. Toxicol.* 15:463-465 (1976).
12. Kenaga, E. E. "Guidelines for Environmental Study of Pesticides: Determination of Bioconcentration Potential," *Residue Rev.* 44:73-113 (1972).
13. Kotin, T. "Dose-Response Relationship and Threshhold Concepts," *Ann. N.Y. Acad. Sci.* 271:22-28 (1976).
14. Hansch, C. "A Computerized Approach to Quantitative Biochemical Structure-Activity Relationships," in *Biological Correlation–The Hansch Approach,* Advances in Chemistry Series 114 (Washington, DC: American Chemical Society, 1972), pp. 20-40.
15. Taylor, A. W. "Post Application Volatilization of Pesticides Under Field Conditions," *J. Air Poll. Control Assoc.* 28:922-927 (1978).
16. Chiou, C. T., V. H. Freed, D. W. Schmedding and R. L. Kohnert. "Partition Coefficient and Bioaccumulation of Selected Organic Chemicals." *Environ. Sci. Technol.* 11:475-478 (1977).
17. Freed, V. H., and C. T. Chiou. "Transport and Distribution of Pesticides," paper presented at the joint symposium of American Chemical Society and Chemical Society of Japan, ACS meeting, Honolulu, Hawaii, April 1979.
18. Chiou, C. T., and V. H. Freed. "Assessment of Volatility and Partition Coefficient from Physical Chemical Properties," Proceedings of Terrestrial Microcosms and Environmental Chemistry Symposium, Corvallis, OR, June 13-17, 1977, NSF/RANN 79-0026, (1977) p. 17.
19. Chiou, C. T., V. H. Freed, L. J. Peters and R. L. Kohnert. "Evaporation of Solutes from Water," (to be published).
20. Hartung, R. "Accumulation of Chemicals in the Hydrosphere," in *Environmental Dynamics of Pesticides,* R. Haque and V. H. Freed, Eds. (New York: Plenum Publishing Corporation, 1975), pp. 185-198.
21. Spencer, W. F., and M. M. Cliath. "Vaporization of Chemicals," in *Environmental Dynamics of Pesticides,* R. Haque and V. H. Freed, Eds. (New York, Plenum Publishing Corporation, 1975) pp. 61-78.
22. Glotfelty, D. E. "The Atmosphere as a Sink for Applied Pesticides," *J. Air Poll. Control Assoc.* 28:917-921 (1978).
23. Kenaga, E. E. "Test Organisms and Methods Used for Early Assessment of Acute Toxicity of Chemicals," *Environ. Sci. Technol.* 12: 1322-1329 (1978).
24. Tulp, M. Th. M., and O. Hutzinger. "Some Thoughts on Aqueous Solubilities and Partition Coefficients of PCB and the Mathematical Correlation Between Bioaccumulation and Physico-Chemico Properties," *Chemosphere* 10:849-860 (1978).
25. Helmer, F., K. Kiehs and C. Hansch. "The Linear Free-Energy Relationship Between Partition Coefficients and the Binding and Conformational Perturbations of Macromolecules by Small Organic Compounds," *Biochemistry* 7:2858-2863 (1968).

26. Hammaker, J. W., and G. M. Thompson. "Adsorption," in *Organic Chemicals in the Soil Environment, Vol. 1* (New York: Marcel Dekker, 1972), pp. 49–144.
27. Sherburne, H. R., and V. H. Freed. "Soil Effects on Herbicides. Adsorption of 3(p-Chlorophenyl)-1,1-Dimethylurea as a Function of Soil Constituents," *J. Agric. Food Chem.* 2:937–939 (1954).
28. Lambert, S. M., P. E. Porter and R. H. Schieferstein. "Movement and Sorption of Chemicals Applied to the Soil," *Weeds* (1965) pp. 185–190.
29. Seba, D. B., and E. F. Corcoran. "Surface Slicks as Concentrators of Pesticides in the Marine Environment," *Pestic. Monit. J.* 3:190–193 (1969).
30. Chiou, C. T., L. J. Peters and V. H. Freed. "A Physical Concept of Soil-Water Equilibria for Nonionic Organics," *Science* (in press).
31. *Handbook of Chemistry and Physics,* 34th ed. (Cleveland, OH: CRC Press, Inc., 19xx).
32. Fujita, R., J. Iwasa and C. Hansch. *J. Am. Chem. Soc.* 86:5175 (1964).
33. Leo, A., C. Hansch and D. Elkins. *Chem. Rev.* 71:525 (1971).
34. Kenaga, E. E. "Partioning and Uptake in Biological Systems," in *Environmental Dynamics of Pesticides,* R. Haque and V. H. Freed, Eds. (New York: Plenum Publishing Corporation, 1975).
35. Hansch, C., and T. Fujita. *J. Am. Chem. Soc.* 86:1616 (1964).
36. Hansch, C., and S. Anderson. *J. Org. Chem.* 32:2583 (1967).
37. Macy, R. *J. Ind. Hyg. Toxicol.* 30:140 (1948).
38. Bowman, M. C., F. Acree, Jr. and M. K. Corbett. *J. Agric. Food Chem.* 8(5):406 (1960).
39. Biggar, J. W., G. R. Dutt and R. L. Riggs. *Bull. Environ. Contam. Toxicol.* 2(2):90 (1967).
40. O'Brien, R. D. In: *Environmental Dynamics of Pesticides,* R. Haque and V. H. Freed, Eds. (New York: Plenum Publishing Corporation, 1975), p. 336.

# CHAPTER 4

# BIODEGRADATION OF ORGANIC CHEMICALS IN THE ENVIRONMENT

**Robert H. Brink**
Office of Toxic Substances
U.S. Environmental Protection Agency
Washington, DC

## INTRODUCTION

The fate of a chemical in natural environments depends on many factors, such as the structure, water solubility, sorptive tendencies, dissociation constant and volatility of the chemical. Other factors include the susceptibility of the chemical transformation processes such as hydrolysis, photolysis, oxidation or reduction, and biodegradation, as well as features of the particular environment, including temperature, rainfall, wind currents, topography or the presence of molecular oxygen.

The transformation of organic compounds by living organisms is a very important factor in the persistence of organic compounds, and degradative processes caused by microoganisms (bacteria, fungi and algae) are the most important degradation mechanisms for organic compounds in nature, with respect to both the mass of material transformed and the extent to which the material is degraded.

This chapter attempts to present an overview of the significance of biodegradation and the major factors involved in the environmental degradation of organic compounds by microorganisms. Some examples of specific kinds of biodegradation processes will be presented and some of the more interesting and puzzling questions faced by those concerned with the environmental fate of chemicals will be noted. The term "biodegradation" will be used to mean degradation resulting from the activity of microorganisms.

## SIGNIFICANCE

Organic chemicals, whether manmade or natural, are found in all of earth's soils, waters and in the atmosphere, in varying degrees. Those organic compounds may be transformed in the environment by chemical and/or biological agents.

Sometimes the transformations are very rapid, e.g., when a readily metabolized compound such as glucose is added to an oxygen-rich river containing a healthy microbial population. Sometimes the degradation processes are very slow, as has been the case for seed grains stored for thousands of years in the dark and arid tombs of Egyptian Pharaohs or for the organic pigments in the frescoes buried at Pompeii. In those cases degradation has been very slow because the environmental conditions were not favorable for degradation, particularly biodegradation.

The rate and extent of transformations of an organic molecule in the environment also are related to the chemical structure of the molecule. Some types of compounds are more susceptible to hydrolytic or photolytic degradations, for example, than other types. Some compounds degrade very slowly under conditions which should favor microbial attack, and such materials may persist and accumulate in nature if not destroyed by some other means. Such persistence and accumulation may be tolerable if the material is nontoxic and esthetically inoffensive. There are, in fact, examples where long-term persistence is highly desirable, as in materials of construction for buildings and highways, or for lignin, which provides a protective coating for the cellulosic structure of woody plants.

On the other hand, resistance to degradation is a problem when chemicals persist and accumulate in or near some organism at toxic levels. Such occurrences may be caused by manmade compounds or natural materials in the environment.

The various environmental transformations of organic compounds may be divided into three categories: (1) biodegradation–produced by living organisms; (2) photochemical–requiring light energy; and (3) degradation by chemical agents–abiotic transformations not requiring sunlight. In nature, all three can occur simultaneously in the same location, e.g., in a sunlit lake, and it frequently is difficult to differentiate clearly between them–especially between biological and chemical oxidations. Nevertheless, it seems clear that biodegradation is the predominant degradation mechanism in soils and water, and that microorganisms account for an overwhelming share of all biodegradations.

Alexander [1] has stated that evidence indicates that microorganisms are responsible for converting to inorganic products many complex organic molecules that cannot be altered significantly by higher life forms. Studies can be cited [2] in which compounds have been found to be degraded by the action of microorganisms but not by higher organisms. The higher life forms, for the most part, have evolved to absorb relatively simple organic molecules.

Two factors which favor microorganisms over other life forms in biodegradation are their relatively rapid reproduction rates (which allow for rapid mutations and enzymatic adaptations) and their metabolic rate per unit mass. In general, the rate of metabolism increases with increasing surface-to-volume ratios. Bacteria and fungi may thus be expected to be immensely more active in metabolism than higher life forms. For example, a lactose-fermenting bacterium can break down 1000–10,000 times its own weight in lactose in one hour, whereas a man would require 250,000 hours to break down 1000 times his own weight in sugar. Dagley [3] has estimated that microbial biomass (including algae) is much greater than that of all combined animal biomass. Overall, the data indicate that bacteria alone account for a large majority of the degradation of organic compounds in soils, and that microorganisms predominate in aqueous systems.

Biodegradation is often the most desirable mechanism for environmental transformations of organic molecules because the enzymatic degradations involved generally proceed to the formation of metabolites used for growth or potential energy storage or to inorganic molecules such as carbon dioxide, methane, water, nitrogen oxides, or ammonium ion and sulfate. In contrast, photochemical and other chemical processes in nature usually do not proceed to the complete "mineralization" of organic substances, and products of unknown toxicity and/or persistence may be generated. However, it must be emphasized that in nature the various transformation processes seldom occur in isolation, and a photolytic or hydrolytic reaction can provide fragments more readily biodegradable than the parent compound. Also, it must be noted that persistent intermediates can result from biodegradations, although this is the exception rather than the rule in the environment, where mixed microbial populations work together to transfrom organic matter into metabolites for growth and energy. In fact, the ability of microorganisms to degrade organic compounds provides the basic element of the modern waste treatment plant.

## GENERAL FEATURES

A chemical compound, in the presence of a microorganism, generally will (1) act as a nutrient in promoting some activity of the organism; (2) have an adverse effect and act as an antimicrobial; or (3) be essentially unreactive with no significant change to either the compound or the microorganism. There are other possibilities which will be covered briefly in this discussion and which may be very important for some chemicals under certain environmental conditions. These include cometabolism, conjugation and accumulation.

## Cometabolism

Cometabolism is a term used to describe the partial transformation of an organic substrate by a microorganism that cannot use the substrate for growth or energy. This phenomenon was first described by Leadbetter and Foster [4], who noted that there was oxidation of ethane to acetic acid, propane to propionic acid and acetone and butane to butanoic acid and methyl ethyl ketone during growth of *Pseudomonas methanica* on methane, the only hydrocarbon which could support growth of the microorganism. They coined the term "cooxidation," but that has now been replaced by "cometabolism," because it is now recognized that the phenomenon is not limited to oxidations. Many other examples have been described by Horvath [5] and Alexander [6]. The name cometabolism comes from the concept that the partially transformed compound is transformed in the presence of another compound which the microbial population can metabolize readily and use for growth and energy purposes. Some workers describe cometabolism as occurring only in the presence of a metabolizable analog of a cometabolized compound. Most researchers now include any example of the partial degradation of a compound by a microorganism which yields no apparent benefit to the microorganism as an example of cometabolism, whether or not there are metabolizable substrates also present.

The significance and extent of cometabolism in the environment remains unclear. Alexander [6] has stated that cometabolism may be fairly common in the environment, particularly with some of the synthetic chemicals released by mankind. He also proposed that the molecule undergoing cometabolism is acted on by an enzyme of broad specificity that normally serves a physiological function and that the products of the reaction cannot be further transformed by any enzymes of the active population present. Most of our knowledge of cometabolism comes from laboratory studies with pure cultures, and it is difficult to assess what really happens in nature. It is likely that many of the laboratory products of cometabolism are actually degraded in the environment by microorganisms not present in the lab culture. For example, DDT has been observed to be cometabolized by lab cultures to *p*-chlorophenylacetic acid (Figure 1), which cannot be degraded further by the lab culture but which is known to be degraded by other organisms found in soil and water. Another example is provided by Raymond et al. [7,8] (Figure 2). In this case, *p*-xylene was transformed to either 2,

5-dimethylmuconic acid or 3-carboxy-6methyl-catechol by *Nocardia* bacteria which were growing on *n*-hexadecane.

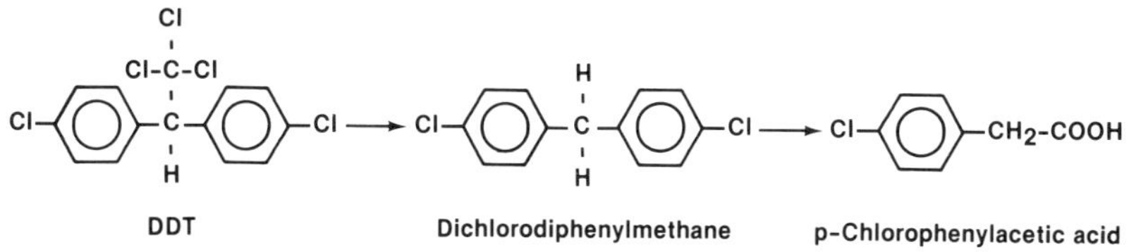


**Figure 1.** Cometabolism of DDT by lab culture.

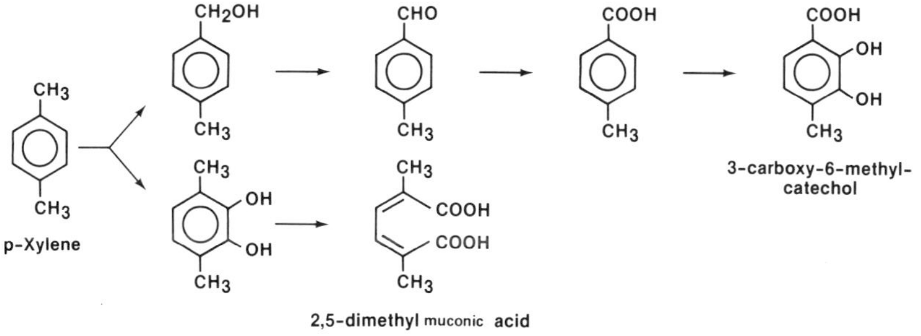


**Figure 2.** Cometabolism of *p*-xylene by *Nocardia* growing on *n*-hexadecane.

Cometabolism is a developing story which is being followed with great interest by those concerned with the environmental persistence of chemicals. Much remains to be learned about what chemicals and products are involved in the environment and which organisms are responsible; why it occurs or how significant it is; and whether or not it might be possible to take advantage of cometabolic reactions either in the degradation of recalcitrant molecules or in the production of some desirable intermediate.

## Conjugation

Conjugation reactions involve the coupling of an organic compound, or an intermediate metabolite of that compound, with an endogenous compound of the microbial cell, resulting in products such as methylated or acetylated versions of the parent compound, amino acid conjugates or glycosides. A related type of synthesis involves the condensation of the parent compound molecules with each other or with degradation intermediates of the parent. Bollag [9] presented examples of these types of reactions; some are shown in Figure 3.

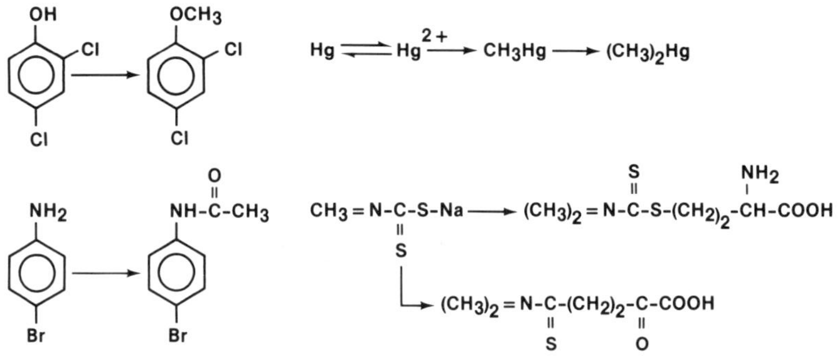


**Figure 3.** Metabolic products resulting from conjugation reactions.

The acetylation of *p*-bromoaniline is interesting because acetylation, although fairly common in mammalian systems, is not commonly observed in microorganisms.

## Accumulation

Accumulation, as the name implies, is the sorption and storage of the unchanged subject chemical. Bioaccumulation of various lipid-soluble persistent compounds, such as DDT and the polychlorinated biphenyls (PCB) and of certain metals or methylated metals, is a well-known problem in higher organisms. There is, however, a tendency to overlook the fact that microorganisms, both living and dead, can sorb significant quantities of foreign compounds and store them, for later release or for a later role in a food chain. The significance of this in the transport of toxic chemicals into food chains, particularly in aquatic habitats, needs to be understood and evaluated more fully.

### Metabolism

Most of the compounds that can be degraded by microoganisms are biodegraded within the microbial cell after passing through the cell wall and the cytoplasmic membrane. In some cases, biodegradation is initiated by extracellular enzymes which lead to the production of fragments that can be transported into the cell. This commonly is associated with the hydrolysis of molecules too large to pass across the cytoplasmic membrane. Typical reactions involve extracellular hydrolysis of polymers such as polysaccharides, proteins, lipids and phospholipids. Most of the enzymes involved in these reactions appear to have relatively low substrate specificity, and it seems possible that these extracellular enzymes may initiate the degradation of those synthetic chemicals which have "natural" attack sites such as glycoside or peptide linkages. Some of the extracellular enzymes are more specific in their activity, and penicillinase is a well-studied example. This enzyme is rather interesting because it is an extracellular enzyme that catalyzes the breakdown of penicillin, a compound which can readily be transported across the cytoplasmic membrane. Of course, from the point of view of the bacterium, this is an excellent arrangement.

Inside the microbial cell, the substrate, if it can be used, is subject to a series of chemical modifications which generally are referred to as metabolism. The starting compound usually will be converted into one or more compounds, known as intermediates, each of which is further metabolized to some ultimate end product of a metabolic pathway. Some examples, many of them common to higher life forms as well as microorganisms, are shown in Figure 4.

Each of the reactions is catalzed by a specific enzyme. Alternative pathways are often available. If a pathway leads to the formation of molecules more complex than the parent compound, the reactions are called "anabolic," If the metabolic pathway leads to a decrease in molecular complexity it is called "catabolic," Catabolic pathways result in the formation of low-molecular-weight compounds that may be excreted as waste products or used as precursors in anabolic pathways leading to the synthesis of new cell constituents. Catabolic reactions also supply the organisms with most of the energy needed to sustain life.

## SOME IMPORTANT VARIABLES

There are a large number of environmental variables that can influence the rate and extent of the biodegradation of an organic compound. Among the more important variables are:

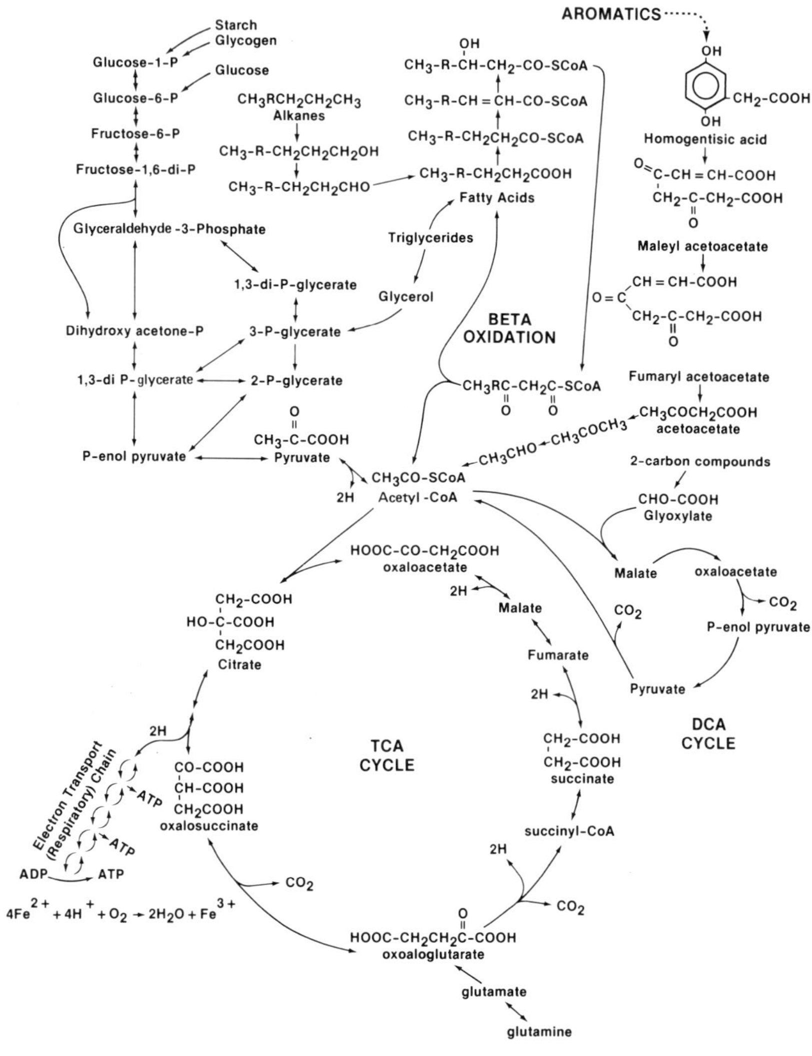


**Figure 4.** Some common metabolic pathways.

1. temperature;
2. hydrogen ion concentration;
3. water and salinity;
4. the quantity and quality of nutrients (other than the organic substrate under consideration), trace metals, vitamins, etc.;
5. dissolved oxygen;
6. the concentration of the organic substrate;
7. the concentration of viable microorganisms;
8. the microbial species composition; and
9. acclimation or adaptation.

In assessing the hazard of a given chemical, it is necessary to be able to predict the concentration of that chemical in the environment. The estimated environmental concentration (EEC) depends on many factors, including the rate at which the compound may be transformed after release to the environment. Methods are now evolving for the calculation of useful reaction rate constants based on laboratory data. What is needed now is a clearer understanding of how environmental variables will influence those rate constants to produce biodegradation rates relevant to a given environment.

## Temperature

Biochemical reactions, including metabolic reactions, follow the general rule that the rate of chemical reaction increases as the temperature increases. Microbial activity, however, requires liquid water, and this limits their reactions to temperatures from about $^-2°C$ (in water of high salinity) to about 100°C. Moreover, most microorganisms contain essential enzymes that will be denatured at temperatures of about 50°C. In work with pure cultures in the laboratory, one can identify temperature ranges over which substrate use and growth of the organism can occur and within that range one usually can identify an optimum temperature range. In the environment, with mixed microbial populations and variations in the physical state of the environment and the chemical composition, optimal temperatures are not so readily determined, although they probably exist for individual species and substrates. A natural population will contain microorganisms adapted to a particular temperature, which may result in more rapid degradation than would be predicted from thermodynamics alone.

## Hydrogen Ion Concentration

Strongly acidic or strongly basic pH will inhibit the activity of most microorganisms, and the majority will thrive best in the pH range 4-9 [10]. Bacteria generally prefer values near 7, and acidic conditions will tend to favor the growth of fungi and yeasts. pH also may influence the products of biodegradation, with lower pH values favoring the synthesis of polysaccharides and the growth of filamentous forms.

pH can have an indirect effect on microbial degradation by its influence on other degradation processes such as hydrolysis and chemical oxidation, as well as on chemical dissociation. In some cases the products of these chemical reactions are biodegradable to a different degree than the parent compound. This may change the rate of mineralization of an organic substrate. For example, the carbamate insecticides pyrolam and dimetiban resist biological oxidation, but their hydrolytic products readily undergo biodegradation in natural waters [11].

## Water and Salinity

For microbial activity to occur, water must be present in its liquid form, but this water may vary considerably with respect to dissolved solids, gases and suspended matter.

One of the more dramatic variables is salinity, with sea water typically containing about 33,000 mg/l dissolved salts, mostly sodium and chloride ions but with appreciable amounts of magnesium, sulfate, calcium and potassium. These ions buffer sea water at a relatively constant pH of 8.0–8.3, somewhat alkaline from an excess of cations. Salinity will vary horizontally and vertically in the oceans, particularly in the vicinity of freshwater inputs. In coastal estuaries receiving fresh water, such as Chesapeake Bay, salinities will range from oceanic levels near the estuary mouth to near freshwater concentrations at river outlets.

Despite the wide ranges in ionic strength, it is not clear why the breakdown of organic matter progresses more slowly in the sea than in inland waters of comparable pH and temperature. Rheinheimer [12] has stated that the slow degradation in oceans is caused chiefly by the inhibitory action of sea water on many nonmarine bacteria, washed into the oceans from the adjoining lands. Reports by Floodgate [13] and Gibbs [14] suggest that nutrient limitations, particularly low nitrogen levels, may be a more important factor. Given sufficient nutrients and a similar inoculum, with many compounds there appears to be little difference in laboratory studies between biodegradation results in saline water and in fresh water. However, this is not always the case. For example, the sequestering agent, nitrilotriacetate (NTA), is known to degrade readily in fresh water and open ocean water, once the microbial population has been adapted to the NTA. But studies have shown that NTA biodegradation does not occur easily in estuarine waters. Bourquin and Przybyszewski [15], however, found that bacteria from estuarine surface layers were easily adapted to the degradation of NTA if the bacteria were transferred to freshwater medium but no adaptations occurred in estuarine water.

Biodegradation of organics in the depths of the sea or in ocean bottom sediments, as might be expected, is not the same as at or near the surface. The same holds true for deep lakes. There is much to be learned about biodegradation in the deeper ocean reaches but, in general, that environment is hostile to microbial activity, partly because of restricted light and oxygen, colder temperatures, limited nutrients, and high pressures. Hydrocarbons from oil tankers, offshore wells or other sources receive deserved notoriety for the floating oil that befouls marine birds and shellfish and coats beaches, but it may be that environmentalists should be even more worried about the heavier fractions of crude oil that will sink below the surface, much of it reaching the bottom and mixing with the sand and sediment. Those heavier fractions of the crude oil consist to a large extent of polycyclics which are biodegraded with difficulty even under favorable circumstances and which may persist for very long periods of time on the ocean floor.

## Nutrients, Trace Metals, Vitamins

Some microorganisms do not have the ability to synthesize sufficient quantities of all the organic compounds (e.g., amino acids, purines, pyrimidines and vitamins) needed for growth, and all microorganisms need nitrogen for growth. Very small amounts of a large number of mineral elements are probably required for the growth of all microbes. Phosphorus, sulfur and, to a lesser extent, magnesium, are required in relatively high concentrations. If one or more of these essential factors is in low supply in a given environment, it may lead to poorer-than-expected biodegradation of added organic matter. This observation may lead to the conclusion that the organic matter is resistant to the microbial attack, whereas, in fact, biodegradation has been limited by a scarcity of one or more essential nutrients, a so-called "limiting nutrient." This is probably not common in fertile soils and most freshwater systems, but it is recognized that nitrogen and phosphorus can be limiting nutrients in the ocean [13,14,16], and in oligotrophic lakes.

## Dissolved Oxygen

Microbial degradations may be aerobic or anaerobic—that is, with or without the use of molecular oxygen as an electron acceptor. Both are significant in nature, and both must be considered in any thorough evaluation of the potential for biodegradation of a chemical. Aerobic oxidation usually involves the incorporation of one atom of the oxygen molecule into the organic substrate [17] and combination of the remaining oxygen with hydrogen to form water. Anaerobic processes include fermentation, bacterial photosynthesis and anaerobic respiration. In this overview of the microbial degradation of organics in the environment, anaerobic respiration in which molecules other than oxygen are used as the final electron acceptor is of principal concern. For example, nitrate can be reduced to nitrite or ammonium, and sulfate and thiosulfate may be used to produce hydrogen sulfide. Anaerobic processes will predominate in environments with low oxygen concentration, as in lakebottom silts, swamps and flooded soils. Poole [18] presented a schematic (Figure 5), which shows the relationship between anaerobic respiration, redox potential and the typical electron acceptors. Methanogenesis, which is the terminal step in a complex series of anaerobic respiration reactions, is an important process in the natural degradation of vegetation, as is known by anyone who has traveled through an actively digesting swamp. It is not clear how significant methanogenesis is in the environmental degradation of synthetic organics, but it seems reasonable to believe that many synthetics, if released to anaerobic environments, will be degraded by anaerobic processes.

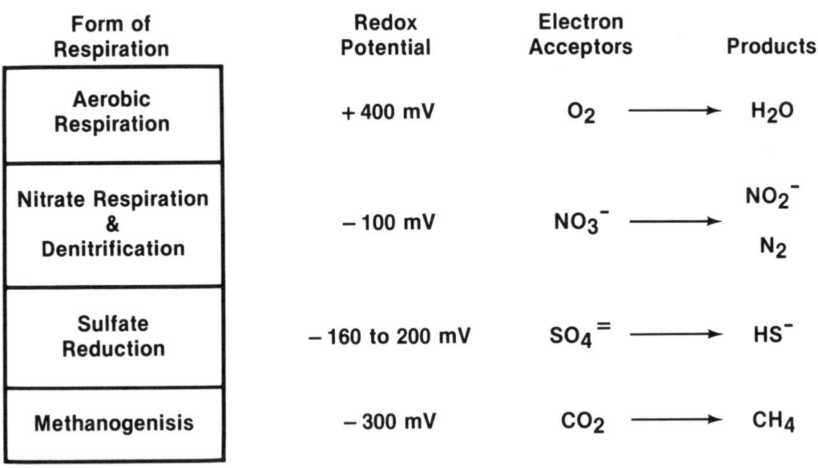


**Figure 5.** Relationship between anaerobic respriation, redox potential and the typical electron acceptors.

## Concentration of Organic Substrate

The concentration of the organic substrate can have a marked effect on its degradation rate. Higher concentrations of some compounds may lead to faster degradation because of reduced acclimation time and/or a rapid increase in the microbial population. On the other hand, some compounds that are readily biodegradable at low concentrations will inhibit microbial activity at higher concentrations.

Of particular interest is the fate of organics present in the environment at very low concentrations (parts-per-billion levels or lower). It had been assumed by many workers in the field that if a compound were readily biodegradable at a moderate concentration, say a few milligrams per liter, then the same compound, if present at nanogram per liter to a few micrograms per liter (which are more realistic environmental concentrations for many chemicals) would also be readily biodegradable. There is uncertainty about this. It may be that when an organic substrate is present at very low concentration, the low concentration may become a limiting factor in the biodegradation of the organic through, perhaps, a lack of enzyme induction. Boethling and Alexander [19,20] have described this phenomenon in studies with substrates such as glucose, *p*-chlorobenzoate and l-naphthyl-N-methylcarbamate. There is a need for research to determine why organics may persist at low concentrations when they are readily biodegradable at higher concentrations. It may be that this persistence is a consequence of the fact that a very low substrate concentration yields a reaction rate so slow that the chemical appears to be nondegrading. For many organics, the fact that a few parts per trillion may persist in nature may not have any practical significance, but there should be serious concern about the persistence of any toxic organics which have a potential for bioaccumulation and biomagnification along food chains.

## Concentration of Viable Microorganisms

The rate (and often the extent and direction) of biodegradation can be related to the density of the microbial population. Organisms that may persist for days or weeks in a sparsely populated natural environment may be degraded in a few hours in an activated sludge treatment plant where the viable microbial population is typically several hundred million per milliliter.

However, as with the effect of substrate concentration, when one considers concentrations of bacteria found in natural soils and waters, the relationships are not so simple. Wright [21], in a report on heterotrophic activity in water, discussed activity as a bacterial population parameter.

Wright studied a river estuary-coastal water system in northeastern Massachusetts, and compared bacterial concentrations with a bacterial activity measurement that is derived from the bacterial count and a measure of activity such as turnover rate or the maximum reaction rate $K_m$ which he calls the specific activity index. In studies on the seasonal, horizontal and vertical variations of bacteria in the water system, Wright found that bacterial numbers varied by about one order of magnitude, and there was no direct correlation between numbers and heterotrophic activity. The acridine orange direct count method (AODC), used by Wright, and more traditional methods to estimate biomass, such as the total plate count, turbidity or volatile suspended solids, do not provide information as to which members of the microbial population are responsible for the observed activity. There is a need to develop methods for identifying the active substrate degraders in environmental samples.

## Microbial Species Composition

The microbial populations in environmental samples can vary considerably in species composition, not only from site to site but also in sequential samples taken from the same site. The species composition and population number are constantly changing in response to changes in, for example, pH, moisture, dissolved oxygen, substrate and nutrient supply, physical mixing, and competition between species. Despite this, to a remarkable degree, a biodegradable organic compound will be degraded at about the same rate and to about the same extent by mixed microbial populations from a wide range of environments, if given sufficient nutrients and dissolved oxygen, and if other variables are controlled. This is quite evident from biodegradation studies conducted by investigators at different locations using different inoculum sources but working with the same substrate and some more-or-less standardized lab procedure such as the biochemical oxygen demand (BOD) test [22] or the Soap and Detergent Association shake flask test [23]. This is partly because some of the most active microorganisms in the degradation of organic compounds, such as the pseudomonads, are ubiquitous, and may be partly caused by the presence in a large number of bacteria of those low-specificity enzymes important in initiating microbial attack on certain synthetic chemicals.

One of the more common causes for the predominance of a bacterial species in a particular environment is the release into that environment of a chemical which the species is able to metabolize. For example, where hydrocarbon spills have occurred there will be found a high percentage of hydrocarbon-utilizing bacteria and fungi. The environment has been "enriched" with respect to the microbial species by presence of the substrate. In some cases the metabolizing species are those whose enzymatic apparatus had to become acclimated to the particular substrate. This is the next variable to be discussed.

### Acclimation or Adaptation

It may be incorrect to call acclimation an environmental variable, but it is an important factor in the biodegradation of many organic molecules, especially those synthetic chemicals released by man, and needs to be considered here.

As noted by Dagley [24], synthetic chemicals will be biodegraded "only when the relevant microbes are able to use the enzymic apparatus acquired during evolution designed to exploit the diverse sources of energy found in nature." Enzymatic attack on synthetic or unfamiliar chemicals will depend on two factors: (1) the ability of the microbial population to accept as substrates those compounds with structures similar but not identical to compounds previously found in nature and degraded by the population; and (2) the ability of the new compound to induce the synthesis of any necessary degradative enzymes through processes referred to as "acclimation" or "adaptation."

As noted in the introduction, this is an attempt to present an overview of environmental biodegradation, and it has been necessary to discuss the above variables in a very rapid and brief fashion, and to ignore some other important factors such as the effects of mechanical mixing and the important role of physical surfaces and boundaries in microbial activities. It is to be hoped that the presentation of these highlights will stimulate the reader to pursue the subject in greater detail to learn more about this complex and fascinating area.

## SPECIFIC DEGRADATION EXAMPLES

This section will present some examples of how microorganisms from natural environments handle the degradation of some specific chemicals. The mechanistic details of these reactions have been obtained largely through laboratory studies with pure cultures which were found to be able to grow on relatively high concentrations of the particular substrate. It is probable that the experimental conditions present a distorted picture of what would actually occur in the environment, particularly because important interspecies relationships such as competition for the substrate or commensalism (the occurrence of two or more organisms living in close proximity where one or more of the organisms may benefit from the association) are not taken into account. Nevertheless, mechanistic studies of biodegradation have provided much interesting information on how environmental degradations might proceed, and have considerably advanced the knowledge of the biochemistry of microbial metabolism.

One approach to a discussion of typical biodegradation reactions is to present examples of the kinds of reactions one may observe; many of these are summarized in Figure 6. Another approach is to describe degradative mechanisms common to certain classes of chemicals, as in the recent review by Chapman [25]. That is the approach that will be followed here.

**Oxidative Reactions**

Hydroxylations

Monohydroxylation $RH \xrightarrow{O_2} R\text{-}OH$

Dihydroxylation

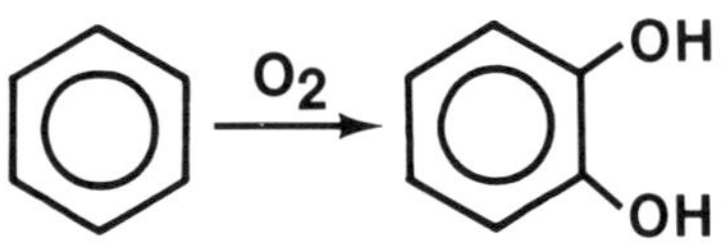


Dealkylation

$\beta$-Oxidation

Cleavage of Ether Linkages

**Reductions**

$RNO_2 \longrightarrow RNH_2$ ; $R\text{-}CO\text{-}COOH \longrightarrow RCHO + CO_2$

**Hydrolysis**

$R\text{-}C(=O)\text{-}X \longrightarrow R\text{-}C(=O)\text{-}OH + H\text{-}X$

$X = \text{-}N(R_2)\text{-}R_1$ , $\text{-}O\text{-}C(R_3)(R_4)$

**Dehalogenation**

| | |
|---|---|
| $R\text{-}X \longrightarrow R\text{-}OH$ | Hydrolytic |
| $R\text{-}CX_3 \longrightarrow R\text{-}CH\text{-}X_2$ | Reduction |
| $RCH_2\text{-}CX_3 \longrightarrow RCH{=}CX_2$ | Dehydrohalogenation |

Figure 6. Some typical biodegradation reactions.

## Aliphatic Hydrocarbons

Figure 7 presents some typical reactions in the oxidative biodegradation of aliphatic compounds. In the first example, the aliphatic hydrocarbon is oxidized at either the terminal or penultimate carbon, to yield a primary or secondary alcohol which is further oxidized to either the acid or ketone followed by splitting off of acetate and a new primary alcohol with two less carbons than the starting material. This is the well known β-oxidation process. The second example illustrates that incomplete degradation will occur with alkanes with a high degree of methyl substitution. In this case 2,2-dimethyl heptane degradation begins at the end of the C-5 chain and continues until the formation of 2,2-dimethylpropionic acid, which is persistent.

## Alicyclic Hydrocarbons

Representative pathways for the microbial degradation of alicyclics are shown in Figure 8. Cyclohexane is oxidized to ϵ-caprolactone and then, with ring opening, is converted to ϵ-hydroxycaproic acid. Cyclohexane carboxylic

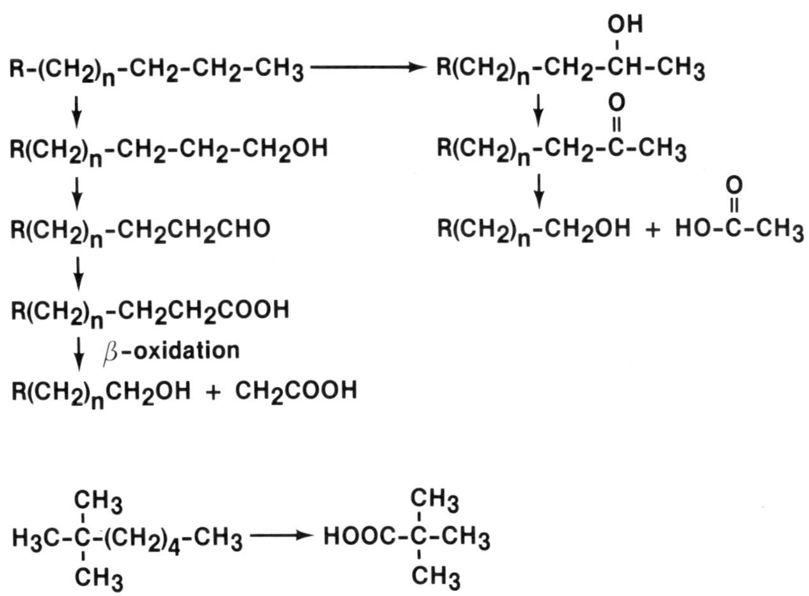


Figure 7. Oxidative biodegradation reactions for aliphatic compounds.

acid is converted to pimelic acid. These ring openings produce structures which are readily degraded further by β-oxidation. Figure 8 also shows an aromatization step which occurs when 9-α-hydroxy-androstadienedione, an intermediate in steroid degradation, is acted on by strains of *Nocardia* and *Pseudomonas* [25]. The resulting phenol is then cleaved by a dioxygenase.

## Benzenoid Compounds

Bacterial attack on benzenoid compounds typically uses molecular oxygen as a cosubstrate in the cleavage of the aromatic ring. The appropriate enzymes, known as dioxygenases, produce reactions such as that described by Gibson et al. [26] and as shown in Figure 9. The presence of functional groups on benzene rings can provide alternative sites for microbial attack. If the substituent is relatively long and linear, the side chain appears to be the preferred site of initial degradation. Compounds with short side chains may be oxidized either on the ring or on the side chain, as shown in Figure 10 [27].

In a review of the degradation of phenolics [28], Chapman showed the role of protocatechuic acid as a central metabolite in the bacterial degra-

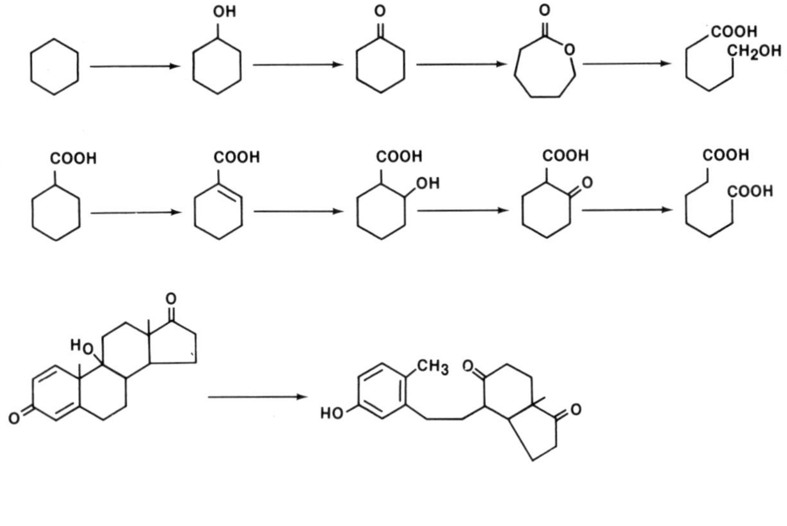


**Figure 8.** Representative pathways for microbial degradation of alicyclics.

dation of cresols (Figure 11). Benzoic acid, phthalic acid and *p*-hydroxy-mandelic acid all feed into this same intermediate. Similar schemes can be presented to show, for example, catechol as a common product from phenanthrene, naphthalene, anthracene, benzene and phenol or gentisic acid as an intermediate in the biodegradation of naphthol, salicylic acid, *m*-hydroxy-benzoic acid and anthranilic acid.

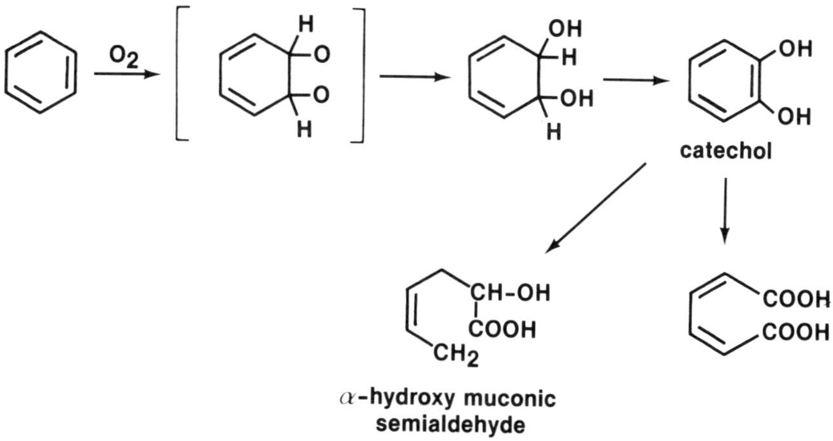


**Figure 9.** Dioxygenase reactions.

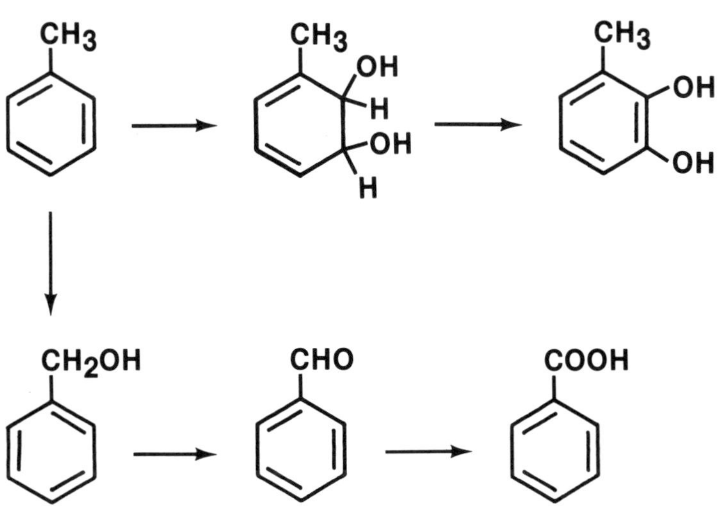


**Figure 10.** Alternative sites for oxidative metabolism.

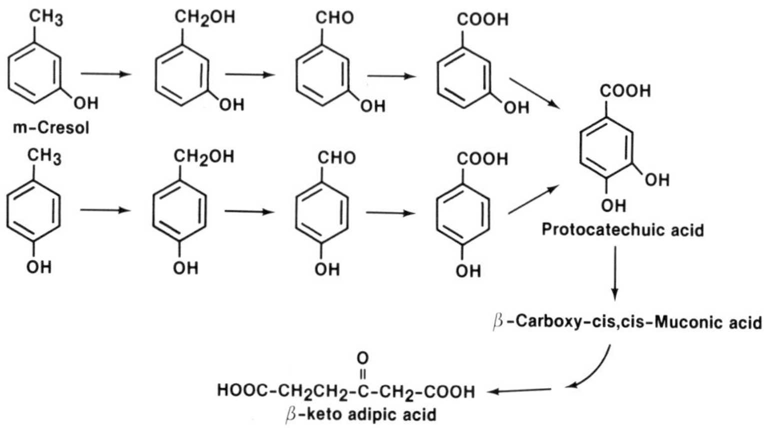


**Figure 11.** Bacterial degradation of cresols to common intermediate.

## Heterocyclic Compounds

Biodegradation involving heterocyclics is not as well studied for the classes of compounds discussed earlier, but for heterocyclics containing an oxygen, a sulfur or a nitrogen in the ring, a common step seems to be hydroxylation of the ring using the hydroxyl group from water and not molecular oxygen. Thus, this step can occur under anaerobic conditions. An example, described by Behrman and Stanier [29] and Hunt et al. [30], as shown in Figure 12, is the hydrolysis of nicotininc acid by *Pseudomonas fluorescens.* The second hydroxyl group, in this transformation, is the result of a monooxygenase reaction which displaces the carboxyl group before ring opening.

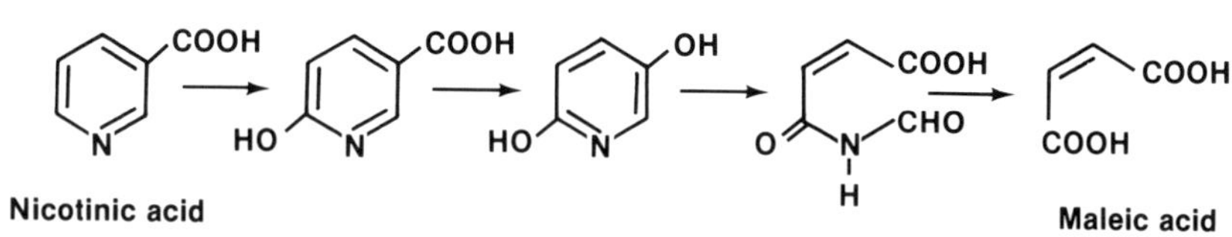


**Figure 12.** Hydrolysis of nicotinic acid by *Pseudomonas fluorescens.*

Another example [31], shown in the first part of Figure 13, is the conversion of furoic acid to the coenzyme A thioester before hydroxylation.

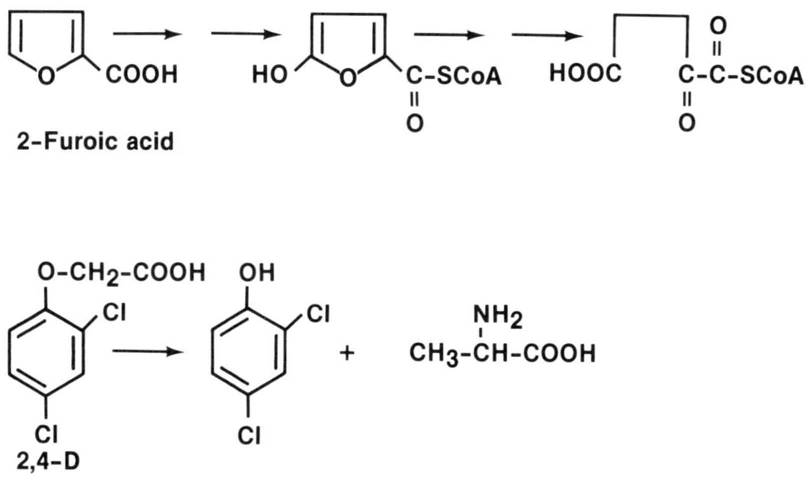


Figure 13. Hydrolysis as a first step in bacterial oxidation of 2-furoic acid and 2,4-D.

## Other Structures

Other types of organic structures which are susceptible to microbial attack include ethers, amines, nitro compounds, sulfonates and halogen-containing organics. The halides have been of particular interest since many of the organohalides are relatively persistent in the environment, and are implicated in bioaccumulation and biomagnification problems. There are a large number of naturally occurring organohalides, and biodegradation processes appear to exist for them and for most of the synthetic organics containing halogens. However, for highly substituted structures or for those with significant steric hindrances because of the location of the halide substituents, biodegradation can be very slow.

## Species Differences

Recent work has begun to show some interesting differences between the degradation pathways used by bacteria and fungi. The lower part of Figure 13 shows the first step in the bacterial oxidation of 2,4-dichlorophenoxyacetic acid (2,4-D), as described by Tiedje and Alexander [32]. This is followed by hydroxylation at C-6 and ring opening. In the presence of the fungus *Aspergillus niger,* however, the 2,4-D ring is hydroxylated at either the C-4 or the C-5 position with no further degradation by the fungus. With hydroxylation at C-4, the C-4 chlorine migrates to the C-5 position.

Of particular interest is the work by Cerniglia et al. [33], which demonstrates that the procaryotic organisms (which includes bacteria and blue-green algae) may oxidize organic compounds by different mechanisms than the eucaryotic organisms (those with a true nucleus and nuclear membrane, such as protozoa, molds, yeasts, green algae and all higher plants and animals, including humans). An example of this difference is shown in Figure 14, with the pathways of oxidation of dibenzofuran by the mold *Cunninghamella elegans,* leading to the formation of the *trans*-dihydrodiol. The same substrate, when acted upon by the bacterium *Beijerinckia,* has a *cis*-diol intermediate. Similar results have been observed for naphthalene, where it is known that in mammalian metabolism the metabolic pathway includes *trans*-1,2-dihydroxyl-1,2-dihydronaphthalene. It appears to be a valid generalization [34] that bacterial oxidation of aromatics will lead to the *cis*-dihydrodiol while higher life forms will oxidize the substrate to the *trans*-dihydrodiol (Figure 15). As these and similar studies proceed, it will be interesting to note whether there are other significant differences in the ways which the bacteria handle organic material as compared to the eucaryotes.

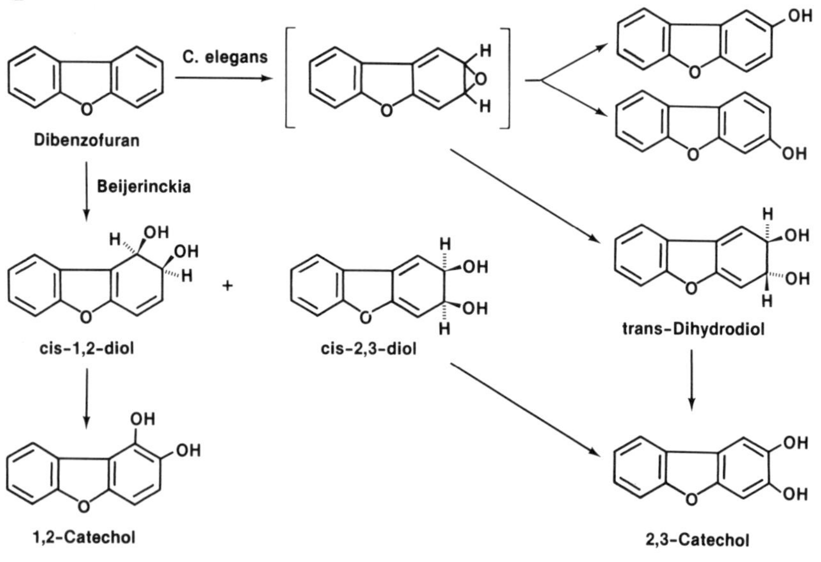


**Figure 14.** Differing oxidative pathways for dibenzofuran by a mold and bacterium.

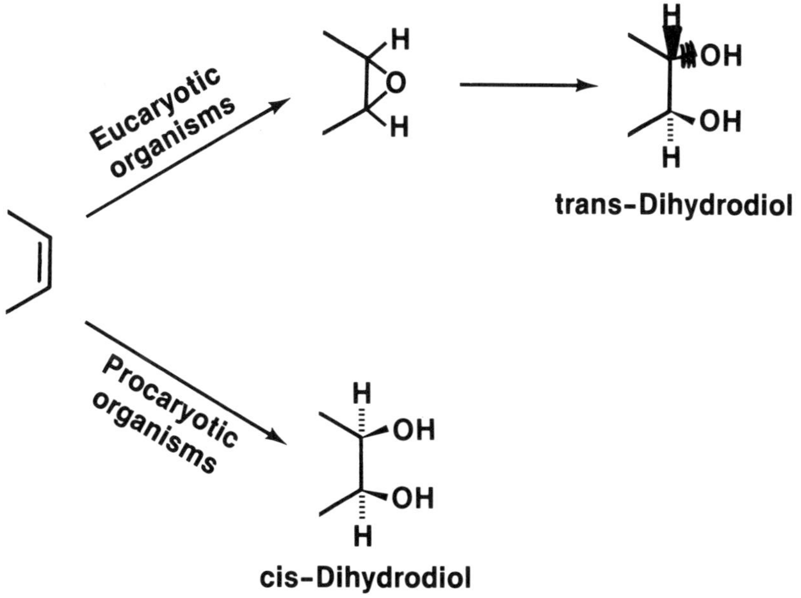


**Figure 15.** General oxidative pathways for bacteria and higher forms of life.

## SUMMARY

It is hoped that this brief overview on biodegradation of organics in the environment will provide some indication of the complexity, variety and fascination available to the researcher in this field. There were many examples of specific mechanisms that might have been chosen in place of those presented here, and it would be wrong to assume that the work not cited is in any way less important. The intent was to provide a sampling and not an extensive or critical review. The interested reader is referred to the reviews by Bollag [9], Dagley [24], Chapman [25,28], Gibson [35] and Goldman [36].

Finally, there is no discussion in this paper of the rate of biodegradation in the environment or the prediction of biodegradation rates and extent on the basis of structure or physicochemical properties of the molecule. Although many workers in this field do make predictions on rates and extent of biodegradation for many types of organics, this is mostly on intuitive grounds. The scientific approach to these questions is still evolving.

## REFERENCES

1. Alexander, M. "Nonbiodegradable and Other Recalcitrant Molecules," *Biotechnol. Bioeng.* 15:611-647 (1973).
2. Howard, P. H., J. Saxena, P. R. Durkin and L. T. Ou. "Review and Evaluation of Available Techniques for Determining Persistence and Routes of Degradation of Chemical Substances in the Environment," U.S. EPA, Publication EPA-560/5-75-006 (1975), p. 37.
3. Dagley, S. "Summary," in *Degradation of Synthetic Organic Molecules in the Biosphere* (Washington, DC: National Academy of Sciences, 1972), p. 338
4. Leadbetter, E. R., and J. W. Foster. "Oxidation Products Formed from Gaseous Alkanes by the Bacterium *Pseudomonas methanica*," *Arch. Biochem. Biophys.* 82:491-492 (1959).
5. Horvath, R. S. "Microbial Co-Metabolism and the Degradation of Organic Compounds in Nature," *Bacteriol. Rev.* 36:146-155 (1972).
6. Alexander, M. "Role of Cometabolism," in *Microbial Degradation of Pollutants in Marine Environments,* U.S. EPA, Publication EPA-600/9-79-012 (1979), pp. 67-75.
7. Raymond, R. L., V. W. Jamison and J. O. Hudson. "Microbial Hydrocarbon Cooxidation. I. Oxidation of Mono- and Dicyclic Hydrocarbons by Soil Isolates of the genus *Nocardia*," *Appl. Microbiol.* 15:857-865 (1967).
8. Jamison, V. W., R. L. Raymond and J. O. Hudson. "Microbial Hydrocarbon Cooxidation: III. Isolation and Characterization of an α, α′-dimethyl-*cis, cis*-muconic acid producing strain of *Nocardia corallina,*" *Appl. Microbiol.* 17:853-856 (1969).
9. Bollag, J. M. "Microbial Transformation of Pesticides," in *Applied Microbiology, Vol. 18,* D. Perlman, Ed. (New York: Academic Press, Inc., 1974), pp. 109-114.
10. Rose, A. H. *Chemical Microbiology,* 2nd ed. (New York: Plenum Publishing Corporation 1968), p. 77.
11. Aly, O. M., and M. A. El-Dib. "Persistence of Some Carbamate Insecticides in the Aquatic Environment," *Adv. Chem. Ser.* 111:210-243 (1972).
12. Reinheimer, G. *Aquatic Microbiology* (New York: John Wiley & Sons, Inc., 1974), p. 158.
13. Floodgate, G. D. "Oil Biodegradation in Oceans," in *Proceedings of the Third International Biodegradation Symposium,* J. M. Sharpley and A. M. Kaplan, Eds. (London: Applied Science Publishers, Ltd., 1975), pp. 87-91.
14. Gibbs, C. F. "Methods of Interpretation in Measurement of Oil Biodegradation Rate," in *Proceedings of the Third International Biodegradation Symposium,* J. M. Sharpley and A. M. Kaplan, Eds. (London: Applied Science Publishers, Ltd., 1975). pp. 127-140.
15. Bourquin, A. W., and V. A. Przybyszewski, "Distribution of Bacteria and Nitrilotriacetate-Degrading Potential in an Estuarine Environment," *App. Environ. Microbiol.* 34:411-418 (1977).

16. Atlas, R. M., and R. Bartha. "Degradation and Mineralization of Petroleum in Sea Water: Limitation by Nitrogen and Phosphorous," *Biotech, Bioeng.* 14:309-318 (1972).
17. Mason, H. S., W. L. Fowlks and E. Peterson. "Oxygen Transfer and Electron Transport by the Phenolase Complex," *J. Am. Chem. Soc.* 77:2914-2915 (1955).
18. Poole, N. J. "The Marine Anoxic Environment," in *Microbial Degradation of Pollutants in Marine Environments.* U.S. EPA, Publication EPA-600/9-79-012 (1979) p. 184.
19. Boethling, R. S., and M. Alexander. "Effect of Concentration of Organic Chemicals on Their Biodegradation by Natural Communities," *Appl. Environ. Microbiol.* 37:1211-1216 (1979).
20. Boethling, R. S., and M. Alexander. "Microbial Degradation of Organic Compounds at Trace Levels," *Environ. Sci. Technol.* 13:989-991 (1979).
21. Wright, R. T. "Natural Heterotrophic Activity in Estuarine and Coastal Waters," in *Microbial Degradation of Pollutants in Marine Environments,* U.S. EPA, Publication EPA-600/9-79-012 (1979).
22. *Standard Methods for The Examination of Water and Wastewater,* 14th ed. (Washington, DC: American Public Health Association, 1975), pp. 543-550.
23. Soap and Detergent Association, Subcommittee on Biodegradation Test Methods. "A Procedure And Standards for the Determination of the Biodegradability of Alkylbenzene Sulfonate and Linear Alkylate Sulfonates," *J. Am. Oil Chem. Soc.* 42:986-993 (1965).
24. Dagley, S. "Microbial Degradation of Stable Chemical Structures: General Features of Metabolic Pathways," in *Degradation of Synthetic Organic Molecules in the Biosphere* (Washington, DC: National Academy of Sciences, 1972), p. 2.
25. Chapman, P. J. "Degradative Mechanisms," in *Microbial Degradation of Pollutants in Marine Environments,* U.S. EPA Publication EPA-600/9-79-012 (1979), pp. 28-66.
26. Gibson, D. T., G. E. Cardini, F. C. Maseles and R. E. Kallio. "Incorporation of Oxygen-18 into Benzene by *Pseudomonas putida,*" *Biochemistry* 9:1631-1635 (1970).
27. Chapman, P. J. "Degradation Mechanisms," in *Microbial Degradation of Pollutants in Marine Environments,* U.S. EPA, Publication EPA-600/9-79-012 (1979), p. 39.
28. Chapman, P. J. "An Outline of Reaction Sequences Used for the Bacterial Degradation of Phenolic Compounds," in *Degradation of Synthetic Organic Molecules in the Biosphere* (Washington, DC: National Academy of Sciences, 1972), p. 21.
29. Behrman, E. J., and R. Y. Stanier. "The Bacterial Oxidation of Nicotinic Acid," *J. Biol. Chem.* 228:923-945 (1957).
30. Hunt, H. L., D. E. Hughes and J. M. Lowenstein. "The Hydroxylation of Nicotinic Acid by *Pseudomonas fluorescens,*" *Biochem. J.* 69:170-173 (1958).
31. Trudgill, P. W. "The Metabolism of 2-Furoic Acid by *Pseudomonas* $F_2$" *Biochem J.* 113:577-587 (1969).

32. Tiedje, J. M., and M. Alexander "Enzymatic Cleavage of the Ether Bond of 2,4-Dichlorophenoxyacetate," *J. Agric Food Chem.* 17:1080-1084 (1969).
33. Cerniglia, C. E., J. C. Morgan and D. T. Gibson. "Bacterial and Fungal Oxidation of Dibenzofuran," *Biochem. J.* 180:175-185 (1979).
34. Cerniglia, C. E., and D. T. Gibson. "Algal Oxidation of *Agmenellum quadruplicatum,* strain PR-6" *Biochem. Biophys. Res. Comm.* 88:50-58 (1979).
35. Gibson, D. T. "Initial Reactions in The Degradation of Aromatic Hydrocarbons," in *Degradation of Synthetic Organic Molecules in the Biosphere* (Washington, DC: National Academy of Science, 1972), pp. 116-136.
36. Goldman, P. "Enzymology of Carbon-Halogen Bonds," in *Degradation of Synthetic Organic Molecules in the Biosphere* (Washington, DC: National Academy of Sciences, 1972), pp. 147-165.

# CHAPTER 5

# GENETICS AND BIOLOGICAL RESPONSE TO ENVIRONMENTAL TOXIC AGENTS

**Howard J. Eisen and Daniel W. Nebert**
Developmental Pharmacology Branch
National Institute of Child Health and Human Development
National Institutes of Health
Bethesada, Maryland

**Allan B. Okey**
Division of Clinical Pharmacology
Department of Paediatrics
Hospital for Sick Children
Toronto, Ontario
Canada

## INTRODUCTION

Many of the molecules that constitute the major environmental toxic chemicals are extremely hydrophobic and, once absorbed by an organism, can be excreted only after metabolic conversion to polar products. For many of these molecules (aromatic hydrocarbons formed by pyrolysis of fuels or insecticides) the initial metabolic step involves reaction with molecular oxygen catalyzed by microsomal monooxygenases [1]. Organisms, from bacteria to humans, have evolved complex mechanisms for adapting to the presence of diverse hydrophobic molecules in the environment. These mechanisms often involve selective increases in monooxygenase activities.

The ability to alter the pattern and extent of metabolic conversion of hydrophobic molecules can have two consequences. An inherently toxic molecule can be converted to an innocuous product and excreted. Alternatively, a nontoxic molecule can be converted into a highly reactive molecule capable of exerting direct toxicity (e.g. hepatic necrosis, or death) or causing fetal malformation or cancer. In any individual, the precise pattern and kinetics of metabolism depends on a complex system of enzymes and regulated responses. It is not surprising that wide individual variations in the metabolism of hydrophobic molecules have been observed in laboratory animals and humans [2]. This chapter will review recent data on the genetic analysis of variation in the monooxygenase system.

## DISCUSSION

### The Cytochrome P-450–Dependent Monooxygenases

These multicomponent systems are embedded in microsomal membranes and comprise NADPH-dependent reductases (flavoproteins), phospholipids and hemoproteins. The intact complex binds substrate and catalyzes the incorporation of one oxygen atom from molecular oxygen into the substrate, the other oxygen atom being incorporated into cellular water (Figure 1.). These enzyme systems are capable of catalyzing reactions with many different classes of molecules. Early in the study of these enzymes [3], it was recognized that two basic patterns of adaptive response occur on exposure to various hydrophobic molecules. Phenobarbital and 3-methylcholanthrene (3-MC) stimulate increases in different forms of cytochrome P-450. These forms can be distinguished by spectrophotometric, electrophoretic and immunological methods. The increase in monooxygenase activities required *de novo* protein synthesis of the hemoprotein moieties involved [4] and hence can be termed an inductive response. The observed increase in hemoprotein synthesis appears to be somewhat selective, in that only those hemoproteins associated with a particular inducer are increased. Even without considering the molecular mechanism of this selective response, genetic approaches can be used to categorize the pattern of inheritance. However, genetics can also be a powerful means for analysis of the molecular events involved in monooxygenase induction. Inductive responses in biological systems can involve different mechanisms of signal recognition, and can affect protein synthesis at different steps.

### Genetic Difference in P-450 Induction

The basis for any genetic analysis is a mutation that affects the phenotypic expression of a characteristic. In the case of phenobarbital-like induction of

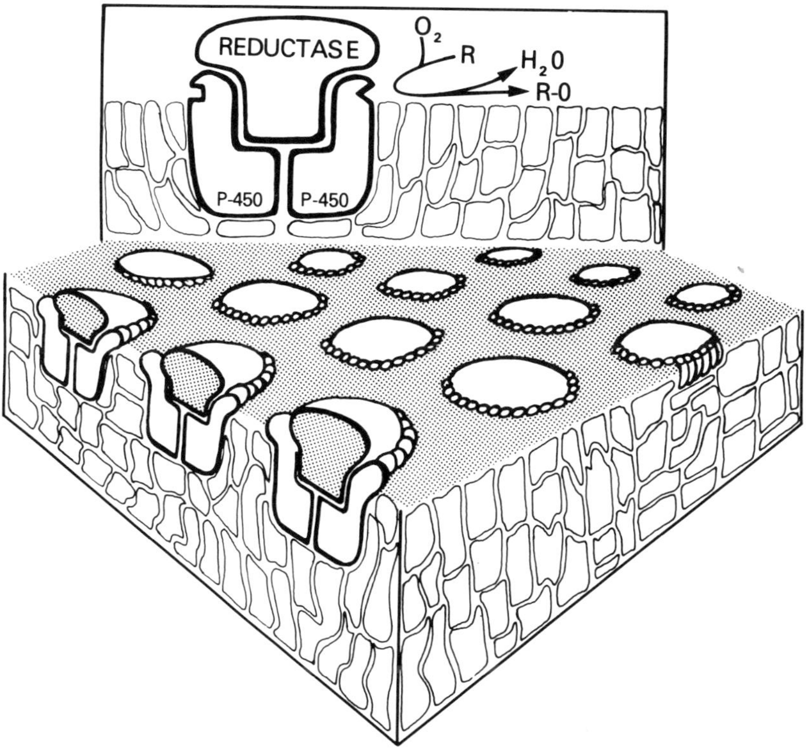


**Figure 1.** Hypothetical diagram of the relationship between flavoprotein reductases and forms of cytochrome P-450 embedded in cellular membranes [2]. R, substrate; R-O, oxygenated intermediate or product. Reproduced with permission from Dr. W. Junk Publishers.

cytochrome P-450, no mutants that alter the induction phenotype have been described. Recent analysis of the coumarin hydroxylase (Coh) locus in the mouse indicates that genetic heterogeneity of the monooxygenase itself exists [5]. In the case of 3-MC-like induction of monooxygenase activities, however, several inbred strains of mice exhibit marked differences in the ability to respond to inducers. These strains were studied by classic genetic techniques to define the pattern of inheritance of these variations [1, 6].

Inbred strains have proven to be extremely valuable for genetic analyses. These strains are produced by many (usually more than 20) generations of brother-sister matings, during which the genotype becomes homozygous for each genetic locus. Thus recessive alleles present in the parents of the strain are expressed in the inbred progeny. A large number of inbred mouse strains exist; although most such strains respond to 3-MC-like inducers, some strains do not.

## The *Ah* locus

In the experiment shown in Figure 2, aryl hydrocarbon hydroxylase (AHH) was used as the genetic marker for an 3-MC–induced monooxygenase activity. The prototype 3-MC–responsive strain (C57BL/6N, also called B6) and the prototype nonresponsive strain (DBA/2N, also called D2) have low basal activities of AHH. Treatment of these mice with 3-MC results in an increase in hepatic and lung AHH in the B6 but not in the D2 parental animals. The $F_1$ hybrid animals show a high level of induction, nearly equal to that of the B6 parent strain. The two backcrosses and the $F_1$ x $F_1$ intercross show a frequency distribution consistent with dominance of the B6 phenotype. A genetic locus can therefore be defined that controls induction of AHH (termed the *Ah* locus for responsiveness to aromatic hydrocarbons). The genetic difference between the two strains appears to involve two alleles: $Ah^b$, responsive (after the prototype B6 strain); and $Ah^d$, nonresponsive (after the nonresponsive D2 strain). The genetic expression of AHH in these two strains can be defined by the simple scheme shown in Figure 3. The presence of a single $Ah^b$ allele is sufficient to promote full expression of AHH induction in all appropriate genetic crosses between B6 and D2 animals. Intermediate levels of induction are not observed in $Ah^b/Ah^d$ heterozygotes. A large body of other experimental evidence supports such a simple genetic scheme for these and other strains [1].

Some other strains of mice show different patterns of dominance and inheritance (Figure 4), however, and it is apparent that other forms of genetic variation exist and affect the expression of the *Ah* locus. In crosses between responsive C3H and nonresponsive D2 (Figure 4, top) the trait is inherited additively. In crosses between responsive B6 and nonresponsive AKR/N (Figure 4, bottom), the lack of AHH induction is expressed as an autosomal dominant trait. In an inbred strain of mice (HS or "heterogenic stock") derived from an original background of eight different inbred strains [10], the induction of AHH by 3-MC varies more than ninefold between individuals [11]. Thus the random distribution of genes that affect the expression of the *Ah* locus can result in wide variations in AHH inducibility in a mouse population derived from a large genetic background.

## Why Are Some Mice "Nonresponsive"?

Two other lines of experimental evidence help to define the genetic basis for nonresponsiveness in the D2 mouse. Perhaps the most obvious explanation for the lack of AHH induction would be a mutation affecting the structural gene for the form of cytochrome P-450 that catalyzes AHH. However,

3-MC is known to induce at least 20 monooxygenase "activities" measured with various (widely differing) substrates in the B6 strain [1]. Furthermore, other enzymes involved in drug metabolism (UDP glucuronosyltransferase, reduced NAD (P): menadione oxidoreductase) and enzymes required for RNA synthesis (ornithine decarboxylase) are also induced by 3-MC. In the D2 animal, all of these responses–involving multiple structural genes–are blocked. The finding that widespread inductive effects (termed pleiotypic effects) [12] are blocked suggests that the genetic defect involves a step in the regulation of induction rather than a defect in a single structural gene.

2,3,7,8-Tetrachlorodibenzo-*p*-dioxin (TCDD) has proved to be a useful "probe" for elucidating the processes involved in this induction. TCDD is an extremely potent inducer of AHH and other activities associated with the murine *Ah* locus [13,14]. TCDD, however, has the unique capacity of stimulating a 3-MC-like pleiotypic response in the D2 strain [14]; the ED50 for induction in the D2 strain is about 15 times higher than in the B6 strain. This observation supplies important information about the integrity of structural genes associated with the *Ah* locus in the D2 animal, and implies that they can be induced by an appropriately potent molecule (TCDD in the intact animal is approximately 50,000 times more potent than inducers such as benzo[a]pyrene.) The defect in the D2 animals therefore appears to be an altered sensitivity to inducers and is reflected in a shifted dose response curve to TCDD.

## A Cytosolic Receptor Associated with the *Ah* Locus

The gene product of the regulatory *Ah* gene is postulated to be a protein that functions as a "receptor" for inducers of the various monooxygenases. An altered receptor in the D2 strain results in decreased interaction with TCDD (reflected by increased ED50) and no detectable interaction with less potent inducers such as 3-MC and benzo[a]pyrene. The pattern of inheritance observed in genetic crosses between the B6 and D2 strains fits such a hypothesis [15]. Recent work with hormones and drugs has resulted in the identification of several classes of receptors that regulate intracellular processes such as induction of specific gene products. The initial reaction between the hormone and its receptor is the formation of a reversible complex. Receptors for peptide hormones and neurotransmitters such as catecholamines are generally localized on the cell membrane. Receptors for steroid hormones are localized in the cell (cytosolic compartment). Receptors for iodothyronines (thyroxin) are localized in the cell nucleus bound to chromatin. The interaction between the ligand and the receptor is generally traced with high-specific radioactive ligands ($^{3}$H and $^{125}$I are the most widely used radionuclides).

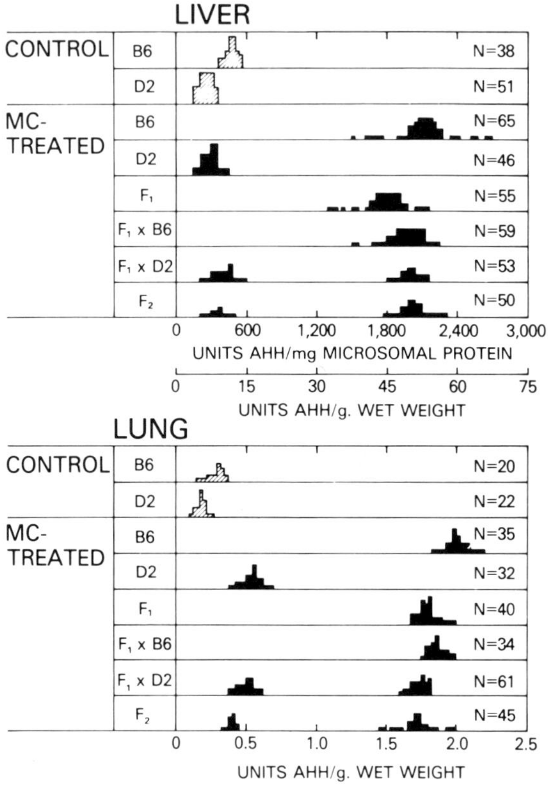


**Figure 2A.** Genetic variance in hepatic (top) and pulmonary (bottom) AHH activity in control and 3-MC-treated offspring from appropriate crosses between B6 and D2 inbred strains and hepatic AHH activity [6]. Histograms for liver samples represent specific AHH activity in control mice and in mice treated intraperitoneally 24 hr beforehand with 3-MC (100 mg/kg body weight); controls received intraperitoneal corn oil. For lung samples, each mouse received intratracheally 24 hr beforehand 3-MC 500 μg in 20 μl of 0.2% gelatin-0.85% NaCl; controls received the sterile vehicle alone. The mice weighed between 15 and 20 g. The number of mice examined individually is given at the right for each group. Reproduced with permission from the Press of Cold Spring Harbor Laboratory.

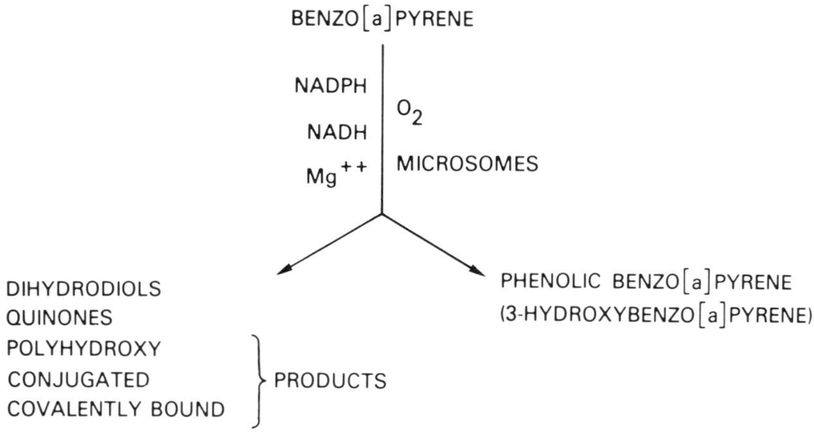


**Figure 2B.** Current concept of the AHH activity [7]. The substrate benzo[a]pyrene is oxygenated to arene oxides which rearrange nonenzymically to phenols or are oxygenated by direct oxygen insertion to phenolic derivatives. The 3- and 9-phenols have the strongest fluorescence in alkali. Other oxygenated derivatives of benzo[a]-pyrene, including dihydrodiols and quinones, are not measured by this assay. One unit of AHH activity is defined as that amount of enzyme catalyzing per minute at 37°C the formation of hydroxylated product causing fluorescence equivalent to that of 1 pmol of 3-hydroxybenzo[a]pyrene. Reproduced with permission from the Press of the Federation Proceedings.

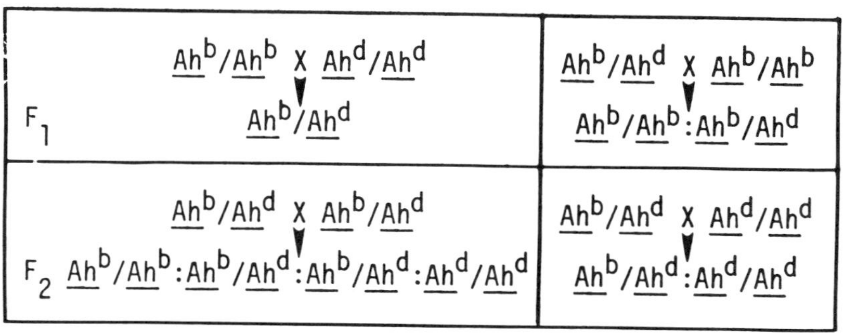


**Figure 3.** Simplified genetic scheme for aromatic hydrocarbon "responsiveness" in the mouse [8]. Reproduced with permission from Plenum Publishing Corporation.

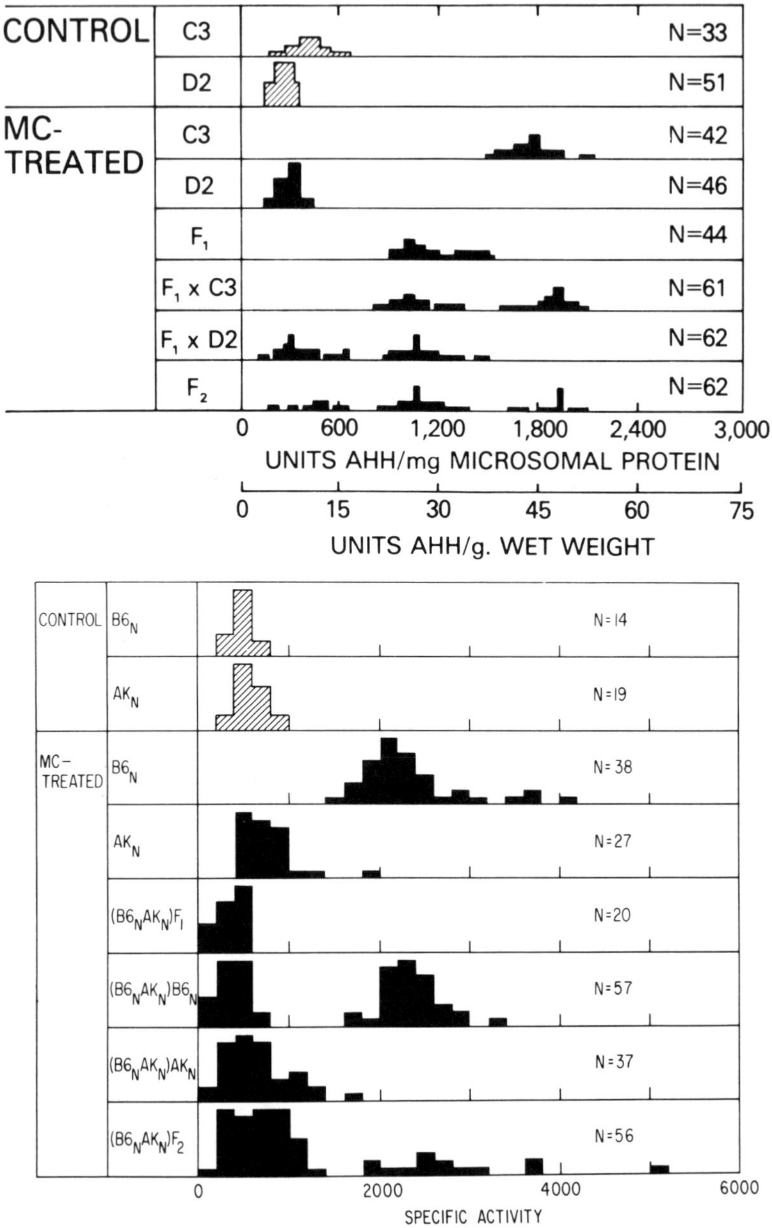


**Figure 4.** Histograms of hepatic microsomal hydroxylase specific activity in control and 3-MC-treated pairs of inbred mice and in 3-MC-treated offspring from genetic crosses involving these pairs [6,9]. Abbreviations of the inbred strains include: $B6_N$, C57BL/6N; $AK_N$, AKR/N; C3, C3H; D2, DBA/2N. Reproduced with permission from Press of Cold Spring Harbor Laboratory and American Society of Biological Chemists, Inc.

Using [$^3$H] TCDD, Poland et al. [16] identified a cytosolic binding moiety whose properties fit both genetic and pharmacological criteria for the putative receptor of AHH induction. From experiments involving in vivo injection of [$^3$H] TCDD and in vitro incubation of cytosol with [$^3$H] TCDD, these investigators showed that hepatic cytosol from B6 mice contained a limited number of "sites" that could bind [$^3$H] TCDD with extremely high affinity ($K_d$ ~1 n*M*). Biologically active congeners of TCDD competed for these binding sites, whereas inactive molecules did not. D2 mouse liver contained no detectable binding sites for [$^3$H] TCDD. A recent extensive structure-activity study [17] showed that certain analogs of biphenyl that can assume coplanar structures (such as TCDD) function as 3-MC–like inducers. Congeners in which the two aromatic rings do not favor coplanar structures can function as phenobarbital-like inducers. Poland et al. [16, 17] showed a good correlation between ED50 of the 3-MC–like inducers (in chick embryo) and competition with [$^3$H] TCDD for binding to the putative receptor.

The studies of Poland and co-workers were based on a technically simple method for separating free [$^3$H] TCDD from macromolecular-bound [$^3$H] TCDD—the dextran charcoal method that is widely used in other areas of receptor research. Recent work by Gustafsson [18] using isoelectric focusing has confirmed the basic aspects of Poland's work with the [$^3$H] TCDD binding protein. The isoelectric focusing assay, however, requires trypsin treatment of cytosol to prevent aggregation, and hence may measure a proteolyzed form of the receptor.

Two important elements of receptor biology were not considered in these pioneering studies: (1) purification and physicochemical characterization of the receptor; and (2) assessment of the biochemical "function" of the receptor. To carry out such studies, it is necessary to define conditions that stabilize the receptor during the various procedures used for rigorous characterization of the molecule. Typically, ion exchange and gel permeaation chromatography, or velocity sedimentation on density gradients are used to separate various binding moieties.

## An Improved Receptor Assay

Rapid assays for the [$^3$H] TCDD receptor, such as the dextran-coated charcoal assay, detect significant amounts of nonsaturable binding in liver cytosol from many mammalian species, and the high affinity [$^3$H] TCDD binding is obscured. The only method that successfully deals with this problem is a combination of dextran-charcoal treatment followed by velocity sedimentation on sucrose gradients. With this assay, a saturable high-affinity binding moiety is detected in liver cytosol from B6 mice that had an $s_{w20}$ of approximately 8S (Figure 5). The high-affinity binding peak can be displaced

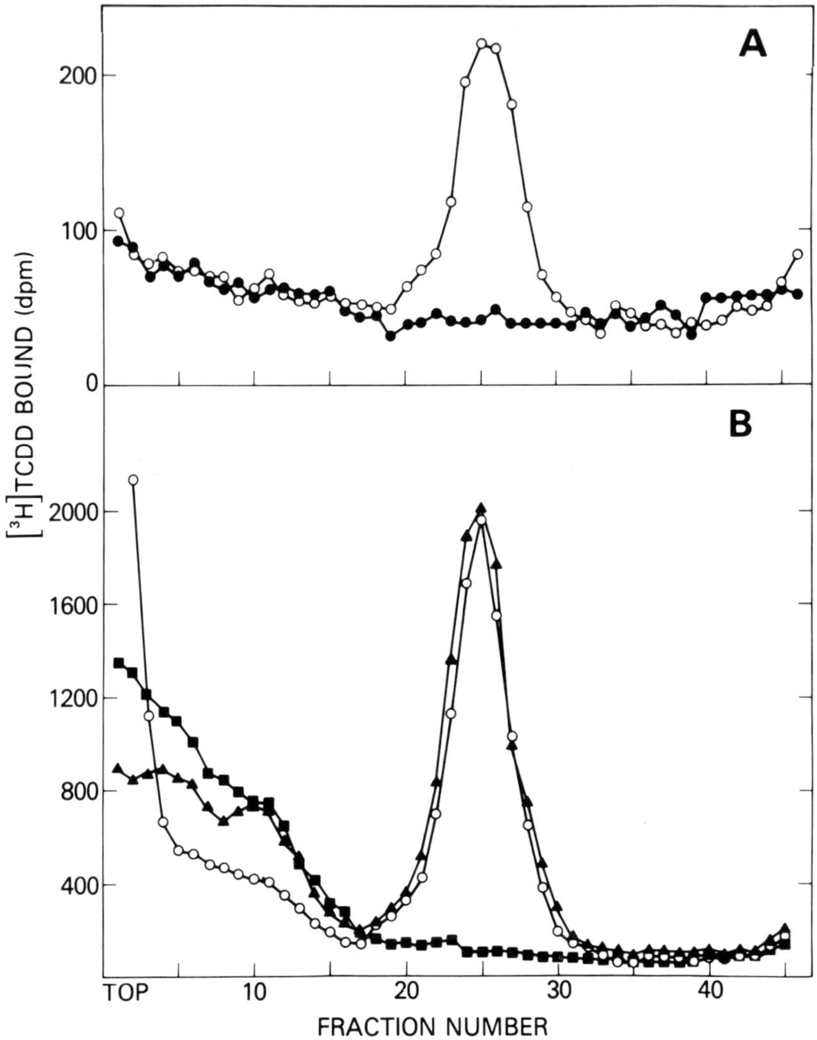


Figure 5. Detection of specific [$^3$H] TCDD binding of a component from B6 hepatic cytosol [15]. (A) Cytosol (1 mg protein/ml) from an eight-week-old B6 male was incubated with 1 n*M* [$^3$H] TCDD in the absence of competitor (○–○) or in the presence of 100 n*M* nonlabeled TCDD (●–●) for 1 hr at 40°C. After dextran-charcoal treatment, gradients were centrifuged and fractionated. (B) Elimination of specific binding peak by 3-MC but not by phenobarbital. Cytosol (5 mg protein/ml) was incubated with 10 n*M* [$^3$H] TCDD in the absence of competitor (○–○), and in the presence of 10 μ*M* 3-MC (■–■) or 10 μ*M* phenobarbital (▲–▲). Reproduced with permission from American Society of Biological Chemists, Inc.

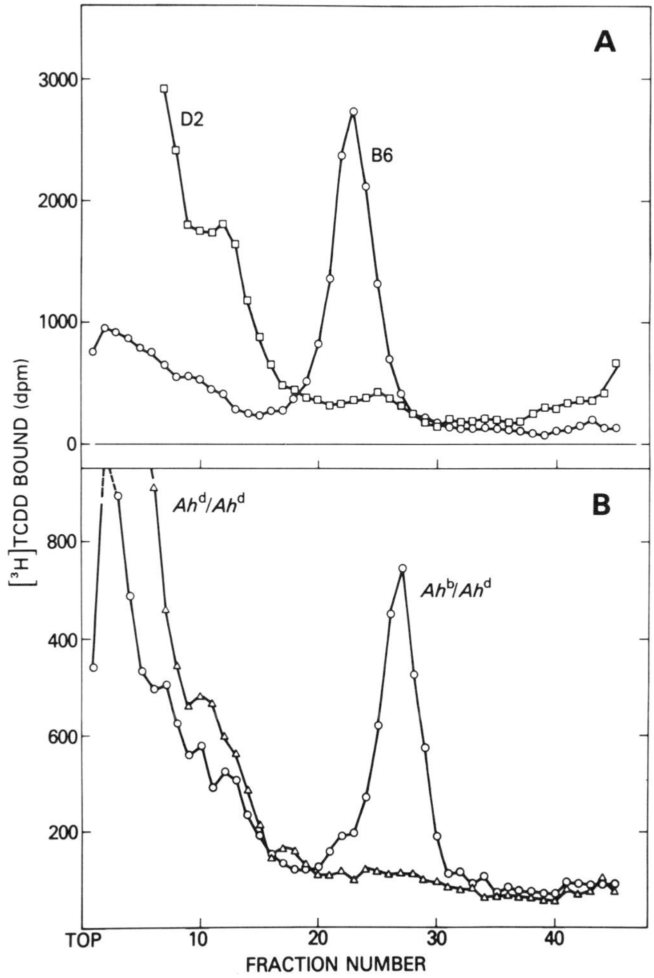


**Figure 6.** Genetic differences in hepatic cytosolic receptor [15]. (A) Hepatic cytosolic fractions (5 mg protein/ml) from responsive B6 or nonresponsive D2 inbred mice were incubated at 4° (with 10 n*M* [$^3$H] TCDD and analyzed as usual by sucrose density gradient separation after dextran-charcoal treatment. (B) Hepatic cytosolic fractions from a phenotypically responsive $Ah^b/Ah^d$ heterozygote (3.1 mg protein/ml) and nonresponsive $Ah^d/Ah^d$ homozygote (3.7 mg protein/ml) were incubated at 4° (with 10 n*M* [$^3$H] TCDD and analyzed as usual. The binding peak in cytosol from the responsive mouse was eliminated by incubation in the presence of 100 n*M* nonlabeled TCDD (data not shown), thus confirming its limited capacity. These progeny from the B6D2F$_1$ x D2 backcross had been phenotyped by the zoxazolamine paralysis test [19] more than one week before this receptor assay. Reproduced with permission from American Society of Biological Chemists, Inc.

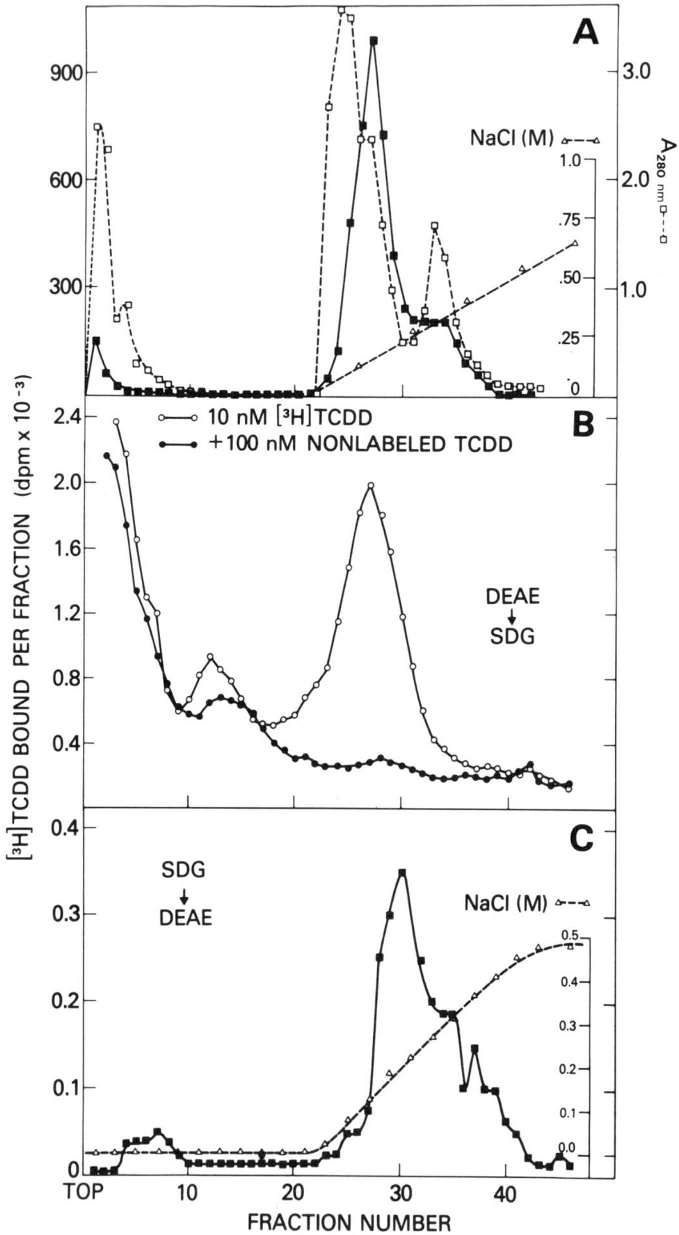


Figure 7. (A) DEAE-cellulose chromatography of $[^3H]$ TCDD-binding moieties (■—■) in B6 hepatic cytosol [15]. The cytosol (5 mg protein/ml) was incubated at 4°C with 10 n$M$ $[^3H]$ TCDD for 1 hr and then applied to a 5-ml column of

DEAE-cellulose that had been equilibrated with HEDG (10 mm Hepes, pH 7.5; 1 mm EDTA, 0.5 mm dithiothreitol, 10% v:v glycerol) buffer. Cytosol (10 ml) was loaded onto the column (total protein applied = 50 mg). The column was washed with HEDG buffer and then eluted with a linear NaCl gradient. The fraction volumes were 3 ml. (B) Sucrose density gradient (SDG) analysis of [$^3$H] TCDD-binding material eluted from the DEAE-cellulose chromatographic column. The cytosol (5 mg protein/ml) was incubated with 10 *nM* [$^3$H] TCDD in the absence (○—○) or presence (●—●) of 100 *nM* nonlabeled TCDD. A 1-ml aliquot of this cytosol was applied to a 1-ml DEAE-cellulose column that had been equilibrated with HEDG buffer; the bound proteins were eluted with 0.5 *M* NaCl. The specific binding detected was 18 fmol (per mg of the original cytosolic protein). (C) DEAE-cellulose chromatography of [$^3$H] TCDD-binding material (■—■) obtained from sucrose density gradients. The cytosol was labeled with 10 *nM* [$^3$H] TCDD and separated after dextran-charcoal treatment as usual on sucrose density gradients. Fractions containing specific [$^3$H] TCDD binding from the appropriate region of the gradient (fractions number 22-30) were pooled and applied to a 1-ml column of DEAE-cellulose equilibrated in HEDG. The column was washed with HEDG buffer and then eluted with a linear NaCl gradient. The fraction volumes were 1 ml. Protein containing 17,000 dpm [$^3$H] TCDD was applied to the column; recovery in the peak from DEAE-cellulose was 2,470 dpm. Reproduced with permission from American Society of Biological Chemists, Inc.

by nonlabeled TCDD or 3-MC, but not by another form of P-450 inducer, phenobarbital. This binding peak is not observed in the prototype nonresponsive strain (D2) (Figure 6). Genetic crosses were carried out to determine if the binding peak correlated with the *Ah* locus. Liver cytosol from $F_1$ hybrids between B6 and D2 mice exhibit the binding protein. Progeny from the B6D2$F_1$ x D2 backcross can be genotyped by a noninvasive method, the zoxazolamine muscle paralysis test [19], and those shown to have the $Ah^b$ allele possess the binding protein in liver cytosol, whereas those that were $Ah^d/Ah^d$ do not have the binding protein (Figure 6).

Extensive competition studies demonstrated that only 3-MC-like inducers competed with [$^3$H] TCDD for binding [15, 16]. The binding activity is completely destroyed by proteolytic enzymes, and is not affected by various nucleases [15]. Further characterization of the binding protein was done using anion exchange chromatography on DEAE-cellulose (Figure 7A). A single major peak of [$^3$H] TCDD binding-protein was observed on elution of DEAE-cellulose columns with an NaCl gradient.

## Nuclear Translocation of Inducer-Receptor Complex

The localization of the TCDD receptor in the cytosol suggests that it might be analogous to a steriod hormone receptor. Steroid hormone receptors bind two types of ligands—the steriod hormones and polynucleotides such as DNA [20, 21]. The DNA binding function is not expressed unless the steroid binding site is first occupied by an agonist ligand. Expression of the DNA binding function generally requires an additional step after steroid binding, termed "activation," which appears to involve a conformational and/or covalent alteration in the steroid-receptor complex. "Activation" of the DNA binding site in vitro and in the intact cell is believed to account for the translocation of the steroid receptor complex into the cell nucleus.

A series of experiments has been carried out to determine if any of these properties of steroid hormone receptors also apply to the TCDD receptor [15]. Nuclei isolated directly from livers of B6 and D2 mice do not contain TCDD receptor, as determined by extraction of nuclei with high ionic strength buffers followed by centrifugation on density gradients. If [$^3$H] TCDD is injected into a B6 mouse, or a mouse known to have the $Ah^b$ allele, a peak of [$^3$H] TCDD binding can be demonstrated in nuclear extracts; injection of [$^3$H] TCDD into a D2 mouse or a nonresponsive $Ah^d/Ah^d$ homozygote does not result in a [$^3$H] TCDD peak (Figure 8). The binding moiety extracted from the nuclei of the $Ah^b$ animals has the same sedimentation properties as cytosolic receptor exposed to a similarly high salt concentration. Furthermore, the accumulation of receptor in the nucleus is accompanied by a decrease in the cytosolic receptor—evidence that supports a "translocation" phenomenon similar to that occurring with steroid hor-

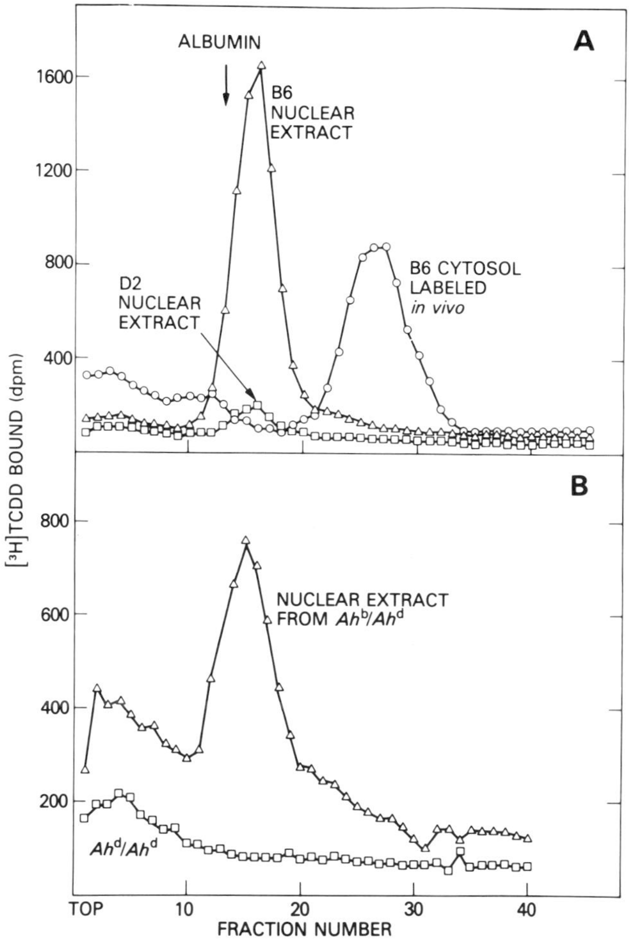


**Figure 8.** Genetic differences in the nuclear binding of [$^3$H] TCDD in vivo [15]. (A) Nuclear extracts (approximately 5 mg protein/ml) from responsive B6 and nonresponsive D2 liver were treated with dextran-charcoal and then centrifuged on sucrose density gradients prepared in HEDG buffer containing 0.4 *M* KCl. B6 cytosol (labeled in vivo, 15 mg protein/ml) was treated with dextran-charcoal and centrifuged as usual on a gradient prepared in HEDG buffer without KCl. (B) Hepatic nuclear extracts from a responsive $Ah^b/Ah^d$ and a nonresponsive $Ah^d/Ah^d$ individual from the B6D2F$_1$ x D2 backcross. The extracts (6 mg protein/ml) after dextran-charcoal treatment were centrifuged on gradients prepared in HEDG buffer containing 0.4 *M* KCl. The B6 and D2 mouse had each received 2 μg of [$^3$H] TCDD (approximately 0.3 μmol/kg body weight) and were killed 2 hr later. The backcross animals had each received 5 μg of [$^3$H] TCDD (about 0.75 μmol/kg body weight) and were killed 3 hr later. These backcross mice had been phenotyped more than one week earlier. Reproduced with permission from American Society of Biological Chemists, Inc.

mone receptors. Currently, the analogy to steroid homone receptors is not complete. Assessment of the function of the receptor and the mechanism of the nuclear translocation observed in vivo requires further experimentation.

## Is the Receptor Detectable in Nonresponsive Mice?

Another problem with current assays for the receptor is that these assays do not detect [$^3$H] TCDD binding in the cytosol of the D2 mouse. Pharmacological studies show that the D2 mouse responds to TCDD. The higher ED50 and hence the lower affinity of TCDD for a receptor in these animals is probably a key factor. Density gradient analysis [15] requires at least 16 hr, during which dissociation of the TCDD receptor complex can take place. It is possible that the receptor complex from D2 animals dissociates more rapidly than the B6 receptor or is unstable for other reasons.

Differing patterns of inheritance of AHH inducibility have been observed in various inbred mouse strains [1]. Can any of these differences be explained by quantitative or qualitative differences in [$^3$H] TCDD binding? [$^3$H] TCDD binding was therefore measured in liver cytosol of several inbred strains and hybrid crosses (Table I). The highest concentrations of receptor are found in the C57BL/6N and C57BL/6J strains. The C3H/HeJ strain contains a lower concentration of receptor, and the nonresponsive AKR and DBA strains contain no detectable receptor. $F_1$ hybrid crosses between B6 and D2 animals contain intermediate levels of receptor. Thus a single $Ah^b$ allele (resulting in a receptor concentration of about 30 fmol/mg) may be adequate to saturate the nuclear sites involved in induction and to produce the maximal response. The C3H mouse liver contains low, but detectable, levels of receptor, and might contain fewer copies of the gene encoding for receptor. Induction is lower in this strain, and shows additive inheritance with the D2 cross (Figure 4). Receptor levels could become limiting in such hybrid crosses between D2 and C3H mice. The AKR mouse is especially interesting because its nonresponsive phenotype is dominant in crosses between AKR and B6 [9]. This phenomenon is difficult to explain, unless one postulates interaction between the *Ah* alleles of the AKR and B6 mouse. A receptor "multimer" formed by subunits from AKR and B6 loci could be inactive because of allosteric interactions. A relevant example is the hemoglobin molecule which contains four subunits. Abnormal alleles, such as $\beta^S$, produce abnormal function (sickling) only under certain conditions. The properties of the molecule differ in homozygous SS and the heterozygous SA or SC states. Gene "dosage" effects and molecular heterogeneity of the receptor could therefore account for the complex patterns of inheritance observed in the murine *Ah* regulatory locus.

Table 1. Concentration of Receptor in Hepatic Cytosol from Various Responsive and Nonresponsive Animals

| Strain | *Ah* Locus Phenotype | N | Specific TCDD Binding[b] (fmol/mg Cytosol Protein) |
|---|---|---|---|
| C57BL/6N | Responsive | 8 | 60 ± 12 |
| C57BL/6J | Responsive | 10 | 34 ± 16 |
| CBA/J | Responsive | p4 | 20 |
| A/J | Responsive | p4 | 16 |
| C3H/HeJ | Responsive | p4 | 12 |
| C3H/HeJ | | 1 | 11 |
| C3H/HeJ | | 1 | 11 |
| DBA/2N | Nonresponsive | 6 | Not detectable |
| DBA/2J | Nonresponsive | 8 | Not detectable |
| AKR/J | Nonresponsive | p4 | Not detectable |
| SWR/J | Nonresponsive | p4 | Not detectable |
| RF/J | Nonresponsive | p4 | Not detectable |
| $Ah^b/Ah^d$ | Responsive[c] | 3 | 35 ± 5 |
| $Ah^d/Ah^d$ | Nonresponsive[c] | 3 | Not detectable |
| Sprague-Dawley rat (Holtzman) | Responsive | 1 | 33 |

[a]Specific binding was measured by sucrose density gradient analysis after dextran-charcoal treatment with the use of 10n*M* [$^3$H] TCDD ± 1000 n*M* nonlabeled TCDD [15]. "N" represents the number of individual animals assayed; "p4" indicates that cytosol from four mice was pooled and used in one assay. The means for C57BL/6N mice and C57BL/6J are significantly different ($P<0.01$ by "t-test"). All animals were males 2–4 months old except RF/J mice (females, 2 months old) and a Sprague-Dawley rat (female, 4 months old). Reproduced with permission from American Society of Biological Chemists, Inc.

[b]Values are expressed as means ± standard deviations when three or more determinations were made separately.

[c]Weanlings from the B6D2$F_1$ x D2 backcross were phenotyped at age 3–5 weeks by the zoxazolamine paralysis test, as previously described [19]. More than 1 week later, these individuals were then assessed for hepatic cytosolic receptor.

## Search for Further Regulatory Mutants

Unfortunately, the only receptor defect observed in inbred mouse strains is a lack of [$^3$H] TCDD binding. Receptor mutants with other types of defect would be extremely useful for establishing the functional significance of nuclear translocation. The nonresponsive HTC and VERO cultured cell lines possess apparently normal levels of TCDD receptor (22); these mutants may therefore reflect a defect in nuclear translocation of the inducer-receptor complex or other defect during the sequence of regulatory events.

Certain cloned cell lines maintained in tissue culture, particularly those derived from hepatocellular tumors, are inducible by 3-MC–like molecules [23]. The toxicity of molecules such as benzo[a]pyrene correlates with the magnitude of AHH induction in these cells. The possibility of using the toxixity of benzo[a]pyrene to select for mutations that affect the inducibility of those cells was recognized several years ago [24].

In a recent study, Hankinson [25] has developed a practical protocol for the selection of nonresponsive mutants from responsive Hepa-1 mouse hepatoma cells. AHH activity in Hepa-1 cells is highly inducible (20-fold) by benzo[a]pyrene or 7,12-dimethylbenzo[a]anthracene. These cells are ordinarily killed by exposure to benzo[a]pyrene for several days—presumably because of the increased production of toxic benzo[a]pyrene metabolites in the induced cells. However, approximately 2 per $10^7$ cells are able to grow in the presence of benzo[a]pyrene, and cultures derived from these cells are found to contain extremely low basal AHH activity and are not inducible by benzo[a]pyrene. Fluctuation analyses (Luria-Delbrück) demonstrate that these resistant cells develop as a result of randomly occurring events and probably represent spontaneous mutations affecting the AHH system. As shown in Figure 9, mutations affecting any one of at least 12 distinct steps in AHH induction might result in benzo[a]pyrene-resistant cells. Some of these mutations may affect the putative receptor for AHH induction.

## Clinical Observations of the *Ah* Polymorphism

The problem of monooxygenase induction is complex; it has proven quite difficult to go beyond studies of the phenotype (based on enzyme assays) to identification of the molecular products of the *Ah* regulatory and structural genes. As described above, characterization of the cytosolic TCDD receptor, the putative product of the *Ah* regulatory gene, is far from complete.

One of the questions raised by this work is whether humans show hereditable differences in AHH induction. All of the studies with human cells to date have dealt with determination of induction phenotype based on enzymatic assays of AHH. Difficulties with this approach emphasize the necessity for identifying the molecular products of the *Ah* regulatory locus [26, 27].

Peripheral circulating lymphocytes are a readily accessible source of human cells and have been used extensively for metabolic and genetic studies. Unfortunately, freshly isolated lymphocytes are not inducible by 3-MC. If the lymphocytes are treated in culture with various mitogens, they develop the ability to respond to 3-MC or other polycyclic aromatic inducers. Initial studies with mitogen-activated lymphocytes indicated a trimodal distribution of AHH inducibility consistent with a hypothesis of two alleles at a single

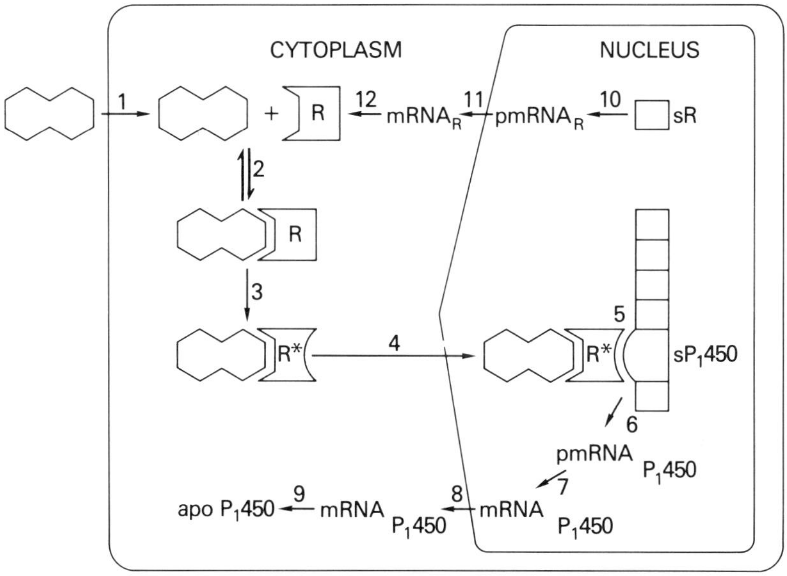


**Figure 9.** A schematic diagram of the molecular events involved in the induction of AHH. An inducer molecule enters the cell (step 1) and binds to a cytosol receptor (step 2); the inducer-receptor complex enters the cell nucleus and effects the transcription of messenger RNA for a specific form of cytochrome P-450 (steps 3-6). Nuclear translocation of the inducer-receptor complex may involve an "activation" step (step 3, R$\longrightarrow$R*) which alters the physicochemical properties of the inducer-receptor complex. The messenger RNA is processed in the nucleus (step 7, pmRNA–precursor messenger RNA), enters the cytoplasm (step 8), and is translated into protein for the P-450 (step 9). The *Ah* locus is represented as the structural gene for the receptor (sR); mRNA transcribed from this gene (step 10) is translated into receptor protein (steps 11, 12).

locus [28] and "additive" inheritance. Several laboratories have been unable to confirm this monogenic, two-allele hypothesis [29-31]. The major difficulty with lymphocyte studies is that inducibility varies as a function of time after mitogen activation, and it is not possible from experiment to experiment to predict the exact time course of inducibility. The ratio of control to induced levels of AHH is often only two-to-three fold and subject to large experimental variation. Carefully controlled studies with human mitogen-activated lymphocytes in this laboratory has demonstrated a bimodal distribution [31], with most ratios of inducibility in a low range. Interestingly, a randomly bred population of mice (derived from many generations of random breeding from parental D2, C3, B6, AKR) shows a similar distribution of AHH inducibility [32].

## CONCLUSIONS

The *Ah* cytosolic receptor is present in all organs, albeit at quite different concentrations (Okey et al. [15], Carlstedt-Duke [33] and unpublished data). It should be possible to measure receptor levels, given sufficient quantities of circulating human lymphocytes. Alternatively, sensitive radioimmunoassays for the forms of cytochrome associated with the *Ah* locus could be used in place of the relatively insensitive enzymatic assays. Recently specific antibodies to the 3-MC-induced $P_1$-450 and P-448 in mouse liver have been developed [11]. The methods used to purify these cytochromes and produce antisera could be applied to human cells [27].

## REFERENCES

1. Nebert, D. W., and N. M. Jensen. " The *Ah* Locus: Genetic Regulation of the Metabolism of Carcinogens, Drugs, and Other Environmental Chemicals by Cytochrome P-450-Mediated Monooxygenases," in *CRC Critical Reviews in Biochemistry,* G. D. Fasman, Ed. (Cleveland, OH: CRC Press, Inc., 1979), p. 401.
2. Nebert, D. W. "Multiple Forms of Inducible Drug-Metabolizing Enzymes. A Reasonable Mechanism by Which Any Organism Can Cope with Adversity," *Mol. Cell. Biochem.* (in press).
3. Conney, A. H. "Pharmacological Implications of Microsomal Enzyme Induction," *Pharmacol. Rev.* 19:317-366 (1967).
4. Haugen, D. A., M. J. Coon and D. W. Nebert. "Induction of Multiple Forms of Mouse Liver Cytochrome P-450. Evidence for Genetically Controlled *de novo* Protein Synthesis in Response to Treatment with β-Naphthoflavone or Phenobarbital," *J. Biol. Chem.* 251:1817-1827 (1976).
5. Wood, A. W. "Genetic Regulation of Coumarin Hydroxylase Activity in Mice. Biochemical Characterization of the Enzyme From Two Inbred Strains and Their $F_1$ Hybrid," *J. Bio. Chem.* 254:5641-5646 (1979).
6. Kouri, R. W., and D. W. Nebert, "Genetic Regulation of Susceptibility of Polycyclic Hydrocarbon-Induced Tumors in the Mouse," in *Origins of Human Cancer,* H. H. Hiatt, J. D. Watson and J. A. Winsten, Eds. (Cold Spring Harbor, NY: Cold Spring Harbor Laboratory, 1977), p.811.
7. Nebert, D. W., and J. S. Felton. "Importance of Genetic Factors Influencing the Metabolism of Foreign Compounds," *Fed. Proc.* 35:1133-1141 (1976).
8. Nebert, D. W., and J. S. Felton. "Evidence for the Activation of 3-Methylcholanthrene as a Carcinogen *in vivo* by Cytochrome $P_1$450 from Inbred Strains of Mice," in *Cytochromes P-450 and* $b_5$, D. Y. Cooper, O. Rosenthal, R. Snyder and C. Witmer, Eds. (New York: Plenum Publishing Corporation, 1975), p. 127.
9. Robinson, J. R., N. Considine and D. W. Nebert. "Genetic Expression

of Aryl Hydrocarbon Hydroxylase Induction. Evidence for the Involvement of Other Genetic Loci," *J. Biol. Chem.* 249:5851-5859 (1974).

10. McClearn, G. E., J. R. Wilson and W. Meredith. "The Use of Isogenic and Heterogenic Mouse Stocks in Behavioral Research," in *Contributions to Behavior-Genetic Analysis: The Mouse as a Prototype,* G. Lindzey and D. D. Thiessen, Eds. (New York: Appleton Century-Crofts, 1970), p. 3.
11. Negishi, M., and D. W. Nebert. "Structural Gene Products of the *Ah* Locus. Genetic and Immunochemical Evidence for Two Forms of Mouse Liver Cytochrome P-450 Induced by 3-Methylcholanthrene," *J. Biol. Chem.* (in press).
12. Kumaki, K., N. M. Jensen, J. G. M. Shire and D. W. Nebert. "Genetic Differences in Induction of Cytosol Reduced-NAD (P): Menadione Oxidoreductase and Microsomal Aryl Hydrocarbon Hydroxylase in the Mouse," *J. Biol. Chem.* 252:157-165 (1977).
13. Poland, A. P., and E. Glover. "Chlorinated Dibenzo-*p*-dioxins: Potent Inducers of δ-Aminolevulinic Acid Synthetase and Aryl Hydrocarbon Hydroxylase. II. A Study of the Structure-Activity Relationship," *Mol. Pharmacol.* 9:736-747 (1973).
14. Poland, A. P., E. Glover, J. R. Robinson and D. W. Nebert. "Genetic Expression of Aryl Hydrocarbon Hydroxylase Activity. Induction of Monooxygenase Activities and Cytochrome $P_1$450 Formation by 2, 3, 7, 8-Tetrachlorodibenzo-*p*-dioxin in Mice Genetically "Nonresponsive" to Other Aromatic Hydrocarbons," *J. Biol. Chem.* 249:5599-5606 (1974).
15. Okey, A. B., G. T. Bondy, M. E. Mason, G. F. Kahl, H. J. Eisen, T. M. Guenthner and D. W. Nebert. "Regulatory Gene Product of the *Ah* Locus. Characterization of the Cytosolic Inducer-Receptor Complex and Evidence For Its Nuclear Translocation," *J. Biol. Chem.* 254: 11636-11648 (1980).
16. Poland, A. P., E. Glover and A. S. Kende. "Stereospecific, High Affinity Binding of 2, 3, 7, 8-Tetrachlorodibenzo-*p*-dioxin by Hepatic Cytosol. Evidence That the Binding Species is the Receptor for the Induction of Aryl Hydrocarbon Hydroxylase," *J. Biol. Chem.* 251:4936-4946 (1976).
17. Poland, A. R., and E. Glover. "Chlorinated Biphenyl Induction of Aryl Hydrocarbon Hydroxylase Activity: A Study of the Structure-Activity Relationship," *Mol. Pharmacol.* 13:924-938 (1977).
18. Carlstedt-Duke, J., G. Elfström, M. Snochowski, B. Högberg and J.-Å. Gustafsson. "Detection of the 2, 3, 7, 8-Tetrachlorodibenzo-*p*-dioxin (TCDD) Receptor in Rat Liver by Isoelectric Focusing in Polyacrylamide Gels," *Toxicol. Lett.* 2:365-373 (1978).
19. Robinson, J. R., and D. W. Nebert. "Genetic Expression of Aryl Hydrocarbon Hydroxylase Induction. Presence or Absence of Association with Zoxazolamine, Diphenylhydantoin, and Hexobarbital Metabolism," *Mol. Pharmacol.* 10:484-493 (1974).
20. Milgrom, E., M. Atger and E.-E. Baulieu. "Acidophilic Activation of Steroid Hormone Receptors," *Biochemistry* 12:5198-5205 (1973).

21. Eisen, H. J., and W. H. Glinsmann. "Maximizing the Purification of the Activated Glucocorticoid Receptor by DNA-Cellulose Chromatography," *Biochem. J.* 171:177-183 (1978).
22. Guenthner, T. M., and D. W. Nebert. "The Cytosolic Receptor for Aryl Hydrocarbon Hydroxylase Induction by Polycyclic Aromatic Compounds. Evidence for Structural and Regulatory Variants Among Established Cell Culture Lines," *J. Biol. Chem.* 252:8981-8989 (1977).
23. Owens, I. S., and D. W. Nebert. "Aryl Hydrocarbon Hydroxylase Induction in Mammalian-Liver-Derived Cell Cultures. Stimulation of "Cytochrome $P_1$450-Associated" Enzyme Activity by Many Inducing Compounds," *Mol. Pharmacol.* 11:94-104 (1975).
24. Benedict, W. F., J. E. Gielen and D. W. Nebert. "Polycyclic Hydrocarbon-Produced Toxicity, Transformation, and Chromosomal Aberrations as a Function of Aryl Hydrocarbon Hydroxylase Activity," *Int. J. Cancer* 9:435-451 (1972).
25. Hankinson, O. "Single-Step Selection of Clones of a Mouse Hepatoma Line Deficient in Aryl Hydrocarbon Hydroxylase, "*Proc. Nat. Acad. Sci., U.S.* 76:373-376 (1979).
26. Atlas, S. A., and D. W. Nebert. "Pharmacogenetics: A Possible Pragmatic Perspective in Neoplasm Predictability," *Sem. Oncol.* 5:89-106 (1978).
27. Nebert, D. W. "The *Ah* Locus. A Gene with Possible Importance in Cancer Predictability." *Arch. Toxicol.* (in press).
28. Kellermann, G., M. Luyten-Kellermann and C. R. Shaw. "Genetic Variation of Aryl Hydrocarbon Hydroxylase in Human Lymphocytes," *Am. J. Human Genet.* 25:327-331 (1973).
29. Kouri, R. E., H. Ratrie, III, S. A. Atlas, A. Niwa and D. W. Nebert. "Aryl Hydrocarbon Hydroxylase Induction in Human Lymphocyte Cultures by 2, 3, 7, 8-Tetrachlorodibenzo-*p*-dioxin," *Life Sci.* 15:1585-1595 (1974).
30. Gurtoo, H. L., N. Bejba and J. Minowada. "Properties, Inducibility, and an Improved Method of Analysis of Aryl Hydrocarbon Hydroxylase in Cultured Human Lymphocytes," *Cancer Res.* 35:1235-1243 (1975).
31. Atlas, S. A., E. S. Vesell and D. W. Nebert. "Genetic Control of Interindividual Variations in the Inducibility of Aryl Hydrocarbon Hydroxylase in Cultured Human Lymphocytes," *Cancer Res.* 36:4619-4630 (1976).
32. Nebert, D. W., and S. A. Atlas. "The *Ah* Locus: Aromatic Hydrocarbon Responsiveness . . . Of Mice and Men," *Human Genet.* 1:149-160 (1978).
33. Carlstedt-Duke, J. M. B. "Tissue Distribution of the Receptor for 2, 3, 7, 8-Tetrachlorodibenzo-*p*-dioxin in the Rat," *Cancer Res.* 39:3172-3176 (1979).

# CHAPTER 6

# ANALYTICAL CHEMISTRY NEEDS FOR ENVIRONMENTAL EPIDEMIOLOGY

**Walter J. Rogan**
National Institute of Environmental Health Sciences
Biometry Branch
Research Triangle Park, NC 27709

## INTRODUCTION

Infectious disease, the traditional habitat of epidemiologists, depends heavily on the laboratory identification of pathogens. Laboratory methods in bacteriology are perhaps best developed, but viral cultures, counter immunoelectrophoresis, fluorescent staining techniques and serology may be used in the investigation of a given outbreak. The clinical pathologist or microbiologist who works with epidemiologists is familiar with the demands that will be made on him or her in the course of an investigation, and can almost always count on using relatively well known and thoroughly standardized techniques. Normal flora are familiar, and methods for minimizing or eliminating contamination are known.

The investigation of disease from chemical exposures or other nonmicrobial agents is very different from the investigation of infectious disease outbreaks in a number of ways, some of which affect chemists. Chemists who are accustomed to analytical procedures for environmental residues may be unaccustomed to clinical material; clinical pathologists may be unfamiliar with the chemicals involved. Pharmacokinetic considerations may confuse the investigator in his choice of the appropriate tissues for analysis, and metabolic characteristics of the particular chemical may make the toxic congener of interest disappear before it can be demonstrated. Although similar problems exist for the infectious disease investigator, most have been worked out for at least the more familiar diseases, whereas in chemical exposures, the disease itself may be poorly characterized or unknown.

This chapter lists some of the demands made on the analytical laboratory by epidemiologists. Most of these investigations have happened in the last few years, which reflects the relative newness of this kind of inquiry. It is likely that such incidents will continue, and probably increase in frequency.

## KEPONE®

Kepone (chlordecone) is a chlorinated hydrocarbon insecticide developed by Allied Chemical Co. in the 1950s. From March 1974 through July 1975, the sole producer of Kepone was the Life Science Products Co., (LSPC), in Hopewell, VA. LSPC produced about 400,000 kg/yr of Kepone, made no other product, and operated out of an abandoned filling station. No human disease (and little animal toxicity) was associated with Kepone exposure until July 1975, when an internist in Hopewell submitted a serum sample to the Center for Disease Control (CDC), and inquired whether his patient's nervousness, irritability and other symptoms might be caused by Kepone absorption. The level of Kepone in the serum was 7.5 ppm. The state health department was notified, and an investigation was begun [1].

The plant had employed 148 persons at some time–33 were currently working. The reason for the rapid turnover was apparently the obvious (to the workers) Kepone-related toxicity, which they referred to as the "Kepone shakes." Of these, 133 participated in an epidemiologic study, answering a questionnaire and giving a sample of venous blood. A total of 270 family members were contacted; 32 samples of blood were taken from them. Additionally, 39 former Allied Kepone production workers participated, and 32 workers in nearby businesses who did not produce Kepone were included. To investigate neighborhood exposure, circles were drawn on a map, and a systematic one-in-five survey of households was done. This netted an additional 214 specimens of blood and questionnaires. An unspecified number of workers from the wastewater treatment plant where LSPC discharges were processed were also included (Table I). In addition to blood samples, stored air sample filters, water, bottom sediments, sludge, fish and shellfish were analyzed.

About 50% of the workers had the syndrome of nervousness, tremor, anxiety, pleuritic chest pain and vision difficulties with or without objective opsoclonus. Two wives who had washed their husbands' work clothes also were diagnosed as having Kepone-related disease. Symptoms were more

**Table I. Whole-Blood Kepone Level, by Group of Exposed Persons[a]**

| Group | No. Tested | No. with Detectable Level | % with Detectable Level | Range of Detectable Level (ppm) | Mean of Detectable Level (ppm) |
|---|---|---|---|---|---|
| Affected LSPC Worker | 57 | 57 | 100 | 0.009–11.8 | 2.53 |
| Unaffected LSPC Worker | 49 | 48 | 99 | 0.003–4.1 | 0.60 |
| Family members, LSPC Worker | 32 | 30 | 94 | 0.003–0.39 | 0.10 |
| Allied Kepone Worker | 39 | 30 | 77 | 0.003–0.45 | 0.06 |
| Neighborhood Worker | 32 | 23 | 72 | 0.003–0.031 | 0.011 |
| Sewage Treatment Plant Worker | 10 | 6 | 60 | 0.004–0.014 | 0.008 |
| Cab Driver | 5 | 1 | 20 | 0.003 | 0.003 |
| Truck Driver | 2 | 1 | 50 | 0.004 | 0.004 |
| Hopewell Resident | 214 | 40 | 19 | 0.005–0.325 | 0.011 |

[a]From Cannon, S. B., J. M. Veazey, Jr., R. S. Jackson, V. W. Burse, C. Hayes, W. E. Straub, P. J. Landrigan and J. A. Liddle. "Epidemic Kepone Poisoning in Chemical Workers," *Am. J. Epidemiol.* 107(6):529-537 (1978) (reprinted by permission).

prevalent in those with higher levels. Illness was not diagnosed in any other groups. The highest blood values were in the 11 ppm range, with a median among the affected workers of 2.53 ppm.

Most epidemiologists would consider clinical trials as within their purview. The demonstration of dose-related human toxicity of Kepone led to a clinical trial of cholestyramine in an attempt to lower body burden of the somewhat persistent toxin and to ameliorate symptoms. Cholestyramine works by binding to bile acids and other substances in the lumen of the intestine, and had decreased the half-life of Kepone in rats. If the excretion of chlordecone was slowed by enterohepatic circulation, i.e., if it was excreted in the bile and then reabsorbed later in the intestine, then cholestyramine would be a reasonable drug to try. First, however, it had to be documented that such circulation occurred.

Cohn [2] and his colleagues at the Medical College of Virginia followed 32 of the LSPC workers. They obtained blood, liver by percutaneous biopsy and fat by subcutaneous biopsy on some or all of these patients. Seven patients were admitted to the clinical research center. Measurements of Kepone in bile, duodenal aspirate and stool were carried out with elaborate maneuvers aimed at quantifying the movement, partitioning, circulation and excretion of the chemical. Once it had been shown to the investigator's satisfaction that enterohepatic circulation was a major factor in the persistence of Kepone, cholestyramine was administered to 11 subjects, placebo to another 11. Cholestyramine decreased by about half the serum half-life of Kepone, from 165 to 80 days, while the placebo group went from 141 to 139.

Thus, the documentation of the etiologic role of Kepone, the elucidation of its pharmacokinetics, and the demonstration of successful treatment all relied heavily on the laboratory. Interpretation of these data from many different tissues and fluids required the absence of strong matrix effects, i.e., endogenously deposited Kepone had to be equally recoverable from all tissues. In only one of the studies—the volume of distribution study—was radiolabeled compound used.

## LEAD

Next to eating lead-based paint, air and dustfall lead are the major sources of lead exposure, particularly to children. Although 98% of lead in air is from vehicular emissions, there are point sources, such as smelters, that have in the past released sufficient particulate lead to pose a hazard to children living nearby. Epidemiologic studies of the relationship between lead in air and the blood lead of children were major evidence in the U.S. Environmental

Protection Agency (EPA) lead-in-air regulation. The analytic support requirements for these studies was extensive, and only the 1972 El Paso study [3] will be reviewed here.

The El Paso smelter emitted 1012 metric tons of lead, 508 metric tons of zinc, 11 metric tons of cadmium and 1 metric ton of arsenic from 1969 to 1971. The CDC El Paso study measured exposure of persons living in El Paso to lead from dust, soil, air, paint, food, water and pottery. Absorption and storage of lead was measured by analysis of blood. Studies of air lead showed a strong relationship between distance from the smelter and lead in air. Analysis of air for lead and bromine allowed construction of a Pb/Br ratio. This ratio is 2.6 in automobile exhaust, and departures from that ratio indicate that the lead source is nonautomobile-related. The ratio was highest near the smelter and fell to 2.6 about 7 km away. Lead content of soil (466 samples) and of household dust (594 samples) was also related to distance from the smelter (Table II). Children's blood lead values were higher in houses where dust lead was high, with higher values seen in younger children (Table III). A total of 1600 paint samples were analyzed for lead; about 30% of houses had one or more samples above 1.0% lead by dry weight. Children living in these houses, however, tended to have blood lead levels similar to other children living in the same area. In all, 758 children were tested. Food and water contamination by lead was negligible; however, 2.8% of homes used pottery with excessive lead release; these children tended to have higher levels. The dose-response relationship between dust lead and blood lead was strong in houses within 1.6 km of the smelter, but not apparent further away. Soil content of lead was not so strongly related to blood lead.

**Table II. Lead Content in Household Dust Samples, El Paso[a]**

| Distance from Smelter (km): | No. of Samples | Lead Content (ppm) | |
|---|---|---|---|
| | | Geometric Mean | Range |
| 0.0–1.6 | 53 | 22,191 | 2,800–103,750 |
| 1.7–3.2 | 219 | 2,124 | 100–84,000 |
| 3.3–6.4 | 209 | 1,552 | 100–29,836 |
| >6.4 | 48 | 973 | 200–22,700 |

[a]From the *New England Journal of Medicine* 292(1):1-6 (1975) (reprinted by permission).

**Table III. Blood Lead by Distance from Smelter and Age[a]**

| Distance | Age | No. Tested | % with Blood Lead 40-59 $\mu$g/100 ml | % with Blood Lead $\geqslant$60 $\mu$g/100 ml |
|---|---|---|---|---|
| $\leqslant$1.6 km | 1-4 | 49 | 55 | 14 |
| | 5-9 | 101 | 34 | 11 |
| | 10-19 | 109 | 25 | 6 |
| | 20+ | 98 | 16 | 0 |
| $>$1.6 km | 1-4 | 83 | 23 | 4 |
| | 5-9 | 124 | 12 | 0 |
| | 10-19 | 292 | 3 | 1 |
| | 20+ | 513 | 3 | 1 |
| Total | | 1369 | | |

[a]From the *New England Journal of Medicine* 292(1):1-6 (1975) (reprinted by permission).

The support needs for this study thus included multiple different substances—food, water, air, soil, dust and blood. The vector by which children were exposed to lead was the primary question—thus, quantitative information of a comparable nature was required of all of these measurements, to allow construction of the various dose-response curves. Because intervention was planned and other smelters were to be investigated, the analytic methodology had to be able to be duplicated at other sites and had to be free of secular trends.

As a result of this study, changes were made in plant emissions. Five years later, children around the smelter were restudied, and the mean values of their blood lead had fallen [4]. The change in blood lead vs the change in air lead—about 2 $\mu$g lead/100 ml blood to 1 $\mu$g lead/$m^3$ of air—became part of the EPA air lead regulation.

## POLYBROMINATED BIPHENYLS

In 1973, two products produced by the Michigan Chemical Company were mixed in shipment. The intended product was Nutrimaster, a $MgO_2$ supplement for dairy cow food. The substitute was Firemaster BP-6, a flame retardant mixture of polybrominated biphenyls (PBB). Many cows and other animals sickened, but the contaminant was not identified until farmers and their customers had consumed contaminated meat, milk and other dairy products. Even the detection of the contaminant had posed analytical problems. Standard tests had been run but were negative; we now think that a gas-liquid chromatograph was eventually left running during a lunch hour, and the very late emerging peaks were found. Identification took the almost chance communication of these results to a chemist at the U.S. Department of Agriculture (USDA) who happened to be familiar with PBB.

Once it was established that the feed grain was contaminated with PBB, and that farmers had eaten animals who had eaten the food, many illnesses that had occurred over the preceding year were attributed to PBB. A questionnaire survey plus blood sampling study was done by the Michigan Department of Public Health (MDPH) in 1974; 298 people participated by filling out the forms—133 from nonquarantined farms; 165 from quarantined farms. A total of 110 blood specimens for PBB were drawn from the quarantined group, 104 from the nonquarantined (Table IV).

**Table IV. Analytic Support Required for Epidemiologic Studies of Human PBB Exposure**

| | Blood | Fat | Breast Milk |
|---|---|---|---|
| MDPH Short-Term Study [5], Fall, 1974 | 214 | | |
| Mt. Sinai, November 1976 [6] | ~1000 | ~300 | |
| MDPH Milk Study [7], 1976 | | | 95 |
| MDPH Long-Term Study [8] 1976-1979 | 3678<br>1000 | ~400 | |
| Mt. Sinai General Population, 1978 | 1750 | 900 | |
| Total Samples | 7642 | 1600 | 95 |

The values ranged from undetectable to 2.26 ppm. Although no specific signs or symptoms were clearly present in the quarantined group and absent in the nonquarantined, a number of the nonquarantined farms were later shown to have quarantinable levels. This would tend to blur any differences that were indeed present.

Over the next three years, several ambitious studies were undertaken, all of which required substantial laboratory support. In November 1976 the Mt. Sinai team performed a medical survey of over 1000 Michigan farmers, their families, Michigan chemical company workers and others. In addition to estimates of PBB in serum, polychlorinated biphenyls (PCB), DDT and DDE were analyzed, and 300 percutaneous fat biopsy specimens were taken [6].

By 1976, concern over widespread contamination of Michigan and the relative insensitivity of serum analysis had resulted in a survey of breast milk for PBB across the entire state [7]. A sample of 95 women was taken—53 from the lower peninsula, 42 from the upper. Of the lower peninsula samples, 51 were positive, and 18 of the upper peninsula samples, with a range of 0-1.2 ppm, on a whole-milk basis. Since this was a probability sample of lactating women, statistical inference could be drawn, and it was concluded that over $9 \times 10^6$ of Michigan's $11 \times 10^6$ citizens had detectable levels of PBB.

Two other major studies have been in the field—the Michigan DPH long-term survey [8], and the Mt. Sinai general population study. The first is a long-term cohort study of 4249 persons, on whom 3678 blood specimens were collected. It has been proposed that this cohort be followed essentially to extinction, to determine what effect, if any, body burden of PBB has on mortality. Although not firm, one proposed plan was to take samples from the entire group initially, and then randomly select one quarter of the families each year for retest. Initially, PBB alone was done; after a thousand or so of the samples had been run, PCB determination was thought biologically important and added. When this decision was made, the samples had already been collected, and thus a fixed volume was available for this analysis. Thereafter, a combined method of analysis for PCB and PBB was developed especially for this study, and had to be made comparable with previous data and then transplanted from the research labs at the CDC to the field labs at MDPH.

Finally, the Mt. Sinai general population study was a medical survey of a stratified random sample of Michigan residents done in separate locations across the state in summer, 1978. This study attempted to confirm the prevalence estimate from the breast milk study, and also to see whether PBB related illness could be detected in the presumed low-exposure nonfarm population. A total of 500 children and 1250 adults participated; all but a very few had blood drawn for PBB, PCB, DDT and DDE in addition to routine clinical tests. Almost 900 fat biopsies were also done, and analyzed for the same chemicals [9].

Thus, over the past six years, a chemical that was an analytic conundrum and required almost accidental identification has become an object of extensive attention, not only qualitatively, but quantitatively. By count, 1600 fat specimens, 7600 sera and about 100 milk specimens have been analyzed in direct support of epidemiological studies. This gives some idea of the effort that may be required when a major environmental contamination takes place; also, the lack of obvious relationship between illnesses and the quantitative levels of PBB has been interpreted as strong evidence against the existence of acute or subacute toxicity, even though the levels have been near the lower end of the analytic range.

## LOVE CANAL

During 1978, residents of a Niagara Falls neighborhood noticed "chemical" odors in their basements, and some found a black sludge in their sumps or welling up to the soil surface nearby. The neighborhood was that surrounding the Love Canal. This canal is a blind segment of a proposed canal that would have allowed water to bypass Niagara Falls and be used to generate electricity. The project was abandoned in 1910, when cheap transmission of power became possible by the invention of alternating current. Until the 1920s, the canal was used by area children as a swimming hole. From then until 1953, it was used as a chemical dumpsite by various chemical companies and municipalities, most notably Hooker Chemical Co. In 1953, the canal was capped, and in the late 1950s homes and ultimately a school were built around the site. Heavy rains during 1977 and 1978 apparently raised the water table sufficiently to bring the chemicals to the surface.

In response to complaints, the New York State Health Department and the Department of Environmental Contamination began investigation in April 1978 [10]. Auger soil, water and air samples were done, and radiation estimates were made. In addition to the fairly obvious visible chemicals, there were levels of 80 compounds, mostly aromatics and chlorinated aromatics, detected in the air of the basements of homes directly adjoining the canal site. Of this potpourri, lists of chemicals were selected as probable indicators, and were searched for at sites more distant. Some of the chemicals found were either known or potential human toxins or carcinogens. A partial list is given in Table V. Many were present at levels that violated occupational exposure guidelines.

**Table V. Selected Chemicals Found at Love Canal Site [9][a]**

| | |
|---|---|
| Benzene | Dibromomethane |
| Toluene | Benzaldehydes |
| Benzoic Acid | Methylene Chloride |
| Lindane | Carbon Tetrachloride |
| Trichloroethylene | Chloroform |

[a]Reprinted by permission of the New York State Health Department.

Although the potential for human toxicity from exposure to these chemicals was clear, exactly what such toxicity might be was enigmatic. Some human and/or animal data were available on some compounds, but obviously nothing was known about such a complex mixture. Some diseases, like cancer, were certainly of interest. However, decisions had to be made in the short run, and the latency period for chemically induced cancer is decades long. The health department decided to investigate three "indicator" conditions that escaped the latency period problem: history of spontaneous abortion, history of birth defects and clinical tests of liver function. Using literature control values, they were able to show that women living in houses along the canal reported rates of spontaneous abortion about twice as high as expected. For women on the south end of 99th Street, this ratio reached statistical significance. In terms of obvious chemical exposure, this was a "follow your nose" hypothesis, and steps were taken to remove people from heavily contaminated houses.

Besides the houses directly adjoining the canal, there were other houses in the area, and residents there believed that they, too, might be at risk from exposure. Interviews were conducted with area residents, but there seemed to be no obvious relationship between distance from the dump site and abortion rates. At that point, i.e., after data on abortions had been collected, the "pond-swale" hypothesis of exposure was formulated. In the canal area, there are ponds that have ditches, or swales, connecting them to each other and to the canal itself. Some of these swales had been filled in, some remained visible, but many had probably carried water at some time, in one direction or another, that could have been contaminated by the canal. About 44% of area houses could be considered "wet" by this vector. When analysis of reported spontaneous abortion rates was done, women in the "wet" areas had spontaneous abortion rates about 1.8 times expected, a value intermediate between those right on the canal and those living in "dry" houses [11]. Epidemiologically, this was persuasive, since the hypothesis had been formed independently and checked with the data. The task was to show that such houses indeed were exposed to greater levels of something that might be the agent, in areas where levels were considerably lower than along the canal. At this writing, considerable attempts to show such elevated exposures at these sites have failed, despite considerable expenditure of person-years and money. The answer to this question is even more important than the validation of the epidemiology—from a public health standpoint, decisions on who moves and who stays must ultimately be made on the basis of exposure, and thus chemical analysis. By the time the epidemiologist can show damage, it is already too late.

## SUMMARY

These investigations illustrate the variety of demands that are made on the chemist in the course of investigating "outbreaks," be they of exposure or of disease, when there is suspicion of a chemical etiology. The following points summarize the main characteristics that will arise in such investigations (Table VI).

The exposure of interest and its vector range widely, from single chemical and obvious source to multiple chemicals and unknown sources. In the Kepone episode, only one chemical was manufactured, and exposure was obvious; in the lead studies, the source and the chemical entity were known, but the precise vector and the relationship between exposure and absorption had to be determined. In the case of PBB, the chemical had to be defined first; the population exposed was very large, and PBB itself is not a single entity, but a mixture of different congeners with differing pharmacokinetics and toxicity. The Love Canal represents a complex mixture of many chemicals, and even the documentation of exposure is problematic.

Multiple matrices or substrates are usual. Analysis of air, water, various foods, soil and multiple biological fluids may be required. Proper identification of the exposure vector will depend on the comparability of data generated from the analysis of many different candidates.

Analytic technology must be transportable to the field or the specimens must be transportable to the analyst or both. Severe difficulties in interpretation arise when different analytical methods are used in different studies, and when the methods in one laboratory cannot readily be duplicated in another. The same is true when analytical tests are sensitive to travel—the outbreak cannot be expected to occur in convenient areas.

The possibility of secular trends in analysis must be minimized. This is particularly true in long-term studies, where conclusions will be drawn from trends in the data which will be assumed to have biological meaning. Thus, a sample analyzed today must be comparable to one analyzed in 20 years.

The methods of analysis must be suitable for large numbers of samples. The detection of relatively subtle effects will almost always require large numbers of observations, as will the construction of dose-response relationships.

The smaller the sample volume required, the better. It can be very hard to get 20 ml of blood from a fat three-year-old. Analysis must be as quantitative as possible. Estimation of risk almost always requires knowledge of a dose-response relationship. The case for a biologically plausible etiologic role of exposure in disease production is considerably strengthened when such a relationship can be shown.

**Table VI. Factors in Chemical Epidemiology**

| | |
|---|---|
| Wide range of exposures and vectors | Many samples |
| Multiple matrices | Small volumes |
| Transport technology | Dose/response |
| Secular trends | Prevention |

Analytical techniques should prevent more epidemiology. Ideally, public health decisions should prevent or limit exposure to hazardous substances. Epidemiology is almost always too insensitive to provide good evidence of safety, and by definition the damage has already occurred.

Despite this last statement, it is likely environmental chemistry will be called on more and more frequently to provide evidence for etiology, rather than occurrence. The examples discussed today illustrate the kinds of problems that arise in such investigations, and some possible solutions.

## REFERENCES


1. Cannon, S. B., J. M. Veazey, Jr., R. S. Jackson, V. W. Burse, C. Hayes, W. E. Straub, P. J. Landrigan and J. A. Liddle. "Epidemic Kepone Poisoning in Chemical Workers," *Am. J. Epidemiol.* 107(6):529-537 (1978).
2. Cohn, W. J., J. J. Boylan, R. V. Blanke, M. W. Farris, J. R. Howell and P. S. Guzelian. "Treatment of Chlordecone (Kepone) Toxicity with Cholestyramine," *New England J. Med.* 298(5):243-248 (1978).
3. Landrigan, P. J., S. H. Gehlbach, B. F. Rosenblum, J. M. Shoults, R. M. Candelaria, W. F. Barthel, J. A. Liddle, A. L. Smrek, N. W. Staehling and J. F. Sanders. "Epidemic Lead Absorption Near an Ore Smelter," *New England J. Med.* 292(1):1-6 (1975).
4. Rosenblum, B. F., R. Kretzschmar, R. Candelaria, J. Hubert, J. Bradley and C. R. Webb. "Follow up on Lead Poisoning–Texas," *Morbid. Mortal. Weekly Rep.* 27(8):1 (1978).
5. "The Short Term Effects of PBB on Health," Michigan Department of Public Health, report of the Subcommittee on PBB, DHEW/CCTRP (1977).
6. Selikoff, I. J. et al. "Health Effects of Exposure to PBB, Results of a Clinical Field Survey, November 4-10, 1976," Interim Summary Report to NIEHS, Environmental Sciences Laboratory, Mt. Sinai School of Medicine of the City University of New York.
7. Brilliant, L. B., K. W. Wilcox, G. Van Amburg, J. Exster, J. Isbister, A. W. Bloomer, H. Humphrey and H. Price. "Breast Milk Monitoring to Measure Michigan's Contamination with PBB," *Lancet* 8091:643-646 (1978).
8. Landrigan, P. J., K. R. Wilcox, J. Silva, H. E. B. Humphrey, C. Kauffman and C. W. Heath. "Cohort Study of Michigan Residents Exposed to PBB: Epidemiologic and Immunologic Findings," *Ann. N.Y. Acad. Sci.* 320:284-294 (1979).
9. Selikoff, J., and H. A. Anderson. "A Survey of the General Population of Michigan for Health Effects of PBB Exposure," New York, Environmental Sciences Laboratory of Mt. Sinai (1979).
10. "Love Canal: Public Health Time Bomb," Special Report to the Governor and the Legislature (1978).
11. Vianna, N., New York State Department of Health. Personal communication.

# SECTION 2

# ENVIRONMENTAL ANALYSIS

CHAPTER 7

# METAL SPECIES IDENTIFICATION IN THE ENVIRONMENT

**Douglas A. Segar**

SEAMOcean
Wheaton, Maryland

**Adriana Y. Cantillo**

National Oceanic and Atmospheric Administration
NOS/OMT Engineering Development Laboratory
Rockville, Maryland

## INTRODUCTION

Since at least the Industrial Revolution, it has been known that many substances released by man into the environment can be hazardous to human health. Among the earliest such substances to be identified as health hazards were various toxic metals and inorganic nonmetals. The impact of synthetic organic compounds is, by contrast, a relatively recent development.

The scientific community and the public at large generally perceive that there is a more complete understanding of the effects of contaminant metals on human health than there is of the effects of synthetic organic compounds. Consequently, there is also a widely held belief that the environmental concentrations and release rates that are considered safe, and which form part of many environmental control regulations, are more firmly based on a good understanding of what the safe levels of metals in the environment are. Furthermore, it is believed that the heavy metal regulatory limits are more effective in ensuring human and ecological safety than are the corresponding regulatory limits for synthetic organic compounds.

These general attitudes to the trace metal environmental hazard are at least partially founded. There is, for example, better information concerning the environmental discharge concentrations of trace elements than there is for many organic compounds because the analytical techniques for metals have historically been better developed and less expensive. Understanding of the role and pathways of trace metals within the atmosphere, biosphere, hydrosphere and geosphere is much broader because it has been possible to study them for a period of decades, compared to the few years that we have been able to study synthetic organics.

In contrast, however, several very important factors about heavy metals are often overlooked. Toxic metals, although few in number, are cycled through the global ecosystem in a multitude of different physicochemical forms, including chemical compounds or associations with natural or synthetic organic compounds. It has been too easy to overlook this in the past because the techniques developed for trace and ultratrace metal analyses have almost exclusively determined the total concentration of the metal in a sample regardless of its original chemical forms. As a consequence, although a great deal is known about the distribution of metals in natural and contaminated ecosystems, relatively poor knowledge exists of the rates, routes and mechanisms of the transfer of metals from one component of the ecosystem to another, or of their controlling factors. This is particularly true of the biosphere, where metals are transported, concentrated, eliminated and utilized by biochemical cycles of great complexity. These biochemical cycles evolved over the eons as organisms developed the capability of controlling the effects of toxic trace metals on their metabolisms. In this regard, it should be noted that several of the metals which appear on the U.S. Environmental Protection Agency (EPA) list of priority aquatic pollutants are known to be essential to the growth of many organisms. It is only when these metals are present in high concentrations and in some instances only when they are present in a specific physicochemical state, that they become toxic or can be concentrated in animal tissue.

The fact that trace metals are a natural part, and that some are even a vital part, of all ecosystems is one of the two most important factors distinguishing trace metals from the vast majority of the organic compounds which are of concern as environmental pollutants. The second factor is that trace metals cannot be degraded or decomposed by waste treatment processes into harmless substances as can organic compounds. Taken together, these two factors indicate that, in the future, a different philosophy should be applied to environmental regulations concerning the release of trace metals than that which is applied to environmental regulations for organic compounds.

The United States and human society in general have only very recently acknowledged the need to prevent uncontrolled release of even small quantities of trace substances into the environment. At present, the United States is only beginning to reach the point where recently passed laws, such as the Federal Water Pollution Control Act; the Toxic Substances Act; the Resource Conservation and Recovery Act; the Federal Air Quality Act; the Marine Protection, Research and Sanctuaries Act; and a host of others have begun to take effect. Through regulation, these laws have forced America to perform what might be described as simple, basic, good housekeeping to prevent the release of toxic substances to the environment. As the worst polluting excesses of our society have been eliminated, the philosophy of the U.S. Congress, which underlies all the relevant laws, has been essentially the "zero discharge" philosophy. Congress recognizes that toxic substances are released to the environment that they are in many documented instances, a hazard to human health and welfare. Congress also recognizes that we do not understand the effects of these substances well enough to establish unequivocally whether or not for any particular toxic substances there is a totally safe rate of release to the environment. Therefore, Congress has determined that the only means at hand to safeguard the biosphere is to eliminate totally the release to the environment of any substance known to be highly toxic to humans or other living things. Congress has realized, of course, that this ideal philosophy was not attainable and, in the various laws that it has enacted, Congress made concessions to reality as typified by the requirement for "best available" technology (BAT) to be used in removing toxic substances from industrial wastewater discharges. The "zero discharge" philosophy was, and still is, adhered to, despite the fact that Congress has been continuously and progressively forced to acknowledge its impracticability, particularly in economic terms. This acknowledgment of impracticability may be exemplified by the modification of the BAT requirement to that of "best practicable technology."

If one examines the present legislative, regulatory and scientific framework from which our future environmental protection goals will be drawn, it is obvious that the "zero discharge" philosophy will come under increasing attack for its total impracticability. At the same time, scientific understanding for the role and behavior of most toxic substances in the environment has not improved sufficiently to invalidate the original reasons for adoption of the "zero discharge" philosophy. Thus, there can be no soundly based laws and regulations which minimize or eliminate harmful effects and, at the same time, minimize social and economic impacts by permitting controlled release of quantities of toxic substances in a manner and amounts proven to be safe. This is a scenario for conflict and controversy that can be minimized or avoided only through development of a sufficient information base concerning toxic substance behavior in the environment to enable management of toxic substances releases in a manner that guarantees safety and yet optimizes the economic and social benefits of using the assimilative capacity of the environment for this purpose. If this is to be the goal, a new philosophy of toxic substance control must be adopted. The "zero discharge" requirements should apply only to substances for which society can find a safe replacement or readily and totally be degraded into harmless substances in waste, effluent or emission treatment processes utilizing "best available" technology. For all other substances, it should be recognized that discharge management will be essentially an imperfect art. For the foreseeable future, the permitted releases will be arrived at by balancing the economic, social and safety factors. These factors will be based on the best available knowledge of toxic substance environmental behavior, even though it will probably be inadequate for the task.

Adoption of this philosophy would dictate that environmental science studies concerning toxic substances be focused more intensively on the study of the biogeochemical cycles of those chemicals for which no substitute is available, and which cannot be readily destroyed and made harmless by treatment. It is interesting to note in this regard that in recent years the level of research effort concerning synthetic organics in the environment has been rising rapidly, whereas that concerning trace metals has been somewhat diminished. This has occurred despite the fact that the vast majority of the synthetic toxic organic compounds are replaceable and degradable, while all of the toxic metals are not. There is, therefore, a strong argument to be made for an enhanced effort to understand the biogeochemical cycles of trace metals.

To gain such an enhanced understanding of toxic metal cycles, two areas must be discussed: (1) the pathways by which metals are transferred into and within the biosphere, and (2) the role of metal compound formation in determining the fate and toxicity of metals in the environment. The remainder of this chapter will describe briefly the importance of metal-organic compound formation in determining the fate and toxicity of metals in the environment and will discuss some of the techniques available to investigate their chemical forms in environmental samples. These include a set of promising new techniques employing atomic spectroscopy detection for various chromatographic separation methods.

## TRACE METAL SPECIES IN THE ENVIRONMENT

Trace metals are present in the environment in many different chemical forms. These chemical forms may be classified broadly into three groups:

inorganic compounds, simple and inorganically complexed ions, and metal-organic compounds. In the environment, inorganic compounds of trace metals are generally found only in solid phases, although these solid phases may exist in colloidal suspension in natural waters. Transport of metals across biological membranes requires the metal to be in solution. Therefore, elements in solid phases must normally be converted chemically to ionic or organically combined form in solution before they can enter the biosphere. Such conversion may take place either in the bulk liquid phase or aquatic systems or in the aqueous phases generated by organisms for this purpose, e. g., the intestinal fluids of vertebrates. Once a metal has been taken up by an organism through its external membrane, the subsequent transport of the metal to other parts of the organism usually also takes place in solution. Each different chemical species of an element has its own characteristic rate of diffusion and spectrum of reactions with the molecules that form living cell tissue. Therefore, the speciation of the element in natural waters and biological fluids such as blood and vacuole solutions is critically important in determining the functions and effects of the metal on the organism. For example, copper [1-4], cadmium [5] and thallium [6] are known to be considerably more toxic to various aquatic organisms when present in ionic form than when combined in most of their metal-organic compounds. Methylmercury is known to be accumulated more readily and is more toxic than inorganic mercury [7].

The simplest form of a metal in solution is the "free" ion. Coordination compounds of the ion will form if suitable ligands, such as hydroxylchloride, and sulfate ions, are present and can replace one or more of the water molecules in the hydrated ion complex (Figure 1). Complexes of this type are generally not strong ion complexes but ion pairs held by weak electrostatic forces. Most of these species will, therefore, be indistinguishable from one another and from the free ions during analyses which use techniques involving acidification or the use of a strong complexing agent. The equilibria existing among these species can, however, be investigated from thermodynamic calculations [8, 9] and by polarographic techniques [10-13].

Many organic compounds have electron donor groups and can, therefore, coordinate with metal ions. In general, these complexes are weak unless the organic molecule has two or more donor groups which can coordinate with the same metal ion, forming stable, closed ring, metal chelates (Figure 1). Many naturally occurring and synthetic organic compounds have chelating ability, and the number of possible metal chelates in the environment is, therefore, very large. The metal chelates have stability constants which can vary over many orders of magnitude. In many instances, because of the stereochemical requirements of complex formation, the stability constant of the complexes of a specific organic molecule may range over many orders of

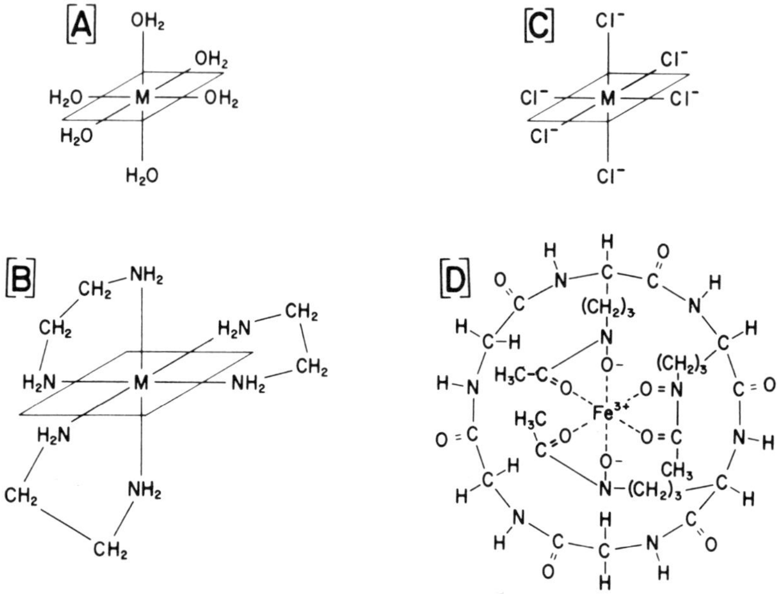


Figure 1. Examples of coordination compounds found in environmental samples. (A) Hydroxy-metal complex; (B) chloro-complex; (C) metal-EDTA chelate complex; and (D) ferrichrome, a ferric ion chelate complex.

magnitude among different metals. Chelates in the environment may be classified into two types, "labile" and "nonlabile." Labile chelates such as ethylene diamine tetraacetic acid (EDTA)-metal complexes are such that small changes of pH may markedly affect the stability of the complex, and the complexed metal ion may readily exchange with uncomplexed ions of the same metal in solution. Nonlabile chelates are those with extremely high stability constants, usually with a large organic molecule forming a cage structure around the metal ion, and whose metal ion is not readily exchangeable with other metal ions in solution. Examples of these "nonlabile" complexes are vitamin $B_{12}$ (cobalamin) and the ferrichromes (Figure 1). The distinction between nonlabile and labile complexes is purely arbitrary. However, as the analytical approach to these two types of complexes will be somewhat different, the distinction has a function value.

In addition to metal chelates, three other types of metal-organic compounds may be found in the environment: those with direct metal-to-carbon bonds (organometallics), salts of organic acids and complexes with $\pi$-electron donating compounds.

Compounds with $\pi$-electron donating systems include such compounds as ferrocene, in which a ferrous ion is sandwiched between two cyclopentadiene molecules (Figure 2) and Zeise's salt, in which a platinum ion is complexed with an ethylene molecule (Figure 2). These compounds are not generally stable, and probably have little importance in the environment, although they may be present in petroleum oils and tars, and are important in some biological processes [14].

Transition metal salts of organic acids are unlikely to be important in natural systems. However, the alkaline earth metal carbamate salts may be important in the calcium/phosphate cycles in the environment. The formation of soluble calcium carbamino-carboxylates (Figure 3) is thought to be responsible for the dissolution of bones and teeth under suitable conditions [15].

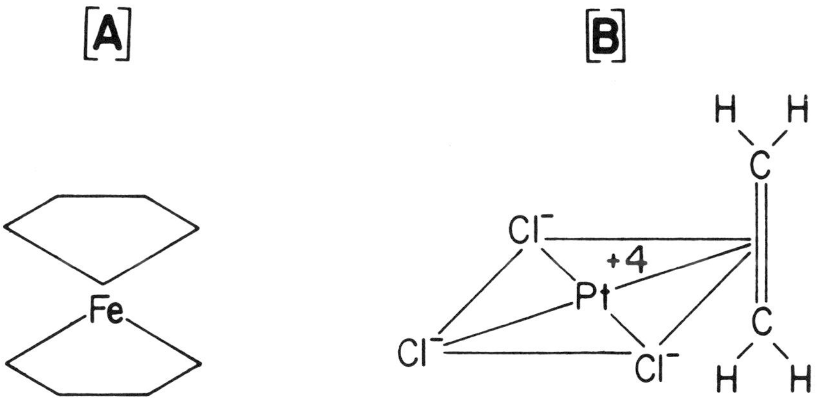


**Figure 2.** Examples of pi electron complexes; (A) Ferrocene, (B) Zeise's salt.

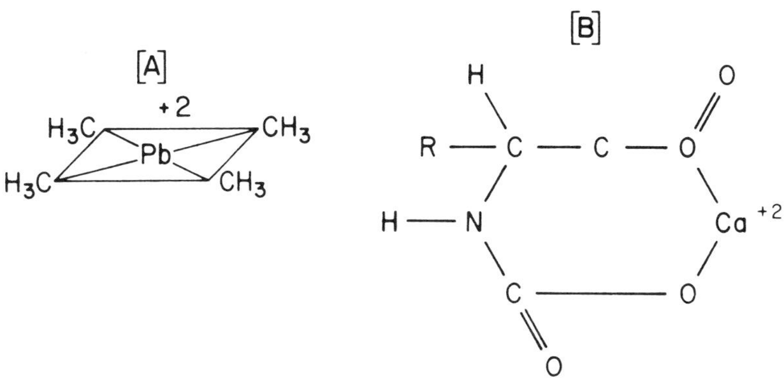


**Figure 3.** Examples of (A) an organometallic compound, tetramethyl lead; and (B) calcium carbamino-carboxylate.

## IMPORTANCE OF METAL SPECIES IN THE ENVIRONMENT

To illustrate the importance of metal species in determining the fate and effects of trace metals introduced into the global environment, a brief review is given of the importance of chemical species present in natural waters in mediating the biology and geochemistry of aquatic ecosystems.

Despite the fact that the nature of metal organic compounds in natural waters has been investigated more extensively than in other components of the biogeosphere, relatively little is known about such compounds, and the effects of these species are not well understood. However, some effects are known, and they can be classed into two areas: the control of solubility, volatility and oxidation state, and the control of availability of toxicity to organisms.

The complexing of metals by organic matter in natural waters will increase the solubility of the metal if the complex itself is soluble. The "solubilization" effect of chelation has been observed for a number of elements [19-22]. There is some doubt, however, whether in natural waters, chelation with naturally occurring organics yields true soluble complexes or colloidal complexes [23], and whether chelation can significantly affect solubility of elements in ocean waters with low dissolved organic matter concentrations [24].

Some chelates are insoluble, in which case chelation of a metal can lead to their precipitation. In natural systems, there is an abundance of particulate matter containing organic compounds which may chelate dissolved metals, and thus remove them from solution [25]. It is also known that the scavenging ability of hydrated oxides for trace metals from solution is strongly affected by the presence of organic chelating agents on the oxide surface or in solution [26].

The factors affecting metal solubility are often critical to the fate of elements in the environment. For example, in water and wastewater treatment processes, chelated contaminant metals may not be removed as easily as the simple metal ions [27, 28]. In addition, the control of solubility of metals may have profound influences upon the corrosion of metals in the environment. A metal surface may either be dissolved more rapidly or stabilized by chelation effects on the surface, and the principal action of fouling organisms in mediating corrosion may be release of extracellular organic chelators.

Some organically combined species of metals are not ionized in solution and are volatile. Such species as tetramethyl lead, methylated selenium compounds [29], methyl iodide [30], elemental mercury [7] and an unknown cadmium species [31] may be transported from aquatic systems into the atmosphere because of this volatility. Speciation thus plays a vital role in contaminant transport processes at the air-water interface, particularly as natural waters generally have surface slicks which tend to concentrate the un-ionized metal-organic compounds. Hydrophobic metal-organic compounds may be responsible for the high concentration of toxic metals found at the air-sea interface [32], and neuston species may well be exposed to a different spectrum of metal species than other aquatic organisms. The formation of alkylated metals by bacterial action may also be important in mobilizing metals in aquatic sediments to the water column and to the biota within the water column [17].

Understanding the subtle effects of metal-organic complexes within aquatic ecosystems is made all the more difficult because the formation of complexes is not instantaneous. Therefore, equilibrium calculations can rarely lead to reliable estimates of the actual concentration of a chelate complex present in a sample. For example, when ionic copper is added to sea water containing EDTA, the formation of the complex has been shown to take several hours [4], and ionic zinc added to sea water does not equilibrate with the zinc in the organically complexed fraction even after one year [33].

In certain instances, chelation of a metal may stabilize a metal in an oxidation state which is not otherwise stable. For example, chelation by natural organic matter can stabilize ferrous iron in aerated natural waters and retard its oxidation to ferric iron [34].

The chemical species of an element is of critical importance in controlling the toxicity and availability of the element to organisms. Many organometallics are considerably more toxic to organisms than are the inorganic metal ions themselves; for example, methyl mercury and methyl arsenic [17]. In addition, the chelation of a metal in solution can change its toxicity to organisms. Copper ions in solution are extremely toxic to a variety of organisms. However, if the copper is chelated, its toxicity is considerably reduced [1, 4]. More subtle effects of chelation on living organisms have been reported by many investigators concerned with understanding the factors which control the productivity of planktonic algae. The presence of a chelating agent such as EDTA is either essential to or accelerates the growth of marine phytoplankton [35, 37]. It is not clear whether the function of such chelation is to reduce the toxicity of the ionic form of some elements to the plankton or, alternatively, to solubilize and make such essential elements as iron and manganese available for uptake. Probably both mechanisms are important for different elements and in different environmental situations.

## IDENTIFICATION AND QUANTITATION OF METAL-ORGANICS

Except for those few compounds such as hemoglobin, which are participants in the major biochemical cycles, reports of the analytical determination of individual metal organic species in environmental samples were virtually nonexistent until recent years. The presence of metal-organic compounds in natural waters has been inferred from differential analysis of metal ions in oxidized samples [38, 43], from various toxicity and growth experiments [1-3, 35-37], and from solubility considerations [19-23, 35, 44]. At least one specific compound, cyanocobalamin (vitamin $B_{12}$), has been determined by biological assays and colorimetric techniques [45]. The reason for the paucity of data can be understood better by considering some of the characteristics of techniques currently used for environmental chemical analysis.

Analytical techniques commonly used for trace metal analyses in environmental samples include neutron activation, atomic absorption and emission, X-ray fluorescence, isotope dilution mass spectrometry (MS), colorimetry and polarography. With the exception of colorimetry and polarography, each of these analytical techniques will normally determine the total quantity of metal present in the determinative step regardless of chemical species. Any deviation from this principle, when a metal compound is present in the determinative step but not included in the analysis, is considered to be a matrix interference in the analysis. Colorimetry and polarography, on the other hand, will normally determine only the concentration of the free ion of the element in one specific oxidation state. In practice, any species in equilibrium with this ionic state with rapid kinetics will affect the determination, since relatively long plating time and anodic stripping techniques are usually necessary for polarographic determination of metals at the concentrations normally encountered in natural waters [46-49], and colorimetric methods usually are allowed to proceed to equilibrium before the determination is completed.

Except for the analysis of a few elements by neutron activation, flameless atomic absorption, polarography and colorimetry, preconcentration and separation of the metal must be carried out before determination in environmental samples, particularly aqueous solutions. This step is necessary because of inadequate analytical sensitivity and matrix interferences, and it involves such procedures as ion exchange and solvent extraction. These procedures are invariably selective for only certain chemical species. Therefore, the total metal is not determined. Often the separation procedure is preceded by an oxidation step to destroy oxidizable metal species and permits the metal in these species to be included in the analytical result.

The general principle behind most analytical procedures for metals in environmental samples is, therefore, to determine the total metal regardless of its chemical form. The problems encountered in intercalibration studies of the determination of trace elements in natural waters may be partly related to the failure of some techniques to achieve this goal. The success of flameless atomic absorption for direct determination of some metals in natural water samples [50, 51] has helped to minimize such problems in recent years.

In the study of organic compounds in natural systems, the limited value of data concerning the concentration of total carbon was recognized many years ago. Therefore, analytical techniques were sought which could determine specific organic molecules. Direct techniques, except bioassay, cannot be used for analysis of individual compounds, and almost all environmental organic analyses involve complex separation procedures to isolate individual compounds for detection and quantitation. The separation procedures are usually highly selective for a particular group of organic compounds and, therefore, normally exclude metal-organic compounds from the fianl determination step. The final determination is usually carried out by some combination of a chromatographic final separation and detection with a nonspecific detector. Gas and liquid column chromatography are the most extensively used of all final separation techniques, although thin layer chromatography (TLC), electrophoresis, field desorption MS and other techniques are used in certain specific analyses. The detection that follows the final separation is usually based upon some general property of the organic molecule itself (e. g., colorimetric reactions, ultraviolet (UV) absorption, combustion energy or ionization, thermal conductivity and molecular mass) and therefore, is not specific to one type of organic molecule. The specificity of the analysis for the type of organic molecule that is being determined is normally introduced in the prior separation procedures.

A number of detection systems that are selective for one type of functional group are widely used, for example, electron-capture (EC) detectors selective for halogen containing compounds, colorimetric reactions such as that of ninhydrin with amino nitrogen groupd, thermionic detectors selective for phosphorus-containing compounds, and mass spectrometers used in the mass fragmentography mode to be selective for compounds containing a fragmenting functional group of known mass. This last system, with a mass spectrometer acting as the detector, is perhaps the most versatile and powerful analytical system currently available to environmental chemists. However, its limitations include very high cost and the difficulty of interfacing mass spectrometers with separation systems other than gas chromatographs.

The enormous success of gas chromatography/mass spectrometry in isolating, identifying and determining specific organic compounds in environmental samples provided the background necessary for the genesis of the first of a new hierarchy of interfaced analytical systems designed for the analysis of individual metal-containing organic and inorganic species. This was the combination of GC with a atomic absorption spectrophotometer as the element specific detector. The first such instruments were developed for analysis of alkyl mercury compounds [52, 53]. Elemental and alkylated mercury compounds were separated in a gas chromatograph. The effluent compounds were reduced to elemental mercury by combusting in a flame or heating in a tube furnace, and the elemental mercury was passed through an absorption cell in the atomizer compartment of the atomic absorption spectrophotometer. Before these applications, spectral detection for gas chromatography had been limited almost entirely to the flame photometric detector [54, 55]. The flame photometric detector is not ideally suited to measure atomic emission because of the wide wavelength band pass of the monochromator used, and the difficulty in compensating for flame background and temperature variations caused by organic and other inorganic species in the column effluent. It has, therefore, been used primarily as a selective detector for phosphorus and sulfur by monitoring broad-band molecular emission. Juvet and co-workers [54, 55] did demonstrate the potential utility of the flame photometric detector for element-specific atomic emission, but little use of their techniques has subsequently been made.

The use of flameless atomic absorption analysis for detection of mercury compounds separated by a gas chromatograph was important because it represented the first use of a truly element-specific detection system for chromatography, with sufficient sensitivity to be used for environmental sample analyses, and with a remarkable degree of freedom from interferences.

Although the GC atomic absorption instrumentation described by Gonzalez and Ross [52] and Longbottom [53] is ideal for mercury compounds, it cannot be used for compounds of other elements. Mercury is the only metal which forms an unreactive monatonic gas with significant vapor pressures at low temperatures. Atoms of other metals formed by thermal or combustive decomposition of their compounds cannot be passed through a low-temperature transfer line and cell for atomic absorption. Segar and Gonzalez [56] described two GC atomic absorption spectrophotometer combinations which overcame this limitation by decomposing the metal compounds to atoms in the atomic absorption spectrophotometer atomizer itself. The simplest system involved the passage of the chromatograph effluent gases through a heated transfer line into a compressed air stream, at the point of its introduction to the nebulizer chamber of a standard flame atomic absorption spectrophotometer (Figure 4). This system, although simple, does not provide very high sensitivity for metal analysis, and a second system was developed [56, 57] in which the gas chromatograph effluent was passed directly into the center of the heated graphite tube of a flameless atomic absorption atomizer, which was maintained at a temperature sufficient to decompose the metal-organic compounds (Figure 5). With this technique,

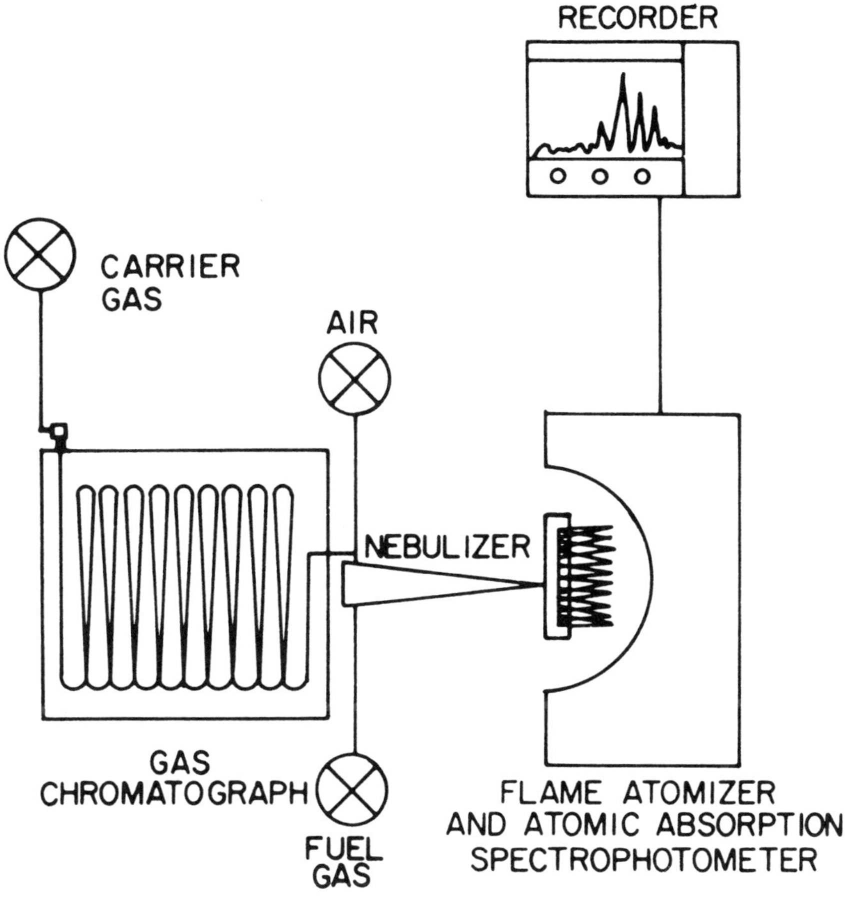


**Figure 4.** Schematic of flame atomic absorption gas-liquid chromatograph.

dilution of the column effluent with air is avoided, and the analytical sensitivity is considerably enhanced. A typical set of chromatograms obtained with this first crudely constructed instrument determining individual lead alkyls in 2-microliter injections of gasoline, with no instrumental scale expansion on the atomic absorption spectrometer readout is shown in Figure 6. Several modifications of this technique have been developed which show promise for use in speciation analyses. A simple, heated quartz tube [58-62] and a T tube furnace [62], in which decomposition of the metal-organic compounds takes place in a heated carbon bed over which the effluent from the gas chromatograph passes before entering the absorption arm

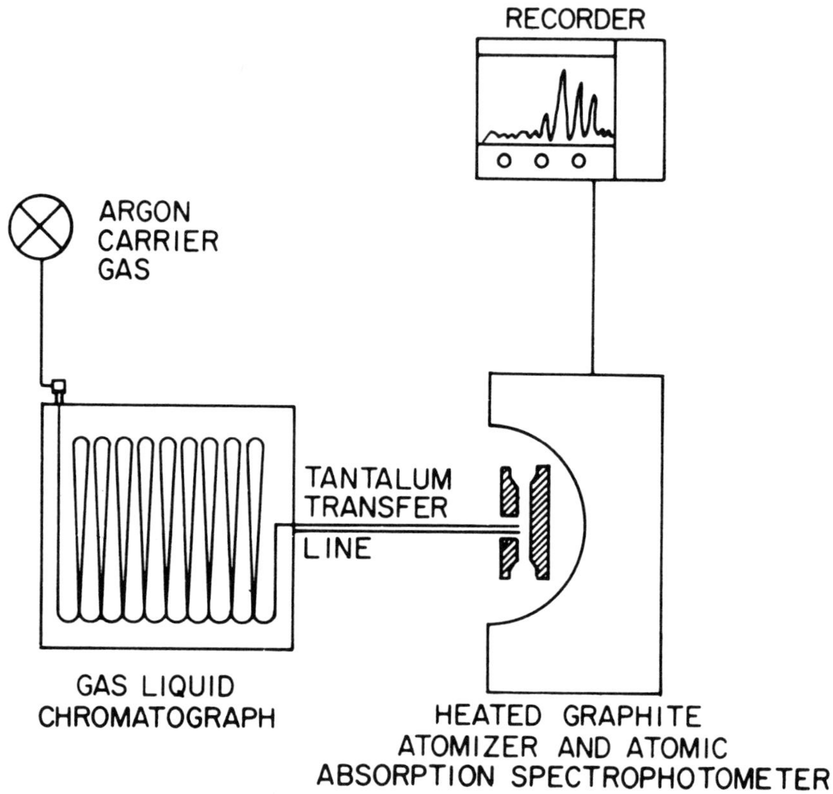


**Figure 5.** Schematic of nonflame atomic absorption gas-liquid chromatograph.

of the tube, have both been used in place of the heated graphite atomizer. In addition, the use of a direct current argon plasma emission spectrometer as a detector has also been investigated [64].

The sensitivity of the GC flameless atomic absorption spectrophotometric technique can be considerably improved by collecting individual chromatographic peaks as they exit the chromatographic column and by atomizing each peak instantaneously in the flameless atomizer. In this mode of operation, the absolute analytical sensitivity is essentially the same as that which can be obtained by the normal mode of individual injections into the flameless atomizer. However, the collection of the metal-organic compounds as they are eluted in separate peaks from the chromatographic column is difficult. At least two methods have been investigated: the use of cold traps by a valve-switching arrangement, the compounds being evaporated by rapid heat-

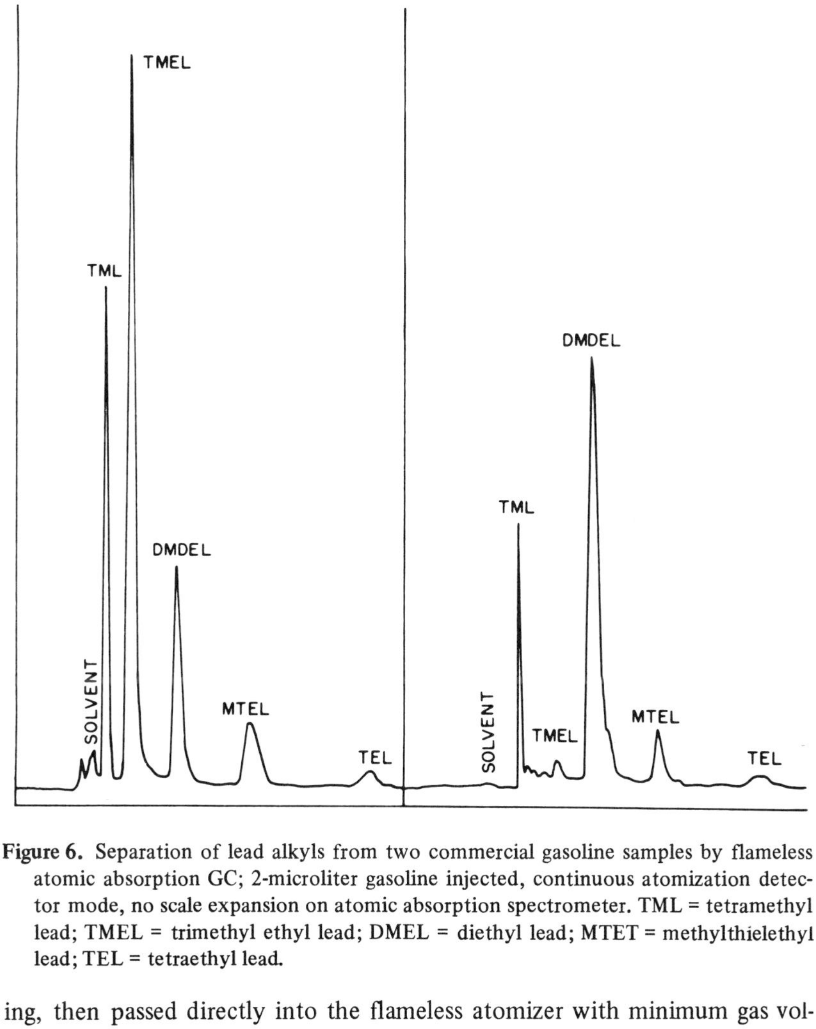


**Figure 6.** Separation of lead alkyls from two commercial gasoline samples by flameless atomic absorption GC; 2-microliter gasoline injected, continuous atomization detector mode, no scale expansion on atomic absorption spectrometer. TML = tetramethyl lead; TMEL = trimethyl ethyl lead; DMEL = diethyl lead; MTET = methylthielethyl lead; TEL = tetraethyl lead.

ing, then passed directly into the flameless atomizer with minimum gas volume. This arrangement is complex and offers only small sensitivity advantages over the continuous mode of detector operation. Alternatively, the flameless atomizer can be temperature programmed so that, during th passage of a chromatographic effluent peak through the atomizer, the temperature is sufficient to decompose the metal-organic compound but not sufficient to volatilize or atomize the metal. The metal, therefore, accumulates on the walls of the atomizer and may be atomized instantaneously by increasing the atomizer temperature for a few seconds immediately after the collection of each chromatographic effluent peak. Many difficulties are inherent in the use of this technique, including memory effects, and it can be used only for those metal-organic compounds which are decomposed at low temperatures relative to the temperature required to volatilize the metal.

Since the introduction of atomic absorption detectors for GC in 1972, the method has been adopted for routine analysis of many organometallics in environmental samples. Alkylated mercury compounds have been routinely determined in fish tissues and other samples [52]. The microbial transformations of mercury in estaurine sediments have also been studied [65]. Interest has also been revived in the use of the microwave emission detector for analysis of mercury and alkyl arsenic acids [66-68] and of metal β-diketone chelates [69, 70] after gas chromatographic separation. The gas chromatograph-microwave emission combination has also been used to determine the total concentrations of selenium, arsenic and antimony in environmental samples after preparation of volatile metal derivatives from metals in the sample [71, 72]. Lead alkyls in gasoline samples have been routinely determined by flame [73] and flameless [57, 63] atomic absorption gas chromatography. Lead and selenium alkyls have been determined in air, water, sediment and fish tissues, and the vapor phase above sediments and cultures, by flameless atomic absorption GC with a simplified heated quartz tube atomizer [74-76]. Volatile mercury and cadmium species in algal cultures have also been determined by flameless atomic absorption GC [77]. Selenium compounds have been determined in plant transpiration gases [61], organoarsenicals in water and air samples [78-80], and tin and organotin compounds in waters, sediments and algae [81].

The combination of gas chromatographic separation with atomic spectral detection is now a well-established analytical technique that enables environmental analysts to investigate, for the first time, many volatile metal species. However, much still remains to be done to optimize the instrumentation and to develop applications, and the degree of progress in these areas since the authors made this statement previously [82] is disappointing.

Very few metal-organic species in the environment are sufficiently volatile that they can be separated by GC. Atomic absorption spectrophotometry, however, can readily be used as a detection technique for liquid chromatography. For flame atomic absorption emission or fluoresence detection, the effluent of the chromatographic column can simply be passed directly into the nebulizer inlet of the flame or plasma atomizer [61, 83-94]. The combination of flame detectors and liquid chromatography suffers from two major drawbacks: the sensitivity is poor, and the flame uses large quantities of sample destructively, prohibiting collection of column effluent fractions for further characterization. Both of these drawbacks may be reduced by interfacing the liquid chromatograph with a flameless atomic absorption spectrophotometer. The flameless atomic absorption high-pressure liquid chromatograph was first described by Segar and Gonzalez [56]. The configuration of the instrumentation is shown schematically in Figure 7. The column effluent is passed through an injection valve, which injects between 5 and 50 microliters of the effluent into a heated graphite furnace atomizer through a tantalum capillary. The tantalum capillary is left permanently in place in the inject port of the atomizer. A sequencer controls the operations of the high-pressure liquid chromatograph atomic absorption spectrophotometer, injection valve and a multiport sampling valve (Figure 7). The multiport sampling valve permits automated injection of standard and blank solutions to calibrate the atomic absorption spectrophotometer at intervals. Two electrically operated on-off valves are provided, before and after the chromatographic column (Figure 7). These valves may be closed during the analysis cycle of the flameless atomic absorption spectrophotometer and reopened to permit only sufficient volume to pass the column for the subsequent injection. In this discontinous mode, almost all of the column effluent is used for injection into the atomic absorption detector, and very high sensitivity and high resolution may be achieved with small samples and small chromatographic columns; analysis time, however, is long. In an alternative mode, the two on-off valves may be left permanently open, and the bulk of the column effluent which passes directly through the injection valve may be collected in a fraction collector. The atomic absorption spectrophotometer analysis sequence time may be set at any value above the minimum required for drying, ashing, atomizing and cool-down cycles of the heated graphite atomizer (usually 30–180 sec depending on the matrix, element determined and sample injection volume). The atomic absorption detector in the continuous flow mode still provides high sensitivity, and the major portion of any metal-containing fraction eluted from the column may be collected for further characterization. However, resolution and precision of peak characterization are poor. Vickrey et al. [95] have recently described a mode of operation that eliminates the problem of long analysis time in the pulsed mode and low resolution in the continuous mode. In this new mode, when the retention times of metal-containing compounds on the chromatographic column are known, the column effluent with each metal-containing fraction is stored temporarily in a capillary loop of suitable length. Each fraction is then analyzed by the atomic spectroscopy detector, as in the high-resolution discontinuous mode, while the remainder of the chromatographic column effluent, which is void of metal fractions, is not analyzed at all by the atomic spectroscopy detector. So long as mixing of the sample along the length of the storage capillary is small, the loss of resolution through using this storage mode is minimal. The applications of this instrumentation to the analysis of metal-organic species in environmental samples promise to be extensive.

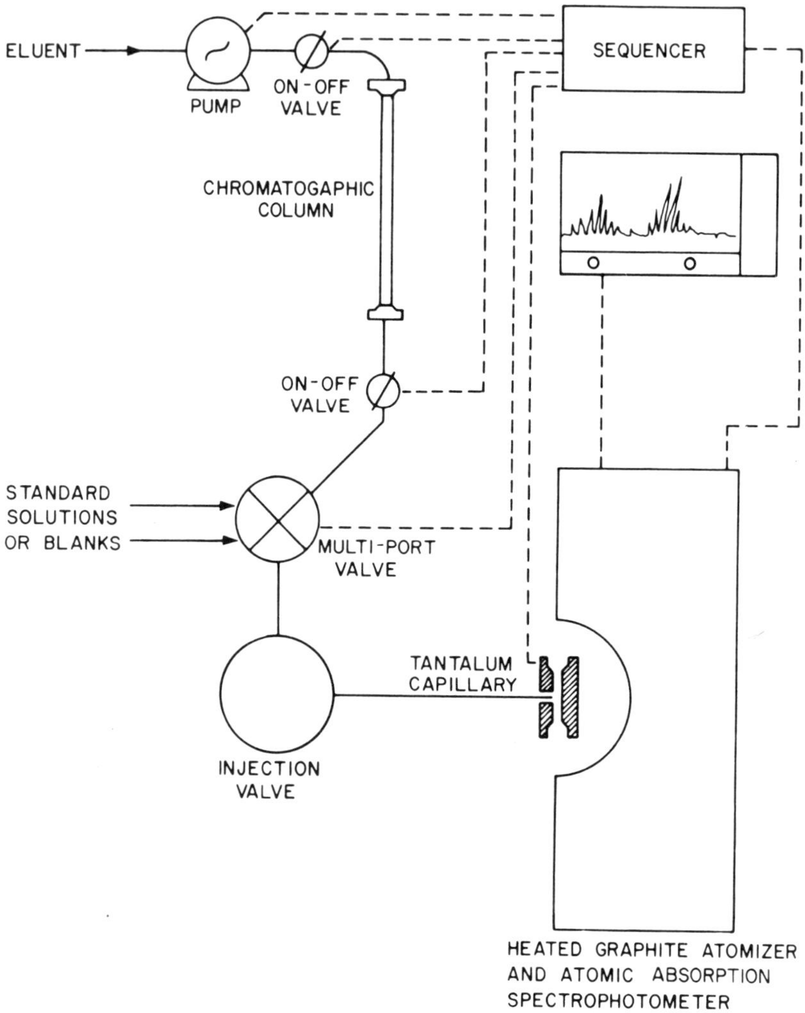


**Figure 7.** Schematic of nonflame atomic absorption high-pressure liquid chromatograph.

Despite the early promise of liquid chromatography-atomic spectroscopy combinations, particularly high-sensitivity flameless atomic spectroscopy, very few applications to environmental samples have yet been reported. The speciation of inorganic arsenicals in aqueous media has been studied [80]. Copper compounds in sea water [96], clinical samples [61] and zinc aryls and alkyls in lubricating oils [61] have also been investigated [59, 61, 77]. Nevertheless, the development of the instrumentation is proceeding in several areas [61, 77, 93-99], and the number of applications should grow rapidly during the next few years.

## SUMMARY

Considerations of the future needs for scientific information in support of safe environmental laws and regulations that are also cost-effective dictate that a better understanding is necessary of the nature, distribution, transformation and effects of the specific compounds and physicochemical forms of trace metals in the environment. The need for such understanding as it relates to synthetic organic compounds in the environment is less critical.

Traditionally, understanding of metal speciation in the environment has been limited by the lack of adequate techniques for the analytical determination of metal species, especially metal-organics. A new family of techniques is emerging, involving various forms of chromatography (e. g., ion exchange, adsorption, gel exclusion and gas-liquid) for the separation of the different species of a metal in an environmental sample and various modes of element-specific atomic spectroscopy (e. g., flame and flameless atomic adsorption, and plasma emission) for the determination of metals in the separated fractions.

The combination of chromatographic separation and atomic spectral analysis is simple and relatively inexpensive. Only minor modifications of equipment already used in most environmental analytical laboratories are required or, alternatively, very simple equipment may be constructed specifically for this purpose. The flameless atomic absorption gas, and high-pressure liquid chromatography, and the modifications of them that are appearing are likely to constitute the major analytical tools with which the environmental analyst meets the challenge of investigating the nature of metal-organic species in the environment, and subsequently determing them in routine manner.

A number of routine applications of chromatography/atomic spectroscopy to metal species determination in environmental samples have already been developed, and have, in some instances, dramatically improved our understanding of the fate and effects of contaminant trace metals in the environment. Nevertheless, the present intensity of research in the area of metal speciation is considerably less than is justified from consideration of the present and/or future needs of environmental regulators and managers. Metal species identification in the environment is indeed one of the keys to rational regulation.

## REFERENCES

1. Steeman N. E., and S. Wium-Anderson. "Copper Ions as Poison in Sea and in Fresh Water," *Mar. Biol.* 6:93-97 (1970).
2. Lewis, A. G., P. Whitfield and A. Ramnarine. "The Reduction of Copper Toxicity in a Marine Copepod by Sediment Extract," *Limnol. Oceanog.* 18(2):324-325 (1973).
3. Morris, O. P., and G. Russell. "Effect of Chelation on Toxicity of Copper," *Mar. Poll. Bull.* 4(10):159-160 (1973).
4. Anderson, D. M., and F. M. M. Morel. "Copper Sensitivity of *Gonyaulax tamerensis,*" *Limnol. Oceanog.* 23(2):283-294 (1978).
5. Sundra, W. G., D. W. Engel and R. M. Thuotte. "Effect of Chemical Speciation on Toxicity of Cadmium to Grass Shrimp, *Palaemonetes Pugio:* Importance of Free Cadmium Ion," *Environ. Sci. Technol.* 12(4):409-413 (1978).
6. Huber, F., V. Schmidt and H. Kirchmann. "Aqueous Chemistry of Organolead and Organothallium Compounds in the Presence of Microorganisms," in *Organometals and Organometalloids,* F. E. Brinckman and J. M. Bellama, Eds., Symp. Series 82, (Washington, DC American Chemical Society, 1978), pp. 65-81.
7. Wood, J. M. "Biological Cycles for Toxic Elements in the Environment." *Science* 183:1049-1058 (1974).
8. Sillen, L. G. "The Physical Chemistry of Seawater," in *Oceanography,* M. Sears, Ed. (Washington DC: American Association for the Advancement of Science, 1961). pp. 549-581.
9. Zirino, A., and S. Yamamoto. "pH Dependent Model for the Chemical Speciation of Copper, Zinc, Cadmium, and Lead in Seawater," *Limnol. Oceanog.* 17(5):661-671 (1972).
10. Baric, A., and M. Branica. "Polarography of Seawater. I. Ionic State of Cadmium and Zinc in Seawater," *J. Polarog. Sci.* 13:4-8 (1967).
11. Zirino, A., and M. L. Healy. "Inorganic Zinc Complexes in Seawater," *Limnol. Oceanog.* 15(6):956-958 (1970).
12. Zirino, A., and M. L. Healy. "pH-Controlled Differential Voltammetry of Certain Trace Transition Elements in Natural Waters," *Environ. Sci. Technol.* 6(3):243-249 (1972).
13. Sugai, S. F., and M. L. Healy. "Voltammetric Studies of the Organic Association of Copper and Lead in Two Canadian Inlets," *Mar. Chem.* 6(4):291-308 (1978).
14. Harris, J., M. Tsutsui and B. L. Van Duuren. "Pi Complexes in Biological Systems," *Science* 158:1701-1708 (1967).
15. Neuberg, C., A. Grauer, M. Kriedl and H. Lowry. "The Role of the Carbamate Reaction in the Calcium and Phosphorus Cycles in Nature," *Arch. Biochem. Biophys.* 70:70-85 (1957).
16. Irukayama, K., T. Kondo, F. Kai and M. Fujiki. "Studies on the Origin of the Causative Agent of Minimata Disease I. Organic Mercury Compounds in Fish and Shellfish from Minmata Bay," *Kumamoto Med. J.* 14:157-169 (1961).
17. Brinckman, F. E., and W. P. Iverson. "Chemical and Bacterial Cycling of Heavy Metals in the Estaurine System," in *Marine Chemistry in the*

*Coastal Environment,* T. M. Church, Ed. (Washington, DC American Chemical Society, Symp. Series 18), pp. 319-322.
18. Saxena, J., and P. H. Howard. "Environmental Transformation of Alkylated and Inorganic Forms of Certain Metals," *Adv. Appl. Microbiol.* 21:185-226 (1977).
19. Koshy, E., M. V. M. Desai and A. K. Ganguly. "Studies on Organo-Metallic Interactions in the Marine Environment, Part 1. Interaction of Some Metallic Ions with Dissolved Organic Substances in Seawater," *Curr. Sci.* 38:555-558 (1969).
20. Koshy, E., M. V. M. Desai and A. K. Ganguly. "Studies on Organo-Metallic Interactions in the Marine Environment, Part 2. Interaction of Metallic Ions with Humic Acid from a Marine Sediment," *Curr. Sci.* 38:582-586 (1969).
21. Park, K., and D. W. Hood "Effect of Organic Material on the Solubility of Calcium Carbonate in Seawater," in *Preprints of the International Oceanographic Congress, New York,* M. Sears, Ed. (Washington, DC American Association for the Advancement of Science, 1959), p. 873-875.
22. Desai, M. V. M., E. Mathew and A. K. Ganguly. "Differential Interaction of Marine Humic and Fulvic Acids with Alkaline Earth and Rare Earth Elements," *Curr. Sci.* 39:429-433 (1970).
23. Shapiro, J. "Effect of Yellow Organic Acids on Iron and Other Metals in Water," *J. Am. Water Works Assoc.* 58:1062-1082 (1964).
24. Duursma, E. K., and W. Sevenhuysen. "Note of Chelation and Solubility of Certain Metals in Seawater at Different pH Values," *Neth. J. Sea Res.* 3(1):95-106 (1966).
25. Pillai, T. N. V., M. V. M. Desai, E. Mathew, S. Ganapathy and A. K. Ganguly. "Organic Materials in the Marine Environment and Associated Metallic Elements," *Curr. Sci.* 40:75-81 (1971).
26. Davis, J. A., and J. O. Leckie. "Effect of Adsorbed Complexing Ligands on Trace Metal Uptake by Hydrous Oxides," *Environ. Sci. Technol.* 12(12):1309-1315 (1978).
27. U.S. Public Health Service. "Interaction of Heavy Metals and Biological Sewage Treatment Processes," Robert A. Taft Sanitary Engineering Center, Publication No. 999-WP-22 (1956).
28. Bender, M. E., W. R. Matson and R. A. Jordan. "On the Significance of Metal Complexing Agents in Secondary Sewage Effluents," *Environ. Sci. Technol.* 4(6):520-521 (1970).
29. Wong, P. T. S., Y. K. Chau, P. L. Luxon and B. Silverberg, "Methylation of Lead and Selenium in the Environment," paper presented at the International Conference on Heavy Metals in the Environment, Toronto, Ontario, Canada, October 27-31, 1975.
30. Lovelock, J. E., R. J. Maggs and R. A. Rasmussen. "Atmospheric Dimethyl Sulphide and the Natural Sulphide Cycle," *Nature* 273:452-453 (1972).
31. Huey, C. W., F. E. Brinckman, W. P. Iverson and S. O. Grim. "Bacterial Volatilization of Cadmium," paper presented at the International Conference on Heavy Metals in the Environment, Toronto, Ontario, Canada, October 27-31, 1975.

32. Duce, R. A., J. G. Quinn, C. E. Olney, S. R. Piotrowicz, B. J. Ray and T. L. Wade. "Enrichment of Heavy Metals and Organic Compounds in the Surface Microlayer of Narragansett Bay, Rhode Island," *Science* 176:161-163 (1972).
33. Piro, A., M. Bernhard, M. Branica and M. Verzi. "Incomplete Exchange Reaction Between Radioactive Ionic Zinc and Stable Natural Zinc in Seawater," Radioactive Contam. Mar. Environ., Proc. Symp., Vienna, Austria, 1973, pp. 29-45.
34. Theis, T. L., and P. C. Singer. "Complexation of Iron (II) by Organic Matter and its Effect on Iron (II) Oxygenation," *Environ. Sci. Technol.* 8(6):569-573 (1974).
35. Johnson, R. "Seawater, the Natural Medium of Phytoplankton. II. Trace Metals and Chelation, and General Discussion," *J. Mar. Biol. Assoc. U.K.,* 44:87-109 (1964).
36. Barber, R. T. "Organic Ligands and Phytoplankton Growth in Nutrient Rich Seawater," in *Trace Metals and Metal-Organics Interaction in Natural Waters,* P. C. Singer, Ed. (Ann Arbor, MI: Ann Arbor Science Publishers, Inc., 1974).
37. Barber, R. T., and J. H. Ryther. "Organic Chelators: Factors Affecting Primary Production in the Cromwell Current Upwelling," *J. Exp. Mar. Biol.* 3:191-199 (1969).
38. Williams, P. M. "The Association of Copper with Dissolved Organic Matter in Seawater," *Limnol. Oceanog.,* 14(1):156-158 (1969).
39. Hood, D. W. "Chemistry of the Oceans: Some Trace Metal-Organic Associations and Chemical Parameter Differences in the Top One Meter of Surface," *Environ. Sci. Technol.* 1(4):303-305 (1967).
40. Slowey, J. F., L. M. Jeffrey and D. W. Hood. "Envidence for Organic Complexed Copper in Seawater," *Nature* 214:377-378 (1967).
41. Stiff, M. J. "The Chemical States of Copper in Polluted Fresh Water and a Scheme of Analysis to Differentiate Them," *Water Res.* 5:585-599 (1971).
42. Alexander, J. E., and E. F. Corcoran. "The Distribution of Copper in Tropical Seawater," *Limnol. Oceanog.* 12(2):236-242 (1967).
43. Foster, P., and A. W. Morris. "The Seasonal Variation of Dissolved Ionic and Organically Associated Copper in the Menai Straits," *Deep Sea Res.* 18(2):231-236 (1971).
44. Pagenkopf, F. K. "Metal-Ion Transport Mediated by Humic and Fulvic Acids," in *Organometals and Organometalloids,* F. B. Brinckman and J. M. Bellama, Eds. (Washington, DC American Chemical Society, Symp. Series 82, 1978), pp. 372-387.
45. Riley, J. P. "Analytical Chemistry of Seawater," in *Chemical Oceanography, Vol. 2,* J. P. Riley and G. Skirrow, Eds. (London: Academic Press, Ltd., 1965), pp. 295-424.
46. Chau, Y. K., and K. Lum-Shue-Chan. "Determination of Labile and Strongly Bound Metals in Lake Water," *Water Res.* 8:383-388 (1974).
47. Guy, R. D., and C. L. Chakrabarti. "Analytical Techniques for Speciation of Trace Metals," in Symp. Proc., International Conference on Heavy Metals in the Environment, Toronto, Ontario, Canada, October 27-31, 1975, Vol. 1. T. C. Hutchinson, Ed., p. 275-294.

48. Guy, R. D., and C. L. Chakrabarti, "Analytical Techniques for Speciation of Heavy Metal Ions in the Aquatic Environment," *Chem., Can.* 28(10): 26-29 (1976).
49. Batley, G. E., and T. M. Florence. "Determination of the Chemical Forms of Dissolved Cadmium, Lead and Copper in Seawater," *Mar. Chem.* 4:347-363 (1976).
50. Ediger, R. D. "A Review of Water Analysis by Atomic Absorption," *Atom. Abs. Newsl.* 12:151-157 (1973).
51. Segar, D. A., and A. Y. Cantillo. "The Direct Determination of Trace Metals in Seawater by Flameless Atomic Absorption," in *Analytical Chemistry in Oceanography,* T. R. P. Gibb, Ed. (Washington, DC: American Chemical Society, Advances in Chemistry Series 147, 1975), pp. 56-81.
52. Gonzalez, J. G., and R. T. Ross. "Interfacing of an Atomic Absorption Spectrophotometer with a Gas-Liquid Chromatograph for the Determination of Trace Quantities of Alkyl Mercury Compounds in Fish Tissue," *Anal. Lett.* 5(10):683-694 (1972).
53. Longbottom, J. E. "Inexpensive Mercury-Specific Gas Chromatographic Detector," *Anal. Chem.* 44(6):1111-1112 (1972).
54. Juvet, R. S., and R. P. Durbin. "Characterization of Flame Photometric Detector for Gas Chromatography," *Anal. Chem.* 38(4):565-569 (1966).
55. Zado, F. M., and R. S. Juvet. "A New Selective-Nonselective Flame Photometric Detector for Gas Chromatography," *Anal. Chem.* 38(4): 569-573 (1966).
56. Segar, D. A., and J. G. Gonzalez. "Vapour Phase Sample Injection for Flame and Flameless Reservoir Atomic Absorption," paper presented at the Fourth International Conference on Atomic Spectroscopy, October 29-November 2, Toronto, Ontario, Canada (1973).
57. Segar, D. A. "Flameless Atomic Absorption Gas Chromatography," *Anal. Lett.* 7(1):89-95 (1974).
58. Chau, Y. K., and P. T. S. Wong. "An Element- and Speciation-Specific Technique for the Determination of Organometallic Compounds," in *Environmental Analysis,* G. W. Ewing, Ed. (New York: Academic Press, Inc., 1977), pp. 215-225.
59. Chau, Y. K', and P. T. S. Wong. "An Element-Specific Technique for the Analysis or Organometallic Compounds," in Proc. of the 8th IMR Symp., Gaithersburg, Maryland, September 20-24, 1976, N.B.S. Spec, Pub. 464, p. 485-490.
60. Van Loon, J. C., and B. Radziuk. "A Quartz "T" Tube Furnace-Atomic Absorption Spectroscopy System for Metal Speciation Studies," *Can J. Spectros.* 21(2):46-50 (1976).
61. Van Loon, J. C., B. Radziuk, N. Kahn, J. Lichwa, F. J. Fernandez and J. D. Kerber. "Metal Speciation Using Atomic Absorption Spectroscopy," *Atom. Abs. Newsl.* 16:79-83 (1977).
62. Chau, Y. K., P. T. S. Wong and P. D. Goulden. "Gas-Chromatography - Atomic-Absorption Spectrometry for Determination of Tetraalkyllead Compounds," *Anal. Chim. Acta.* 85(2):421-424 (1976).
63. Robinson, J. W., E. L. Kiesel, J. P. Goodbread, R. Bliss and R. Marshall. "Development of Gas Chromatography-Furnace Atomic Absorption

Combination for Determination of Organic Lead Compounds–Atomization Processes in Furnace Atomizers," *Anal. Chim. Acta.* 92(2):321-328 (1977).

64. Lloyd, R. J., R. M. Barnes, P. C. Uden and W. G. Elliott. "Direct Current Atmospheric Pressure Argon Plasma Emission Echelle Spectrometer as a Specific Metal Gas Chromatographic Detector," *Anal. Chem.* 50(14): 2025-2029 (1978).
65. Blair, W., W. P. Iverson and F. E. Brinckman. "Application of a Gas Chromatograph-Atomic Absorption Detection System to a Survey of Mercury Transformations by Chesapeake Bay Microorganisms," *Chemosphere* 3:167-174 (1974).
66. Talmi, Y. "The Rapid Sub-Picogram Determination of Volatile Organo Mercury Compounds by Gas Chromatography; with a Microwave Emission Spectrometric Detector System", *Anal. Chim. Acta.* 74:107-117 (1975).
67. Talmi, Y., and D. T. Bostick. "Determination of Alkylarsenic Acids in Pesticides and Environmental Samples by Gas Chromatography with a Microwave Emission Spectrometric Detection System," *Anal. Chem.* 47(13):2145-2150 (1975).
68. Talmi, Y., and V. E. Norvell. "A Rapid Method for the Determination of Methylmercury Chloride in Water Samples by Gas Chromatography with a Microwave Emission Spectrometric Detector," *Anal. Chim. Acta.* 85: 203-208 (1976).
69. Kawaguchi, K., T. Sakamoto and A. Mizuike. "Emission Spectrometric Detection of Metal Chelates Separated by Gas Chromatography," *Talanta* 20:321-326 (1973).
70. Dagnall, R. M., T. S. West and P. Whitehead. "The Determination of Volatile Metal Chelates by Using a Microwave Excited Emissive Detector," *Analyst* 98:647-654 (1973).
71. Talmi, Y., and V. E. Norvell. "Determination of Arsenic and Antimony in Environmental Samples Using Gas Chromatography with a Microwave Emission Spectrometric System," *Anal. Chem.* 47(9):1510-1515 (1975).
72. Talmi, Y., and A. W. Andren. "Determination of Selenium in Environmental Samples Using Gas Chromatography with a Microwave Emission Spectrometric Detection," *Anal. Chem.* 46(14):2122-2130 (1974).
73. Coker, D. T. "Determination of Individual and Total Lead Alkyls in Gasoline by a Simple Rapid Gas Chromatography/Atomic Absorption Spectrometry Technique," *Anal. Chem.* 47(3):386-389 (1975).
74. Chau, Y. K., P. T. S. Wong and P. D. Goulden. "Gas Chromatography-Atomic Absorption Method for the Determination of Dimethyl Selenide and Dimethyl Diselenide," *Anal. Chem.* 47(13):2279-2281 (1975).
75. Chau, Y. K., P. T. S. Wong and H. Saitoh. "Determination of Tetralkyl Lead Compounds in the Atmosphere," *J. Chromatog. Sci.* 14(3):162-164 (1976).
76. Chau, Y. K., P. T. S. Wong, G. A. Bengert and O. Krammar. "Determination of Tetraalkyllead Compounds in Water, Sediment and Fish Samples," *Anal. Chem.* 51(2):186-188 (1979).
77. Huey, C. W., F. E. Brinckman, W. P. Iverson and S. O. Grim. "Bacterial Volatilization of Cadmium," paper presented at the International Con-

ference on Heavy Metals in the Environment, Toronto, Ontario, Canada, October 27-31, 1975.
78. Andreae, M. O. "Determination of Arsenic Species in Natural Waters," *Anal. Chem.* 49(6):820-821 (1977).
79. Johnson, D. L., and R. S. Braman. "Alkyl- and Inorganic Arsenic in Air Samples," *Chemosphere* 6:333-338 (1975).
80. Brinckman, F. E., G. E. Parris, W. R. Blair, K. L. Jewett, W. P. Iverson and J. M. Bellama. "Questions Concerning Environmental Mobility of Arsenic: Needs for a Chemical Data Base and Means for Speciation of Trace Organoarsenicals," *Environ. Health Persp.* 19:11-24 (1977).
81. Hodge, V. F., S. L. Seidel and E. D. Goldberg. "Determination of Tin (IV) and Organotin Compounds in Natural Waters, Coastal Sediments and Macro Algae by Atomic Absorption," *Anal. Chem.* 51(8):1256-1259 (1979).
82. Segar, D. A., and A. Y. Cantillo. "Metal Species Identification in the Environment. A Major Challenge for the Analyst," in Symp. Proc., International Conference on Heavy Metals in the Environment, Toronto, Ontario, Canada, October 27-31, 1975, Vol. 1, T. C. Hutchinson, Ed., p. 183-204.
83. Manahan, S. E., and D. R. Jones. "Atomic Absorption Detector for Liquid-Liquid Chromatography," *Anal. Lett.* 6(8):745-753 (1973).
84. Umebayashi, M., and K. Kitagishi. "Direct Attachment of Atomic Absorption Spectrometer to a Liquid Chromatograph for the Identification, Estimation, and Continuous Monitoring of Metal Ions and Metal Chelates," paper presented at Fifth International Conference on Atomic Spectroscopy, Monash University, Melbourne, Australia, August 25-29, 1975.
85. Freed, D. J. "Flame Photometric Detector for Liquid Chromatography," *Anal. Chem.* 47(1):186-187 (1974).
86. Yosa, N., and S. Ohashi. "Application of Atomic Absorption Method as a Flow Detector to Gel Chromatography," *Anal. Lett.* 6(7):595-601 (1973).
87. Jones, D. R., and S. E. Manahan. "Atomic Absorption Detector for Chromium Organometallic Compounds Separated by High Speed Liquid Chromatography," *Anal. Lett.* 8(8):569-574 (1975).
88. Jones, D. R., and S. E. Manahan. "Aqueous Phase High-Speed Liquid-Chromatographic Separation and Atomic-Absorption Detection of Amino Carboxylic-Acid-Copper Chelates," *Anal. Chem.* 48(3):502-505 (1976).
89. Cassidy, R. M., M. T. Hurteau, J. P. Mislan and R. W. Ashley. "Preconcentration of Organosilicons on Porous Polymers and Separation by Molecular-Sieve and Reversed-Phase Chromatography With an Atomic Absorption Detection System," *J. Chromatog. Sci.* 14(9):444-447 (1976).
90. Botre, C., F. Cacace and R. Cozzani. "Direct Combination of High-Pressure Liquid-Chromatography and Atomic-Absorption for Analysis of Metallorganic Compounds," *Anal. Lett.* 9(9):825-830 (1976).
91. Van Loon, J. D., J. Lichwa and B. Radziuk. "Non-dispersive Atomic Fluorescence Spectroscopy, a New Detector for Chromatography," *J. Chromatog. Sci.* 136(2):301-305 (1977).

92. Van Loon, J. C., and B. Radzuik. "Evaluation of the Non-dispersive Atomic Fluorescence as Detector for Chromatography," in *Environmental Analysis,* G. W. Ewing, Ed. (New York: Academic Press, Inc., 1977), pp. 117-133.
93. Uden, P. C., and I. E. Bigley. "High-Pressure Liquid Chromatography of Metal Diethyldithiocarbamates with UV and DC Argon-Plasma Emission Spectroscopic Detection," *Anal. Chim. Acta.,* 94:29-34 (1977).
94. Uden, P. C., B. D. Quimby, P. M. Barnes and W. G. Elliott., "Interfaced D.C. Argon-Plasma Emission Spectroscopic Detection for High-Pressure Liquid Chromatography of Metal Compounds," *Anal. Chim. Acta.,* 101(1):99-109 (1978).
95. Vickrey, T. M., H. E. Howell and M. T. Paradies. "Liquid Chromatogram Storage and Analysis by Atomic Absorption Spectrometry," *Anal. Chem.* 51(11):1880-1883 (1979).
96. Segar, D. A., and A. Y. Cantillo. "Chromatography-Atomic Spectroscopy Combinations. Applications to Metal Species Identification and Determination," in proc. of the 8th IMR Symp., Gaithersburg, Maryland, September 20-24, 1976, N.B.S. Spec. Pub. 464, p. 491-493.
97. Vickrey, T. M., and H. E. Howell. "Simple and Inexpensive Interface Between a Liquid Chromatrograph and a Flameless Atomic-Absorption Spectrometer Detector," *Anal. Lett.* 11(12):1075-1095 (1978).
98. Koizumi, H., R. D. McLaughlin and T. Hadeishi. "High Gas Temperature Furnace for Species Determination of Organometallic Compounds with a High-Pressure Liquid Chromatograph and Zeeman Atomic Absorption Spectrometer," *Anal. Chem.* 51(3):387-392 (1979).
99. Brinckman, F. E., W. R. Blair, K. L. Jewett and W. P. Iverson. "Application of a Liquid Chromatograph Coupled with a Flameless Atomic Absorption Detector for Speciation of Trace Organometallic Compounds," *J. Chromatog. Sci.* 15(11):493-503 (1977).

# CHAPTER 8

# VALIDATION OF EXTRACTION AND CLEANUP PROCEDURES FOR ENVIRONMENTAL ANALYSIS

**Phillip W. Albro**

Laboratory of Environmental Chemistry
National Institute of Environmental Health Sciences
Research Triangle Park, North Carolina

## INTRODUCTION

Environmental analysis commonly involves four steps: (1) sample collection and storage; (2) extraction; (3) cleanup; and (4) determination. Validation of the determination step, a traditional function of analytical chemists, is accomplished through experimental approaches and by statistical methods that are widely accepted and to be found in any good textbook of analytical chemistry. Problems associated with sample collection and storage have been addressed recently [1], and the validation of sampling procedures in a statistical sense is also an established procedure whose principles are widely accepted and to be found in textbooks.

The other two aspects of environmental analysis, extraction and cleanup, are less likely than the sampling and determination steps to be validated adequately by accepted principles, simply for lack of widely accepted principles specifically applicable to these operations. The purpose of this chapter is to discuss a collection of recent experiments relating to modeling of extraction and cleanup procedures. The results of these experiments, it is to be hoped, allow something to be said about the design of practical validation studies on extraction and cleanup procedures in general.

Validation of extraction procedures involves the need to take into consideration several complications:

1. The recovery of the compound(s) of interest by a given method often differs depending on the sample matrix (e.g., blood vs serum, plasma vs milk, liver vs heart, or clay soil vs sandy soil, etc.). This has been discussed previously [1].
2. The recovery from a given type of sample matrix often differs for very similar compounds (e.g., polychlorinated biphenyls vs polybrominated biphenyls), which is especially troublesome when one wishes to use an internal standard in the procedure [1].
3. The reproducibility of the recovery during extraction is often observed to be less than that of the determination step when the two are validated separately. Since the reliability of a final analytical result, taken as the mean ± confidence limits of a set of replicates, cannot be greater than the reproducibility of the least reproducible step in the overall analytical procedure, the variances for each step should be, but seldom are, taken into consideration in discussing the significance of analytical results.
4. Because most extraction and cleanup procedures are evaluated through the use of "spiked" (fortified) samples, that is, samples to which "known" amounts of the compound(s) of interest have been added, it is absolutely essential that the spiking procedures themselves be both adequately validated and described in detail. Validation and detailed description of the spiking procedures are probably the most neglected aspects of method evaluation in the literature.

Validation of a cleanup procedure involves determining the recovery, reproducibility and the degree of remaining contamination at each step in the procedure. Because there will be inevitable handling losses at each step, each step must be empirically justified by showing that it reduces the level of interfering contaminants more than it reduces the recovery of the compound(s) of interest. Whether or not a given contaminant does in fact interfere depends on the method to be used in the determination step, thus, some measure of relevant interference is essential. Finally, some attempt must be made to show that a proposed cleanup procedure will not create interfering artifacts (false positives) from other, noninterfering, components potentially present in the sample matrix or extract.

To validate a spiking procedure, one must demonstrate that the spiked compound equilibrates with, or distributes in the sample matrix in the same way as the corresponding endogenous compound. Alternatively, one can provide evidence that the recovery of spiked compound is the same as the recovery of endogenous compound over the full range of concentrations concerned in the analytical study, and for each type of sample matrix to be studied. The technical difficulties involved in either of the two approaches will be apparent, and account for the relative dearth of such studies in the current literature. In what follows, experimental data will be used to illustrate the principles discussed above.

## VALIDATION OF SPIKING PROCEDURES

### Comparison of "Spiked" to "Endogenous" Distribution Patterns

A method has been published for spiking plasma or serum with di-(2-ethylhexyl)phthalate (DEHP) by allowing the biological fluid to extract the DEHP from Celite [2]. The method consisted of pretreating Celite by washing with concentrated HCl, then with distilled, deionized water until the washings were neutral, extracting with acetone and methylene chloride, allowing the Celite to air-dry, and finally drying at 105°C in a convection oven. The clean Celite was slurried with a solution of DEHP in *n*-hexane (200 $\mu$g DEHP/100 mg Celite); the slurry was air-dried in a hood overnight and finally dried in a vacuum desiccator over Carbowax 20M. The amount of DEHP on the Celite was accurately determinable because it contained a tracer concentration of $^{14}$C-labeled DEHP. The thoroughly mixed, coated Celite was shaken at 200 rpm with plasma or serum, at 100 mg Celite/ml, for 30 min at room temperature, then incubated at 4°C overnight. The Celite was centrifuged out at 1700 rpm twice and the uptake of DEHP into the serum or plasma was measured by radioassay of the $^{14}$C.

"Endogenous" DEHP in this study was DEHP leached from plastic blood bags during storage of whole blood in a hospital blood bank. Plasma was separated by centrifugation, and the distribution of phthalate among lipoprotein classes, albumin and other carriers determined by standard fractionation procedures and gas chromatography (GC). A comparison of the distributions seen for "spiked" and "endogenous" DEHP is shown in Table I. In contrast to these results, DEHP added to plasma or serum using a small amount of an organic solvent (acetone, methanol or DMSO) was found to be mainly adsorbed to albumin. One would expect extraction procedures to treat Celite-spiked DEHP the same as "endogenous" DEHP, while organic solvent-spiked DEHP might not necessarily correspond to the other preparations in relative recovery.

### Spiking Linearity

Coated Celite can be "diluted" by admixture with uncoated Celite as desired, keeping the ratio of Celite to serum or plasma constant. This procedure was employed with $^{14}$C-labeled dieldrin; *p,p*-DDT; 2,3,7,8-tetrachlorodibenzo-*p*-dioxin (TCDD) and a mixture of polychlorinated biphenyls (PCB) similar in composition to Aroclor 1254. The Celite method was suitable for spiking serum, plasma or milk with all of the above except TCDD, which bound to

**Table I. Distribution of DEHP Among Plasma Components[a]**

| Component | Percentage of DEHP | |
|---|---|---|
| | Spiked | Endogenous |
| Nonlipoproteins | 16 | 18 |
| Chylomicrons | 6.4 | 6.8 |
| VLDL | 22 | 28 |
| LDL | 36 | 39 |
| HDL | 19 | 7 |

[a]Total plasma load = 120 μg DEHP/ml.

Celite too tightly for the biological fluids to extract it. Levels of pesticides and other lipophilic compounds from parts-per-billion (ppb) to 200 parts per million (ppm) may be spiked into serum, plasma or milk in this way.

The uptake of $^{14}$C-dieldrin into serum as a function of the amount added is shown in Figure 1. The regression line shows a slope of 1.01 and a correlation coefficient of 0.9978. A similar test with $^{14}$C-DDT gave a slope of 0.97 and correlation coefficient of 0.9976.

## Spiking Reproducibility

Spiking reproducibility may be illustrated from an experiment in which $^{14}$C-PCB in DMSO solution was used. Three rat livers were made into 50% aqueous homogenates using a Teflon®-glass tissue homogenizer. Each homogenate (5 g) was placed in an ultrasonic cleaner bath, and while the samples were sonicated they were "injected" with 20 microliters of DMSO containing 133.7 ng of $^{14}$C-PCB. Each sample was next shaken at 300 rpm on a rotary shaker for 20 min at room temperature. Five 0.2-ml aliquots were removed from each sample, transferred to scintillation vials, digested with 2 ml of NCS tissue solubilizer (Amersham/Searle) each and radioassayed. The results are shown in Table II. Analysis of variance by the ANOVA procedure showed no significant differences between or within samples. The mean "recovery" (uptake) of PCB was 99.6 ± 3.9% of the amount spiked. Thus, at this level, 53.5 ng/g liver, this spiking procedure gave a uniform, known (predictable) level of PCB incorporation suitable for providing a set of blind quality control samples to other laboratories for analysis.

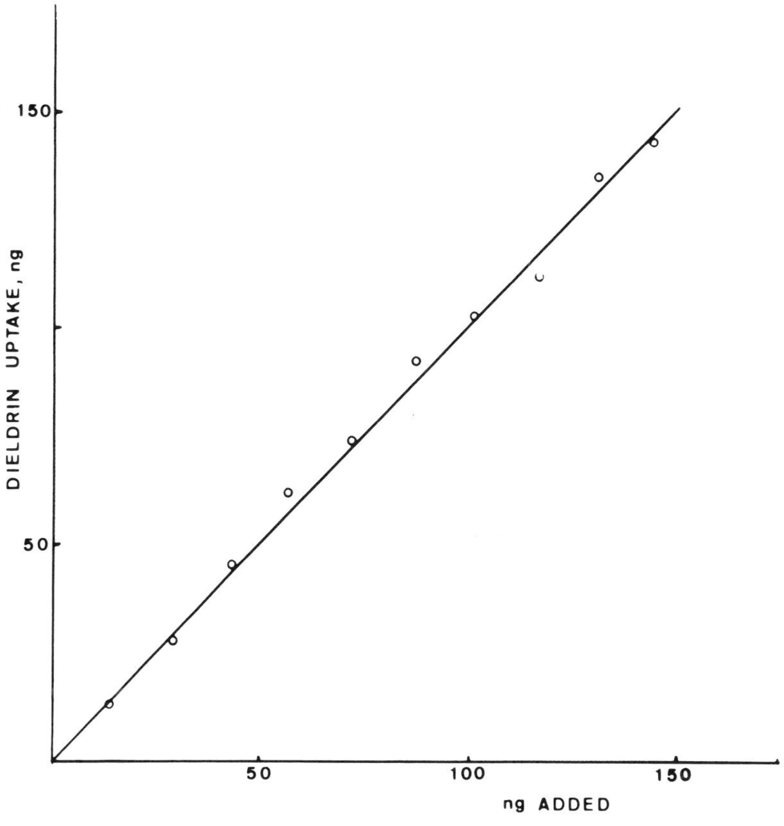


**Figure 1.** Amount of $^{14}$C-dieldrin extracted into fetal calf serum from acid-washed celite, relative to the amount added.

## Positive Interferences

In cases where radiolabeled samples cannot be used or are not available, recovery studies may be confounded by the occurrence of endogenous levels of the compound of interest in the sample matrix used for the preparation of spiked "knowns." Positive interference in the analysis resulting from components other than the actual compound of interest would have an equivalent misleading effect. Such situations can be dealt with by employing the method of constant additions.

Table II. Uniform Spiking of Liver for Quality Assurance Studies

| Sample | ng/g | Sample | ng/g | Sample | ng/g |
|---|---|---|---|---|---|
| A1 | 52.7 | B1 | 50.0 | C1 | 57.4 |
| A2 | 53.3 | B2 | 52.2 | C2 | 56.4 |
| A3 | 53.1 | B3 | 53.5 | C3 | 52.0 |
| A4 | 48.2 | B4 | 52.7 | C4 | 52.8 |
| A5 | 52.3 | B5 | 57.0 | C5 | 55.1 |
| Mean | 51.9 | | 53.1 | | 54.8 |
| SD | 1.9 | | 2.3 | | 2.0 |
| RSD, % | 3.65 | | 4.30 | | 3.75 |
| Grand Mean | 53.3 ± 2.1 | | | | |
| Mean Uptake, % | 99.6 ± 3.9 S.D. | | | | |
| F | 1.8687 | | | | |
| P | 0.1965 | | | | |

Table III. Method of Constant Additions[a]

| Sample | Spike (ng)[b] | Found (ng) |
|---|---|---|
| 1 | 56.87 | 60.6 |
| 2 | 113.7 | 120.4 |
| 3 | 170.6 | 175.6 |
| 4 | 227.5 | 232.2 |
| 5 | 284.4 | 272.1 |

[a] Regression line; found (Y) = A + B x spike (X).
[b] 10-g portions of rat adipose spiked with N x 56.87 ng of *p,p'*-DDT, extracted, cleaned and analyzed by GLC with an electron capture detector.

For illustration, five 1-g samples of rat adipose tissue were separately ground using glass mortars and pestles, with 8 g of anhydrous sodium sulfate and 10 mg of Celite coated with various increments of *p,p*-DDT. The increments were whole multiples of 56.87 ng of DDT. The dry powders were transferred to separatory funnels that had been plugged at the outlets with glass wool. Ethyl acetate (25 ml) was used to rinse each mortar and passed through the adipose-$Na_2SO_4$-Celite. This was followed by 50 ml of methylene chloride. The extracts were concentrated in vacuo, cleaned by partitioning between $H_2SO_4$ and benzene, and analyzed for *p,p*-DDT by gas chromatography using an electron capture detector (EC/GC). The results are shown in Table III. A regression line, Y = a + bX, was calculated where Y = amount of DDT recovered in nanograms per gram adipose, X = amount of DDT spiked. The line Y = 11.78 + 0.940X had a correlation coefficient of 0.9977. The slope indicated a mean recovery of 94.0%, while a/0.94, or 12.53 ng/g, would represent the amount of endogenous DDT that would cause the positive interference seen. If the [amount spiked + 12.53 ng] values for each sample are compared with the corresponding amounts measured, it can be seen that the overall recoveries had a coefficient of variation of ± 4.2%. The apparent recoveries, neglecting to take positive interference into consideration, averaged 102.6 ± 4.3%. Had the endogenous level been just slightly lower, simple and direct calculation of recoveries would have given no hint that positive interference was occurring.

In contrast to these fairly successful experiments, Table IV gives the results of attempts to validly spike rat skin with PCB. Labeled PCB ($^{14}$C) similar to Aroclor 1254 were fed orally in cottonseed oil. The rat was killed 24 hr later and the depilated (shaved) skin was removed. The endogenous level of PCB was determined by digesting eight pieces of skin in NCS tissue solubilizer and assaying the radioactivity. (It was previously shown that PCB metabolites contributed negligible radioactivity to the skin under these conditions.) Skin from control rats was spiked with $^{14}$C-PCB either from hexane or DMSO. Each sample processed was spiked separately; 12 pieces of skin were spiked from hexane (~10 μl/g) and 12 from DMSO. Two extraction procedures that differed as to recovery of endogenous PCB were employed, as shown in the table. In each case, either the mean recovery or the recovery variance for the spiked samples differed significantly from the corresponding value for the "endogenous" samples. However, this discrepancy would not have been realized if nothing but spiked samples had been studied. These results suggest that spiking of solid tissue samples will only be valid when the recovery of endogenous compound is essentially quantitative in the extraction, and perhaps not even then.

**Table IV. Recovery of PCB From Rat Skin**

| Spiking Solvent | Percentage Recovered ± SD | |
|---|---|---|
| | Method A[a] | Method B[b] |
| None[c] | 20.3 ± 5.6 (3) | 95.6 ± 24.6 (7) |
| Hexane | 98.3 ± 2.8 (3) | 81.8 ± 4.2 (3) |
| DMSO | 52.8 ± 6.1 (3) | 92.4 ± 4.0 (3) |

[a]Method A = boiling briefly in benzene. Number of replicates in parentheses.
[b]Method B = Polytron homogenization in benzene:methanol, 3:1 (v/v).
[c]Endogenous PCB.

## VALIDATION OF EXTRACTION PROCEDURES

Because, as has been mentioned above, a given extraction procedure must be validated separately for each type of sample matrix as well as for each compound of interest, few if any extraction procedures may presently be used in analytical studies without some preliminary evaluation. That a method has been extensively validated for PCB in blood does not mean it will have the same characteristics when applied to the extraction of polybrominated biphenyls (PBB) from blood, or of PCB from milk [1]. Thus, no 100% complete set of validation data can be provided at any one time for any "general purpose" extraction procedure.

The extraction procedure for adipose tissue described above (elutriation with ethyl acetate and methylene chloride, spiking with compounds adsorbed to Celite) has the advantage of speed and the use of smaller volumes of solvent than are required by most comparable procedures. Five 1-g samples of rat adipose were extracted by the new procedure, and five others, similarly ground with sodium sulfate, were each extracted overnight in a Soxhlet apparatus with refluxing methylene chloride. Aliquots (1/10) of each extract were dried to constant weight under nitrogen to determine the apparent lipid content of the tissue. The Soxhlet procedure gave 862 ± 3.0 mg/g tissue (RSD = 0.35%), while the simple elutriation procedure gave 879 ± 4.5 ng lipid per gram of tissue (RSD = 0.51%). These means did not differ significantly by a two-tailed t-test. Validation by direct comparison with an established procedure may be necessary, as was done here, when there is no direct means to determine the "right" answer.

Additional 1-g portions of adipose were spiked by including $^{14}$C-TCDD-coated Celite during the grinding with sodium sulfate. The levels of TCDD tested ranged from 2.0 to 50 ng/g adipose. Over this range, the mean recovery of TCDD was 99.0 ± 0.7%, with less than 0.3-1.0% of the spike either lost on the glass surfaces or remaining in the solid residue.

Five portions of adipose were spiked with 200 ppm of $^{14}$C-labeled DEHP (again on Celite, here 20 mg/g adipose) and extracted by elutriation. The extracts were analyzed in triplicate for lipid content and radioactivity. Lipid weights (N = 5) had a coefficient of variation of ± 1.7%; the mean lipid content was 856 mg/g tissue. The recovery of DEHP was 98.6 ± 0.26%, using the equation $SD = \bar{X}_1/\bar{X}_2(V_1{}^2 + V_2{}^2 - 2r_{12}V_1V_2)^{1/2}$ because recovery is a ratio [3].

For this extraction procedure to actually be used in an analytical study of endogenous levels of some environmental agent, it would be necessary to show that recovery of the particular agent from spiked samples correlates with recovery of endogenous material, over the range of concentrations seen applicable to the study. The "validation" data shown above can indicate that the procedure is promising, but additional validation would be needed for any particular application.

### Effect of Pollutant Concentration on Confidence Interval

To illustrate this effect, fifteen 5-g portions of well-mixed and screened clay soil were spiked with $^{14}$C-DDT in acetone. Three soil samples were spiked at each of five levels, ranging from 11 ppb to 1.1 ppm. The acetone was evaporated overnight in a chemical hood, and the samples were extracted by shaking for 1 hr at 200 rpm at room temperature in 25 ml of 1,2-dimethoxyethane. The soil settled out rapidly on stopping the shaker, and aliquots of the supernate were subjected to radioassay by scintillation counting.

The data were checked for homogeneity by Bartlett's procedure, then analyzed by ANOVA. The mean recoveries were not statistically significantly different (grand mean = 81.7 ± 2.9%), so there was no apparent dependence of recovery on concentration. However, the coefficients of variation (relative standard deviations) and 95% confidence limits increased exponentially as the spiking level decreased. The coefficients of variation fit the equation: CV = a-b ($\log_{10}$ DDT concentration), gave a linear correlation coefficient of $r = 0.9329$ and probability that r does not differ significantly from zero of $P < 0.025$.

In this illustration, the number obtained for mean recovery could be used as a correction factor in the analysis of "unknowns," because it did not depend on concentration. However, the confidence limits that would have to be reported were highly sensitive to the level of DDT found, and would have to be calculated for each sample from the exponential equation. Mere knowledge of the determinative analytical precision would be a misleading indicator of the reliability of any value reported.

## VALIDATION OF CLEANUP PROCEDURES

To illustrate some of the principles discussed in the introduction relative to validation of cleanup procedures, homogenates of rat liver were spiked with TCDD at 100 parts per trillion (pg/g) and with Aroclor 1254 as a potential interference at 1 ppm (μg/g). All samples (10 g of liver each) were extracted as described previously [4], and the extracts were cleaned up by one of three different procedures. The product of each cleanup step was assayed for TCDD by EC/GC on an OV-210, and for total residual mass either by weighing on a microbalance or as described by Amenta [5]. The ratio of "non-TCDD" to TCDD on a mass basis was designated "total contamination factor," while the ratio of TCDD apparently present by EC/GC to that actually present by high resolution GC-mass spectrometry [6] was designated "EC/GC contamination factor." The latter would be a relevant factor if EC/GC were to be used in an actual analytical study, while the "total contamination factor," related to the "degree of enrichment" sometimes reported, is of little relevance and only shown for comparative illustration.

The first cleanup procedure is briefly summarized in Table V, and its results in Table VI. This procedure was evaluated before "relevance" was sought, and EC/GC data were not obtained. The procedure was eliminated from further consideration because a point of diminishing returns was reached at Step 5, after which loss of TCDD was not accompanied by additional decrease in contaminants.

**Table V. Effect of Multiple Cleanup Steps, with Repeats**

| | |
|---|---|
| Step 1: | Separation of Extract |
| Step 2: | Partition between $H_2SO_4$ and $CCl_4$ |
| Step 3: | Chromatography on Florisil |
| Step 4: | Chromatography on Basic Alumina |
| Step 5: | Chromatography on Acidic Alumina |
| Step 6: | Repeat Step 5 |
| Step 7: | Repeat Step 4 |

**Table VI. Results of Procedure in Table V**

| | TCDD Lost (%) | | |
|---|---|---|---|
| Step | This Step | Overall | Contamination Factor, Total |
| 1 | 11 | 11 | $8.4 \times 10^6$ |
| 2 | 16 | 25 | $1.0 \times 10^6$ |
| 3 | 5 | 29 | $4.2 \times 10^4$ |
| 4 | 6 | 33 | $8.5 \times 10^2$ |
| 5 | 10 | 40 | $4.5 \times 10^2$ |
| 6 | 20 | 52 | $4.9 \times 10^2$ |
| 7 | 30 | 66 | $5.7 \times 10^2$ |

Table VII outlines a more satisfactory cleanup procedure yielding a product acceptable for analysis by EC/GC (Table VIII). Its two disadvantages were the relatively poor recovery, which limited sensitivity, and the amount of time and effort required per sample.

**Table VII. Effect of Multiple Cleanup Steps, None Repeated**

| Rat Liver, 10 g, with TCDD @ 100 ppt | |
|---|---|
| Step 1: | Saponification of the extract |
| Step 2: | Partitioning, Hexane vs Acetonitrile |
| Step 3: | Partitioning, $H_2HO_4$ vs $CCl_4$ |
| Step 4: | Chromatography on Florisil |
| Step 5: | Chromatography on Basic Alumina |
| Step 6: | Chromatography on Acidic Alumina |
| Step 7: | Reversed-Phase Chromatography |

**Table VIII. Results of Procedure in Table VII**

| | TCDD Recovered (%) | | Contamination | |
|---|---|---|---|---|
| Step | This Step | Overall | Factor, Total | EC/GC |
| 1 | 89 | 88 | $8.5 \times 10^6$ | Inf. |
| 2 | 70 | 62 | $3.2 \times 10^6$ | Inf. |
| 3 | 84 | 52 | $3.6 \times 10^5$ | 970 |
| 4 | 92 | 48 | $3.1 \times 10^4$ | 877 |
| 5 | 94 | 45 | $3.3 \times 10^3$ | 812 |
| 6 | 90 | 40 | $3.7 \times 10^2$ | 88 |
| 7 | 56 | 23 | $3.3 \times 10^2$ | 0 |

Table IX shows a much simpler cleanup procedure yielding a high recovery of TCDD, and a degree of cleanup in three steps (Table X) that required six steps in the previous example. Indeed the three-step method was found adequate for EC/GC determination of TCDD if a capillary column (25 m x 0.25 mm glass, OV-215) was substituted for the packed column used in this experiment (details of the capillary column method will be published later).

**Table IX. Effect of Simple Cleanup, Optimized**

| | |
|---|---|
| Step 1: | Partition, $H_2SO_4$ vs $CCl_4$ |
| Step 2: | Chromatography on Basic Alumina |
| Step 3: | Chromatography on Acidic Alumina |

**Table X. Results of Procedure in Table IX**

| | TCDD Recovered (%) | | Contamination Factor | |
|---|---|---|---|---|
| Step | This Step | Overall | Total | EC/GC |
| 1 | 86 | 85 | $5.3 \times 10^6$ | 2500 |
| 2 | 98 | 83 | $1.2 \times 10^5$ | 629 |
| 3 | 97 | 81 | $6.1 \times 10^3$ | 98[a] |

[a] Zero with capillary column.

No data on reproducibility of the various cleanup steps are given here, because these procedures are not seriously proposed for actual use but were simply examined as illustrations. Considered as illustrations then, one would conclude that some of the reasonable-seeming cleanup steps or step sequences are unjustified, because they cause major losses of the compound of interest without commensurate elimination of interferences. In any serious effort to develop a cleanup procedure for some specific application, the demonstration that spiking was valid, the extraction method was suitable and the preparation of a table such as those (VI, VIII or X) shown here (including reproducibility for each step and extending the study to various concentrations) would constitute one acceptable approach to validation. Doubtless other approaches could be imagined using the same general principles.

## SUMMARY

Validation data for a given extraction/cleanup procedure apply only to the particular compounds and sample matrices studied, and can not be extrapolated to "closely related" compounds or "similar" types of matrices.

The reproducibility of the extraction and cleanup procedure must be taken into consideration along with the reproducibility of the determination step in calculating confidence limits on final analytical results.

When spiked samples are used to determine recoveries, it must be demonstrated that recovery of spiked compound correlates with recovery of the corresponding endogenous compound. This can not be assumed, as it is often found not to be the case.

Validation of a cleanup procedure involves determining the recovery, reproducibility, and level of remaining interferences at each step in the procedure. Any step causing greater loss of the compound of interest than decrease in interference is unjustified and should be omitted.

## REFERENCES

1. Albro, P. W. "Problems in Analytic Methodology: Sample Handling, Extraction, and Cleanup," *Ann. N.Y. Acad. Sci.* 320:19-27 (1979).
2. Albro, P. W., and J. T. Corbett. "Distribution of Di- and Mono-(2-Ethylhexyl) Phthalate in Human Plasma," *Transfusion* 18:750-755 (1978).
3. Pearl, R. *Medical Biometry and Statistics*, 3rd ed. (Philadelphia: W. B. Saunders Co., 1940), p. 370.
4. Albro, P. W., and B. J. Corbett. "Extraction and Clean-up of Animal Tissues for Subsequent Determination of Mixtures of Chlorinated Dibenzo-*p*-Dioxins and Dibenzofurans," *Chemosphere* (7):381-385 (1977).
5. Amenta, J. S. "A Rapid Chemical Method for Quantification of Lipids Separated by Thin-Layer Chromatography," *J. Lipid Res.* 5:270-272 (1964).
6. Hass, J. R., M. D. Friesen, D. J. Harvan and C. E. Parker. "Determination of Polychlorinated Dibenzo-*p*-dioxins in Biological Samples by Negative Chemical Ionization Mass Spectrometry," *Anal. Chem.* 50: 1474-1478 (1978).

# CHAPTER 9

# CONTAMINANT ENRICHMENT MODULES AND APPROACHES TO AUTOMATION OF SAMPLE EXTRACT CLEANUP

**D. L. Stalling, J. D. Petty, L. M. Smith and G. R. Dubay**

Columbia National Fisheries Research Laboratory
U.S. Fish and Wildlife Service
Columbia, Missouri

## INTRODUCTION

Recent advances in electronics have greatly facilitated the interfacing of analytical instrumentation with computers, as, for example, in the gas chromatography/mass spectrometry (GC/MS)/data system. Computerized instrumentation, improved instrument sensitivity and selective residue enrichment combine to make possible more comprehensive contaminant analysis. Current analytical methods research at the Columbia National Fisheries Research Laboratory (CNFRL) stresses development of a comprehensive approach for the analysis of environmentally persistent pollutants [1]. This approach should be well suited to the analysis of pollutants in the three major compartments of the aquatic environment: water, sediment and biota. Analytical methods developed to meet these needs should be structured to take full advantage of the developments taking place in analytical instrumentation.

A comprehensive approach to multiclass residue analysis must include the collection and preparation of samples, enrichment (including fractionation), identification and quantitation of contaminants. The modular approach being developed will significantly reduce the sample manipulations, thereby minimizing losses and reducing man-hours, materials and space requirements.

These modular chromatographic units will provide the enrichment needed before trace level contaminants can be identified and quantified. Factors emphasized in designing chromatography modules are primarily their selectivity for structural features, functional groups and chemical classes, and secondarily their potential for sequential application and mechanization. Contaminant enrichment is the main goal of these modules.

In this chapter contaminant enrichment refers to the process of concentrating environmental contaminants relative to biogenic material or other interfering chemicals. A contaminant enrichment process is defined as a procedural unit designed to provide a general contaminant enrichment capability. Further, a contaminant enrichment module is a process unit that has specifically been designed or adapted for direct coupling to other units to permit continuous, sequential operation.

A means of quantitatively assessing the performance of enrichment modules is defined as the contaminant enrichment factor (CEF):

$$\text{CEF} = \frac{(\text{weight of material to be processed})(\%\ \text{contaminant recovery})}{(\text{weight of residual matrix after processing})(100)}$$

Research at CNFRL has yielded a number of highly efficient and versatile enrichment processes that can be directly coupled in several combinations to provide for continuous processing of a sample [1]. Performance characteristics of the modular enrichment units are summarized in Tables I and II. Contaminant enrichment factors for the modules are presented in Table III.

Normally, the percent recovery of specific contaminants is the feature most frequently stressed in describing a cleanup procedure. Use of both recovery data and CEF will facilitate comparison of procedures for enrichment of complex environmental residues, thus enabling analysts to evaluate more accurately alternative procedures.

Herein is summarized progress toward a programmable contaminant enrichment chromatography system that incorporates the following chromatographic enrichment modules: (1) gel permeation, (2) alkali metal silicate, and (3) dispersed carbon. The utility of integrating enrichment modules was previously

**Table I. Attributes of Contaminant Enrichment Modules**

| |
|---|
| Should sequentially link to at least one other module, i.e., GPC + carbon/foam chromatography |
| Should provide selective contaminant fractionation, i.e., planar vs nonplanar aromatics or GPC molecular weight separations |
| Should provide selective concentration of a chemical class, i.e., acidic compound isolation with cesium-silicate chromatography |
| When combined, modules form the basis for mechanized or automated system |

**Table II. Contaminant Enrichment Modules Investigated at CNFRL**

| Modules | Features |
|---|---|
| GPC | Quantitative recovery of neutral contaminants; 98–99.5% removal of biogenic contaminants; reusable and suitable for automation; stand alone module or cleanup procedure; molecular weight fractionation |
| Cesium Silicate | Isolates acidic contaminants; limited reuse of adsorbent; no retention of neutral or basic contaminants; suitable for automation |
| Carbon/Biobeads | Combines GPC and carbon adsorption selectivity; requires multiple solvent and/or reverse elution; reuseable and suitable for automation; permits isolation of non-*ortho* chlorine substituted PCB; requires further development; suitable for chlorinated dibenzofurans and dibenzo-*p*-dioxins |
| Carbon/Foam | Requires multiple solvent and/or reverse elution; reusable and suitable for automation; permits isolation of non-*ortho* chlorine substituted PCB; suitable for chlorinated dibenzofurans and dibenzo-*p*-dioxins |

**Table III. Contaminant Enrichment Factors**

| Modules | CEF | Contaminant and Sample Matrix |
|---|---|---|
| GPC | 50–100 | For majority of contaminants in fatty tissue |
| Carbon Coated Biobeads | $2.3 \times 10^3$ | For 3,4,3′,4′-TCB and TCDD in fish oil |
| GPC + Carbon Foam | $5\text{–}10 \times 10^3$ | For TCDD in fish oil |

demonstrated by processing an extract of a whole fish sample spiked at 100 $\mu g/g$ with 39 representative environmental contaminants [1]. Special emphasis has also been placed on the application of the dispersed carbon module to the enrichment of planar aromatic contaminants, particularly chlorinated dibenzofurans (CDF) and dibenzo-*p*-dioxins (CDD).

## EXPERIMENTAL

### Chromatography Apparatus

A 2.5-cm i.d. Chromaflex chromatography column (Kontes, Inc., Vineland, NJ), fitted with adjustable plungers, was connected to a polytetrafluoroethylene, six-port, two-position, rotary valve (Rheodyne, Berkley, CA) using four of the six ports in such a manner that the column flow could be reversed by changing the position of the valve.

The column was connected to a thick-walled 300-ml glass reservoir, which served as a reservoir for both the sample and solvent. The glass reservoir was fitted with a 24/40 standard taper joint adapter, which was connected to a low-pressure nitrogen regulator. Nitrogen pressure (0.5–6.0 psi) controlled solvent flow through the column.

### Adsorbent Preparation

#### *Potassium Silicate*

Potassium silicate was used to remove acidic biogenic compounds and contaminants before adsorption of planar contaminants by carbon dispersed on glass fibers. In a 1-liter erlenmeyer flask, 100 g of SiliCar CC-7 silica gel (Mallinckrodt, Inc., St. Louis, MO) was mixed with a solution of 56 g KOH (Fischer Scientific, St. Louis, MO) dissolved in 400 ml of absolute methanol. The flask, after addition of a magnetic stirring bar, was covered with a small beaker and placed in a hood on a magnetic stirring hot plate. The flask was warmed to approximately 60°C and stirred for 1 hr. After the suspension was cooled, it was transferred to a glass chromatography column, which contained a glass wool plug in the bottom. The adsorbent was then washed with 200 ml of anhydrous methanol and 200 ml of methylene chloride. After solvent removal, the adsorbent was dried overnight at 130°C and stored in a screw-capped bottle.

*Carbon on Glass Fiber*

Approximately 600-mg glass fiber filters (Toyo GA200, Nuclepore Corp., Pleasanton, CA) were cut into small pieces and shredded briefly with a Polytron homogenizer (Brinkman Instruments, Westbury, NY). Methylene chloride was used as the suspending solvent. Then, 50 mg AMOCO PX-21 carbon (AMOCO, Inc., Chicago, IL) was added to the stirred suspension of the glass fibers. The carbon and glass fibers were mixed thoroughly, and the adsorbent mixture was packed, in small portions, into a glass chromatography column.

## Column Preparation

Two discs, 2.5 cm in diameter, of Toyo GA 200 glass filter pads, were placed in the bottom of the chromatography column. The carbon glass fiber adsorbent was slurry packed in such a way that the carbon/glass fiber occupied 1.0 cm of the column. After packing the column, two additional pieces of filter pad were placed on the top of the column, and the plunger was fitted to the top of the adsorbent bed. The column was subsequently washed with 200 ml of solvent A (methylene chloride:methanol: benzene 75:20:5 v/v/v), followed by 50 ml of toluene, and finally by 100 ml of solvent A. For use in enrichment of CDD and CDF, a low nitrogen pressure (0.5-6.0 psi) in the solvent reservoir or a solvent pump was required to maintain solvent flow through this carbon/glass fiber adsorbent. Prepassage of lipid extracts (in methylene chloride) through potassium silicate columns was required to remove acidic components that would have been adsorbed on the carbon, thus reducing the solvent flow.

## Contaminant Enrichment

The fish oil sample was initially dissolved in methylene chloride at a lipid concentration of less than 200 mg/ml and was passed through a column containing potassium silicate (6 cm x 1.8 cm i.d.) to remove phenolics, free fatty acids and other acidic biogenic compounds.

The potassium silicate was washed with 50 ml of methylene chloride after passage of the lipid solution through the column. This rinse was combined with the eluate from the potassium silicate adsorbent. Solvent flow through the column was no more than 5 ml/min. After removal of acidic components, the sample solution was passed through the carbon/glass fiber adsorbent column. After emptying the reservoir of sample solution, the reservoir was washed with four 5.0-ml portions of solvent A, and the washings were passed through the carbon adsorbent column. Next, the carbon (with planar components adsorbed) was washed with 100 ml of solvent A. TCDD and related compounds were recovered from the carbon by reverse elution with toluene. These compounds were eluted with toluene and collected in the 5- to 25-ml portion of the toluene eluate. The carbon was washed with an additional 25 ml of toluene in an attempt to remove more strongly adsorbed compounds. This last 25-ml fraction of the eluate was discarded.

## Auxiliary Enrichment Modules

After recovery of the contaminants adsorbed by the carbon, further cleanup of the sample was required. The use of sulfuric acid/silica gel adapted from the procedure published by Lamparske et al. [2] proved very effective in removing residual biogenic compounds. Alumina was used to separate PCB, chlorinated naphthalenes and other interfering substances from the CDF and CDD by a modification of the procedure described by Porter and Burke [3].

### *Combined Cesium Silicate and Sulfuric Acid/Silica Gel Cleanup*

Composite columns of cesium silicate and sulfuric acid/silica gel were prepared in Pasteur pipettes, each adsorbent occupying a 3-cm length of the column supported by a small plug of glass wool. Silica gel treated with cesium hydroxide was packed above 40% sulfuric acid on silica gel, with the two adsorbents separated by about 0.5 cm of anhydrous sodium sulfate.

The toluene solution from the reverse elution of the carbon was evaporated to less than 0.1 ml by using nitrogen flow and a 60°C water bath. The residue was transferred to the combined cesium silicate/sulfuric acid silica gel column with five 0.2-ml washes of hexane. Next, 4 ml of hexane was added to the column; the 1- to 5-ml eluate volume was collected. This eluate contained the chlorinated naphthalenes, dibenzofurans, and dibenzo-*p*-dioxins. This solution was analyzed by electron capture/gas chromatography (EC/GC) to determine if additional cleanup or fractionation was required.

*Alumina Chromatography*

BioRad acid Alumina AG4 (BioRad, Inc., Richmond, CA) was Soxhlet-extracted with methylene chloride and activated overnight at 190°C. A volume of 3.5 ml of alumina was packed in a 5-ml graduated transfer pipette and washed with hexane, and the eluate from the composite cesium silicate/ sulfuric acid silica gel adsorbent was applied to the column of alumina after evaporation to 0.1 ml. The following elution scheme was used to fractionate the planar constituents:

1. 10 ml hexane;
2. 15 ml 2% methylene chloride in hexane;
3. 15 ml 5% methylene chloride in hexane; and
4. 15 ml 8% methylene chloride in hexane.

TCDD eluted in the 39- to 49 ml-portion of the eluate volume. The elution of other components is illustrated in Figure 1. Chlorinated naphthalenes eluted in the 12- to 24-ml portion, and polychlorinated dibenzofurans eluted in the 23- to 52-ml portion.

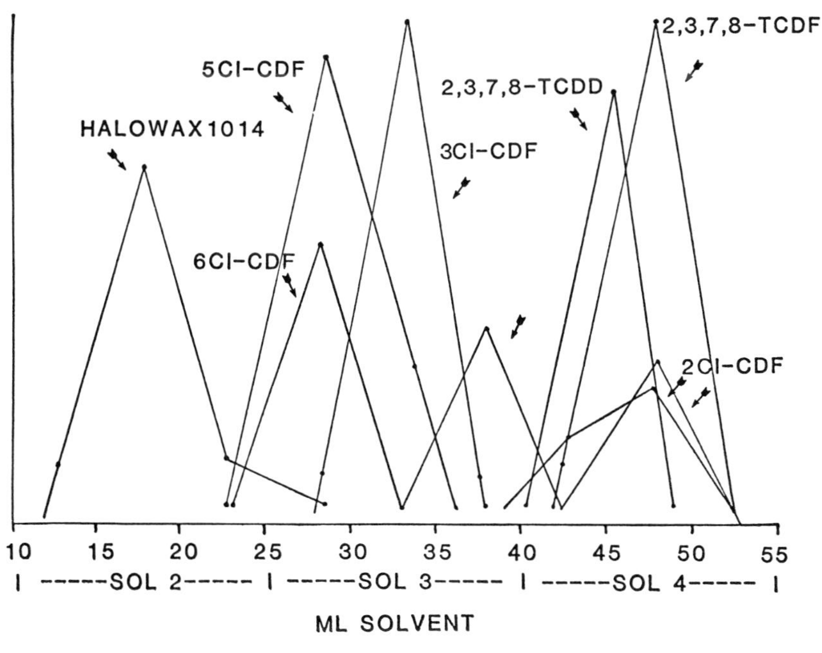


**Figure 1.** Chromatographic separation of chlorinated planar aromatics on alumina. Reference experimental section for column dimensions and solvent elution scheme.

## RESULTS

### Recovery Studies

Salmon oil was spiked with a mixture of CDD and CDF to determine the recovery and cleanup efficiency of this sequential contaminant enrichment scheme. The composition of the spiking mixture was as follows: 2,8- and 3,6-dichloro-, 2,4,6-trichloro-, 2,3,7,8-tetrachloro-, 1,2,4,7,8-pentachloro-, 1,2,4,6,7,9-hexachloro-, 1,2,3,4,6,7,9-heptachloro- and octachlorodibenzofurans and 2,3,7,8-tetrachloro-, 1,2,3,4,7,8-hexachloro- and octachlorodibenzo-*p*-dioxins. Four replicate samples of salmon oil were spiked at three levels of contamination: 25, 100 and 250 pg/g. Samples spiked at the high and low levels corresponded to 100 g of fish having a 10% lipid content (10 g of oil). The fish oil samples were weighed and dissolved in methylene chloride, and the contaminants were added to the oil solution. The contaminant standard solutions were prepared in toluene at a concentration of either 0.1 or 1.0 μg/ml. The toluene solutions of standards were added to the fish oil solution with a 10 μl syringe.

After processing the samples with both of the combined silica gel adsorbents, potassium silicate/carbon-glass fiber and cesium silicate/sulfuric acid, the samples were analyzed by temperature-programmed EC/GC. Figures 2 through 5 are representative of these analyses. Recovery data for the sample series are presented in Table IV.

The EC/GC analysis revealed that the processed extracts were remarkably free of interfering materials, and that recoveries of 70-100% could be expected for CDD and CDF congeners containing four or more chlorines. These preliminary results have demonstrated that sequentially combining chromatographic modules in a continuous flow system is feasible for enrichment of trace levels of CDF and CDD residues from tissue. Extension of this contaminant enrichment technique to additional matrices is in progress.

### Automatic Chromatography System

To use the described chromatographic modules for contaminant enrichment more fully, a chromatography system is being developed which is controlled by a microprocessor [1]. The operator will control the system through a display panel and programmable keyboard. The system will incorporate an interpretive language enabling the operator to program the separation pathway and operational functions to effect the desired sample processing steps.

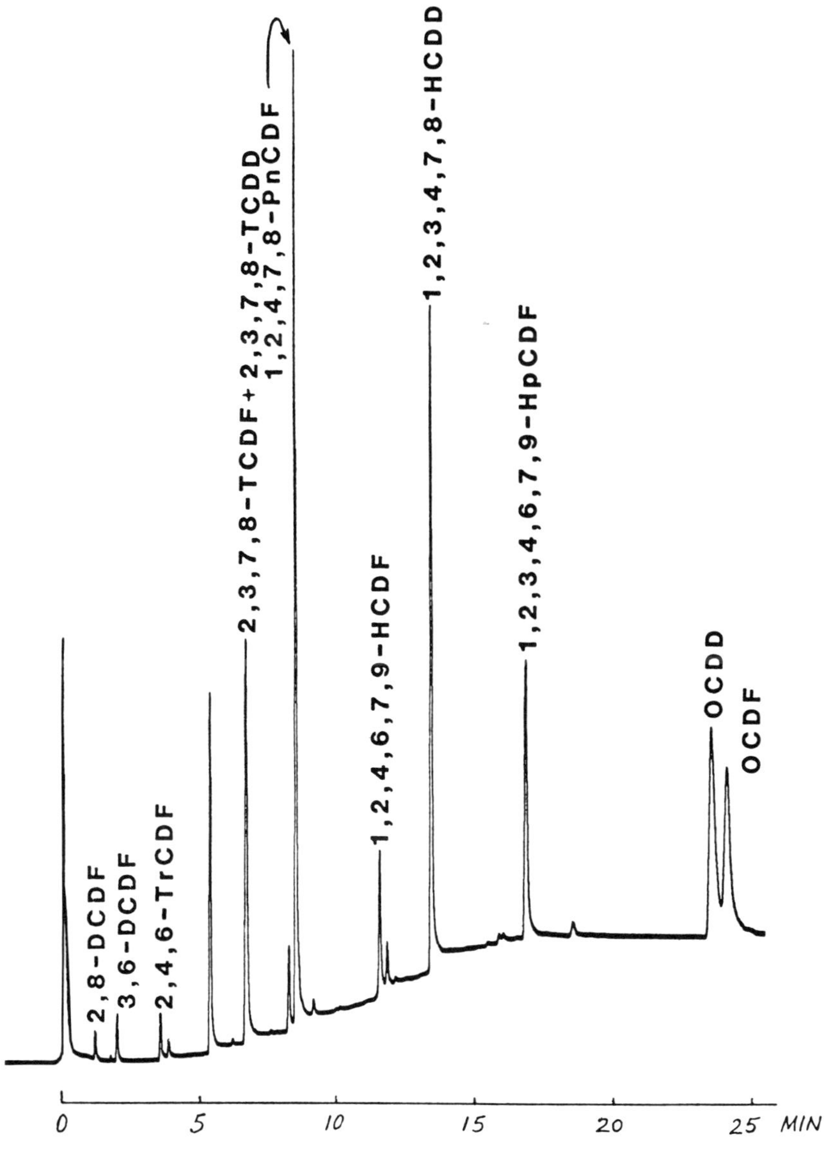


**Figure 2.** Standard solutions of chlorinated dibenzofurans and dioxins. Gas chromatographic conditions: 12-m WCOT glass column coated with OV-17, 50 cm/sec helium carrier flow; temperature program: 190°C isothermal for 2 min, programmed to 240°C at 4°C/min with 15 min final temperature hold, EC detector.

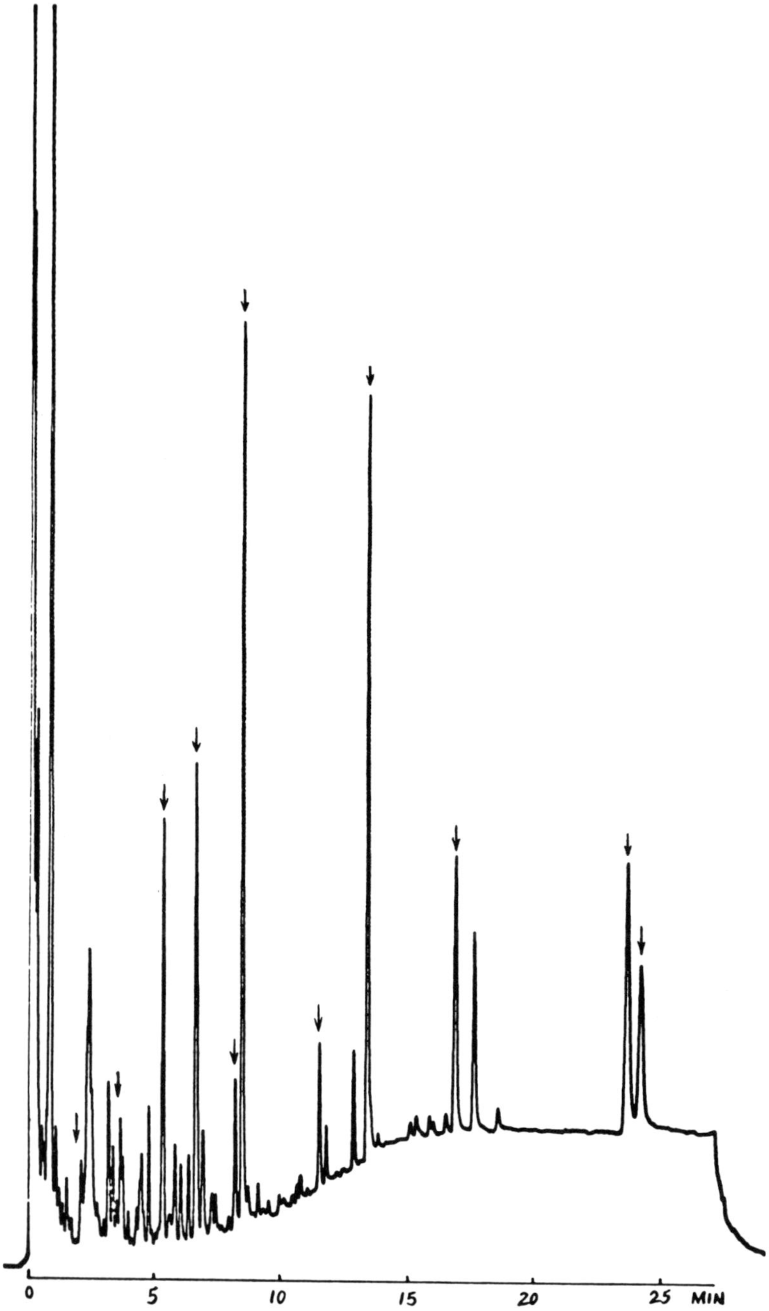


**Figure 3.** 25-ppt spike of CDF and CDD in salmon oil after enrichment by potassium silicate, carbon-glass fiber, cesium silicate/sulfuric acid-silica gel chromatography. GC conditions described in Figure 1.

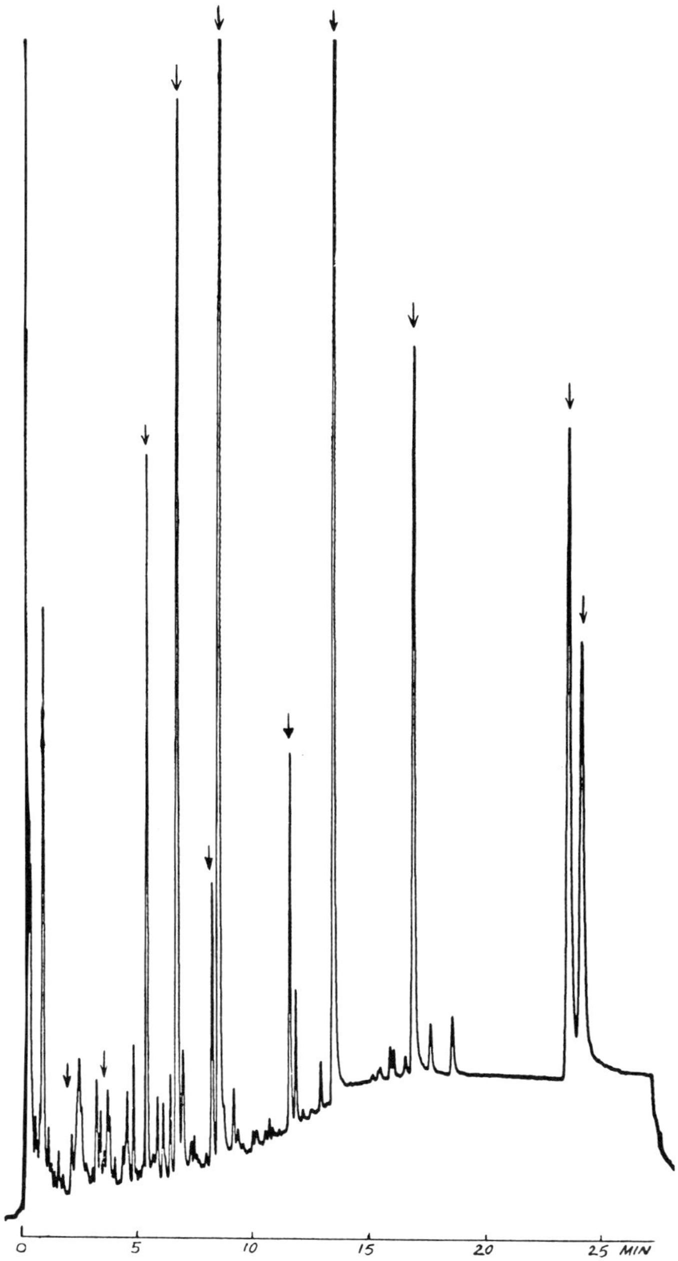


**Figure 4.** 100-ppt spike of CDF and CDD in salmon oil after enrichment by potassium silicate, carbon-glass fiber, cesium silicate/sulfuric acid-silica gel chromatography. GC conditions described in Figure 1.

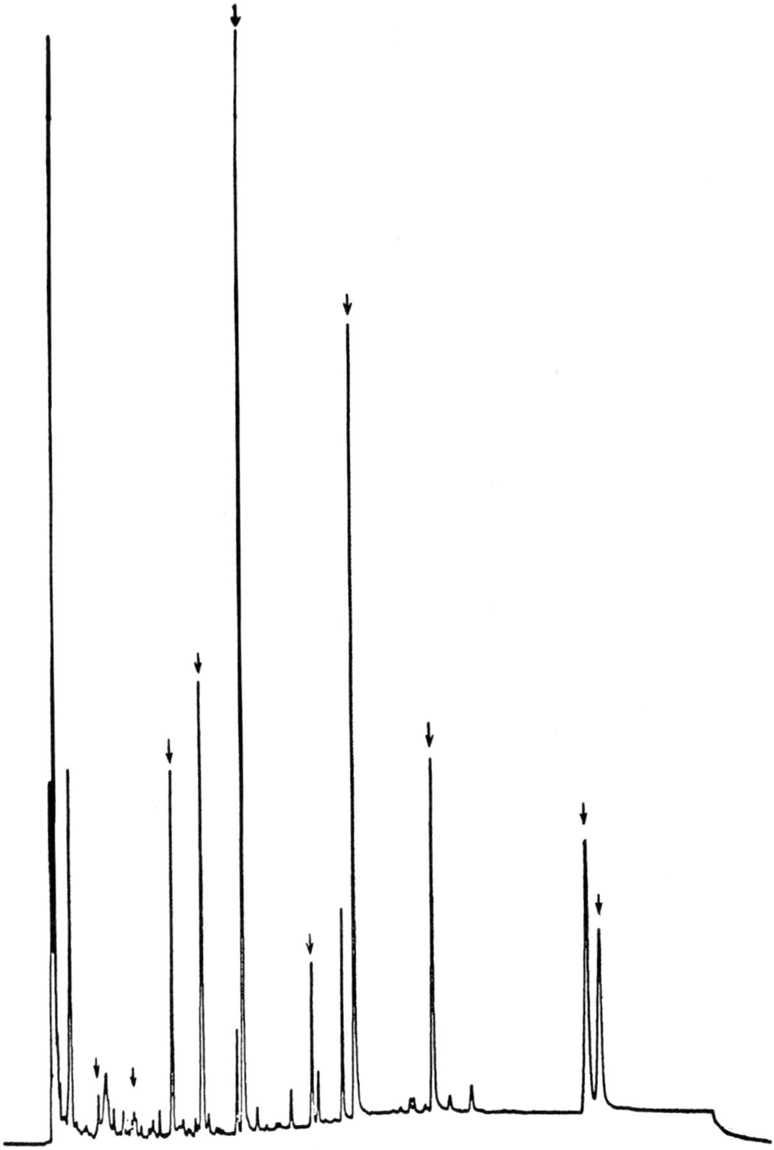


**Figure 5.** 250-ppt spike of CDF and CDD in salmon oil after enrichment by potassium silicate, carbon-glass fiber, cesium silicate/sulfuric acid-silica gel chromatography. GC conditions described in Figure 1.

**Table IV. Recovery of Chlorinated Dibenzofurans and Chlorinated-Dibenzo-*p*-dioxins in Salmon Oil by Combined Cleanup Techniques of Potassium Silicate/Carbon-Glass Fibers and Cesium Silicate/Sulfuric Acid-Silica Gel**

| | Compound[a] | | | | | | |
|---|---|---|---|---|---|---|---|
| Sample Spike | 2,3,7,8-TCDF+TCDD[b] | 1,2,4,7,8-PnCDF | 1,2,4,6 7,9-HCDF | 1,2,3,4,6,7,9-HCDD | 1,2,3,4 6,7,8,9-HpCDF | OCDD | OCDF |
| 2.5 ng Each | 76 | 73 | 83 | 86 | 80 | 90 | 78 |
| in 10 g Oil | 96 | 72 | 79 | 83 | 83 | 96 | 81 |
| | 77 | 75 | 73 | 81 | 71 | 77 | 70 |
| | 78 | 65 | 71 | 80 | 74 | 87 | 72 |
| Mean %(s) | 81(9) | 70(5) | 75(5) | 82(3) | 77(5) | 87(7) | 75(5) |
| 10 ng Each | 98 | 94 | 79 | 95 | 80 | 78 | 75 |
| in 20 g Oil | 103 | 97 | 84 | 98 | 84 | 73 | 67 |
| | 103 | 96 | 83 | 99 | 93 | 79 | 78 |
| | 103 | 102 | 88 | 100 | 92 | 73 | 75 |
| Mean %(s) | 102(2) | 97(3) | 84(4) | 98(2) | 87(6) | 76(3) | 74(5) |
| 25 ng Each | 65 | | 71 | | 79 | 68 | 77 |
| in 10 g Oil | 69 | 76 | 79 | 79 | 78 | 70 | 65 |
| | 64 | 85 | 64 | 72 | 60 | 59 | 44 |
| Mean %(s) | 66(2) | 80(–) | 68(3) | 76(–) | 72(8) | 66(3) | 62(14) |

[a] Analytical measurements were made by using a 12-m OV-17 WCOT glass column and an electron capture $^{63}$Ni detector. Helium was used as the carrier gas at a linear velocity of 50 cm/sec. The temperature program used follows: 190°C for 2 min, then increased to 240°C at 4°C/min, then held at 240°C for 15 min.

[b] 2,3,7,8-Tetrachloro-dibenzo-*p*-dioxin and -dibenzofuran were not separated on the OV-17 column. The combined peak response was used to calculate recovery. The following designate degree of chlorine substitution: T = tetra-; Pn = penta-; H = hexa-; Hp = hepta-; and O = octa-.

Through the microprocessor controller, the user can perform a wide variety of separations. Single-column gel permeation chromatography may be performed either manually or by stored programs on as many as 23 samples. Adsorption chromatography with a carbon module can be implemented and the carbon adsorbent can be regenerated, usually without removal of the column. Provisions have also been made to process up to two groups of 24 individual adsorption columns. This capability enables a separate column to be used for each sample. Gel permeation and carbon chromatography are examples of two of the many types of separations that can be performed sequentially. The design and operation of the controller is the subject of a doctoral dissertation [4].

## DISCUSSION

Gel permeation chromatography (GPC) provides a means of separating contaminants from coextracted biogenic compounds. The development of an automated GPC system led to expanded contaminant enrichment by sequential linkage of additional enrichment modules to the GPC effluent [1]. A new chromatographic enrichment module was developed which used alkali metal silicates, based on a method published by Ramljak et al. [5]. In this procedure, silica gel was treated with a saturated solution of KOH in isopropanol, producing an adsorbent capable of retaining most phenols and carboxylic acids and effectively separating them from neutral compounds. However, this adsorbent proved limited in isolating certain acidic compounds of interest, e.g., U.S. EPA consent decree phenols. Consequently, silica gels treated with hydroxides of the alkali metal (Li, Na, K and Cs) were evaluated, and cesium silicate proved superior for retention of acidic compounds [1].

A third chromatographic procedure, carbon-foam chromatography, has been investigated extensively at CNFRL. This modular procedure in which a dispersed carbon adsorbent is used, is readily coupled to the GPC or cesium silicate module, thus forming the basis of a more efficient and comprehensive enrichment scheme.

For neutral aromatic compounds, coplanarity of closely situated aromatic systems in the molecule appears to be the most important prerequisite for strong adsorption on carbon. Previous studies of the interaction of aromatic compounds with carbon established that the strength of adsorption increases as the number and coplanarity of the aromatic centers increases. Additionally, the adsorptive forces are increased by electronegative substituents (Cl, Br, and $NO_2$) on the aromatic systems [1].

Because CDF, CDD and chlorinated naphthalenes are strongly sorbed on carbon, recovery of this type of compound from granular carbon is difficult

[6]. The use of columns containing small amounts of finely divided carbon (50 mg) was found experimentally to be impractical because of limited solvent flow, even though recovery of these strongly adsorbed compounds was satisfactory.

The discovery of a method for dispersing finely divided carbon on the surface of shredded polyurethane foam [7] overcame this problem. The carbon particles strongly adhere to the foam and are not dislodged during chromatography. The increased porosity of this support and the resulting increase in solvent flow greatly facilitated the use of carbon as an adsorbent. Although shredded urethane foam is an excellent support for carbon, ultraviolet (UV) degradation of the foam can occur. Purification of the foam requires effort, and background EC/GC peaks are occasionally encountered.

Because of problems encountered with solvent swelling of the copolymer and the finding that sample background could be improved by dispersing carbon on glass fibers, attention was directed toward development of a large-capacity carbon-glass fiber contaminant enrichment module for CDD and CDF. In addition, the combination of this module with other auxilliary cleanup procedures that could be readily incorporated into a sequential configuration was explored.

Recently, the evaluation of the modular approach for the enrichment of CDF and CDD from extracts of aquatic organisms has been emphasized. Detection of these compounds in fish was sought because several members of this class have been shown to be highly toxic to mammals [8]. Chlorinated dibenzofurans are produced when PCB are heated to high temperatures in the presence of oxygen, as in open burning or pyrolysis [9]. One CDF isomer, 2,3,7,8-tetrachlorodibenzofuran, exhibits aryl hydrocarbon hydroxylase enzyme induction activity comparable to that of 2,3,7,8-tetrachlorodibenzo-*p*-dioxin (TCDD), the most toxic organic contaminant yet studied [10].

Because CDF were suspected of being environmental contaminants, their enrichment from low concentrations with a module in which dispersed carbon is used should greatly facilitate their detection. One additional goal of this study was to provide samples for analysis of CDF and CDD by direct probe chemical ionization high resolution negative ion mass spectrometry (HRNICI-MS). Chemical ionization HRNICI-MS has proved to be a very powerful tool for detecting the presence of chlorinated pesticides and dibenzo-*p*-dioxins [11,12]. Fish samples for CDF and CDD analysis were selected from past and current fish collections at CNFRL from the National Pesticide Monitoring Program.

The mass spectrometric analysis of CDF and CDD residues in selected fish, turtle and seal fat samples were performed by Kuehl et al. [13]. For the first time, CDF (having 4–8 chlorines) were detected in aquatic environmental samples. Additionally, chlorinated naphthalenes were detected in the samples examined; all samples analyzed had PCB residues in excess of 10 $\mu g/g$.

Although CDF and CDD were detected in some fish by HRNICI-MS, considerable effort was required to process the sample extracts, and no isomer identification was possible with this technique. To explore other possibilities for analyzing CDF, some of these extracts were examined by EC/GC; however, the resulting chromatograms were unsatisfactory for screening the compounds. For EC/GC analysis, the samples required additional cleanup with alumina and sulfuric acid on silica gel. This auxilliary cleanup removed essentially all of the interferences to EC/GC and presented an additional means of screening for the presence of CDF in environmental samples.

In the preliminary evaluation of alternative supports for carbon dispersion, it was determined that carbon could also be dispersed on a copolymer of styrene-divinyl benzene, as well as on shredded glass fibers. These modifications offered a means of extending the utility of the dispersed carbon module. Although carbon dispersed on this copolymer offered some interesting properties for contaminant enrichment, its application has not been pursued beyond isolating PCB components without chlorine substitution in the *ortho, ortho'* positions of the biphenyl rings from PCB mixtures.

## SUMMARY

Assessment of hazardous organic environmental contaminants usually requires analysis at trace levels in complex biological matrices. These analyses demand rigorous contaminant enrichment before analysis. Further, optimum use of sophisticated analytical instrumentation is facilitated by contaminant enrichment processes that are also specific for chemical classes.

Space and manpower limitations reinforce the need for greater automation and instrumental analysis. A series of chromatographic enrichment procedures (modules) has been developed, designed to be incorporated sequentially into an automated, microprocessor-controlled chromatography system for enrichment of complex residues extracted from environmental samples. Also, improved routine purification capabilities made possible by such automation broaden the scope of contaminants amenable to more extensive analysis, e.g., glass capillary GC or GC/MS.

The utility of an integrated approach to contaminant enrichment has been demonstrated for acidic and neutral planar aromatics, concomitant with rejection of biogenic coextractives. Many additional chromatographic modules can be developed, and it is believed that this approach warrants greater emphasis in environmental contaminant analysis.

## REFERENCES


1. Stalling, D. L., L. M. Smith and J. D. Petty. "Approaches to Comprehensive Analysis of Persistent Halogenated Environmental Contaminants," in *Measurement of Organic Pollutants in Water and Wastewater,* STP 686, C. E. Van Hall, Ed., (Philadelphia, PA: American Society for Testing and Materials, 1979), pp. 302-323.
2. Lamparski, L. L., T. J. Nestrick and R. H. Stehl. "Determination of Part-per-Trillion Concentrations of 2,3,7,8-Tetrachloro-p-dioxin in Fish," *Anal. Chem.* 51:1453-1458 (1979).
3. Porter, M. L., and J. A. Burke. "Separation of Three Chlorodibenzo-*p*-dioxins from Some Polychlorinated Biphenyls by Chromatography on Aluminum Oxide Column," *J. Assoc. Off. Anal. Chem.* 54:1426-1428 (1971).
4. Hartley, J. W. "A Programmable Chromatographic Separation System: Specifications and Design," PhD Thesis, University of Missouri–Columbia, MO (1979).
5. Ramljak, Z., A. Sole, P. Arpino, J. M. Schmitter and G. Guiochon. "Separation of Acids from Asphalts," *Anal. Chem.* 49:1222-1225 (1977).
6. Stalling, D. L., J. L. Johnson and J. N. Huckins. "Automated Gel Permeation-Carbon Chromatographic Cleanup of Dioxins, PCB, Pesticides, and Industrial Chemicals," in *Environmental Quality and Safety, Supplement Vol. III, Pesticides Lectures of the IUPAC, Third International Congress of Pesticide Chemistry* F. Coulson and F. Korte, Eds. (Stuttgart, Germany, G. Thieme Publ., 1975), pp. 12-18.
7. Huckins, J. N., D. L. Stalling and W. A. Smith. "Foam-Charcoal Chromatography for Analysis of Polychlorinated Dibenzodioxins in Herbicide Orange," *J. Assoc. Off. Anal. Chem.* 61:32-38 (1978).
8. Moore, J. A., J. A. Morre, E. E. McConnell, D. W. Dalgard and M. W. Harris. "Comparative Toxicity of Three Halogenated Dibenzofurans in Guinea Pigs, Mice, and Rhesus Monkeys," *Ann. N.Y. Acad. Sci.* 320:151-163 (1979).
9. Rappe, C., H. R. Buser and H. P. Bosshardt, "Dioxins, Dibenzofurans and Other Polyhalogenated Aromatics: Production, Use, Formation, and Destruction," *Ann. N.Y. Acad. Sci.* 320:1-18 (1979).
10. Poland, A., W. F. Greenlee and A. S. Kende. "Studies on the Mechanism of Action of the Chlorinated Dibenzo-p-dioxins and Related Compounds," *Ann. N. Y. Acad. Sci.* 320:214-230 (1979).
11. Hass, J. R., M. D. F. Friesen, D. J. Haruan and C. E. Parker. "Determination of Polychlorinated Dibenzo-*p*-dioxins in Biological Samples by Negative Chemical Ionization Mass Spectrometry," *Anal. Chem.* 50:1474-1479 (1978).
12. Dougherty, R. C. and K. Piotrowska. "Multiresidue Screening by Negative Chemical Ionization Mass Spectrometry of Organic Polychlorides," *J. Assoc. Off. Anal. Chem.* 59:1023-1027 (1976).
13. Kuehl, D. W., R. C. Dougherty, Y. Tondeur, D. L. Stalling, L. M. Smith and C. Rappe. "Negative Chemical Ionization Studies of Polychlorinated Dibenzo-*p*-dioxins, Dibenzofurans and Naphthalenes in Environmental Samples," Chapter 12, this volume.

# CHAPTER 10

# STATE-OF-THE-ART INSTRUMENTAL ORGANIC ANALYSIS IN ENVIRONMENTAL CHEMISTRY

**E. D. Pellizzari**

Research Triangle Institute
Research Triangle Park, North Carolina

## INTRODUCTION

The need to know what chemicals may escape into the environment and at what level they may be harmful leads one to rather quickly realize that until compounds are identified with certainty and are accurately measured, effective control of these chemicals is essentially impossible [1]. Society has become increasingly aware of the presence of trace (and sometimes far more than just trace) quantities of hazardous organics which have entered the environment, inadvertently or otherwise. There is scarcely any edition of a newspaper or a new magazine that does not contain a report of some new environmental mishap. Awareness has steadily increased that the ecological balance is an extremely fragile thing, which can very readily be disturbed by the introduction of manmade products in a wide variety of areas. The commerical production and use of synthetic organic chemicals certainly constitutes a possible major source of insult to the ecological balance.

Synthetic organic chemical production in the United States alone has increased over the last 30 years at an annual average rate of 11% [2]. Types of direct chemical introduction are exemplified by the widespread use of pesticides, fungicides, herbicides and insecticides, to name just a few of the organic chemicals used extensively in today's society.

This fact of environmental contamination coupled with federal regulation to protect the environment from toxic chemicals has certainly placed a great burden on the analytical chemist [3,4]. In analytical organic analysis, the analyst is called on to both identify and measure organic substances in the environment. This may span a tremendous range of different matrices from air, water, soil, sediment, solid wastes, commercial products and biota to human tissue and biological fluids. Indeed, there has been a tremendous burden placed on separation sciences as well as the requirements for better instrumental methods of analysis.

A brief general overview is presented here for a selected few new instrumental techniques which promise to be significant additions to the analyst's arsenal of tools.

## INSTRUMENTAL METHODS

The detection limits and dynamic range for several instrumental techniques are given in Table I. The detection mode and whether the method is selective for certain chemical classes are indicated. The thermal energy analyzer is regarded as a very sensitive and selective detector for N-nitrosamines, with detection limits in the subpicogram range. The dynamic range is approximately six orders of magnitude. Another detection mode receiving considerable attention during the past few years is photoionization, particularly when coupled with gas chromatography (GC). This particular detector, as it is currently designed, is capable of picogram sensitivity with more than six orders of magnitude of linear dynamic range. The electron capture detector (ECD), fluorescence, flame ionization, thermal conductivity and ultraviolet (UV) are all very well-known and established techniques. Also, electron-impact positive-ion mass spectrometry (MS) has been a widely used tool for characterization as well as quantitation of organics. The detection limit is generally a few nanograms in the electron-impact mode and in the low picogram area for multiple-ion detection. The linear dynamic range, however, is primarily limited by the data system associated with the mass spectrometer. A relatively new form of MS is negative chemical ionization. Similar to ECD in principle, negative chemical ionization provides a new sensitive dimension to MS. Finally, gas chromatography coupled with Fourier transform infrared (GC/FT/IR) spectrophotometry has been a welcomed instrumental method for characterization of organic compounds in environmental samples.

The thermal energy analyzer, photoionization, negative chemical ionization MS and GC Fourier infrared spectrophotometry will be further examined as to their principle of operation. Examples of their application to environment analysis will be also presented.

**Table I. Detection Limits/Dynamic Range for Several Instrumental Methods**

| Detection Mode | Selectivity | Grams |
|---|---|---|
| Thermal Energy Analyzer | + | |
| Photoionization | ± | |
| Electron Capture | + | |
| Mass Spectrometry | | |
| Electron Impact | − | |
| Multiple Ion Det. | + | |
| Neg. Chemical Ion. | + | |
| Fluorescence | + | |
| Flame Ionization | − | |
| Thermal Conductivity | − | |
| FT/IR | ± | |
| UV | − | |

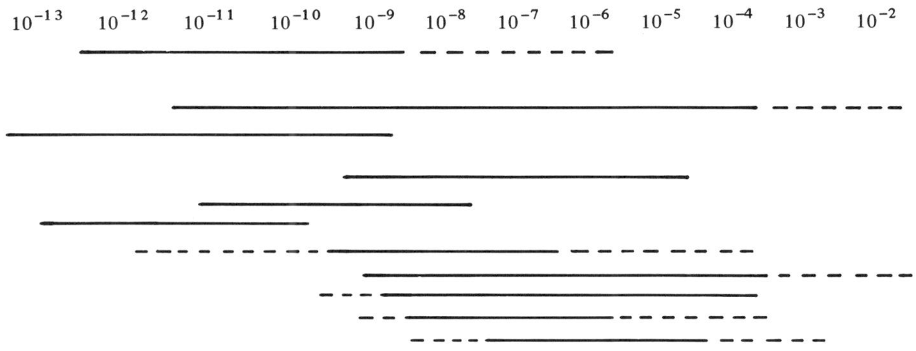

## Thermal Energy Analyzer

The thermal energy analyzer detector was specifically designed by Fine and co-workers for the analysis of N-nitrosamine compounds in a wide variety of sample matrices [5-9]. The thermal energy analyzer detector has been interfaced to a gas chromatograph and to a high-performance liquid chromatograph (HPLC) [9]. These systems permit identification and quantification of volatile and nonvolatile N-nitrosamines.

The N-NO bond, which is approximately 6–10 kcal/mol in most N-nitroso compounds, is a relatively weak bond. Taking advantage of this phenomenon, the thermal energy analyzer employs catalytic pyrolysis to cleave the N-NO bond and release the NO radical (Figure 1). Pyrolysis is generally performed at a temperature of approximately 350–550°C. The effluent from the pyrolysis chamber is then swept by an inert gas such as argon or helium through a set of traps maintained between -70 and -150°C (Figure 1). Most organic materials condense in these traps. The nitrosyl radical, however, remains gaseous and is carried through the traps into a reaction chamber (Figure 1). In this chamber the nitrosyl radical reacts with ozone to form electronically excited nitrogen dioxide. The excited nitrogen dioxide returns to its ground state with the emission of light in the near IR. A sensitive photomultiplier detects this light, and the resulting signal is amplified and displayed in a conventional manner such as on a strip chart recorder.

Although the design of this detector provides for enhanced selectivity for N-nitroso compounds, several other classes of organic compounds may also effect a detector signal. False positive responses can arise from certain olefins, organic nitrites, organic nitrates, C-nitro, C-nitroso, N-nitro, S-nitro and S-nitroso compounds [10-12]. Nevertheless, the high selectivity of the thermal energy analyzer detector does provide for accurate quantitation of N-nitroso compounds at the picogram levels.

The majority of literature references dealing with nitrosamine analysis have used GC. Detectors such as the Hall, Coulson, alkali flame ionization and mass spectrometer have been employed in combination with GC. A thermal energy analyzer response from a sample or its extracts does not automatically signify the presence of a nitrosamine in the sample itself. Confirmation is generally relatively simple and includes the analysis on several different types of GC column packings, a combination of GC and HPLC or confirmation by GC/MS using the appropriate detection mode.

The trace analysis for volatile and nonvolatile N-nitroso compounds has become an area of intense interest and concern for many laboratories around the world. These materials are potential human carcinogens and/or mutagens and have been found at significant levels in a wide variety of environmental and consumer product samples. The thermal energy analyzer system coupled

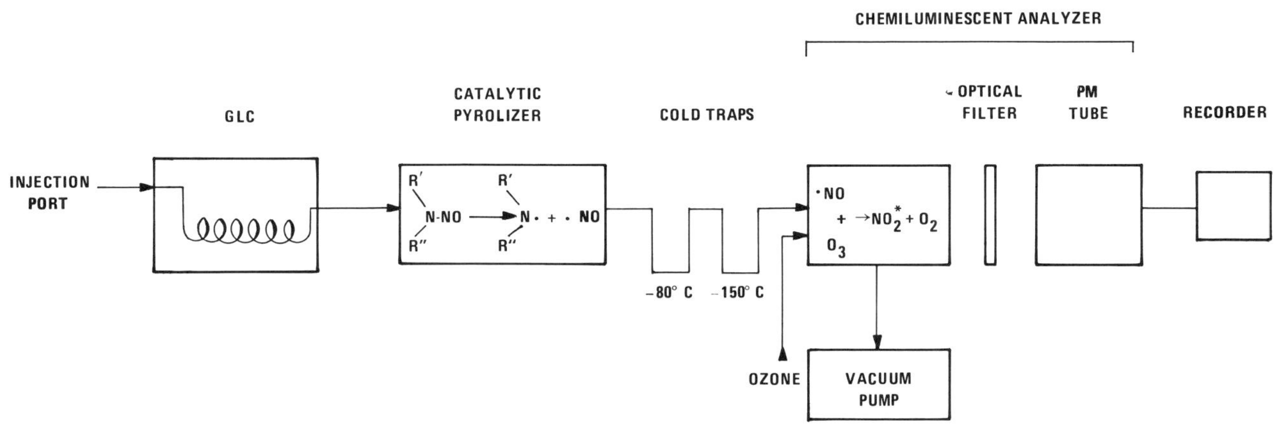


**Figure 1.** Gas chromatograph-thermal energy analyzer system.

with GC or HPLC has been used for analysis of samples from a number of different matrices. Figures 2 and 3 depict a thermal energy analyzer response for an ambient air sample containing N-nitrosodimethylamine or dimethylnitrosamine (DMN) and diethylnitrosamine (DEN) [13]. Figure 4 depicts a GC chromatogram obtained with the thermal energy analyzer for an extract from fried bacon [5]. This sample contained N-nitrosodimethylamine as well as N-nitrosopiperidine (PYRN). Figure 5 depicts two GC chromatograms; the upper tracing is for a canned tuna extract which was spiked with DMN, DEN, dibutylnitrosamine (DBN) and N-nitrosopiperidine [5]. The bottom chromatogram is an unspiked extract of canned tuna showing the nitrosamines of dimethylamine and piperidine.

**Photoionization Detection**

The photoionization detector in combination with GC has become increasingly popular during the past few years. Photoionization and the recombination reactions are believed to occur in this detector using nitrogen as a carrier gas with traces of oxygen present (Figure 6) [14-16]. Essentially, the organic molecule is irradiated with UV light at a specific electron-volt intensity, which cleaves the molecule into positive ions and thermal electrons. Because the ionization potentials for organic substances vary considerably depending on the substitution in the organic molecule, it is possible to choose the appropriate UV lamp which provides the necessary energy to either detect or discriminate organics with certain ionization potentials.

Table II lists the ionization potentials for alkanes and alkenes [17]. In general, these classes of compounds have higher ionization potentials and thus yield a low response when a UV lamp of 10.5 eV or less is used as the source of irradiation. In contrast to the alkanes, the ionization potentials for halogenated hydrocarbons and aromatics are given in Table III [17]. The aromatics have considerably lower ionization potentials than for the alkanes and halogenated hydrocarbons and thus the use of a UV 9.5-eV lamp would allow more sensitive detection of aromatics compared to the other compounds. Thus, the photoionization detector can be deemed as a somewhat specific detector for organics. This instrumental method of detection has been applied to sensing chlorinated aromatics as well as oxygenated compounds in environmental matrices. It has received recent attention for the analysis of these chemical classes in ambient air [17].

**Mass Spectrometry–Negative Chemical Ionization**

Electron capture is a relatively old detection mode that has been well studied. Figure 7 depicts the series of dissociative reactions that can occur

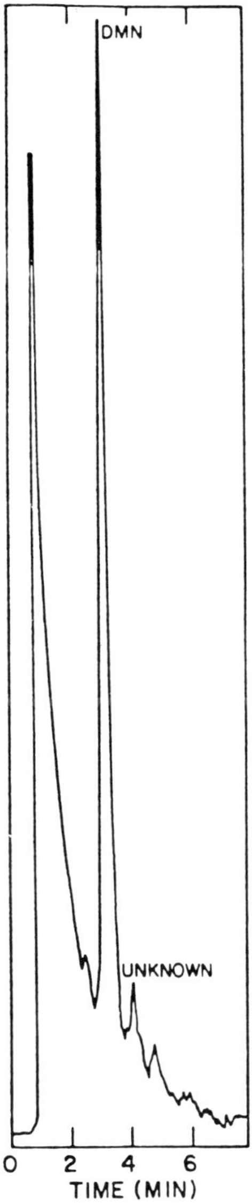


**Figure 2.** TEA-GC of air from 12:38 to 1:38 PM on November 25, 1975 at playground on Northbridge and Cannery Road, Fairfield, MD. DMN = 18 $ng/m^3$.

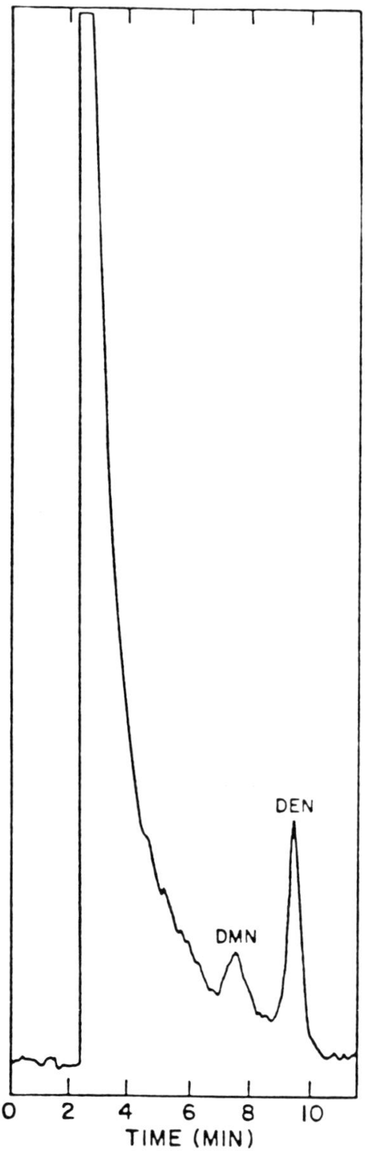


**Figure 3.** TEA-GC of air sample from 12:40 to 1:40 PM on December 12, 1975 at Fourth Street and Highland Ave. in Arundel Village, MD. DMN = 50 ng/$m^3$, DEN = 200 ng/$m^3$ (both confirmed by TEA-HPLC).

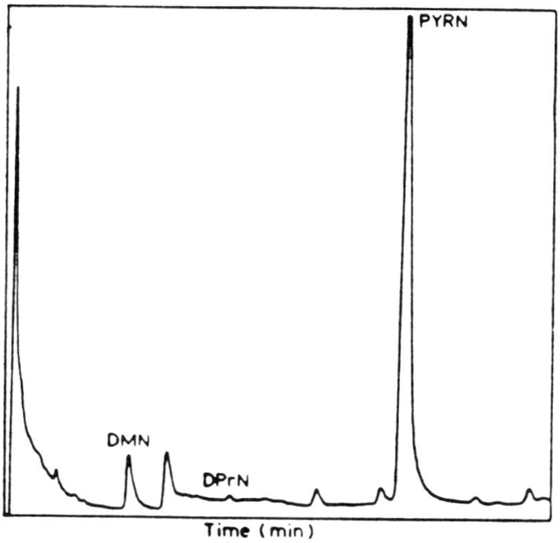


**Figure 4.** Chromatogram of a fried bacon extract, showing DMN (4.9 μg/kg) and PYRN (52 μg/kg). Dipropylnitrosamine was added as an internal standard (0.5 μg/kg); the recovery was 95%.

**Table II. Ionization Potentials for Alkanes and Alkenes**

| Alkanes | IP (eV) | Alkenes | IP (eV) |
|---|---|---|---|
| Ethane | 11.65 | Ethylene | 10.52 |
| Propane | 11.07 | Propene | 9.73 |
| *n*-Butane | 10.63 | 1-Butene | 9.58 |
| *n*-Pentane | 10.35 | 1-Pentene | 9.50 |
| *n*-Hexane | 10.18 | | |

**Table III. Ionization Potential for Halogenated Hydrocarbons and Aromatics**

| Halogenated Hydrocarbons | IP (eV) | Aromatics | IP (eV) |
|---|---|---|---|
| Fluorocarbon-12 | 12.31 | Benzene | 9.25 |
| Fluorocarbon-11 | 11.77 | Toluene | 8.82 |
| Methyl Chloride | 11.28 | *m*-Xylene | 8.56 |
| Chloroform | 11.42 | *p*-Xylene | 8.45 |
| Carbon Tetrachloride | 11.47 | Ethylbenzene | 8.76 |
| Perchloroethylene | 9.34 | *m*-Propylbenzene | 8.72 |
| | | *n*-Butylbenzene | 8.69 |

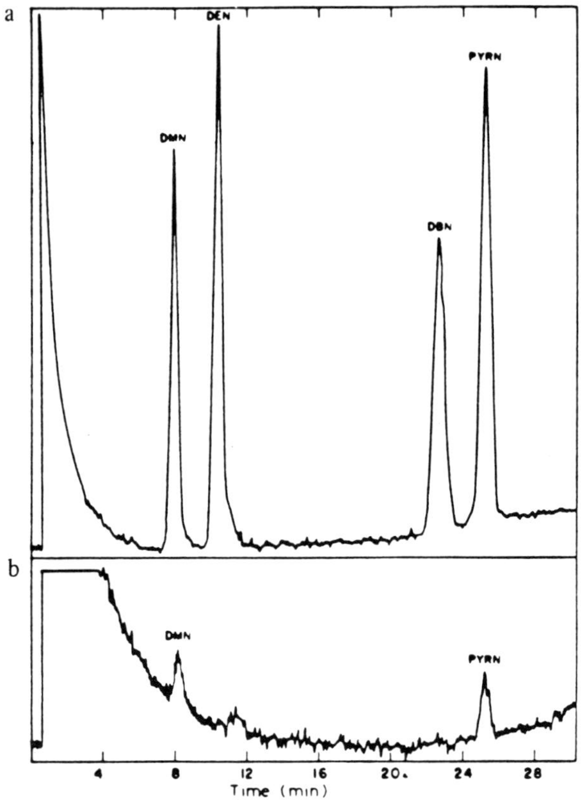


**Figure 5.** Chromatogram of canned tuna extract; (a) after recovery of a mixture of DMN, DEN, DBN and PYRN, each at 5 μg/kg; (b) showing the presence of DMN (0.2 μg/kg) and PYRN (0.45 μg/kg).

between a thermal energy electron and an organic molecule possessing an appreciable electron capturing affinity [18]. These reactions are extremely important not only to the understanding and utilization of the electron capture detector as a detector for GC but also in negative chemical ionization/MS. Whether the mechanism of electron capture is dissociative or nondissociative, as shown in Figure 8, depends upon the ability of the molecule to distribute the electron charge via a resonance mechanism in the parent molecule or via resonance in a product ion [18]. In general, molecules which undergo dissociative electron capture exhibit higher sensitivity than those which are nondissociative. Furthermore as one increases the temperature, the sensitivity also increases for those molecules which undergo a dissociative mechanism

$$R + h\nu \longrightarrow R^+ + e^- \qquad (1)$$

$$N_2 + h\nu \longrightarrow N_2^* \qquad (2)$$

$$N_2 + R \longrightarrow N_2 + R^+ + e^- \qquad (3)$$

$$R^+ + e^- \longrightarrow R \qquad (4)$$

$$O_2 + e^- \longrightarrow O_2^- \qquad (5)$$

$$O_2^- + R^+ \longrightarrow R + O_2 \qquad (6)$$

**Figure 6.** Photoionization and recombination reactions.

[18]. Conversely; the temperature-sensitivity relationship is inversely proportional for nondissociative mechanisms.

Negative chemical ionization/MS has great potential in the analysis of environmental samples [19-23]. A case-example exhibiting its utility is exemplified by the analysis of vapor-phase organics in ambient air (collected on Tenax GC sampling cartridges) using electron impact and negative chemical ionization. Figure 9 depicts a GC/MS/COMP profile obtained by thermal desorption of the Tenax GC cartridge using electron impact. Over 100 compounds were observed. However, when a corresponding duplicate sample was analyzed utilizing the same technique except for operating the mass spectrometer in a negative chemical ionization mode, the results shown in Figure 10 were obtained. These results represent a sample taken upwind from an industrial area in Deer Park, TX. Represented on this chromatogram are the reconstructed ion intensities for $^{35}Cl$, $^{37}Cl$, $^{79}Br$ and $^{81}Br$. By examining the profiles at specific retention times, the number and combination of Cl and Br atoms in a molecule are clearly evident as well as the number of halogenated organics in this sample. Figure 11 depicts an ambient air sample taken downwind from the same industrial area in Deer Park, TX. In addition to the compounds which were detected in the upwind samples, several new compounds are also detected in the downwind sample.

The power of this technique is exemplified in the specificity and sensitivity which is not afforded in electron impact mode. As can be seen from these data, the intensity of each of the peaks which correspond to hal-

*Dissociative:*

$$e^- + AB \xrightarrow{k_{1,2}} A\cdot + B^- \pm \text{energy} \qquad 1$$

$$e^- + AB \xrightarrow{k_1} AB^- \pm \text{energy} \qquad 2$$

$$AB^- + CH_4 \xrightarrow{k_{-1}'} AB + e^- + CH_4 \qquad 3$$

$$AB^- + CH_4 \xrightarrow{k_2'} A\cdot + B^- + CH_4 \qquad 4$$

$$AB^- + P^+ \longrightarrow \begin{cases} \to AB + R\cdot \\ \to A\cdot + B\cdot + R' \end{cases} \qquad 5$$

$$AB^- + R\cdot \xrightarrow{k_{R_1'}} \begin{cases} \to ABR^- \\ \to AB + R^- \\ \to AR + B^- \end{cases} \xrightarrow{+P^+} \text{neutrals} \qquad 6$$

$$B^- + P^+ \longrightarrow \begin{cases} \to BP \\ \to B\cdot + R\cdot \end{cases} \qquad 7$$

$$B^- + R\cdot \xrightarrow{k_{R_2'}} BR + e^- \qquad 8$$

$$A\cdot + e^- \xrightarrow{k_3} A^- \qquad 9$$

$$A^- + P^+ \xrightarrow{k_{N_4'}} AP \text{ or } A\cdot + P\cdot \qquad 10$$

$$A^- + R\cdot \xrightarrow{k_{R_4'}} AR + e^- \qquad 11$$

$$A\cdot + AB^- \xrightarrow{k_{F_{-4}}} AB + A^- \qquad 12$$

$$e^- + P^+ \xrightarrow{k_N'} R\cdot \qquad 13$$

$$e^- + R\cdot \xrightarrow{k_R'} R^- \qquad 14$$

$$A^- + AB \longrightarrow AB^- + A\cdot \qquad 15$$

$$B^- + AB \longrightarrow AB^- + B\cdot \qquad 16$$

$$A\cdot + AB \longrightarrow A_2 + B\cdot \qquad 17$$

$$B\cdot + AB \longrightarrow B_2 + A\cdot \qquad 18$$

where

AB = capturing solute molecule;
$AB^-$ = negative ion;
$A\cdot$ and $B^-$ = products of dissociation;
$P^+$ = positive ions: $Ar^+$, $ArH^+$, $ArCH^+$, $ArCH_2^+$, $ArCH_3^+$, $ArCH_4^+$, $CH_4^+$, $CH_3^+$, etc.;
$R\cdot$ = radical: $H\cdot$; $CH_3\cdot$, etc.

**Figure 7.** Dissociative electron capture reactions.

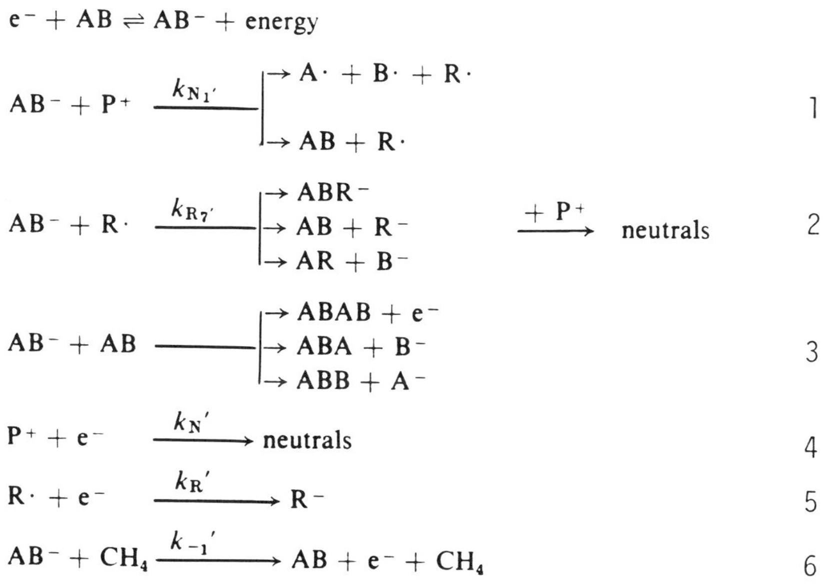

**Figure 8.** Nondissociative electron capture reactions.

ogenated hydrocarbons are much more intense than they were in the electron impact mode. The technique is on an average 2-3 orders of magnitude more sensitive than electron impact. Furthermore, negative chemical ionization/MS provides considerable specificity, which is mandatory for analysis of environmental samples if elaborate purification methods are to be circumvented. For example, analysis of ambient air samples, precludes the use of extensive purification.

## GC/FT/IR Spectrophotometry

Fourier transform infrared spectroscopy measures the interferogram resulting from a Michelson interferometer as shown in Figure 12 [24]. An interferogram is a plot of the infrared intensity vs time recorded as the optical path through one arm of the interferometer is changed by a moving mirror. The recombined beam from the two arms of the interferometer may be in or out of phase depending on the optical path difference. Each frequency comes out of phase at a characteristic optical path difference and the superposition of all frequency produces the observed interferogram.

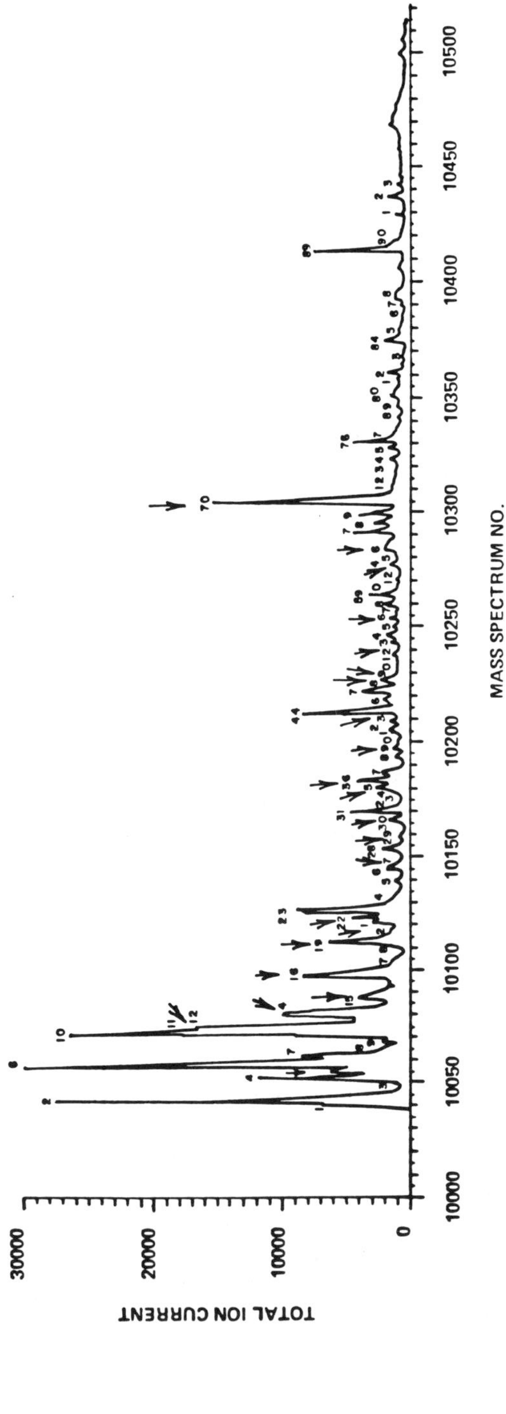


**Figure 9.** Electron impact GC/MS/COMP profile taken downwind of industrial area in Houston, TX.

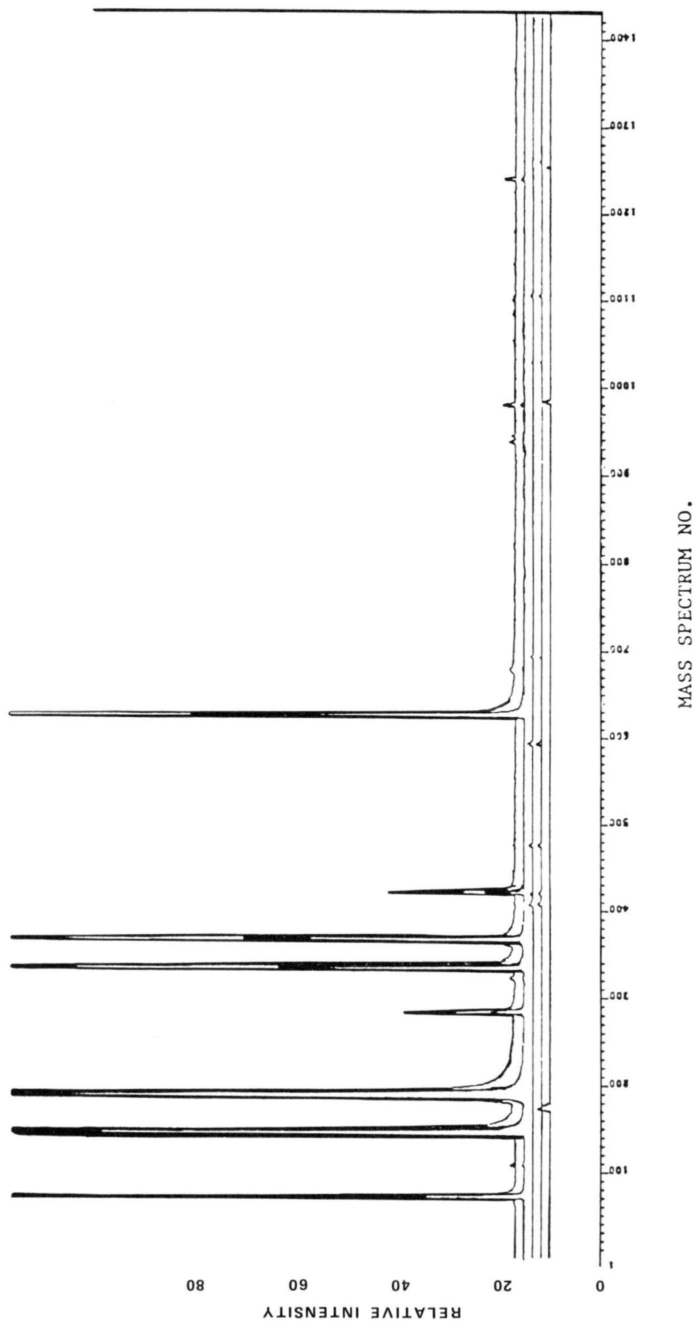


**Figure 10.** Negative chemical ionization GC/MS/COMP profile of upwind ambient air sample for Deer Park, TX.

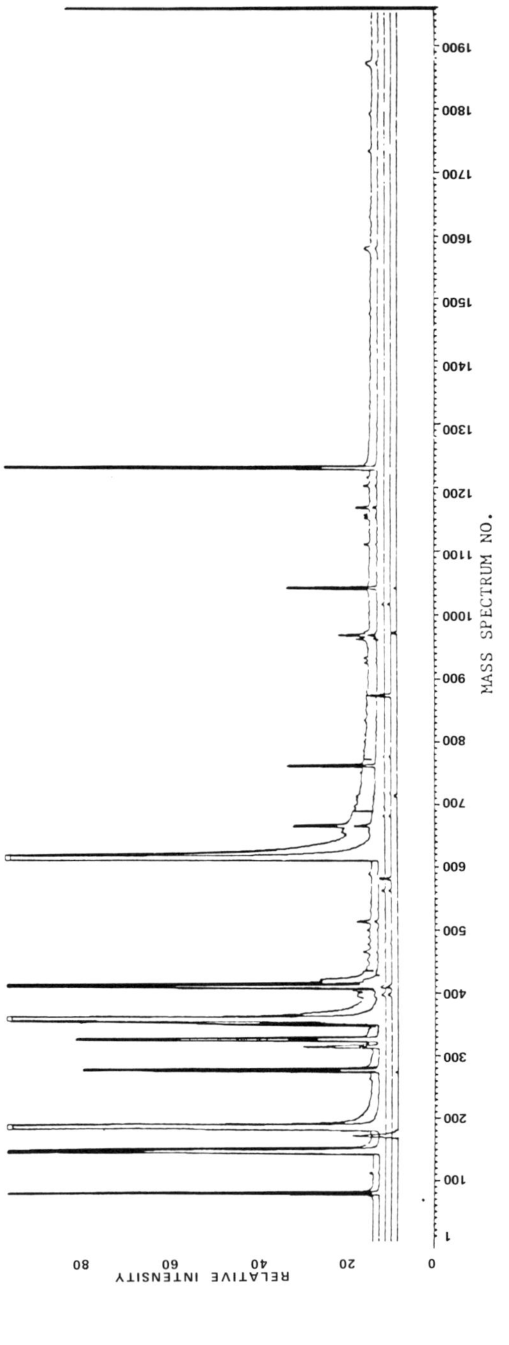


**Figure 11.** Negative chemical ionization GC/MS/COMP profile of downwind ambient air sample in Deer Park, TX.

After the data are collected and stored in a computer, the dedicated computer executes a Fourier transform of the data into a single-beam spectrum which may be then ratioed against a background to produce the customary transmittance or absorbance vs wave number IR spectrum. There are four fundamental advantages of FT/IR over dispersive instruments. These advantages may be summarized by the way they are manifested in the GC/FT/IR system itself. The instrument is fast enough to obtain several scans over chromatographic peaks so that all peaks of a chromatogram may be observed and multicomponent peaks may be deconvoluted. Scanning rates for the IR region is generally 0.5-1.5 sec. Because of the throughput advantage of the intensity from the laser light beam, the sensitivity is much better than dispersive systems permitting analysis of trace components. Detection of 10 ng of isobutyl methacrylate has been reported, and routine sensitivities in the 100-1000 ng range can be expected from most compounds even in real samples with interferences.

In addition to the basic system, light pipes have currently become available which consist of gold-coated glass tubes with KBR windows affixed to the ends (Figure 13) [24]. The GC effluent thus flows into one end through the pipe and then exits. The light pipe and transfer line are heated to prevent condensation of the compound eluting from the GC column. The volume is optimized for the anticipated average GC peak volume. The length to diameter ratio is calculated to give the best signal-to-noise ratio. The detector of choice is the mercury cadmium telluride detector for use in the GC mode. This detector offers an increase in signal-to-noise by about a factor of 5-50 over the more commonly used triglycine sulfate detector.

During the past few years, such a system has been used for the characterization of organics in effluents from energy-related sources as well as other environmental samples [24]. This particular instrumentation is useful in assisting and complementing GC/MS data for characterizing organics. GC/FT/IR is particularly useful in discerning isomeric forms of organics where MS fails. Figure 14 shows the flame ionization detection (FID) profile for an acid sample obtained from product water during coal gasification chromatographed on a packed Carbowax 20M column. The IR spectrum for peaks 14 and 22 are shown in Figures 15 and 16. Peak No. 14 was identified as methyl nonanoate (Figure 15). The quantity which was injected onto the chromatographic column was approximately 175 ng. The infrared spectrum for peak 22 which is 3,5-dimethylphenol is given in Figure 16. This corresponds to about 80 ng.

In addition to the ability to generate a FID or thermal conductivity profile as well as IR spectra, some commercial systems have software programs which can provide what are called "chemigrams" [24]. Figure 17 shows a chemigram for the organic acid fraction from a coal gasification sample. In

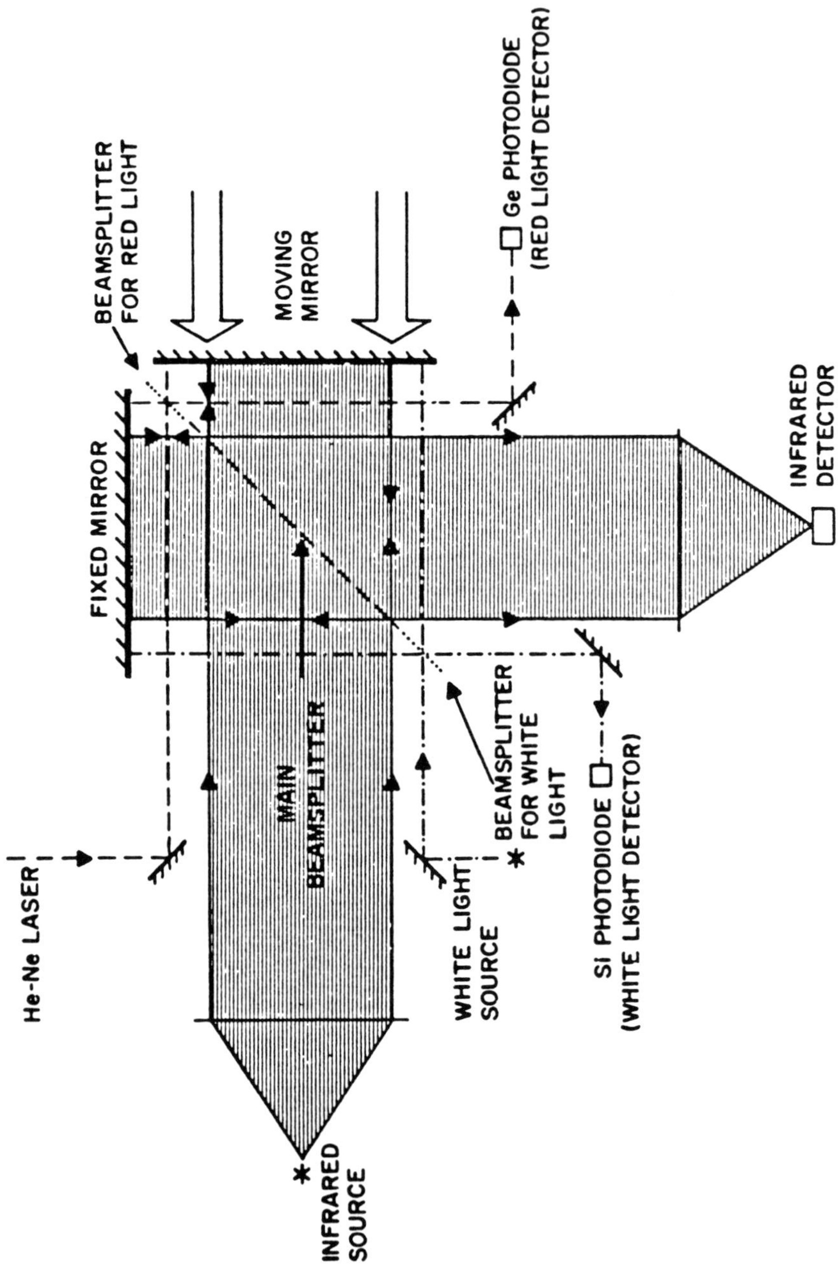


Figure 12. Michelson interferometer.

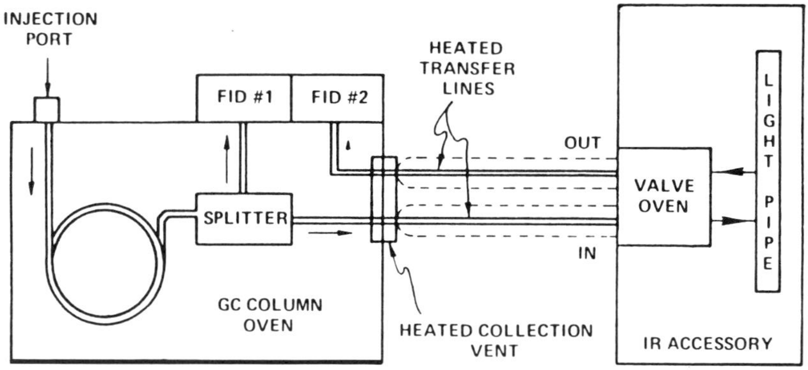


**Figure 13.** Interface between GC and FT/IR systems.

this case in contrast to the previous data, the analysis was conducted on a glass support coated tubular column coated with Carbowax 20M. Depicted here are five IR bands. These tracings are generated in the dynamic mode, i.e., on-the-fly during acquisition of data by performing a 2K transform on the interferograms. From the bottom to top tracings, the IR wavenumbers 800-4000, 1130-1175, 1700-1750, 1320-1380 and 2900-3100 $cm^{-1}$ are described. Any IR window can be set up for observation using computer software. This allows real-time information to be presented to the operator.

## SUMMARY

Interesting new developments in detection methods exhibit great promise in the analysis of environmental samples. In general, it can be said that the techniques are providing higher sensitivity and more specificity. Both are certainly needed for characterization and quantification of organics in the environment.

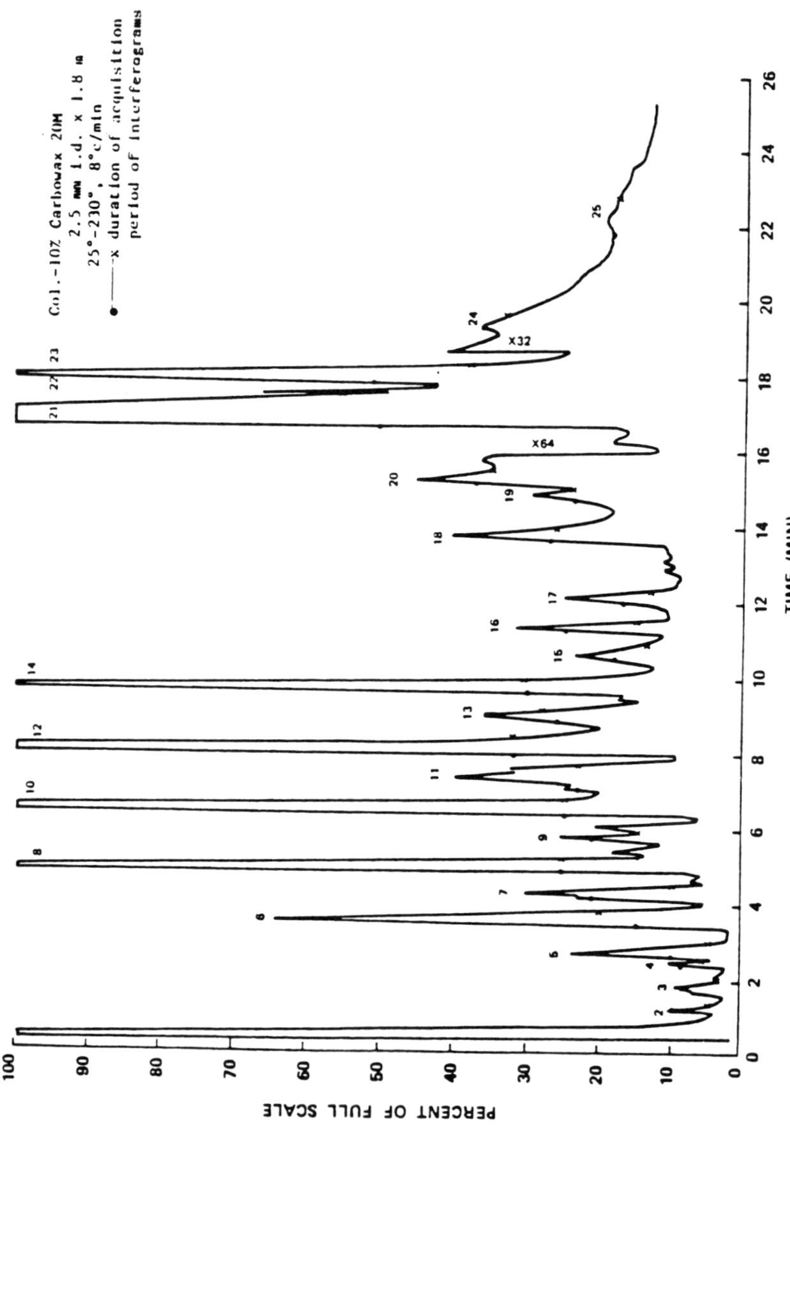


**Figure 14.** GLC (FID) of methylated acid fraction of product water obtained from in situ coal gasification.

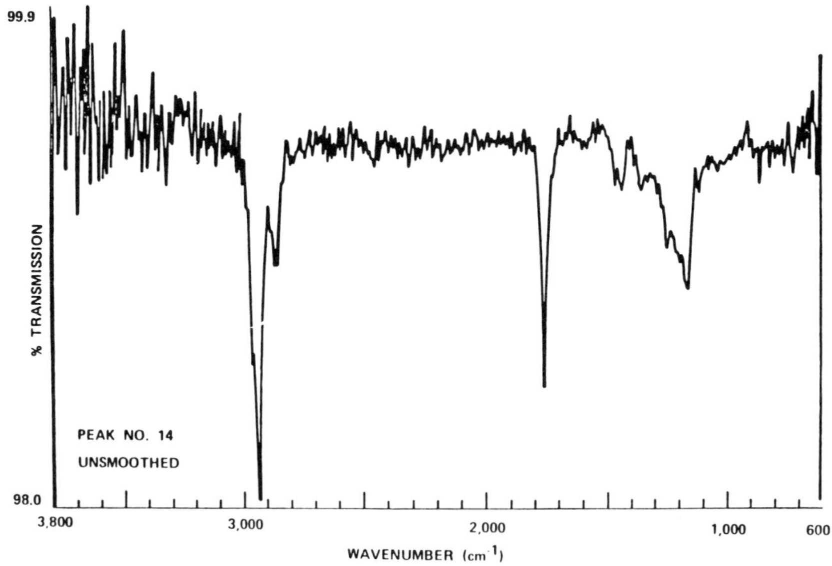


**Figure 15.** IR spectrum of peak No. 14 in Figure 14 identified as methyl nonanoate.

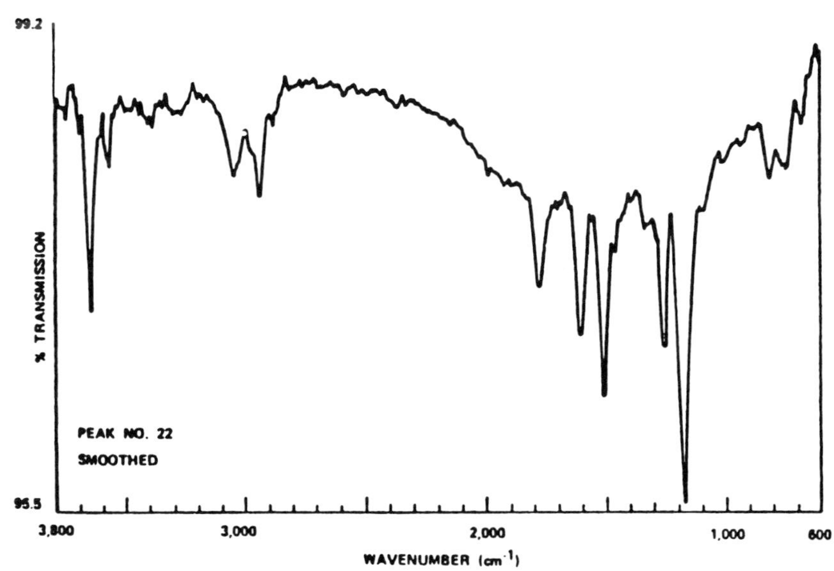


**Figure 16.** IR spectrum of peak No. 22 in Figure 14 identified as 3,5-dimethylphenol.

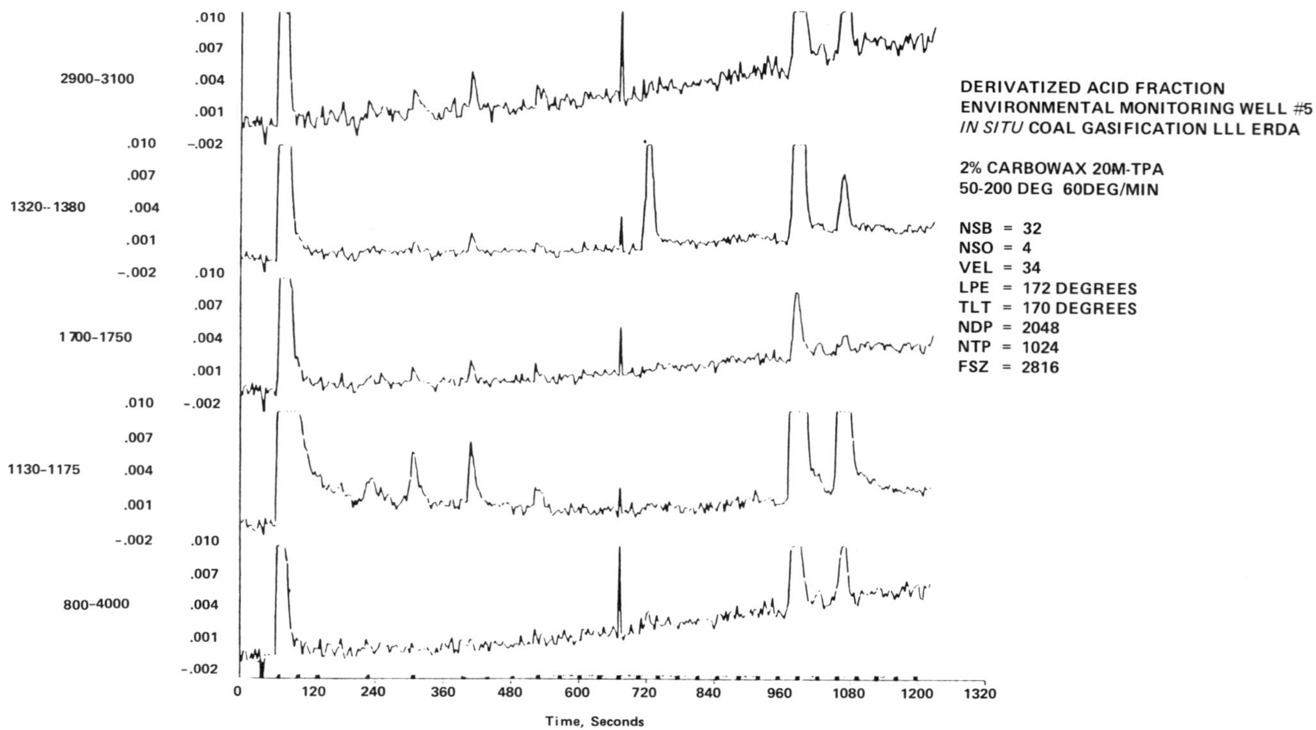


**Figure 17.** "Chemigrams.. of methylated acids in water from environmental monitoring well during in situ coal gasification burn (IR windows: 800–4000, 1130–1175, 1700–1750, 1320–1380 and 2900–3100 $cm^{-1}$).

## REFERENCES

1. National Academy of Sciences. "Principles for Evaluating Chemicals in the Environment," Report of the Committee for the Working Conference on Principles of Protocols for Evaluating Chemicals in the Environment, Washington, DC (1976), p. 299.
2. Commoner, B. In: *Identification and Analysis of Organic Pollutants in Water*, L. H. Keith, Ed. (Ann Arbor, MI: Ann Arbor Science Publishers, Inc., 1976), p. 51.
3. Ritch, J. B. "Protecting Public Health From Toxic Chemicals," *Environ. Sci. Technol.* 13:922 (1979).
4. Horwitz, W. "Practicability in Regulatory Analytical Chemistry," *Anal. Chem.*, 51:741A (1979).
5. Fine, D. H., D. P. Rounbehler and P. E. Oettinger. "A Rapid Method for the Determination of Subpart-Per-Billion Amounts of N-Nitroso Compounds in Foodstuff," *Anal. Chim. Acta.* 78:383-389 (1975).
6. Fine, D. H., and D. P. Rounbehler. "Trace Analysis of Volatile N-Nitroso Compounds by Combined Gas Chromatography and Thermal Energy Analysis," *J. Chromatog.* 109:271-279 (1975).
7. Fine, D. H., F. Rufeh, D. Lib and D. P. Rounbehler. "Positive and Negative Chemical Ionization Mass Spectra of Some Aromatic Chlorinated Pesticides," *Anal. Chem.* 47:1188 (1975).
8. Fine, D. H., F. Huffman, D. Rounbehler and N. M. Belcher. "Analysis of N-Nitroso Compounds by Comparing High Performance Liquid Chromatography and Thermal Energy Analysis," Fourth IARC Meeting on N-Nitroso Compounds, Tallinn, Estonia, USSR, October 1975.
9. Krull, I. S., and M. H. Wolf. "Thermal Energy Analysis for N-Nitroso Compounds," *Am. Lab.* (May 1979) p. 84.
10. Krull, I. S., and D. H. Fine. "Chemical Trace Analysis," in *Handbook of Carcingoens and Other Hazardous Substances*, M. C. Bowman, Ed. (New York: Marcel Dekker, 1979).
11. Krull, I. S., T. Y. Fan and D. H. Fine. "Problems of Artifacts in the Analysis of N-Nitroso Compounds," *Anal. Chem.* 50:698 (1978).
12. Krull, I. S., U. Goff, G. Hoffman and D. H. Fine. *Anal. Chem.* (in press).
13. Fine, D. H., D. P. Rounbehler, E. Sawicki, K. Krost and G. A. DeMarrais. "N-Nitroso Compounds in the Ambient Community Air of Baltimore, MD," *Anal. Lett.* 9:595-604 (1966).
14. Ostojic, N., and Z. Sterberg. "A New Photoionization Detector of Gas Chromatography," *Chromatographia* 7:3 (1973).
15. Driscoll, J. N., and F. F. Spaziani. "PID Development Gives New Performance Levels," *Res. Dev.* 27:50 (1976).
16. Driscoll, J. N., J. Ford, L. F. Jaramillo and E. T. Gruber. "Gas Chromatographic Detection and Identification of Aromatic and Aliphatic Hydrocarbons in Complex Mixtures by Coupling Photoionization and Flame-Ionization Detectors," *J. Chromatog.* 158:171 (1978).
17. Pellizzari, E. D. "Electron Capture Detection in Gas Chromatography," *Chromatog. Rev.* 98:323 (1974).
18. Dougherty, R. C., J. D. Roberts and F. J. Biros. "Positive and Negative Chemical Ionization Mass Spectra of Some Aromatic Chlorinated Pesticides," *Anal. Chem.* 47:54 (1975).

19. Dougherty, R. C., and K. Piotrowska. "Screening by Negative Chemical Ionization Mass Spectrometry for Environmental Contamination with Toxic Residues: Application to Human Urine," *Proc. Nat. Acad. Sci., U.S.* 73:1777 (1976).
20. Dougherty, R. C., J. Dalton and F. J. Biros. "Negative Chemical Ionization Mass Spectra of Polycyclic Chlorinated Insecticides," *Org. Mass Spectrom.* 6:1171 (1972).
21. Busch, K. L., M. M. Bursey and J. R. Hass. *Appl. Spectros.* in press).

# CHAPTER 11

# RECENT MASS SPECTROMETRIC TECHNIQUES FOR THE ANALYSIS OF ENVIRONMENTAL CONTAMINANTS

**J. Ronald Hass, Marlin D. Friesen and Michael K. Hoffman**

Laboratory of Environmental Chemistry
National Institute of Environmental Health Sciences
Research Triangle Park, North Carolina

## INTRODUCTION

Chlorinated aromatic compounds represent a class of chemicals that includes some of the most toxic environmental contaminants in the biosphere. Polychlorinated dibenzo-*p*-dioxins (PCDD) have been found to be highly toxic [1,2,3] and teratogenic [1,4,5] in animal studies as well as the etiologic agent in a number of animal [6,7,8] or human [9,10] diseases. Polychlorinated biphenyls (PCB) are among the most widely distributed contaminants known [11]. These compounds and their associated impurity, the polychlorinated dibenzofurans (PCDF) [12,13,14,15] have been implicated in a human disease syndrome [16]. The closely related polychlorodiphenyl ethers (PCDE) have also been found in used transformer fluid [17]. The determination of PCDD in environmental and biological samples has been the subject of considerable interest, and has recently been reviewed [18]. Several types of interferences have been recognized in attempts to determine the levels of PCDD or PCDF in such samples by glas chromatography/mass spectroscopy (GC/MS). These interferences may come from the sample matrix which itself is under analysis or it may take the form of "contamination" of the sample by the widely distributed polyhalogenated aromatic compound types. Before meaningful quantitative data may be obtained concerning a specific PCDD or PCDF, both of these interferences–matrix and chemical contamination–must be dealt with.

In general, interferences resulting from the matrix can be recognized by means of isotope ratio ($^{35}Cl/^{37}Cl$) measurements during the GC/MS analysis. Greater difficulties result from the similarities of the mass spectra of the chlorinated aromatics which are often found as a contaminant within the sample. For example, the ($M\text{-}Cl_2$) ion found in the EI spectrum of a hexachlorobiphenyl ether has exactly the same elemental composition as the molecular ion of a tetrachlorodibenzofuran. Analyses are further complicated because the numerous isomers of the PCB and PCDE which may be present in a sample, along with the suspected PCDD or PCDF, have GC retention times similar to the compounds of interest.

Negative chemical ionization mass spectrometry (NCI-MS) has been reported to give increased sensitivity and selectivity for the determination of halogenated aromatic compounds [19]. This chapter discusses interferences which arise through the use of NCI techniques for the determination of PCDF and PCDD in the presence of PCDE and PCB. The positive and negative ion Cl mass spectra of 14 PyCDD have been recently published [20]. In this study, interferences from 8 PCDF (Figures 1-8), 5 PCDE (Figures 9-13) and 8 PCB (Figures 14-21) are presented.

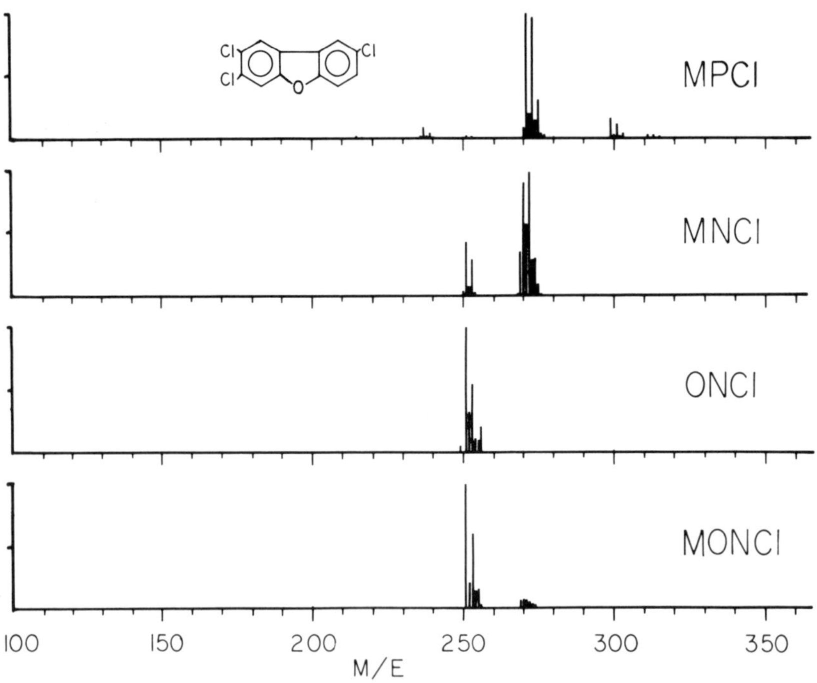


**Figure 1.** 2,3,8-Trichlorodibenzofuran.

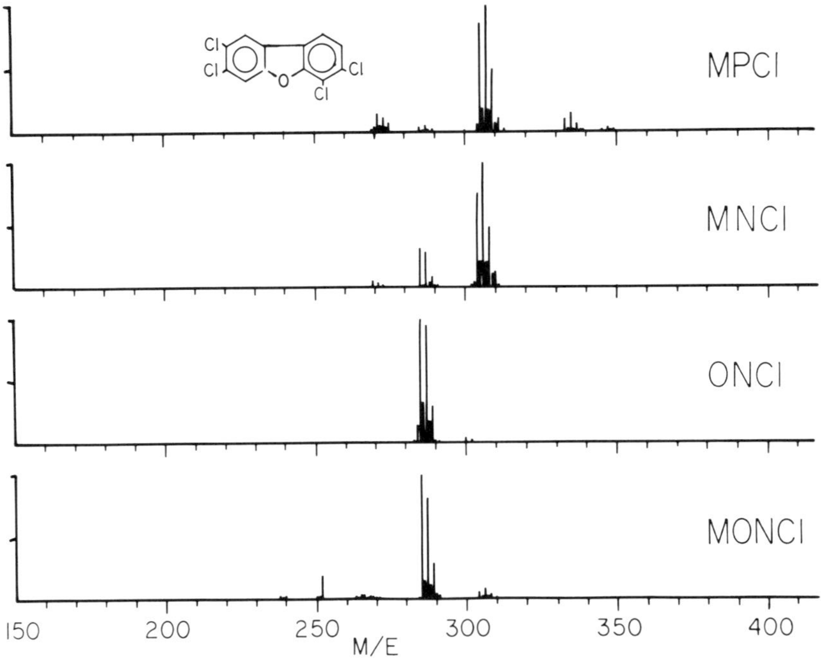


**Figure 2.** 2,3,6,7-Tetrachlorodibenzofuran.

## EXPERIMENTAL

Positive and negative chemical ionization mass spectra were obtained with a Finnigan 3300 mass spectrometer, modified as described previously [19]. Spectrometer control and data acquisition were accomplished by a Finnigan 6110 data system. All mass spectra were corrected for instrumental background. Oxygen, methane and methane/oxygen negative CI (ONCI, MNCI and MONCI) as well as methane positive CI (MPCI) mass spectra were acquired under the conditions previously described [20]. Chemicals were obtained from either commercial (RFR Corp., Hope, RI) or previously described sources [20].

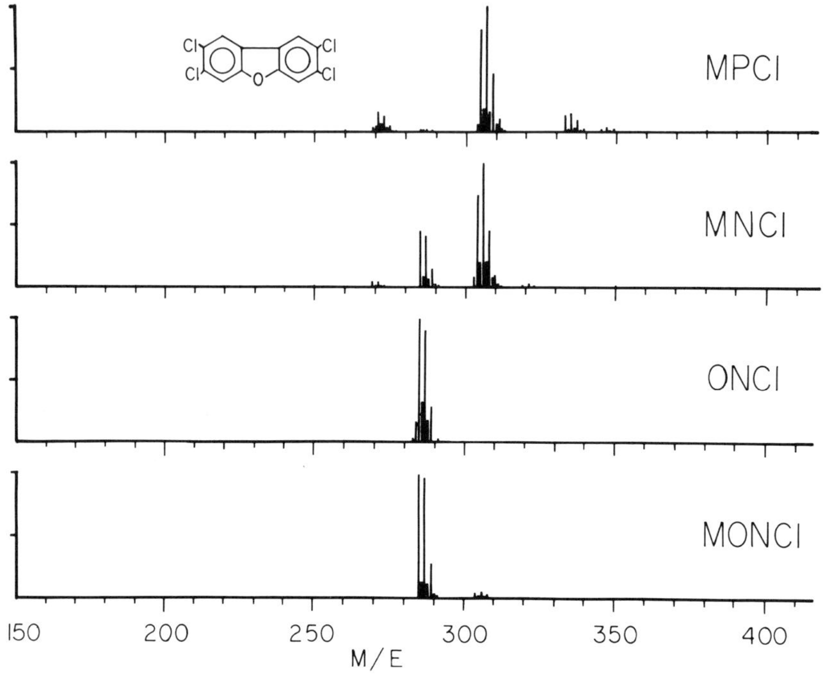


**Figure 3.** 2,3,7,8-Tetrachlorodibenzofuran.

## SUMMARY OF MASS SPECTRAL CHARACTERISTICS

### Methane Positive Ion Chemical Ionization (MPCI)

The MPCI spectra of the PCDD, PCDF, PCDE and PCB all have as base peak the protonated molecular ion $(MH)^+$. The single known exception to this generalization is decachlorodiphenylether which exhibits a base peak at m/z 263. This ion (m/z 263), the pentachlorophenoxy cation, represents cleavage of the ether linkage with charge remaining on the oxygen containing fragment. Also present in all cases are smaller peaks resulting from the addition of $C_2H_5$ $(M+29)^+$ and $C_3H_7$ $(M+41)^+$ cations to the molecular ion.

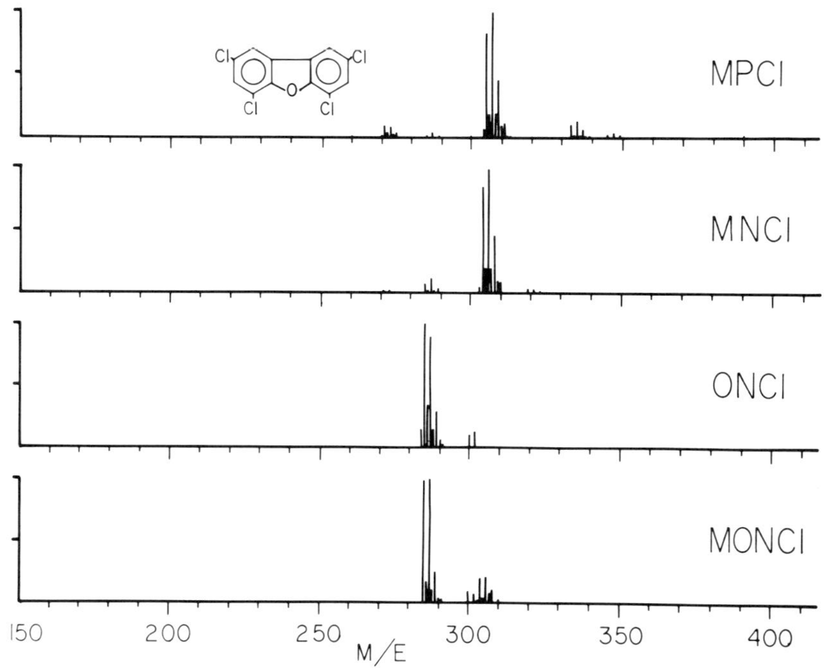


**Figure 4.** 2,4,6,8-Tetrachlorodibenzofuran.

*Polychlorinated Dibenzo-p-Dioxins*

In addition to the peaks mentioned above, dioxins exhibit minor peaks under MPCI conditions which can be rationalized by loss of Cl•, H• or combinations of the two from the protonated molecular ion [20].

*Polychlorinated Dibenzofurans*

Furans show no loss of Cl•, $(M\text{-}35)^+$; however, peaks are present for $(M\text{-}19)^+$ and $(M\text{-}33)^+$. The former is probably the result of exchange of oxygen for chlorine on the molecular ion, while the latter, as indicated by its chlorine isotope pattern, must in some way result from the loss of Cl• and the addition of the elements of hydrogen to the molecular ion.

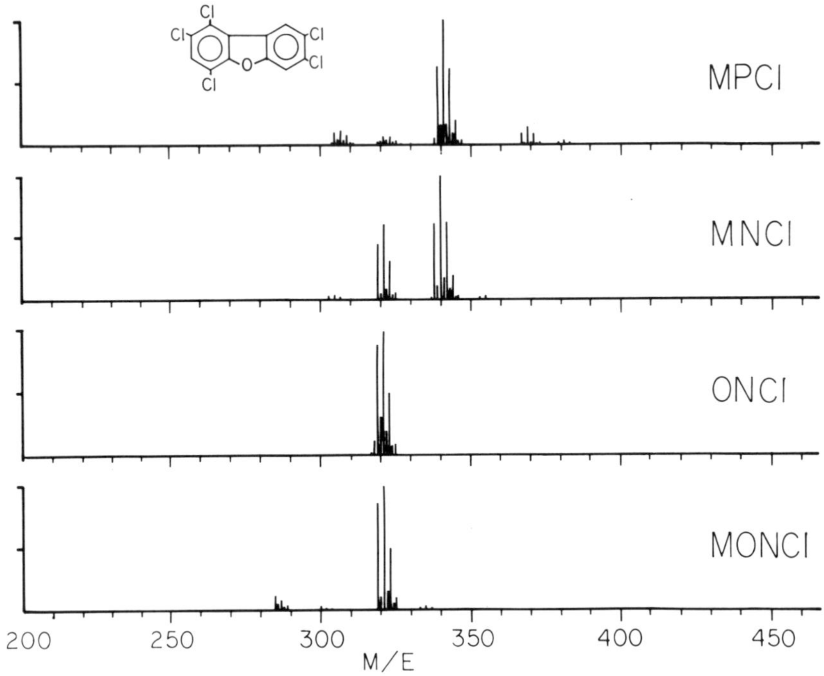


**Figure 5.** 1,2,4,7,8-Pentachlorodibenzofuran.

*Polychlorinated Diphenyl Ethers*

Diphenyl ethers have significant peaks from the formation of chlorinated phenoxy cations (m/z 127, 161, 195, 229 and 263). These peaks are surprisingly intense and for the decachloro isomer, the pentachlorophenoxy cation (m/z 263) is the base peak.

*Polychlorinated Biphenyls*

Biphenyls exhibit few fragment peaks of any intensity. The tetrachloro isomer studied does, however, give a small peak at $(M\text{-}35)^+$.

**Methane Negative Chemical Ionization Mass Spectra (MNCI)**

The MNCI mass spectra are complicated by the fact that it is nearly impossible completely to exclude oxygen from the chemical ionization

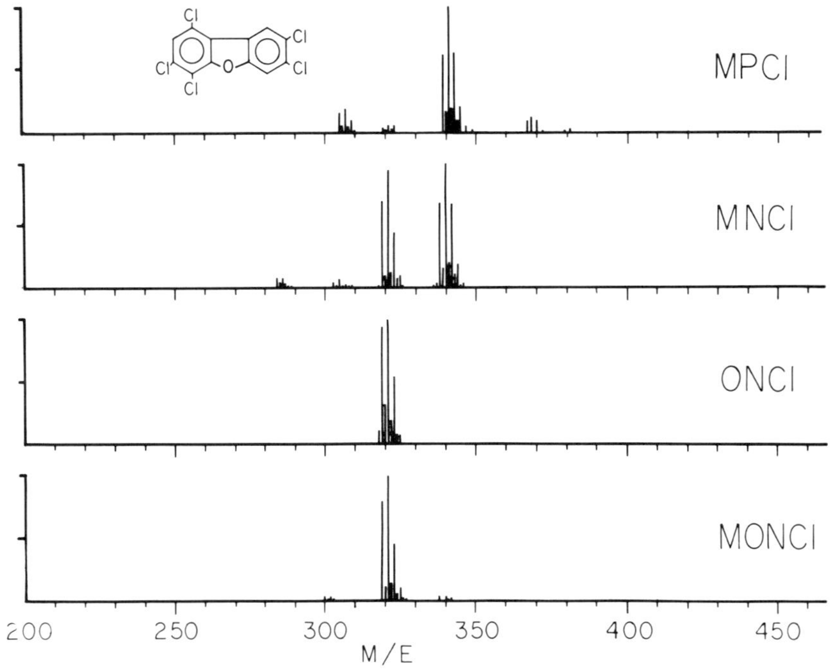


**Figure 6.** 1,3,4,7,8-Pentachlorodibenzofuran.

source. This is especially true if a gas chromatograph is used to introduce the sample into the mass spectrometer. For this reason, MNCI mass spectra consist of a composite of peaks resulting from resonance electron capture and dissociative electron capture processes (characteristics of operation in pure methane) and ion-molecule reactions (characteristic of operation in pure oxygen).

### *Polychlorinated Dibenzo-*p*-dioxins*

The dichlorodioxins produce mass spectra in which the base peak at $(M-1)^-$ results from loss of H• from the molecular anion [20]. For all other PCDD except the tetrachloro isomers, dissociative resonance capture predominates and results in a base peak at $(M-35)^{\bar{\cdot}}$. Further, a small peak consistent with the loss of $Cl_2$ is observed at $(M-70)^{\bar{\cdot}}$. Indeed, this peak is the base peak for the symmetrical 2,3,7,8-tetrachloro isomer.

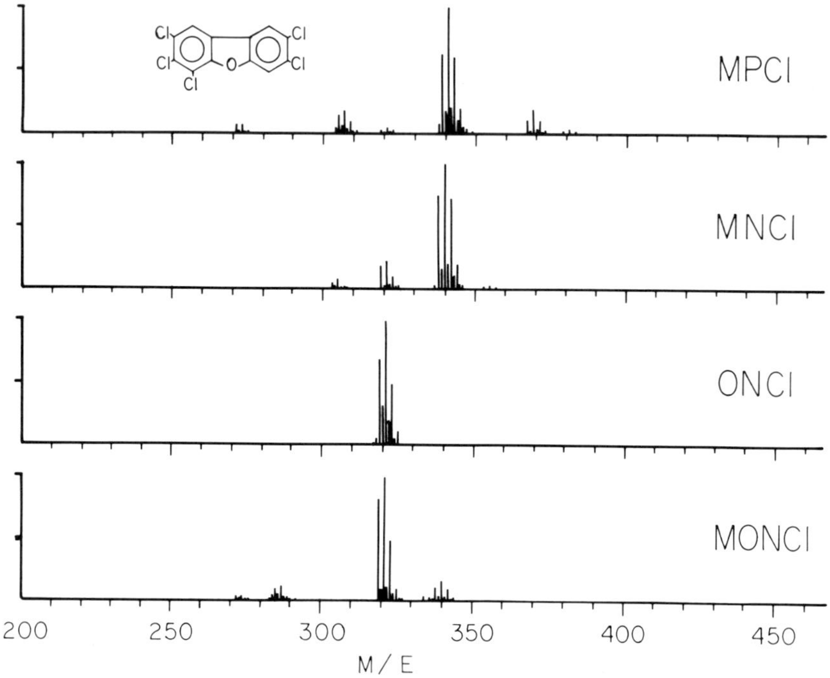


**Figure 7.** 2,3,4,7,8-Pentachlorodibenzofuran.

Other observed peaks are caused by oxygen impurity in the methane reagent plasma. These peaks, which are discussed in the following section on oxygen negative chemical ionization (ONCI), represent exchange of oxygen for chlorine $(M\text{-}19)^-$ on the molecular anion and formation of chloro-*ortho*-quinone (CloQ) radical anions. The peak at $(M\text{-}19)^-$ is the base peak in the spectrum of the highly unsymmetrical 1,2,3,4-tetrachloro isomer, whereas the chloro-*ortho*-quinone radical anion at m/e 176 is characteristic of the 2,3,7,8-tetrachloro isomer.

*Polychlorinated Dibenzofurans*

Under MNCI conditions, furans exhibit molecular anion base peaks, $M^{\overline{\cdot}}$, resulting from resonance electron capture. In addition, small peaks caused by loss of Cl· or $Cl_2$ from the molecular anion are observed. As with the dioxins, the presence of trace amounts of oxygen can give rise to significant peaks at $(M\text{-}19)^-$.

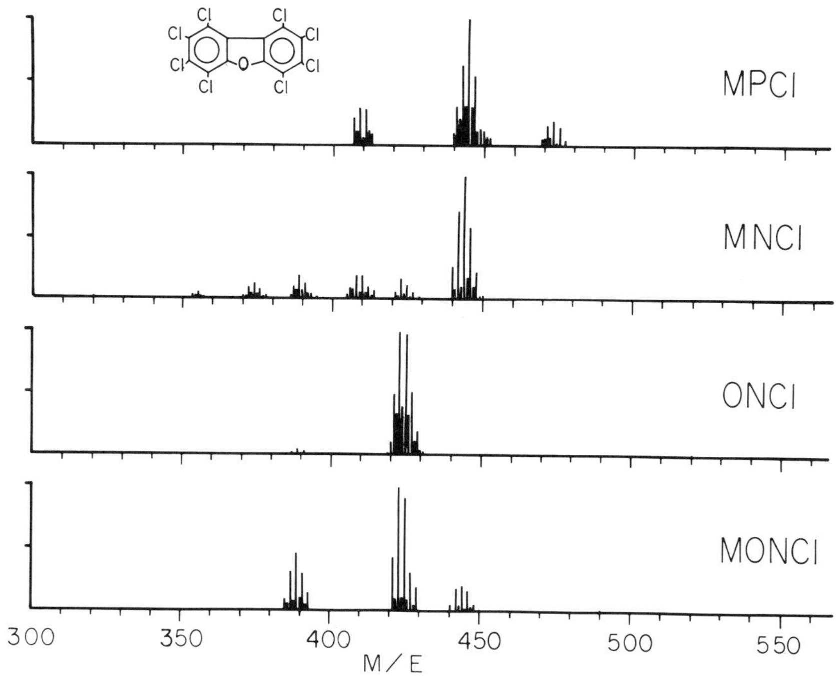


**Figure 8.** 1,2,3,4,6,7,8,9-Octachlorodibenzofuran.

*Polychlorinated Diphenyl Ethers*

Fragmentation reactions of chlorodiphenyl ethers closely resemble those of dioxins in that loss of Cl. from the molecular anion $(M\text{-}35)^-$ is the base peak for most isomers. Exceptions include the decachloro isomer, which fragments preferentially to produce the pentachlorophenoxy radical anion (m/z 263) and the 3,3′,4,4′-tetrachloro isomer for which the molecular ion, $M^{\overline{\cdot}}$, is the base peak. It should be noted this isomer is the one diphenyl ether studied which had no chlorine substitution *ortho* to the oxygen atom.

The inability to remove all oxygen leads to significant peaks at $(M\text{-}19)^-$ and $(M\text{-}55)^{\overline{\cdot}}$. The latter peak implies exchange of oxygen for chlorine and loss of HCl from the molecular anion. In addition, small peaks are observed in all cases for chlorophenoxy radical anions resulting from cleavage of phenyloxygen bond. These peaks are useful in determining the number of chlorines present on each of the two phenyl rings of the parent diphenyl ether molecule.

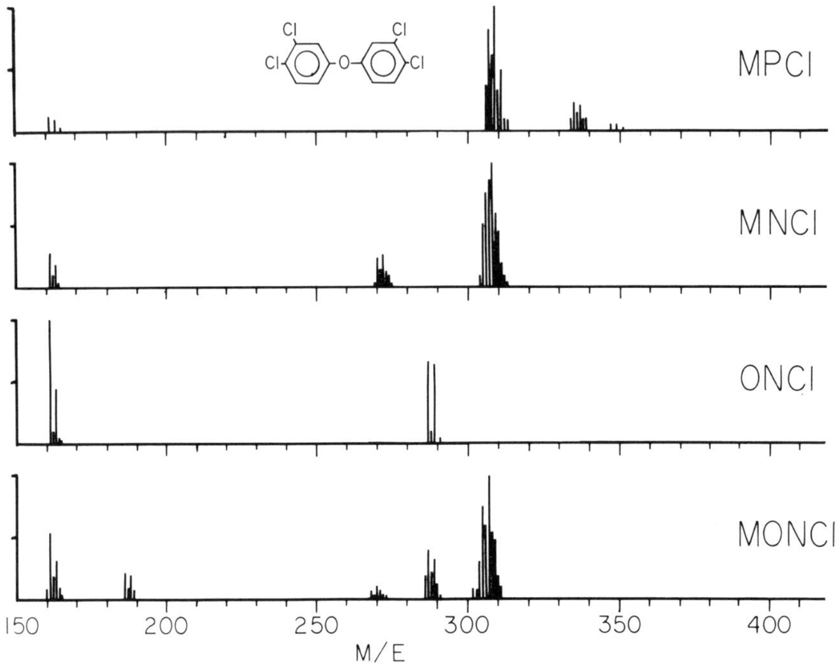


**Figure 9.** 3,3′,4,4′-Tetrachlorodiphenyl ether.

*Polychlorinated Biphenyls*

Biphenyls exhibit the molecular anion, $M^{\overline{\cdot}}$, as the base peak under MNCI conditions. A small $(M\text{-}35)^-$ peak is also observed, as well as significant peaks at $(M\text{-}19)^-$ resulting from ion-molecular reactions involving oxygen.

## Oxygen Negative Chemical Ionization (ONCI) Mass Spectra

ONCI mass spectra are of special interest because most of the peaks observed result from ion-molecule reactions between oxygen and negatively charged sample ions. Such reactions lead to fragment ions which can often be very helpful in determining the structure of the sample molecule.

*Polychlorinated Dibenzo-*p*-dioxins*

The ONCI spectra of polychlorodibenzo-*p*-dioxins have been described previously [20], and will be summarized briefly. Most of the negative ion

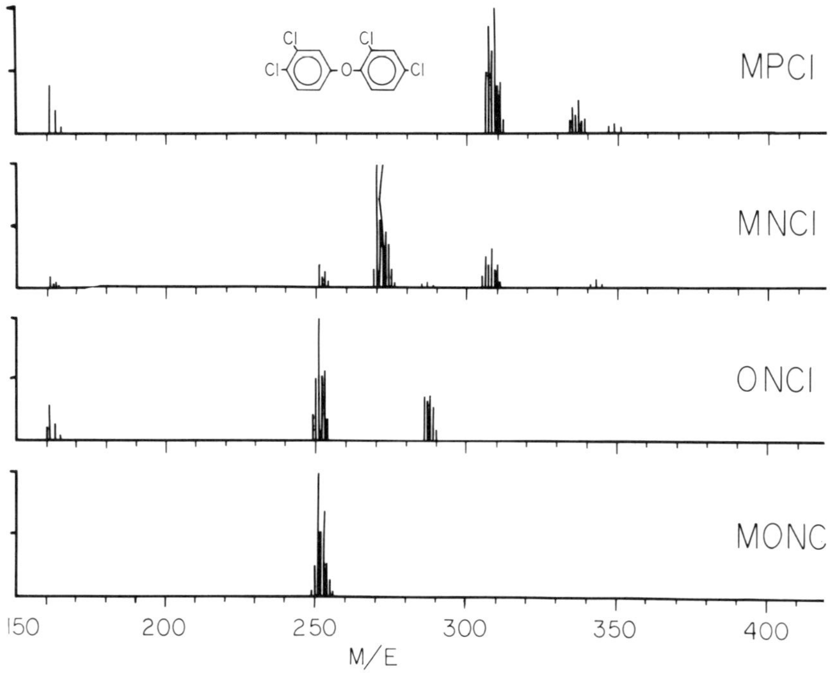


**Figure 10.** 2,3′,4,4′-Tetrachlorodiphenyl ether.

current is carried by either an ion resulting from the displacement of chlorine by oxygen $(M\text{-}19)^-$ or by the reaction of the dioxin molecular anion with oxygen to give the two possible chloroquinoxide anions. The formation of the CloQ anion is a major process in the absence of Cl adjacent to the ether oxygen. Additional peaks are observed in the ONCI mass spectra of certain dioxins corresponding to exchange of oxygen for hydrogen on the chloro-*ortho*-quinone radical anion $(\text{CloQ} + 15)^{\overline{\cdot}}$, exchange of oxygen for chlorine from the radical anion fragment $(\text{CloQ} - 19)^-$ or the M-19 anion $(M\text{-}38)^-$ and exchange of oxygen for HCl $(M\text{-}20)^{\overline{\cdot}}$. In addition, many dioxins give peaks for loss of hydrogen $(M\text{-}1)^-$ and for exchange of oxygen for HCl $(M\text{-}4)^{\overline{\cdot}}$.

*Polychlorinated Dibenzofurans*

The ONCI mass spectra of all dibenzofurans examined are dominated by the exchange of oxygen for chlorine to give $(M\text{-}19)^-$ as the base peak. Small peaks are also present in the mass spectra of certain isomers because of the

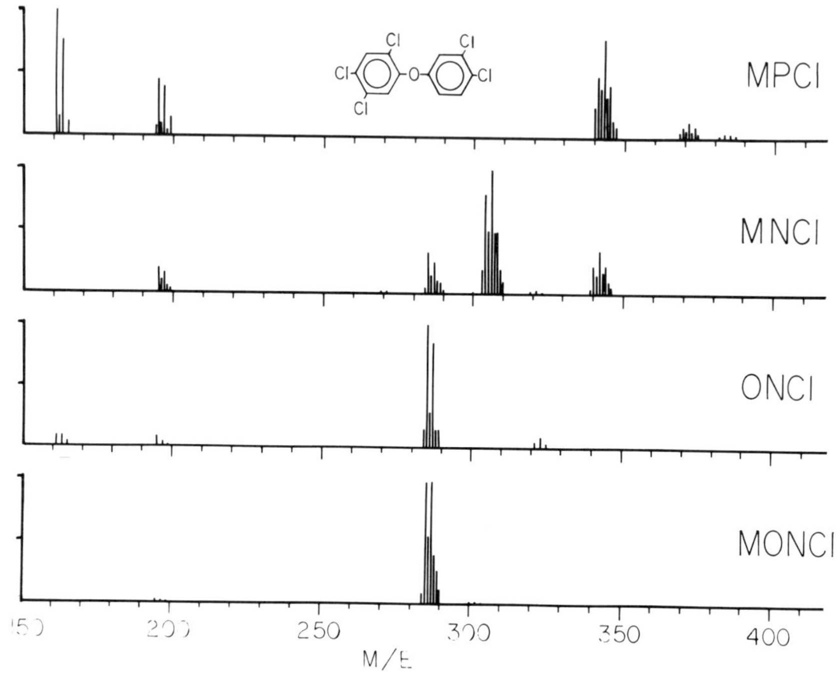


**Figure 11.** 2,3′,4,4′,5-Pentachlorodiphenyl ether.

exchange of the elements of oxygen for HCl $(M\text{-}4)^{\bar{\cdot}}$. Octachlorodibenzofuran exhibits a small peak at $(M\text{-}54)^-$ because of the loss of the elements of chlorine in exchange for oxygen.

*Polychlorinated Diphenyl Ethers*

The principal reactions of chlorodiphenyl ethers under ONCI conditions are outlined in Figure 22. In general, those isomers with at least one chlorine group *ortho* to oxygen yeild a base peak $(M\text{-}55)^-$ representing the displacement of chlorine by oxygen with the additional loss of HCl. A peak at $(M\text{-}19)^-$ is also present and, for those isomers with no chlorine substitution *ortho* to oxygen, it becomes significant in comparison to $(M\text{-}55)^{\bar{\cdot}}$. Important peaks representing chlorophenoxy anions are also observed, becoming the base peak in the case of the decachloro and the 3,3′,4,4′-tetrachloro isomers. In addition, decachloro diphenyl ether exhibits no peaks resulting from ion-molecule reactions with oxygen, i.e., $(M\text{-}19)^-$ or $(M\text{-}55)^-$ are absent. It does, however, yield a significant peak for loss of Cl• from the molecular anion.

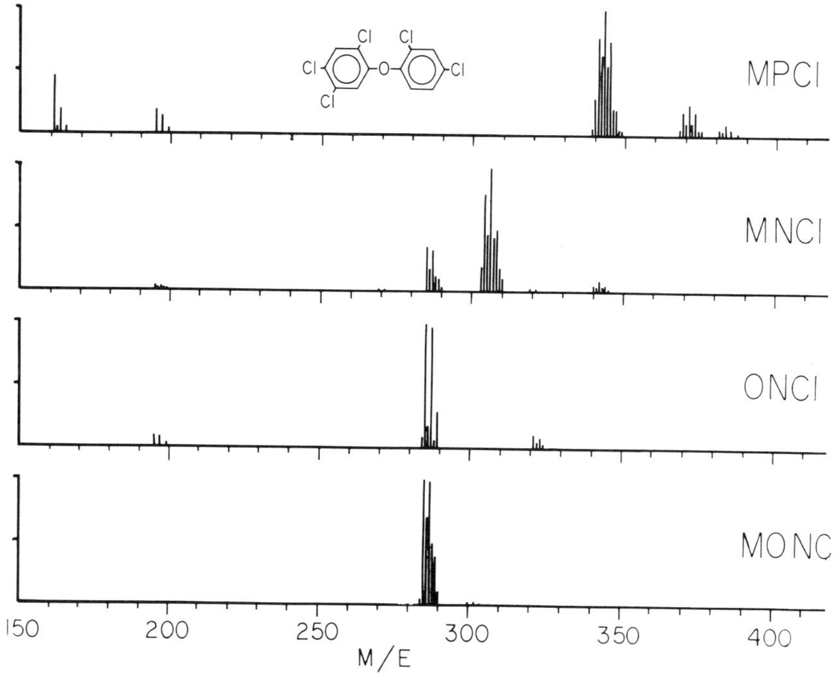


**Figure 12.** 2,2′,4,4′,5-Pentachlorodiphenyl ether.

*Polychlorinated Biphenyls*

All ONCI mass spectra of polychlorinated biphenyls exhibit $(M\text{-}19)^-$ as the base peak. Small peaks are observed for the molecular anion $M^{\overline{\cdot}}$.

## Methane/Oxygen Negative Chemical Ionization (MONCI) Mass Spectra

In an effort to avoid the problems associated with the Townsend discharge ion source, while retaining the useful information obtained with oxygen as the reagent gas, spectra were run under conditions where the methane:oxygen ratio was about 10:1. The MONCI mass spectra thus obtained are expected to resemble a mixture of ONCI and MNCI related peaks.

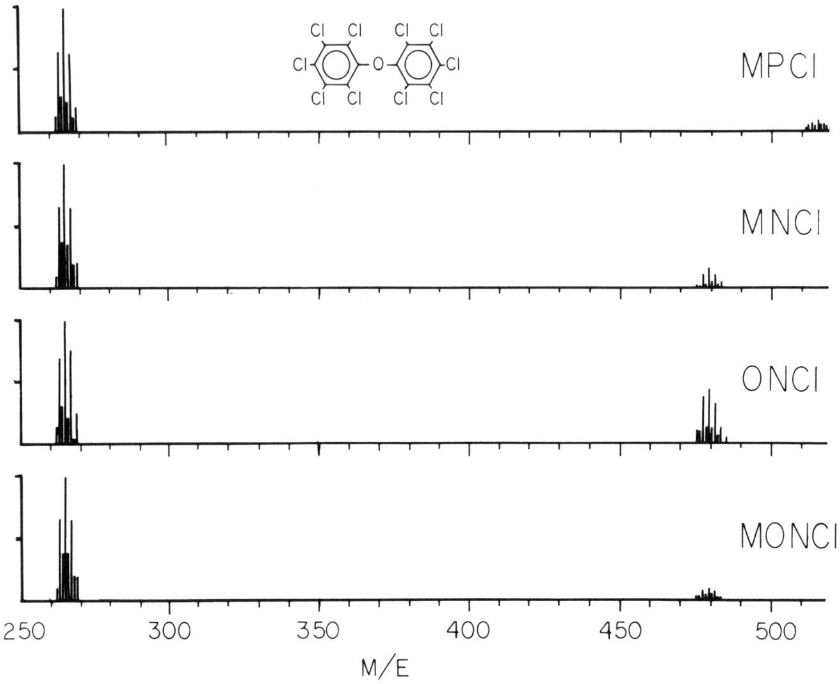


**Figure 13.** 2,2′,3,3′,4,4′,5,5′,6,6′-Decachlorodiphenyl ether.

*Polychlorinated Dibenzo-*p*-dioxins*

For the dioxins, peaks observed under MNCI conditions predominate. In general, however, chloro-*ortho*-quinone radical anions were more intense than under MNCI conditions. In addition, the two tetrachloro isomers gave MONCI mass spectra similar to their ONCI spectra.

*Polychlorinated Dibenzofurans*

The MONCI mass spectra of furans were nearly identical to their ONCI mass spectra. Small peaks were also observed for $M^{\overline{\cdot}}$ and $(M\text{-}35)^-$.

*Polychlorinated Diphenylethers*

The MONCI mass spectra of chlorodiphenyl ethers closely resembled their ONCI mass spectra. An exception was the spectrum of the 3,3′,4,4′-tetrachloro isomer (Figure 9).

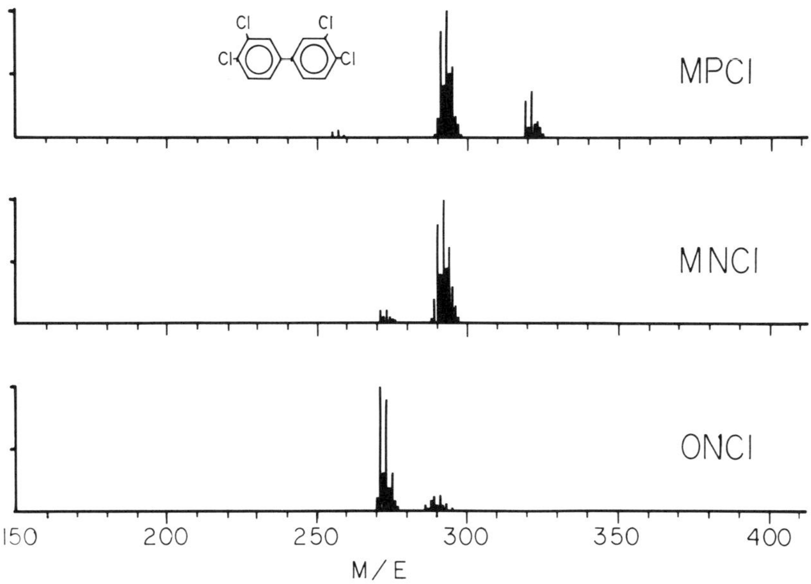


**Figure 14.** 3,3′,4,4′-Tetrachlorobiphenyl.

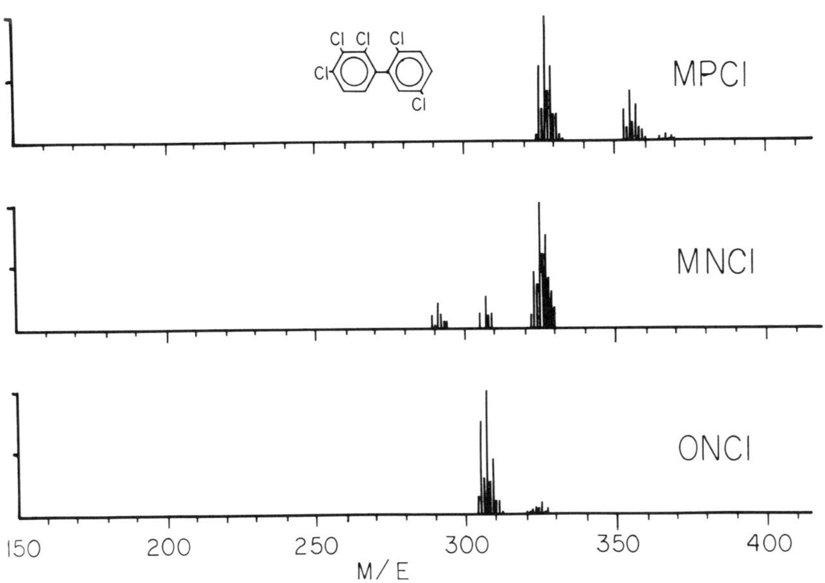


**Figure 15.** 2,2′,3,4,5′-Pentachlorobiphenyl.

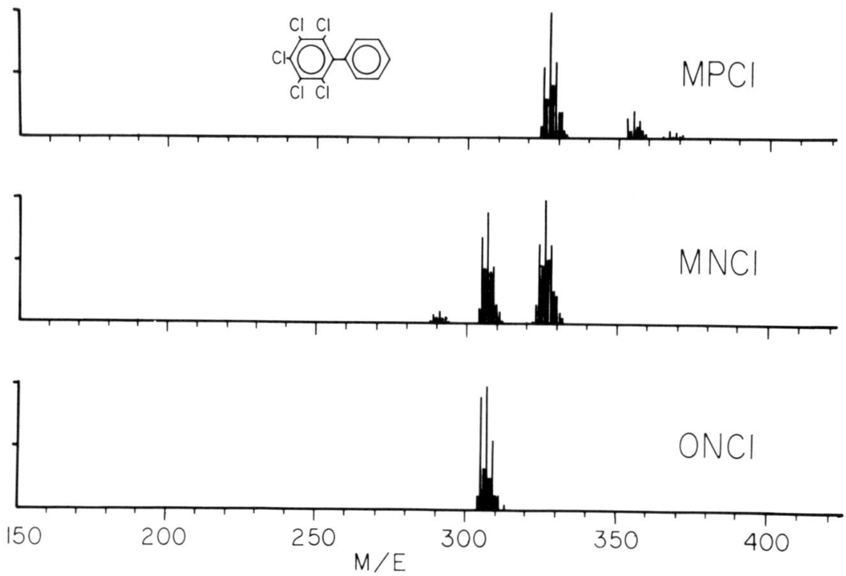


**Figure 16.** 2,3,4,5,6-Pentachlorobiphenyl.

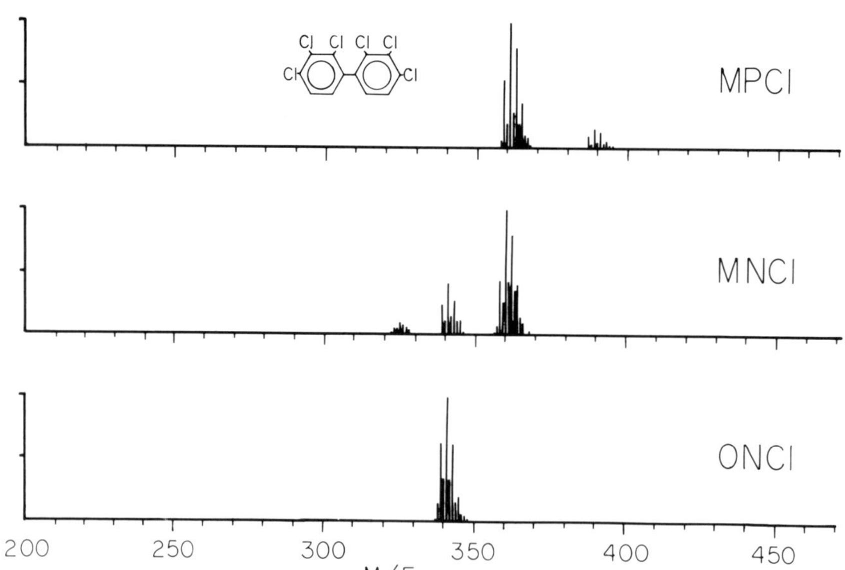


**Figure 17.** 2,2′,3,3′,4,4′-Hexachlorobiphenyl.

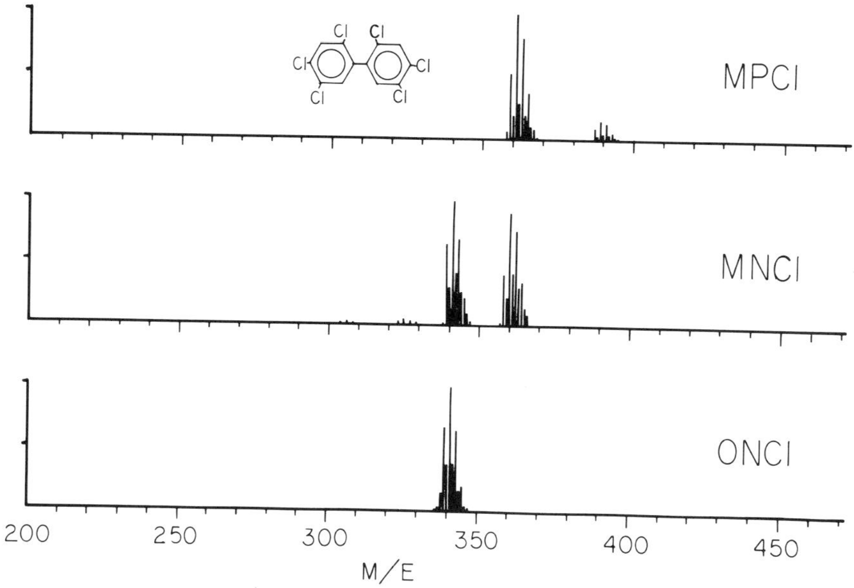


**Figure 18.** 2,2′,4,4′,5,5′-Hexachlorobiphenyl.

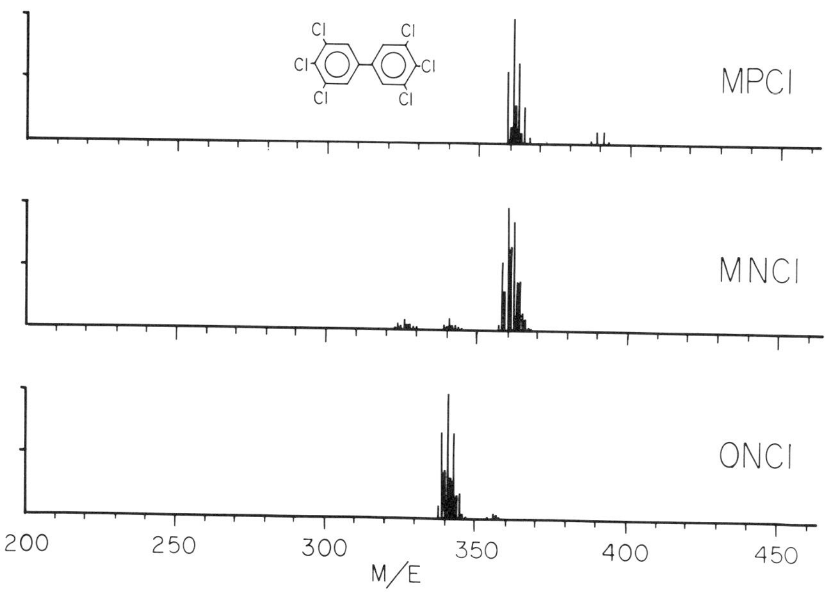


**Figure 19.** 3,3′,4,4′,5,5′-Hexachlorobiphenyl.

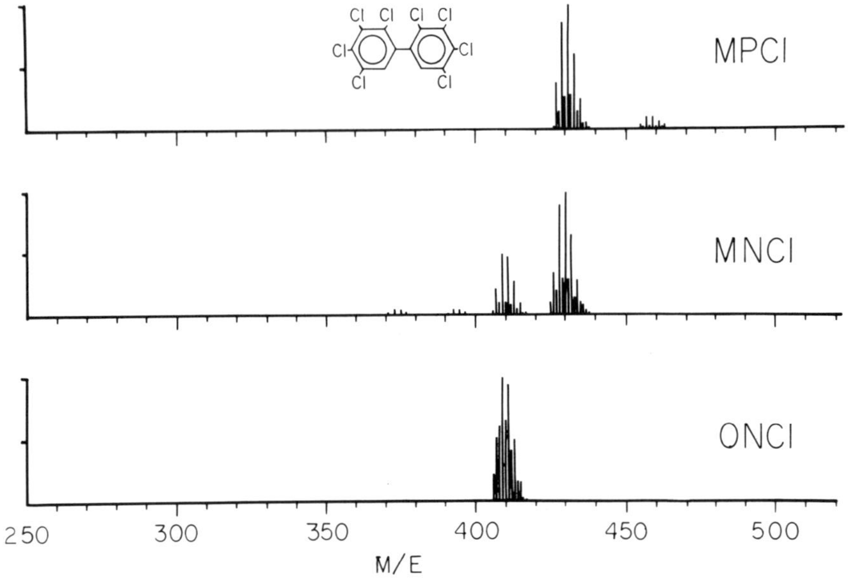


**Figure 20.** 2,2′,3,3′,4,4′,5,5′-Octachlorobiphenyl.

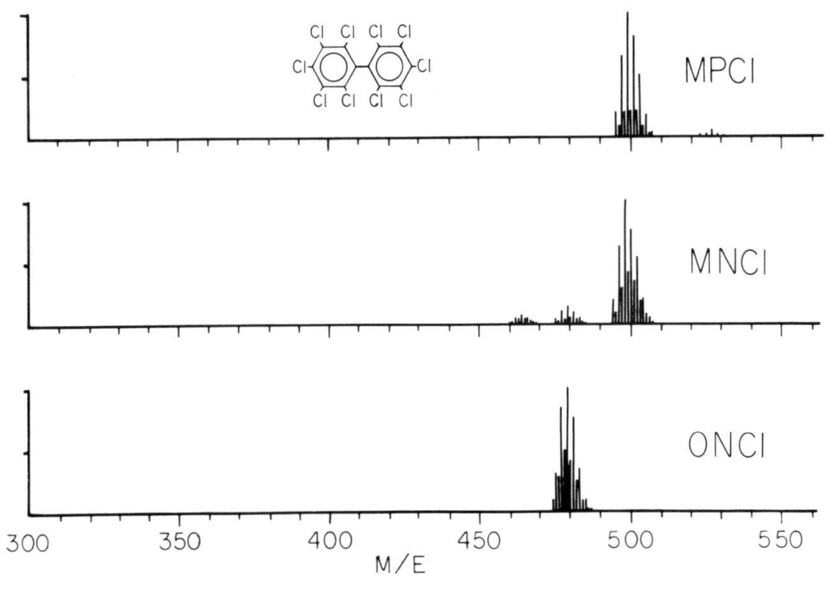


**Figure 21.** 2,2′,3,3′,4,4′,5,5′,6,6′-Decachlorobiphenyl.

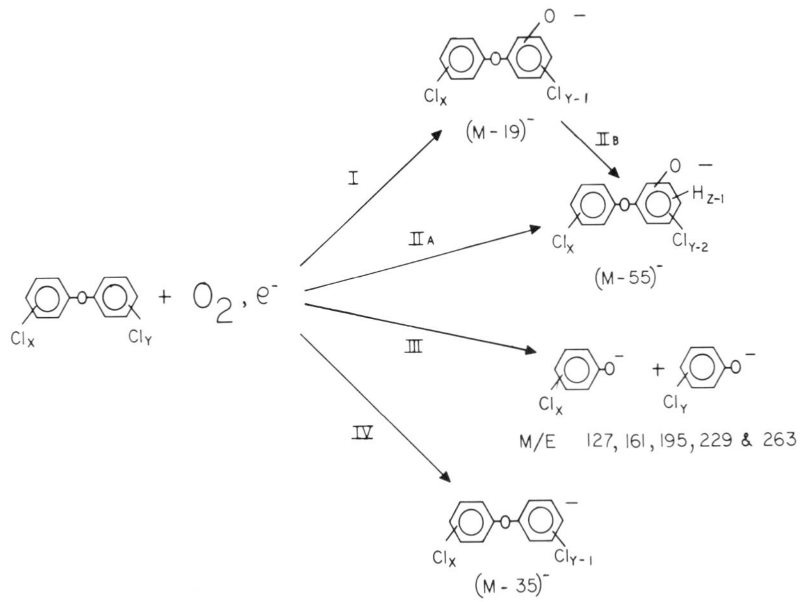


**Figure 22.** Reactions of chlorodiphenyl ethers under oxygen negative chemical ionization conditions.

## DISCUSSION

### Analytical Implications

Major peaks exhibited by the four groups of compounds studied under negative chemical ionization conditions are summarized in Table I. In general, one observes that oxygen-containing compounds react differently than non-oxygen-containing compounds. In addition, among the reagent gases studied, the greatest amount of structural information is gained with the use of oxygen or methane mixed with oxygen.

Of apparent analytical importance is the observation that for dioxins and diphenyl ethers under ONCI or MONCI conditions, chlorine substitution at the ring positions *ortho* to oxygen dictates whether cleavage or chlorine substitution will predominate. For example, 2,3,7,8-TCDD, with no such *peri* chlorines gives a base peak at m/e 176, representing the dichloro-*ortho*-quinone radical anion whereas 1,2,3,4-TCDD with 2 *peri* chlorines gives

**Table I. Major Peaks in the Mass Spectra of PCDD, PCDF, PCDPE and PCB**

| | PCDD | PCDF | PCDPE | PCB |
|---|---|---|---|---|
| MPCl | $(M + 1)^+$ | $(M + 1)^+$ | $(M + 1)^+$ | $(M + 1)^+$ |
| MNCl | $(M - 35)^-$ | $(M)^-$ | $(M - 35)^-$ | $(M)^-$ |
| ONCl | $(M - 19)^-$ | $(M - 19)^-$ | $(M - 19)^-$ | $(M - 19)^-$ |
| | | | $(M - 55)^-$ | |
| | 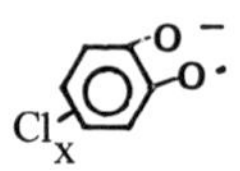 | | 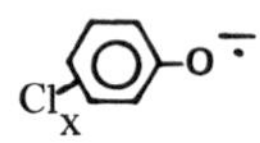 | |

predominantly $(M\text{-}19)^-$. Assuming this observation to be general, one has a means of determining the number of chlorines per ring and the presence of *peri* chlorines in an unknown dioxin by monitoring the proper ions. For example, 2,3,7,8-TCDD is the only tetrachlorodioxin isomer which has no *peri* chlorines. It could be uniquely identified by monitoring dichloro-*ortho*-quinone radical anion isotope peaks at m/e 176 (intense) and the $(M\text{-}19)^-$ chlorine displacement isotope peaks at m/e 301 (weak). In fact, this technique can provide a more positive identification of a specific dioxin than is possible with GC/EIMS using either low or high resolution techniques since any information provided by GC retention times is still available, and interference from dioxin exact mass equivalents such as chlorophenylbenzoquinones, or fragment ions from the other chemically interfering compounds, will not be encountered.

Similar information is available in the case of chlorodiphenyl ethers under ONCI conditions. Here, however, *ortho*-chloro substitution seems to lead to a preference for formation of $(M\text{-}55)^-$ anions rather than $(M\text{-}19)^-$ anions. Clearly, too few compounds were analyzed to make sweeping generalizations; however, such reactions do show analytical promise. As with the dioxins, fragment anions indicative of chlorine substitution are observed. Their importance is diminished somewhat, however, because the same information can be gained with more sensitivity under positive chemical ionization conditions.

## Specificity

The cleanup procedure which precedes MS must assure that only a narrow range of compound types will be present in the final analysis. The cleanup procedure presently in use in the authors' laboratory has been described previously [21]. The initial chloroform:methanol extraction effectively removes the compounds of interest from the bulk of the tissue matrix. The sulfuric acid cleanup step is necessary to separate the compounds of interest from lipids carried along in the initial extraction. Such highly acidic conditions do not favor generation or destruction of dioxins; however, a finite amount of carbon tetrachloride is soluble in concentrated sulfuric acid, and a corresponding loss of dioxin or furan will be noted. An appropriate correction for any such loss can be applied by noting the volume of carbon tetrachloride before and after extraction with $H_2SO_4$, as confirmed by radiolabel experiments.

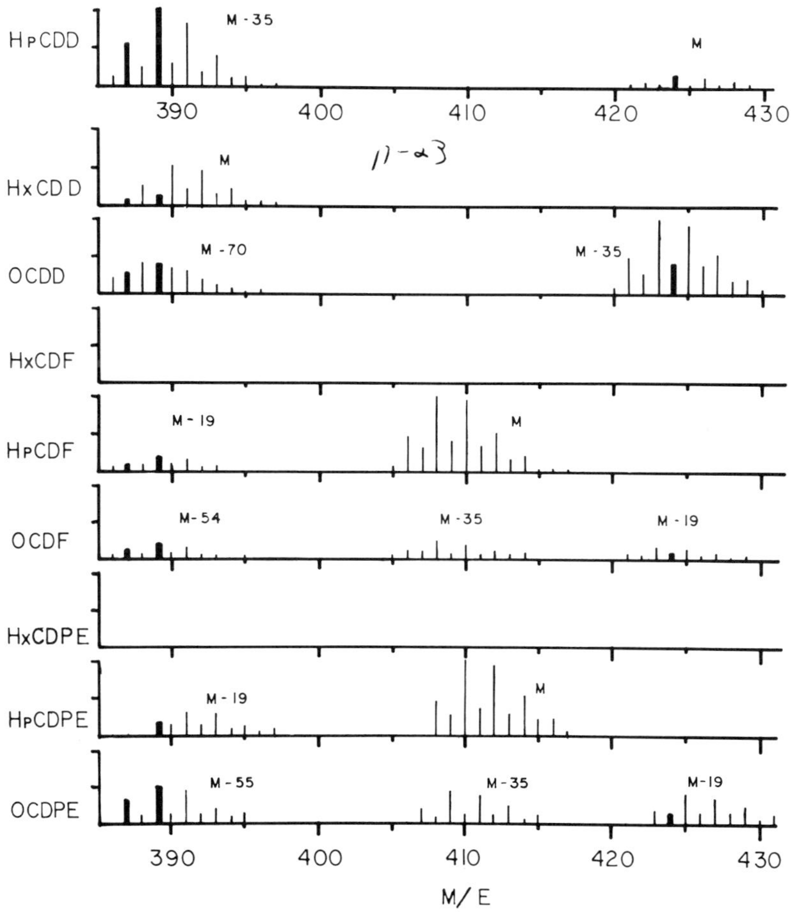


**Figure 23.** MNCI mass spectra of compounds expected to interfere with a heptachlorodibenzo-*p*-dioxin (HpCDD). Hx = hexa, O = octa.

The fractionation step involving column chromatography is very important in the overall analysis. It has been shown that reactions can and do take place in the heated injection port of a gas chromatograph which can produce interfering species. For example, *ortho*-hydroxychlorodiphenylethers (predioxins) react to form dioxins at high temperatures. Chlorophenols and "predioxins," however, are more polar than dioxins and furans, and are not eluted in the 20% methylene chloride:hexane fraction. Polychlorinated biphenyls are less polar and are removed as potential interferences in the 3% methylene chloride:hexane fraction. Ideally, the fraction of interest is left with only the chlorinated dioxins, furans and, possibly, chlorodiphenyl ethers to interfere with each other.

GC adds a measure of added specificity over introduction of the entire sample into the mass spectrometer ion source from a heated probe cup. However, even with capillary column techniques [22], interfering compounds can coelute with the compounds of interest. Obviously, the problem will be most severe for tetrachloro, pentachloro and hexachloro isomers where more possible interfering isomers exist.

We can look at one compound in detail to examine the possible interferences. Figure 23 shows the spectrum of a heptachlorodibenzo-*p*-dioxin obtained under methane negative chemical ionization mass spectrometric conditions. Below it are displayed the spectra of dioxins, furans and diphenyl ethers which would be expected to interfere under conditions where GC separation is inadequate. Note that peaks at masses 387 and 389 in the $(M\text{-}35)^-$ fragment ion cluster and at 424 in the $M^-$ molecular anion cluster have been emphasized to indicate that they were the ions monitored in the actual selective ion monitoring analysis.

HxCDD are seen to interfere only with the fragment ion peaks at m/z 387 and 389. OCDD, with one more chlorine than HpCDD, is more troublesome because its fragmentations produce interferences at both m/z 387 and 389 in $(M\text{-}35)^-$ and at m/z 424 in the molecular anion of HxCDD. A well-chosen set of GC conditions should help to eliminate this problem by separating families of dioxins with equivalent numbers of chlorines into distinct bands.

Chlorodibenzofurans elute from 3% OV210 in approximately the same time span as the chlorodibenzodioxins having the same number of chlorines. Again, however, it is seen that only furans with chlorine substitution greater than or equal to that of the dioxin in question will interfere. Interfering peaks (M-19 cluster from HpCDF overlaps with the M-35 cluster from HpCDF as would the M-54 cluster from OCDF; the M-19 cluster from OCDF will interfere in the molecular anion region of HpCDD) result from ion-molecule reactions involving oxygen and could conceivably be eliminated by operating under conditions where oxygen was completely excluded from the methane

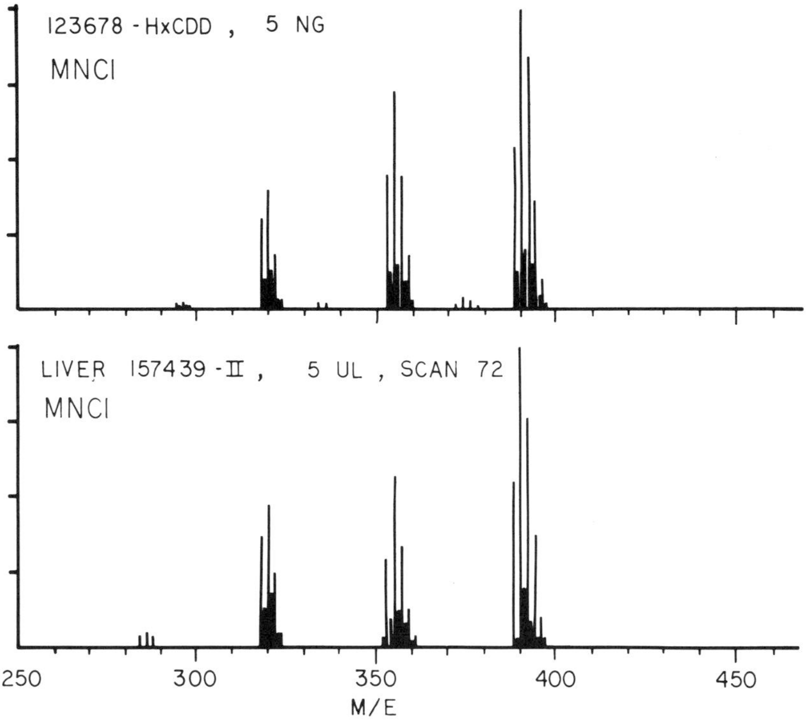


**Figure 24.** MONCI mass spectrum of the peak identified as 1,2,3,6,7,8-HxCDD in liver 157439-II.

reagent plasma. Unfortunately, this has not been practical in the case of GC/MS.

was completely excluded from the methane reagent plasma. Unfortunately, this has not been practical in the case of GC/MS.

Peaks causing interference in dioxin spectra because of chlorodiphenyl ethers are also a result of oxygen-related ion-molecule reactions. Only chlorodiphenyl ethers which have at least two more chlorines than the dioxin in question interfere at both $(M\text{-}35)^-$ and $M^-$. On 3% OV210, chlorodiphenyl ethers elute faster than like-substituted dioxins and as an example, an octachlorodiphenyl ether conceivably could interfere with a hexachlorodioxin. Any possibility of interference by chlorodiphenyl ethers can be eliminated by monitoring the $C_6H_{4-n}Cl_nO_2$ ion using MONCI.

As noted in an earlier publication [19], negative chemical ionization techniques are generally more sensitive than positive ion techniques for the analysis of these chlorinated aromatic compounds. This improved sensitivity of NCI can result in improved specificity by permitting one to obtain full mass spectra rather than just the ratio of a few ion intensities. This is illustrated in Figure 24, which shows easily interpreted MONCI spectrum of an HxCDD obtained from a cow liver sample (compare with standard). This particular sample contained insufficient levels of these compounds for their detection even by selected ion monitoring techniques when EI ionization was employed. Obviously, the availability of full mass spectra greatly reduces the probability of interference in measurement steps of an analysis.

## CONCLUSIONS

Potential interferences arising from the analysis of PCDD, PCDF, PCDE and PCB mixtures by NCI techniques have been examined. Interference resulting from EI ionization such as $(M\text{-}Cl_2)^{+\cdot}$ ion from a PCDE occurring at the same mass and $M^{+\cdot}$ from a PCDF initially containing two fewer chlorines are avoided by use of NCI techniques. However, a new potential interferenence arises from oxygen displacement of chlorine reactions in PCB. Thus, reliable determinations should be based upon both EI and NCI measurements for each sample.

## REFERENCES

1. Courtney, K. D., and J. A. Moore. "Teratology Studies with 2,4,5-Trichlorophenoxyacetic Acid and 2,3,7,8-Tetrachlorodibenzo-*p*-dioxin," *Toxicol. Appl. Pharmacol.* 20:396-403 (1971).
2. McConnell, E. E., J. A. Moore, J. K. Haseman and M. W. Harris. "The Comparative Toxicity of Chlorinated Dibenzo-*p*-dioxins in Mice and Guinea Pigs," *Toxicol. Appl. Pharmacol.* 44:335-356 (1978).
3. McConnell, E. E., J. A. Moore and D. W. Dalgard. "Toxicity of 2,3,7,8-Tetrachlorodibenzo-*p*-dioxin (TCDD) in Rhesus Monkeys (*Macaca mulatta)* Following a Single Oral Dose," *Toxicol. Appl. Pharmacol.* 43:175-187 (1978).
4. Courtney, K. D., D. W. Gaylor, M. D. Hogan, H. L. Falk, R. R. Bates and I. Mitchell. "Teratogenic Evaluation of 2,4,5-T," *Science* 168:864-866 (1970).
5. Emerson, J. L., D. L. Thompson, D. J. Streibing, C. G. Gerbig and V. G. Robinson. "Teratogenic Studies on 2,4,5-Trichlorophenoxyacetic Acid in the Rat and Rabbit," *Food Cosmet. Toxicol.* 9:395-404 (1971).
6. Firestone, D., W. Ibrahim and W. Horowitz. "Chick Edema Factor. III. Application of Microcoulometric Gas Chromatography to Detection of Chick Edema Factor in Fats or Fatty Acids," *J. Assoc. Offic. Anal. Chem.* 46:384 (1963).
7. Flick, D. F., D. Firestone and J. P. Marliac. "Studies of Chick Edema Disease. Preparation and Biological Effects of a Crystalline Chick Edema Factor Concentrate," *Poultry Sci.* 44:1214 (1965).

8. Cantrell, J. S., N. C. Webb and A. J. Mabis. "Identification and Crystal Structure of Hydropericardium Producing Factor: 1,2,3,7,8,9-Hexachloro-*p*-dioxin," *Acta Cryst.* B25:150 (1969).
9. Kimmig, J., and K. H. Shultz. "Occupational Acne (So-Called Chloracne) Due to Chlorinated Aromatic Cyclic Ethers," *Dermatologia* 115:540-546 (1957).
10. Jones, E. L., and H. Krizek. "A Technique for Testing Acnegenic Potency in Rabbits Applied to the Potent Acnegen, 2,3,7,8-Tetrachlorodibenzo-*p*-dioxin," *J. Invest. Dermatol.* 39:511-517 (1962).
11. Wasserman, M., D. Wasserman, S. Cucos and H. J. Miller. "World PCBs Map: Storage and Effects in Man and His Biologic Environment in the 1970s," *Ann. N.Y. Acad. Sci.* 320:69-124 (1979).
12. Vos, J. G., J. H. Koeman, H. L. Van der Mass, M. C. ten Noever de Brauw and R. H. de Vos. "Identification and Toxicological Evaluation of Chlorinated Dibenzofuran and Chlorinated Naphthalene in Two Commercial Polychlorinated Biphenyls," *Food Cosmet. Toxicol.* 8:625-633 (1970).
13. Roach, J. A. G., and I. H. Pomerantz. "The Finding of Chlorinated Dibenzofurans in a Japanese Polychlorinated Biphenyl Sample," *Bull. Environ. Contam. Toxicol.* 12:338-342 (1974).
14. Bowes, G. W., M. J. Mulvihill, M. J. De Camp and A. S. Kende. "Gas Chromatographic Characteristics of Authentic Chlorinated Dibenzofurans: Identification of Two Isomers in American and Japanese Polychlorinated Biphenyls," *J. Agric. Food Chem.* 23:1222-1223 (1975).
15. Buser, H. R., C. Rappe and A. Gara. "Polychlorinated Dibenzofurans (PCDFs) Found in Yusho Oil and in Used Japanese PCB," *Chemosphere* 7:439-449 (1978).
16. Nagayama, J., M. Kuratsune and Y. Masuda. "Determination of Chlorinated Dibenzofurans in Kanechlor and Yusho Oil," *Bull. Environ. Contam. Toxicol.* 15:9-13 (1976).
17. Albro, P. W., C. Parker and J. Corbett. "General Approach to the Fractionation and Class Determination of Complex Mixtures of Chlorinated Hydrocarbons," *J. Chromatog.* (in press).
18. Hass, J. R., and M. D. Friesen. "Qualitative and Quantitative Methods for Dioxin Analysis," *Ann. N.Y. Acad. Sci.* 320:28-42 (1979).
19. Hass, J. R., M. D. Friesen, D. J. Harvan and C. E. Parker. "Determination of Polychlorinated Dibenzo-*p*-dioxins in Biological Samples by Negative Chemical Ionization Mass Spectrometry," *Anal. Chem.* 50: 1474-1479 (1978).
20. Hass, J. R., M. D. Friesen and M. K. Hoffman. "The Mass Spectrometry of Polychlorinated Dibenzo-*p*-dioxins," *Org. Mass Spectrom.* 14:9-16 (1979).
21. Albro, P. W., and B. J. Corbett. "Extraction and Clean-up of Animal Tissues for Subsequent Determination of Mixture of Chlorinated Dibenzo-*p*-dioxins and Dibenzofurans," *Chemosphere* 7:381-385 (1977).
22. Buser, H. R. "Determination of 2,3,7,8-Tetrachlorodibenzo-*p*-dioxin in Environmental Samples Using High Resolution Gas Chromatography and Low Resolution Mass Spectrometry," *Anal. Chem.* 49:918-922 (1977).

## CHAPTER 12

# NEGATIVE CHEMICAL IONIZATION STUDIES OF POLYCHLORINATED DIBENZO-*p*-DIOXINS, DIBENZOFURANS AND NAPHTHALENES IN ENVIRONMENTAL SAMPLES

**D. W. Kuehl**

U. S. Environmental Protection Agency
Environmental Research Laboratory–Duluth
Duluth, Minnesota

**R. C. Dougherty and Y. Tondeur**

Department of Chemistry
Florida State University
Tallahassee, Florida

**D. L. Stalling and L. M. Smith**

U.S. Department of the Interior
Columbia National Fishery Research Laboratory
Columbia, Missouri

**C. Rappe**

Department of Chemistry
University of Umeå
Umeå, Sweden

## INTRODUCTION

This chapter describes an advance in the analytical procedures for the isolation and identification of planar polychlorinated aromatic organic chemicals, such as dibenzo-*p*-dioxins (PCDD), dibenzofurans (PCDF) and naphthalenes (PCN), and demonstrates the utility of the methods by examining a series of environmental samples which includes 13 fish samples from various U.S.

rivers, Lake Michigan sediment sampled near Waukeegan, WI, a snapping turtle from the Hudson River, NY and a seal from the Baltic Sea. There are over 1000 toxic chemicals registered for use as pesticides in the United States and many thousands of other toxic chemicals enter the environment as a result of industrial uses, metabolism, photochemical conversions, etc. One of these classes of chemicals, the planar-polychlorinated aromatic compounds, contains one of the most toxic synthetic chemicals known to man, 2, 3, 7, 8-tetrachlorodibenzo-*p*-dioxin (TCDD) [1]. Dibenzo-*p*-dioxins originate as a by-product during the preparation of chlorophenols and chlorophenoxy-containing chemicals such as 2, 4-dichlorophenoxy acetic acid (2, 4-D) and 2, 4, 5-trichlorophenoxy acetic acid (2, 4, 5-T). Dibenzofurans originate as by-products in the preparation of polychlorinated biphenyl (PCB) mixtures. Naphthalenes are both a by-product in PCB production and a commercial product by themselves. Because of the extreme toxicity of TCDD and related chemicals, much effort has been put forth to evaluate the biological activity of PCDD and to develop methodologies for their analysis. Baughman and Meselson [2] have estimated that 1-pg sensitivity is required to detect TCDD in 1-g samples for environmental monitoring. This value was determined by providing a 100X factor for nonlethal toxicity and a 10X safety factor from the lethal single oral dose (LD50) for guinea pigs of 1 ppb [3].

The analysis of TCDD in environmental samples generally has been done by either high resolution mass spectrometry (HRMS) or gas chromatography/mass spectrometry (GC/MS), in which both techniques use electron-impact as the ionization mode. Multiple ion detection (MID) is used to monitor M, M+2 and M+4 of TCDD at m/z 320, 322 and 324, respectively, during GC/MS [4], while the high-resolution method uses an averaging computer to monitor peaks at m/z 322 ± 0.3 amu [2]. In this case, high resolving power was required to separate TCDD from DDE and a pentachlorobiphenyl isomer which also produce ions at m/z 322. Scan-averaging was then required to increase the sensitivity lost to resolving power. With this system, Baughman and Meselson observed a significant change in TCDD response when squalene, a hydrocarbon, was added to TCDD-spiked samples. This led them to state "that in order not to cause a significant loss of sensitivity the total sample size should be kept under 5 $\mu$g" [2]. It is most necessary, then, to use highly efficient cleanup procedures.

Sample cleanup procedures used for PCDD and PCDF analyses have generally followed traditional methods. The elution of octachlorodibenzo-*p*-dioxin (OCDD) from a florisil column was characterized by Mills et al. [5] in the pesticide elution scheme. Other procedures have included treatment by presulfuric acid/alumina/sulfuric acid [6]; alcoholic potassium hydroxide/sulfuric acid/alumina [7]; alcoholic potassium hydroxide/silica gel/alumina

[8]; alcoholic potassium hydroxide/sulfuric acid/silica gel/alumina [9]; and various combinations of these procedures. Generally good recoveries have been observed for all of these procedures; however, it has been noted that digestion with alkali can result in the loss of as much as 90% of OCDD [10] and 60% of octachlorodibenzofuran (OCDF) [11]. More recently, an alternative cleanup procedure used with GC/MS has been described [12]. This procedure, however, is quite complex, involving six basic steps before analysis:

1. alcoholic KOH digestion;
2. solvent extraction of the digestion;
3. chromatography on a 44% $H_2SO_4$/silica gel column;
4. chromatography on a basic alumina column;
5. chromatography on a 10% $AgNO_3$/silica gel column; and
6. chromatography on a second basic alumina column.

This procedure is very lengthy, subject to contamination and very costly.

It appeared that the overall dioxin analytical procedure needed to be reevaluated and perhaps revised. Any new procedure must be highly selective and highly sensitive. In addition, the procedure must: (1) eliminate interferences from other polychlorinated pesticides; (2) eliminate interferences from extraneous compounds found in environmental samples; and (3) be as simple as possible to avoid losses and contamination. The procedure evaluated here combines gel permeation chromatography, carbon-coated polyurethane foam chromatography and negative chemical ionization (NCI) mass spectrometry.

The use of gel permeation chromatography (GPC) for the separation of lipids from pesticides was initially demonstrated by Stalling et al. [13] and subsequently automated [14] for large numbers of samples. Initially, this system was designed to isolate nonpolar chemicals, but later was extended to the polar compounds by Kuehl and Leonard [15, 16]. The advantages of GPC were combined with selective adsorption by passage of the GPC effluent through a carbon-coated polyurethane foam column. The carbon chromatography further enriches the cleanup by adsorbing planar aromatics, which include PCDD, PCDF and PCN.

Carbon-coated polyurethane foam chromatography (CFC) was initially developed [17] to remove polychlorinated dibenzodioxins from Herbicide Orange, a mixture of *n*-butyl esters of 2, 4-D and 2, 4, 5-T. The mixture was used extensively as a defoliant in Southeast Asia until a ban on the military use of 2, 4, 5-T was ordered by the U.S. Department of Defense. More recently, elution characteristics for a wide variety of polychlorinated hydrocarbons and polynuclear aromatic hydrocarbons (PAH) have been determined by CFC using a six-step elution profile [18]. After elution with the fifth solvent mixture (1:1 benzene/ethyl acetate), all interfering chemicals such as DDT and PCB have been removed, and only the planar molecules, such as the polychlorinated dibenzo-*p*-dioxins, dibenzofurans and naphthalenes, remain on the carbon/foam column. These chemicals may be easily removed from the carbon/foam by reversing the direction of solvent flow and eluting with toluene. The sample may then be concentrated for analysis.

The method of analysis we have used in this study is NCI mass spectrometry, a technique originally developed by Dougherty et al. [19]. The analytical application of NCI mass spectrometry is broader, but quite similar to that of gas chromatography with electron capture (EC/GC) detection. Compounds that give intense EC responses will virtually always be sensitive to NCI mass spectra. Moreover, mass resolution in NCI spectra serves the same function as time resolution in GC. However, by using a HRMS, it is possible to obtain mass resolution on the order of one part per billion, which is considerably higher than is available with conventional GC. The reduction in chemical noise by mass analysis also contributes to the lower detection limit for the NCI system as compared to GC.

NCI spectra are obtained by operating a chemical ionization mass spectometer (ion source pressure ~1 torr) in the negative ion mode. Under these conditions, five major negative ion forming reactions occur, assuming that the ion source contains oxygen and organochlorine compounds. These reactions are the following

$$M + e_s^- \rightarrow M^{*\dot{-}} \xrightarrow{N} M^{\dot{-}} \tag{1}$$

$$M + Cl^- \rightarrow (M{+}Cl)^- \tag{2}$$

$$M + Cl^- \rightarrow (M{-}H)^- + HCl \tag{3}$$

$$M + O_2^{\dot{-}} \rightarrow (M{-}Cl + O)^- + ClO\cdot \tag{4}$$

$$M + e_s^- \rightarrow A^- + B\cdot \tag{5}$$

The dominant ion in the NCI spectra of aromatic polychlorides is $(M{-}Cl{+}0)^-$ (Equation 4).

NCI mass spectrometry is especially suited for screening samples of environmental substrates, because spectra of toxic substances such as chlorinated pesticides and PCB can be obtained at high sensitivity and with less background interferences than electron impact mass spectra. The difference in sensitivity of polychlorinated chemicals to nonhalogenated biogenic molecules is often three or four orders of magnitude. This differential sensitivity can be explained on the basis of two observations.

1. The spectral intensity for biochemical compounds is highly reduced. With the exception of free carboxylic acids and some of the prosthetic groups from the electron transport chain, the biomolecules are virtually transparent to negative chemical ionization. These molecules have negative electron affinities and only weakly attach gas phase nucleophiles.
2. In contrast, the polychlorinated chemicals have generally positive electron affinities and will readily attach an electron or attach gas phase nucleophiles to form intense negative ions.

Applications of NCI screening of environmental and human samples have been demonstrated in several papers by Dougherty [20-23]. In these papers, substrates such as samples of human urine, seminal fluid, blood, milk and breast fluid, as well as chocolate candy bars, beef fat and fish, have been screened for a wide variety of pesticides, herbicides and industrial chemicals. The use of NCI for dioxin analysis has recently appeared in the literature. Both Hunt et al. [24] and Hass et al. [25] have reported an increase in sensitivity for TCDD using oxygen NCI rather than methane chemical ionization (CI). In addition, Hass et al. [25, 26] have investigated spectra of a series of PCDD by positive methane CI (MPCI), methane NCI (MNCI), methane/oxygen NCI (MONCI) and oxygen NCI (ONCI), and have concluded that MNCI is best suited for quantitative analysis of the more halogenated congeners and MONCI is best suited for qualitative confirmation of the presence of PCDD.

## EXPERIMENTAL

### Sample Extractions

Aliquots (25-, 50-, or 100-g) of composites of ground whole fish were blended with enough anhydrous sodium sulfate to dry the sample. The samples were then Soxhlet-extracted for 8 hr with 1:1 hexane/acetone. The hexane/acetone was evaporated with a Kuderna-Danish apparatus fitted with a three-ball Snyder column. The resulting oil was weighed and diluted to 100 mg/ml with methylene chloride for GPC. The seal oil, sediment and turtle samples were subjected to extraction with methylene chloride in glass columns.

### Gel Permeation Chromatography

The GPC system was similar to that previously described [12]. A 50 x 2.5 mm column of BIO-RAD SX-2 was eluted at 3.5 ml/min with a 1:1

mixture of cyclohexane and methylene chloride. The chromatogram was monitored with a Varian Areograph Ultraviolet detector operating at 254 nm. Injections (5-ml) were made into the system and the 160- to 225-ml fraction was allowed to pass into the carbon/form column.

## Carbon/Foam Chromatography

The CFC procedure is similar to that previously described [15]. The carbon coated foam is generated by adding 0.5 g Amoco PX-21 carbon ($\leqslant 44\ \mu$) to 10.0 g. polyurethane in 250 ml $CHCl_3$ and blending for 2-5 min in a Waring blender. The carbon-coated foam is then dried and Soxhlet-extracted for 12 hr with toluene. Carbon/foam (1g) is then packed into a 1.0 x 8.5 cm column for use.

After a sample has been loaded onto the CFC it is eluted with 35 ml of 50% benzene/ethyl acetate. The column is then washed with 50 ml of toluene in a reverse-flow direction. The toluene fraction is concentrated for NCI analysis of polychlorinated dibenzo-*p*-dioxins, dibenzofurans and naphthalenes.

## Negative Chemical Ionization Mass Spectrometry

NCI mass spectra were obtained by direct probe introduction, using an AEI-902 mass spectrometer equipped with a SRIC chemical ionization source. Ionization was initiated with 470-V electrons with a regulated emission current of 0.25 mamp. Source pressures were monitored by use of a MKS Beratron which was operated at the source potential (-8 kV) and isolated from earth. Spectral quality methylene chloride, distilled before use, and Matheson research grade isobutane (1:1) with the addition of 2% oxygen was used as the reagent gas. Spectra were obtained with a source temperature of 150°C and source pressures of 0.5 torr, 30, 60 and 90 sec after sample introduction.

# RESULTS AND DISCUSSION

A listing of all samples used in this study is given in Table I. GPC/CFC/NCI analysis of 13 composite fish samples is summarized in Table II. Thirteen samples contained some polychlorinated naphthalenes, four to seven chlorines; five samples contained some polychlorinated dibenzofurans, four to seven chlorines; and only two samples contained polychlorinated dibenzo-*p*-dioxins, four to eight chlorines. Figures 1 and 2 are NCI mass spectra of the Ohio River fish caught at Marietta, OH in 1971 and Connecticut River fish caught at Wilson, CT in 1970, respectively, each showing a series of PCDF and PCN. PCDF are identified as oxygen-chloride exchange reaction products (M-19 Equation 4) at m/z 285, 319 and 353 for the penta- through heptachloro isomers and PCN, also oxygen-chloride exchange products, at m/z 279, 313 and 347 for the penta through heptachloro isomers. In addition, the spectra show ions at m/z 305, 339, 373 and 407 which correspond to penta through octachloro PCB.

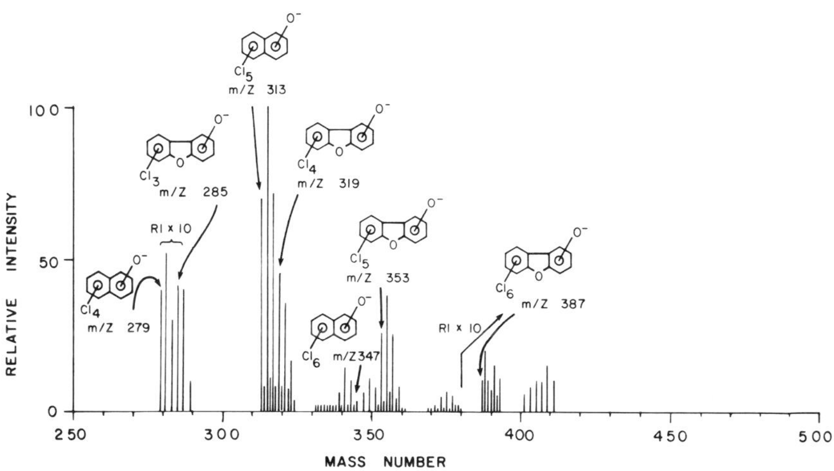


**Figure 1.** Negative chemical ionization mass spectra of an extract from Ohio River carp caught near Marietta, OH.

Figures 3 and 4 are NCI spectra of Tittawabassee River fish caught in 1977 at Dow Dam and Emerson Park. These samples also contained penta and hexachloronaphthalenes as well as tetra- to octachlorodibenzo-*p*-dioxin isomers. The dioxins are identified as oxygen-chloride exchange reaction products at m/z 301, 335, 369, 403 and 437 respectively for tetra- to octachloro isomers. In addition, both samples show an unidentified octachloro compound at m/z 471.

Table II also contains a summary of findings in the sediment, seal and turtle samples for which NCI spectra are shown in Figures 5, 6 and 7, respectively. No PCDD were observed in these samples. Naphthalenes were

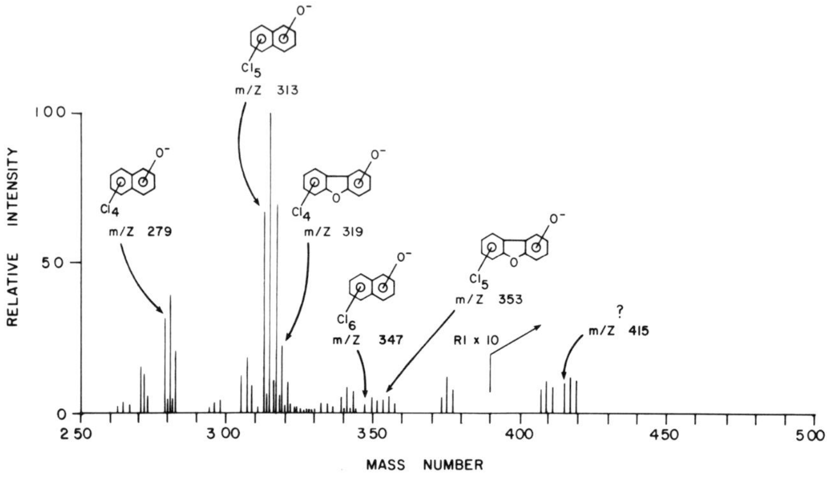


**Figure 2.** Negative chemical ionization mass spectra of an extract from Connecticut River perch caught near Wilson, CT.

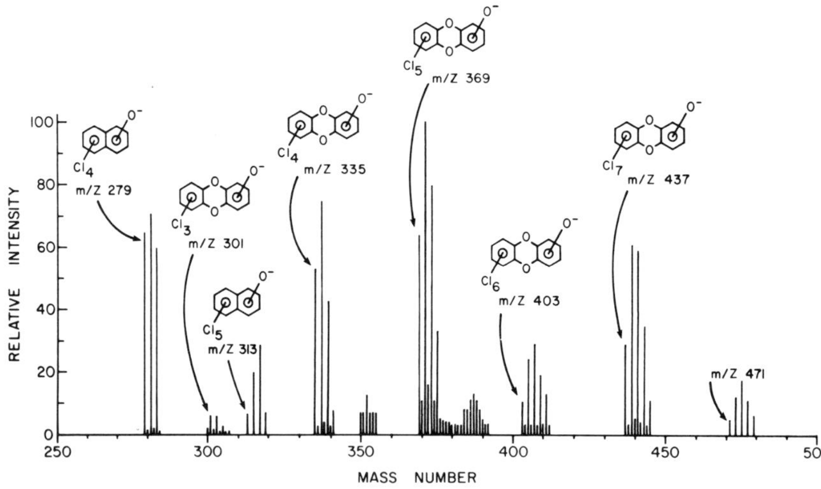


**Figure 3.** Negative chemical ionization mass spectra of an extract from Tittabawassee River bass caught near Dow Dam, MI.

**Table I. Identification of Samples Analyzed for Polychlorinated Dibenzo-*p*-dioxin, Dibenzofurans and Naphthalenes by NCI**

| Sample | Origin | Amount (g) |
|---|---|---|
| Carp | Ohio River at Cincinati, OH, 1970 | 100 |
| Carp | Ohio River at Marietta, OH, 1971 | 100 |
| Carp | Ohio River at Cincinnati, OH. 1974 | 100 |
| Lake Trout | Lake Michigan at Saugatuck, MI, 1974 | 25 |
| Channel Catfish | Ohio River at Marietta, OH, 1970 | 100 |
| Perch | Connecticut River at Wilson, CT, 1974 | 25 |
| Perch | Connecticut River at Wilson, CT, 1970 | 25 |
| Largemouth Bass | Hudson River at Wappinger Falls, NY, 1974 | 100 |
| Carp | Ohio River at Marietta, OH, 1974 | 50 |
| Bloater | Lake Michigan at Sheboygan, WI, 1974 | 50 |
| Goldfish | Hudson River at Wappinger Falls, NY, 1976 | 75 |
| Bass | Tittabawassee River at Midland (Dow Dam), MI, 1977 | 100 |
| Bass | Tittabawassee River at Midland (Emerson Park), MI, 1970 | 100 |
| Seal | Baltic Sea, Gulf of Bothmita, 1976 | 100 |
| Sediment | Lake Michigan at Waukegan, IL, 1979 | 100 |
| Turtle | Hudson River, NY, 1979 | 100 |

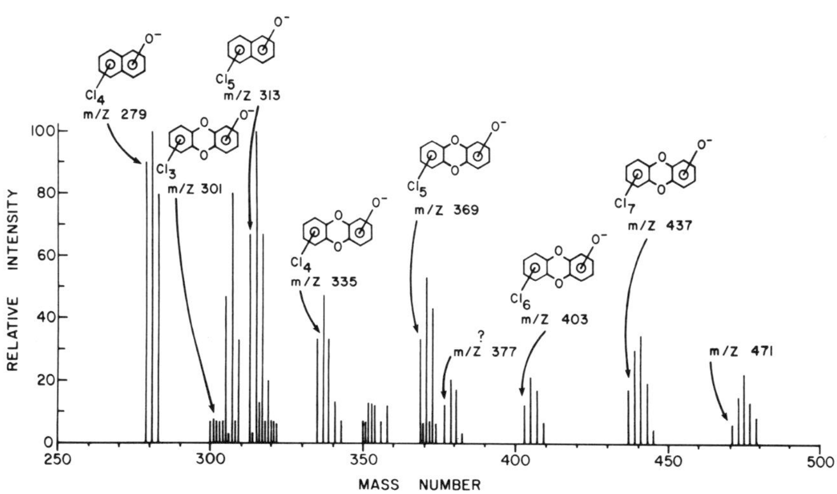


**Figure 4.** Negative chemical ionization mass spectra of an extract from Tittabawassee River bass caught near Emerson Park, MI.

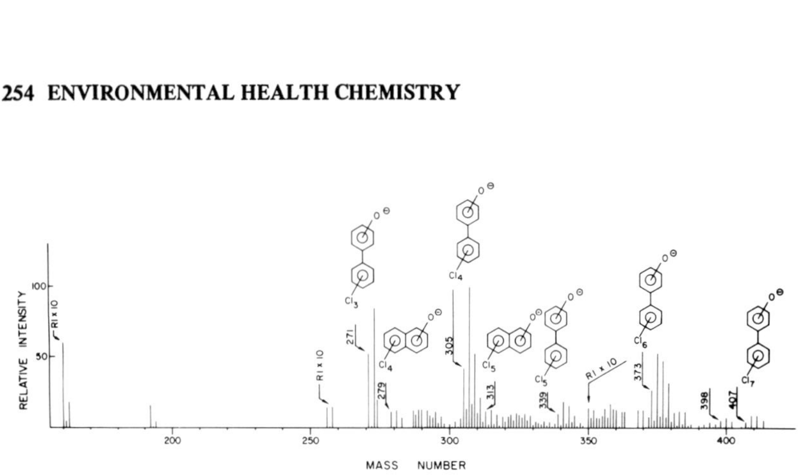


**Figure 5.** Negative chemical ionization mass spectra of a Waukeegan area Lake Michigan sediment extract.

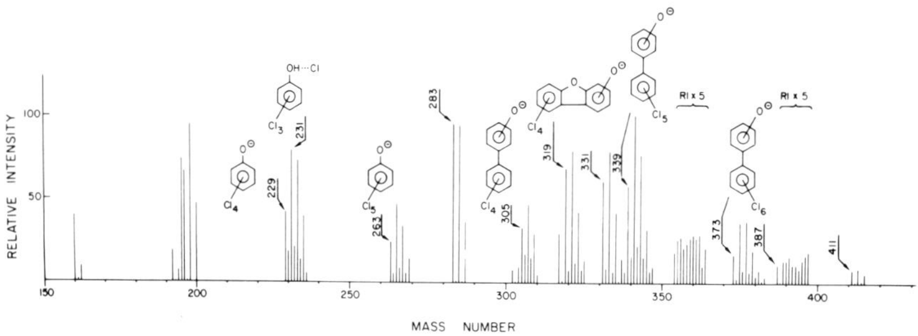


**Figure 6.** Negative chemical ionization mass spectra of a Baltic Sea seal extract.

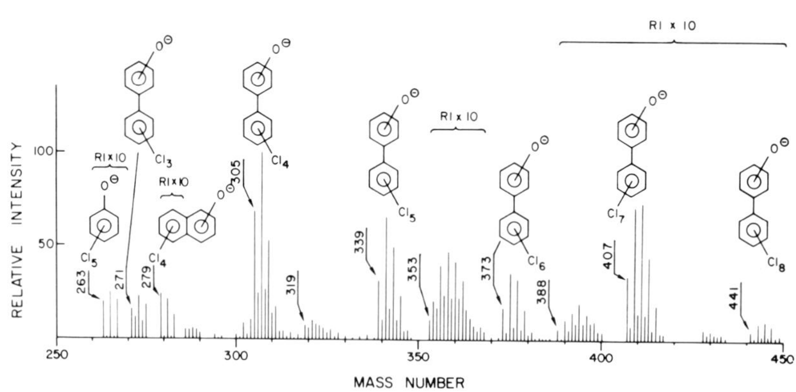


**Figure 7.** Negative chemical ionization mass spectra of a turtle caught in the Hudson River, NY.

Table II. Summary of Results of Negative Chemical Ionization Studies of Fish, Sediment, Seal and Turtle Samples Identification is Denoted by an o)

| Chemical | 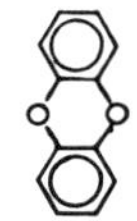 | | | | | 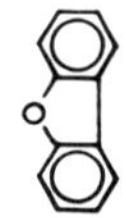 | | | | | 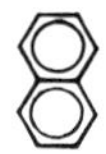 | | | | |
|---|---|---|---|---|---|---|---|---|---|---|---|---|---|---|---|
| | 4 Cl | 5 Cl | 6 Cl | 7 Cl | 8 Cl | 4 Cl | 5 Cl | 6 Cl | 7 Cl | 8 Cl | 4 Cl | 5 Cl | 6 Cl | 7 Cl | 8 Cl |
| Fish - Ohio R., Cinc., '70 | | | | | | o | o | o | | | o | o | o | o | |
| Fish - Ohio R., Marietta, '71 | | | | | | o | o | o | o | | o | o | o | o | |
| Fish - Ohio R., Cinc., '74 | | | | | | | | | | | o | o | o | | |
| Fish - Lk. Mich., Saug., '74 | | | | | | o | o | o | | | o | o | o | o | |
| Fish - Ohio R., Marietta, '70 | | | | | | | | | | | o | o | o | | |
| Fish - Conn. R., Wilson, '74 | | | | | | | | | | | | o | o | | |
| Fish - Conn. R., Wilson, '70 | | | | | | o | o | o | | | o | o | o | o | |
| Fish - Hudson R., W. Falls, '74 | | | | | | | | o | | | o | o | o | | |
| Fish - Ohio R., Marietta, '74 | | | | | | | | | | | o | o | o | | |
| Fish - Lk. Mich., Shebo., '74 | | | | | | | | | | | | | o | o | |
| Fish - Hudson R., W. Falls, '76 | | | | | | | | | | | o | o | | | |
| Fish - Tittaba. R., Dow Dam, '77 | o | o | o | o | o | | | | | | | o | o | | |
| Fish - Tittaba. R., Emerson Park, '77 | o | o | o | o | o | | | | | | | o | o | | |
| Turtle - Hudson R., '79 | | | | | | | o | o | | | | o | | | |
| Sediment - Lk. Mich., '79 | | | | | | | o | o | | | | o | o | | |
| Seal - Baltic Sea, '79 | | | | | | | o | | | | | | | | |

observed in the sediment and turtle but not the seal. Pentachlorodibenzo furan(s) is (are) predominant in the seal sample and possibly in the sediment and turtle samples.

Environmental contamination with PCDF and PCN has previously been discussed in terms of the global distribution of contaminated PCB [27-29], and most investigations have been initiated because of obvious signs of stress in animals, birds or fish [30]. Although finding PCN in this study was not unexpected, the occurrence of the large number of PCDF in these samples was unexpected. It should be noted that although PCDF toxicity has been well documented, the toxicity of PCN has also been established [31]. In each of the samples containing PCDF the pentachloro isomers dominate. This correlates with the observation that the pentachloro isomers were most abundant in 13 of 17 Japanese, American and German PCB mixtures. Perhaps even more significant from an environmental health point of view was the observation that human liver samples from patients intoxicated by Kanemi Rice Oil ("Yusho" disease) from Japan were also more highly contaminated with two pentachlorodibenzofuran isomers [32, 33]. Although PCDF are known contaminants in PCB, their concentrations can be increased on heating. Morita et al. [32] found a fourfold increase of PCDF in PCB which had been used in a heat exchange system during a two-year period. Dibenzofuran concentrations in PCB can be increased to percent levels under pyrolytic conditions (500-700°C) [34]. Particular importance is attached to finding of PCDF because of the large inventory of PCB which yet remains to enter the global ecosystem and the possibility of transformation of PCB into PCDF at high yields. Moreover, certain PCDF are similar in toxicity to the most toxic dibenzo-*p*-dioxin congeners.

The finding of PCDD only in the Tittawabassee River samples appear to indicate a point-source discharge. Because PCDD are known contaminants in chlorophenols and chlorophenoxy acetic acid ester type of herbicides [1, 35], the Tittabawassee River PCDD are probably caused by industrial activity associated with these products. However the finding of PCDD and PCDF in municipal incinerator fly ash [36, 37] and subsequent papers showing the formation of PCDD by burning chlorophenates [38] and chlorobenzenes [39] has led to the correlation of their formation with combustion, and subsequently to the hypothesis that the distribution of PCDD in the environment is a result of combustion and the transport of combustion products [40, 41]. This hypothesis has since been the subject of controversy [42, 43]. The transport pathway of the PCDD found in the Tittabawassee fish is uncertain; however, whatever the pathway, the PCDD, as analyzed by these techniques, are unique to this watershed.

In addition to the identification of PCDD, PCDF and PCN, the spectra contain many unidentified compounds. A summary of their mass and chlorine content data is shown in Table III. A similar summary was published by Bowes [30] in a study of herring gulls, *Larus argentatus*, in which the PCDD/PCDF fraction of florisil chromatography contained 16 unidentified polychlorinated chemicals. Several polychlorinated biphenyl ethers, which can form dibenzofurans, the phenoxyphenols, which can pyrolyze to dibenzo-*p*-dioxins, have been identified as additional contaminants of PCDD and PCDF [44-46], perhaps these or similar chemicals may eventially be correlated with the currently unidentified compounds.

**Table III. Unidentified Planar Polychlorinated Aromatic Compounds as Observed in NCI Spectra and Listed by m/z Values and Number of Chlorines Observed**

| m/z | No. of Chlorines | Sample |
|---|---|---|
| 283 | 3 | Baltic Sea seal |
| 331 | 4 | Baltic Sea seal |
| 377 | 6 | Tittabawasse River fish |
| 398 | 5 | Lake Michigan sediment |
| 415 | 5 | Connecticut River fish |
| 471 | 8 | Tittabawassee River, Dow Dam, fish |
| 471 | 8 | Tittabawassee River, Emerson Park, fish |

## SUMMARY

An analytical procedure based on gel permeation chromatography, carbon-coated polyurethane foam chromatography and negative chemical ionization mass spectroscopy has been developed to isolate and identify planar polychlorinated aromatic hydrocarbons in environmental samples. This technique provides a rapid qualitative screen for these compounds, but no attemp was made to accurately quantify the individual compounds present. The GPC/CFC procedure for planar molecule isolation, in addition to being highly efficient, has several advantages over previously used digestion and adsorption chromatography methods. First, the method is very simple, involving one continuous chromatographic system that is easily reversed in flow to remove planar molecules. This simplicity reduces the possibility of contamination by excess solvent and lab equipment, as well as keeping the overall analysis time down. Second, the method is very mild; no strong acid or base digestion step is used that would destroy or alter molecules of interest. Third, the GCP/CFC system can be solvent-washed, blanked and reused to keep the cost of analysis low. Also, NCI mass spectrometry offers several advantages over previously used electron impact. First, polychlorinated molecules have much more sensitivity in NCI than EI; therefore, overall detectability will be much lower. Second, NCI offers a very large sensitivity differential of polychlorinated molecules over biomolecules, which makes many interferences transparent to NCI. The analysis described in this chapter shows that this method works very well, and may become the analytical procedure of choice for this class of most toxic chemicals.

Future development that may yet improve this method would be the use of high resolution glass capillary gas chromatography interfaced to a positive-negative pulsed chemical ionization mass spectrometer. Such experiments are now underway.

## REFERENCES

1. NIEHS Conference on Chlorinated Dibenzodioxins and Dibenzofurans. Research Traiangle Park, N.C., April 2-3, 1973. *Environ. Health Persp.* Vol. 5 (1973).
2. Baughman, R., and M. Meselson, *Chlorodioxins–Origin and Fate,* Adv. Chem. Ser. 120 (Washington, DC: American Chemical Society 1973), p. 92.
3. "Report on 2, 4, 5-T," A report of the Panel on Herbicides of the President's Science Advisory Committee, Executive Office of the President, Office of Science and Technology (1971).
4. Crummett, W. B., and R. H. Stehl. "Determination of Chlorinated Dibenzo-*p*-dioxins and Dibenzofurans in Various Materials," *Environ. Health Persp.* 5:15-25 (1973).
5. Mills, P. A. et al. "Electron Solvent Systems for Florisil Column Clean-up in Organochlorine Pesticide Residue Analyses," *J. Assoc. Off. Anal. Chem.* 55:39-34 (1972).
6. Ress, J., G. R. Higginbotham and D. Firestone "Methodology for Chlorinated Aromatics in Fats, Oils and Fatty Acids," *J. Assoc. Off. Anal. Chem.* 53:628-634 (1970).
7. Baughman, R., and M. Meselson. "An Analytical Method for Detecting TCDD: Levels of TCDD in Samples from Viet Nam," *Environ. Health Persp.* 5:27-35 (1973).
8. Mahle, N. H., H. S. Higgins and M. E. Getzendamer "Search for the Presence of 2, 3, 7, 8-Tetrachlorodibenzo-*p*-dioxin in Bovine Milk," *Bull. Environ. Contam. Tox.* 18:123-130 (1977).
9. Hammel, R. "Clean-up Techniques for the Determination of Part-Per-Trillion Residues Levels of 2, 3, 7, 8-TCDD," *J. Agric Food Chem.* 25:1049-1053 (1977).
10. Albro, P. W. and B. J. Corbett, "Extraction and Clean-up of Animal Tissue for Subsequent Determination of Mixtures of Chlorinated Dibenzo-*p*-dioxins and Dibenzofurans," *Chemosphere* 7:381-385 (1977).

11. Firestone, D. "Determination of Polychlorinatedibenzo-*p*-dioxins and Polychlorinated Dibenzofurans in Commercial Gelatins by Gas-Liquid Chromatography," *J. Agric. Food Chem.* 25:1274-1280 (1977).
12. Lamparski, L. L., T. J. Nestrick and R. H. Stehl. "Determination of Part-Per-Trillion Concentrations of 2, 3, 7, 8-Tetrachlorodibenzo-*p*-dioxin in Fish," *Anal. Chem.* 51:1953-1958 (1979).
13. Stalling, D. L., R. C. Tindle and J. L. Johnson. "Cleanup of Pesticide and Polychlorinated Biphenyl Residues in Fish Extracts by Gel Permeation Chromatography," *J. Assoc. Off. Anal. Chem.* 55:32-38 (1972).
14. Tindle, R. C. and Stalling, D. L. "Apparatus for Automated Gel Permeation Cleanup of Pesticide Residue Analysis," *Anal. Chem.* 44: 1768-1773 (1972).
15. Kuehl, D. W. and E. N. Leonard. "Isolation of Xenobiotic Chemicals from Tissue Samples by Gel Permeation Chromatography," *Anal. Chem.* 50:182-185 (1978).
16. Kuehl, D. W., G. D. Veith and E. N. Leonard. "Brominated Compounds Found in Waste Treatment Effluent and Their Capacity to Bioaccumulate," in *Water Chlorination: Environmental Impact and Health Effects, Vol. 2* (Ann Arbor, MI: Ann Arbor Science Publishers, Inc., 1978), pp. 175-192.
17. Stalling, D. L., J. N. Huckins, J. L. Johnson and A. Smith. "Adsorption of Chlorinated Dibenzo-*p*-dioxins on Charcoals: Cleanup of Herbicide Orange and Analytical Application," Presented at 89th annual meeting of the Assoc. of Official Analytical Chemists, Washington, DC, 1975.
18. Stalling, D. L., L. M. Smith and J. D. Petty. "Approaches to Comprehensive Analyses of Persistant Halogenated Environmental Contaminants," Presented at the ASTM Committee D19 on Water symposium Measurement of Organic Pollutants in Water and Wastewater, Denver, CO, June 19-20, 1978.
19. Dougherty, R. C., J. Dalton and F. J. Biros. "Negative Chemical Ionization Mass Spectra of Polycyclic Chlorinated Pesticides," *Org. Mass Spectrom.* 6:1171-1181 (1972).
20. Dougherty, R. C., and K. Piotrowska. "Multi-residue Screening by Negative Chemical Ionization Mass Spectrometry of Organic Polychlorides," *J Assoc. Off. Anal. Chem.* 59:1023-1027 (1976).
21. Dougherty, R. C., and K. Piotrowska. "Screening by Negative Chemical Ionization Mass Spectrometry for Environmental Contamination with Toxic Residues: Applications to Human Urines," *Proc. Nat. Acad. Sci. U.S.* 73:1777-1781 (1976).
22. Dougherty, R. C., and E. A. Hett. "Negative Chemical Ionization Mass Spectrometry: Applications in Environmental Analytical Chemistry," in *Pentachlorophenol,* K. Ranga Rao, Ed. (New York, Plenum Publishing Corp., 1978), pp. 339-350.
23. Dougherty, R. C., M. J. Whitaker, L. Smith, D. L. Stalling and D. W. Kuehl. "Negative Chemical Ionization Studies of Human and Food Chain Contamination with Xenobiotic Chemicals," *Environ. Health Persp.* (in press).
24. Hunt, D. F., T. M. Harvey and J. W. Russell. "Reagent Gases for Chem-

ical Ionization Mass Spectrometry," *J. Chem. Soc. Chem. Commun.* 152-154 (1976).
25. Hass, J. R., M. D. Friesen, D. J. Harvan and C. E. Parker. "Determination of Polychlorinated Dibenzo-*p*-dioxins in Biological Samples by Negative Chemical Ionization Mass Spectrometry," *Anal. Chem.* 50: 1474-1479 (1978).
26. Hass, J. R., M. D. Friesen and M. K. Hoffman. "The Mass Spectrometry of Polychlorinated Dibenzo-*p*-dioxins," *Org. Mass Spectrom.* (in press).
27. Bowes, G. W., M. J. Mulvihill, B. R. T. Simoncit, A. L. Burlingame and R. W. Risebough. "Isolation and Identification of Chlorinated Dibenzofurans from Polychlorinated Biphenyls and from Yusho Oil Containing PCB," in *Dioxin: Toxicological and Chemical Aspects,* F. Cattabeni, A. Cavallaro and G. Galli, Eds. (Jamaica, NY: Spectrum Publishers, 1978), p. 79.
28. Vos, J. G., J. H. Koeman, H. L. Van der Mass, M. C. ten Noever de Brau and R. H. de Vos. "Identification and Toxicological Evaluation of Chlorinated Dibenzofuran and Chorinated Naphthalene in Two Commercial Polychlorinated Biphenyls," *Food Cosmet. Toxicol.* 8:625-633 (1970).
29. Roach, J. A. G., and I. H. Pomerant. "The Finding of Chlorinated Dibenzofurans in a Japanese Polychlorinated Biphenyl Sample," *Bull. Environ. Contam. Toxicol.* 12:338-342 (1974).
30. Bowes, G. W., B. R. Simoneit, A. L. Burlingame, B. W. de Lappe, D. B. Peakall and R. W. Risebrough. "The Search for Chlorinated Dibenzofurans and Chlorinated Dibenzodioxins in Wildlife Populations Showing Elevated Levels of Embryonic Death," *Environ. Health Persp.* 5:191-198 (1973).
31. Kimbrough, B. D. "Toxicity of Chlorinated Hydrocarbons and Related Compounds," *Arch. Environ. Health* 25:125-131 (1972).
32. Morita, M., J. Nakagawa, K. Akiyama, S. Mimura and N. Isono. "Detailed Examination of Polychlorinated Dibenzofurans in PCB Preparation and Kanemi Yusho Oil," *Bull. Environ. Contam. Toxicol.* 18:67-73 (1977).
33. Rappe, C., H. R. Buser, H. Kuroki and Y. Masuda. "Identification of Polychlorinated Dibenzofurans (PCDFs) Retained in Patients with Yusho," *Chemosphere* 4:259-266 (1979).
34. Buser, H. R., H. P. Bosshardt and C. Rappe. "Formation of Polychlorinated Dibenzofurans (PCDFs) from the Pyrolysis of PCBs," *Chemosphere* 7:109-119 (1978).
35. Buser, H. R., and H. P. Bosshardt. "Determination of Polychlorinated Dibenzo-*p*-dioxins in Commercial Pentachlorophenol by Combined Gas Chromatography-Mass Spectrometry," *J. Assoc. Off. Anal. Chem.* 59:562-569 (1976).
36. Olie, K., P. L. Vermeulen and O. Hutzinger. "Chlorinated-*p*-dioxins and Chlorodibenzofurans are Trace Components of Fly Ash and Flue Gas of Some Municipal Incinerators in the Netherlands," *Chemosphere* 8:455-459 (1977).
37. Buser, H. R., H. P. Bosshardt and C. Rappe. "Identification of Poly-

chlorinated Dibenzo-*p*-dioxin Isomers Found in Fly Ash," *Chemosphere* 1:165-172 (1978).
38. Rappe, C., S. Marklund, H. R. Buser and H. P. Bosshardt. "Formation of Polychlorinated Dibenzo-*p*-dioxins and Dibenzofurans by Burning or Heating Chlorophenates," *Chemosphere* 3:269-281 (1978).
39. Buser, H. R. "Formation of Polychlorinated Dibenzofurans and Dibenzo-*p*-dioxins from the Pyrolysis of Chlorobenzenes," *Chemosphere* 6:415-424 (1979).
40. "Dioxins Formed by Normal Combustion," *Chem. Eng. News* (November 20, 1978) p. 7.
41. "The Trace Chemistries of Fire—A Source of and Route for the Entry of Chlorinated Dioxins into the Environment," Chlorinated Dioxin Task Force, Michigan Division, Dow Chemical Co., Midland, MI (1978).
42. "Dow Finds Support, Doubt for Dioxin Ideas," *Chem. Eng. News* (February 12, 1978) p. 23.
43. "EPA Disputes Dow's Dioxin Theory," *Chem. Eng. News* (February 26, 1978) p. 6.
44. Jensen, S., and L. Renberg. "Contaminants in Pentachlorophenol: Chlorinated Dioxins and Pre-dioxins," *Ambio*. 1:62-68 (1972).
45. Shadoff, L. A., W. W. Blaser, C. W. Kocher and H. G. Fravel. "Chlorinated Benzylphenylethers: A Possible Interference in the Determination of Chlorinated Dibenzo-*p*-dioxins in 2,4,5-Trichlorophenol and its Derivatives," *Anal. Chem.* 50:1586-1588 (1978).
46. Buser, H. R. PhD. Dissertation, University of Umea, Sweden (1978).

# CHAPTER 13

# SPERM DENSITY AND TOXIC SUBSTANCES: A POTENTIAL KEY TO ENVIRONMENTAL HEALTH HAZARDS

**Ralph C. Dougherty, Michael J. Whitaker, Sheng-Yuh Tang, Rosemary Bottcher and Michael Keller**

Department of Chemistry
Florida State University
Tallahassee, Florida

**Douglas W. Kuehl**

U. S. Environmental Protection Agency
Environmental Research Laboratory
Duluth, Minnesota

## INTRODUCTION

The "Atlas of Cancer Mortality" [1] provides the strongest evidence yet available for the association of human cancer with environmental factors. The association between areas of high cancer mortality and chemical or metallurgical industrial sites can hardly be a mere chance phenomenon. The objective of the research reported here is to develop techniques that will make it possible to identify the specific compounds in the environment which pose a threat to human health, and to provide the analytical data that will be required for proper regulation of these substances. The basic strategy in this research is to attempt to relate quantitative human health parameters to an exposure index or body burden for specific toxic substances. This approach is complementary to microbiological screening techniques [2] which assess the mutagenicity risk associated with specific chemicals that may be released into the environment. Mutagenicity screening tests readily identify highly reactive toxic materials such as dichloroethane [2]. The analytical screening procedure reported here tends to identify toxic materials that have long half-lives in the environment, such as polyhalogenated aromatic and aliphatic compounds.

Sperm density and other male fertility parameters were examined as one indicator of human health that might be correlated with a body burden for persistent toxic substances. The reasons for this choice are twofold. Spermatogenesis in humans requires a succession of between eight and ten cell division steps (Figure 1). Substances that inhibit cell division and are capable of crossing the blood testicular barrier will have an effect on sperm density that is considerably larger than their effect on the rate of an individual cell division. If the rate of cell division were decreased by 10%, sperm density would decrease by a minimum of 57% because of geometric magnification

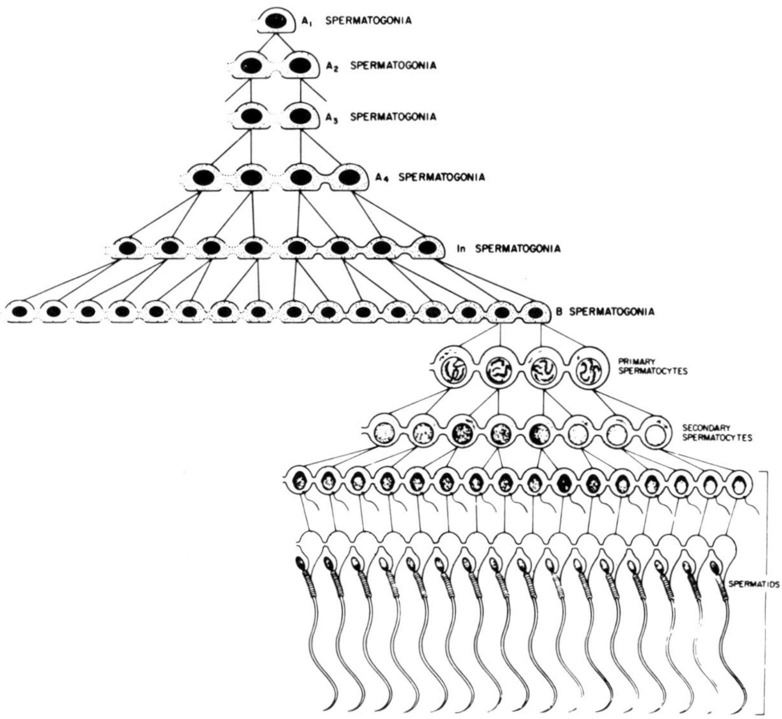


**Figure 1.** Schematic view of spermatogenesis in humans. A minimum of eight cell division steps are required to produce a sperm cell.

of the effect on the cell division sequence. Substances that inhibit cell division are very often mutagenic, carcinogenic or both; thus, sperm density may reflect, at least for some classes of compounds, low-level exposure to compounds that may contribute to the cancer burden in the population.

The second reason for studying sperm density and toxic substances stems from a series of literature reports which indicate the relationship between exposure to toxic materials and fertility parameters [3, 4] and a series of reports which strongly suggest that sperm densities in U.S. males have significantly declined over the last 30 years [5-13]. With regard to the effect of toxic substances on sperm density and fertility parameters, it is particularly interesting that smoking appears to correlate linearly with decreasing sperm density and increasing numbers of sperm abnormalities [4]. The data which illustrate the apparent decline in sperm density in U.S. populations over the last 30 years are indicated in Table 1. Before 1950, average sperm densities in a number of populations always exceeded 100 million cell/ml. Average sperm densities subsequent to 1970 have been in the range of 50–80 million cell/ml. There has been a corresponding decrease in the median sperm densities for the populations studied. The causes for this apparent decrease in sperm density are certain to be complex. Changing patterns in sexual behavior, increased use of drugs and increased stress could all conceivably contribute to a decrease in sperm density. It is also true that toxic substances in the environment may be a contributor to declining male fertility parameters.

**Table I. Sperm Density in U.S. Males as a Function of Time**

| Year | Number of Cases | Mean Sperm Density ($10^6$ cell/ml) | Comments | Reference |
|---|---|---|---|---|
| 1929 | 271 | 100[a] | | 7 |
| 1938 | 200 | 120[a] | 0.5% had $<20 \times 10^6$/ml<br>25.% had $<60 \times 10^6$/ml | 8 |
| 1949 | 49 | 145 | Range = 50–321 x $10^6$/ml | 9 |
| 1950 | 100 | 101 | | 10 |
| 1951 | 1,000 | 107 | 29% had $<60 \times 10^6$/ml<br>44% had $>100 \times 10^6$/ml | 9 |
| 1974 | 386 | 48 | | 12 |
| 1975 | 1,300 | 79 | Median = 65 x $10^6$/ml | 5 |
| 1975 | 100 | 81 | Median = 61 x $10^6$/ml | 12 |
| 1977 | 4,122 | 70 | Median = 50 x $10^6$/ml<br>23% had $<20 \times 10^6$/ml | 6 |
| 1979 | 22 | 62 | | 13 |
| | 24 | 22[b] | | |

[a]Wives were pregnant at the time.

[b]Occupational dibromochloropropane exposure for 60 days or more in current year.

The technique that is used here for assessment of exposure levels or body burdens for specific toxic substances is direct screening using negative chemical ionization mass spectrometry [14-17]. Negative chemical ionization (NCI) mass spectrometry is uniquely suited to screening environmental samples for contamination with toxic substances. This suitability stems from the fact that the molecules of biology are largely highly reduced and have many high-energy electrons. Biomolecules characteristically produce very weak responses to negative ion MS because, in general, their electron affinities are negative. With few exceptions, proximal cancer-causing substances are either oxidizing agents, alkalating agents or both. Molecules in this class have low-energy vacant orbitals, and generally they produce intense negative ion beams. The selectivity of negative ion MS for compounds that are toxic allows for less-than-perfect cleanup procedures in an analytical screening scheme. By using less-than-perfect cleanup procedures it is possible to maintain recoveries for broad classes of toxic substances at high levels.

NCI mass spectra are obtained by operating a high-pressure (1 torr) mass spectrometer ion source in the negative mode. The primary electron beam (470 eV) is rapidly degraded in energy by interaction with the dominant gas molecules in the ion source. The degraded primary electrons and secondary electrons that result from the formation of positive ions form an electron swarm that is part of the low-density ionic plasma in the source. Under NCI conditions there are five major anion-producing reactions that are important in the analysis of toxic substances [14-17]. These are:

1. resonance capture of a thermal electron;
2. disassociative capture of a thermalized electron;
3. anion association;
4. proton abstraction; and
5. oxygen exchange for either halides or hydrogen atoms.

$$M + e^- \rightarrow M^{\cdot -*} \xrightarrow{N} M^{\cdot -} \tag{1}$$

$$A\text{-}B \xrightarrow{e^-} A^- + B\cdot \tag{2}$$

$$M + X^- \rightarrow MX^- \tag{3}$$

$$AH + B^- \rightarrow A^- + BH \tag{4}$$

$$AY^{\cdot -} + 0_2 \rightarrow AO^- + YO\cdot \tag{5}$$

In NCI mass spectrometry the reagent gas is present in the source at concentrations between $10^4$ and $10^5$ times the concentration of the substrate. Under these conditions the ion-forming reactions are controlled by the nature of the reagent gas and the substrates in the source. The reagent gas used in this study was a mixture of isobutane (50%), methylene chloride (48%) and oxygen (25). Chloride ions are produced by dissociative capture of an electron by methylene chloride. Chloride attachment gives the best results for screening for aliphatic polyhalogen compounds such as chlordane and nonachlor. The oxygen exchange reaction gives the best results for screening for polychloro polynuclear aromatic hydrocarbons (PAH). Isobutane is part of the reagent gas mixture to extend the filament lifetime.

At least half of the battle in analytical toxicology is preparation of samples before the final analytical step. The following guidelines have been used in the development of cleanup procedures for screening seminal fluid samples for contamination with toxic substances.

1. The cleanup procedures must be exceptionally simple. If high recoveries and reproducibility are to be maintained, it is the authors' experience that the cleanup procedure must be limited to no more than three steps.
2. Every step in the cleanup procedure should remove major components of the unwanted matrix while passing broad classes of chemical compounds.
3. The number of solvent evaporation steps in each cleanup procedure should be restricted to one. This restriction minimizes problems associated with contaminated solvents and their contributions to blank analyses.
4. Gas chromatography (GC) and adsorption chromatography are not used in these screening designs. Many toxic substances will not survive GC or adsorption chromatography without appropriate derivatization. For screening applications, derivatization is more or less prohibited.

The cleanup procedure used in this study is based on continuous liquid-liquid extraction (CLLE) steam distillation [18, 19]. Toxic substances that migrate in the environment and are not water-soluble virtually all have significant vapor pressures over water. Toxic substances that are significantly water soluble are generally not bioaccumulated, and thus are not expected to appear in the samples examined. The steam distillation procedure [19] is a micromodification of the CLLE distillation system developed by Veith and Kiwus [18].

The following sections of this chapter discuss the experimental procedures used, the result for both toxic substance screening and sperm density analysis, and a statistical evaluation of the relationship (if one exists) between the presence of persistent toxic substances and low sperm densities.

## EXPERIMENTAL

### Mass Spectral Screening

NCI mass spectra were obtained by direct probe introduction into an AEI MS-902 mass spectrometer equipped with an SRIC chemical ionization source. Ionization was initiated with 470-V electrons with a regulated emission current of 0.25 mamp. Source pressures were monitored with a MKS Beratron which was operated at the source potential (-8 KV). The reagent gases used in these experiments were distilled methylene chloride (48%), Matheson research grade isobutane (50%) and air. Source temperatures were maintained at 150°C. Spectra were recorded using ultraviolet (UV) oscillograph at 30 sec after introduction of the sample and at 30-sec intervals for 2.5 min. Electron multiplier responses were maintained at the same value throughout the series of experiments so that relative ion intensities could be used as a qualitative guide to concentrations of the substrates in the sample. Instrument sensitivity was maintained at a constant level and was checked by examining the sensitivity of the spectrometer to standard test compounds, in particular "ultramark."

## Steam Distillation Clean-Up

In a typical experiment, 2 ml of human seminal plasma was added to 35 ml of 10% sulfuric acid in water in a 50-ml flask. The contents of the flask were digested at 80°C for 30 min and subjected to CLLE steam distillation for an additional 30 min. The CLLE solvent was 2, 2, 4-trimethylpentane (isooctane). The steam distillation head used is illustrated in Figure 2. The isooctane layer was drawn off and decanted using a Pasteur pipette. The solvent was then dried (with magnesium sulfate) and reduced in volume using a Snyder column. Final volume reduction was accomplished with a stream of nitrogen. The 0.1-ml concentrate was divided into two portions; 5% of the sample was used for electron capture gas chromatography (EC/GC) and 95% of the sample for direct probe NCI mass spectrometry.

## Sample Collection And Sperm Density Determination

Volunteer donors were recruited from the Florida State University student population. Volunteers were requested to observe a 48-hr period of continence before collection of a seminal plasma sample. Samples were collected into chemically cleaned glass vials. Similar vials were also used in conducting procedural blanks. Samples were frozen within 12 hr of collection and stored in a sample freezer that had not been used for storage of chemical or toxic substance standards. When a sufficient number of samples had been collected, they were allowed to thaw. Ejaculate volumes were determined by measurement with a standard pipette. Sperm densities were determined by diluting 0.1 ml of the liquefied seminal plasma to 1 ml with distilled water. The

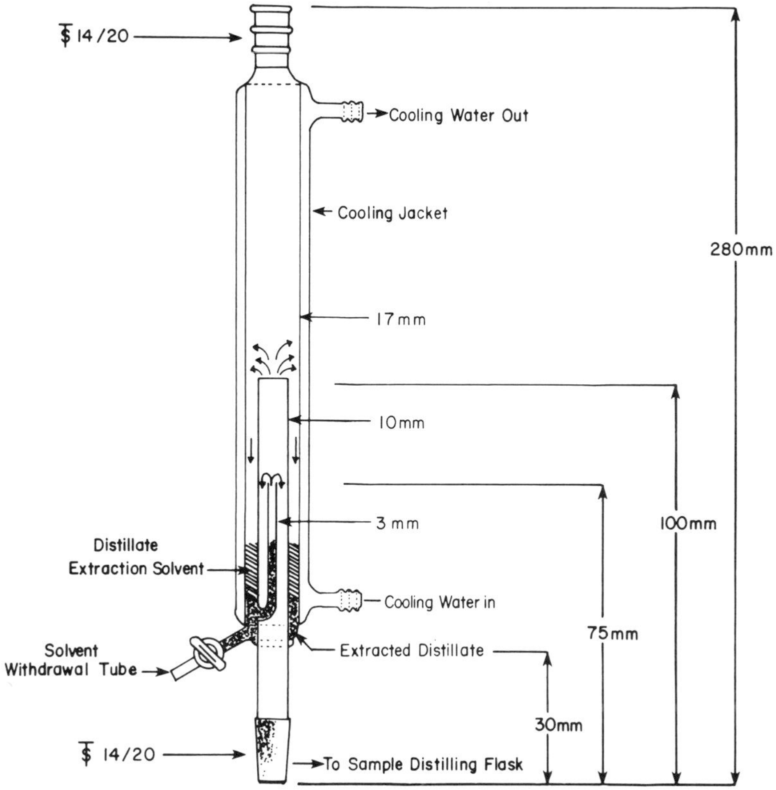


**Figure 2.** Micro steam distillation apparatus used for sample clean up.

samples were counted by counting five fields in a standard hemocytometer. Replicate counts were conducted for every seven samples. Reproducibility in replicate counts was better than 10%.

## RESULTS AND DISCUSSION

The specific reason for examining sperm density as a function of the presence of specific toxic substances stems from the fact that these compounds decrease the cell division rate by causing DNA damage. Exposure of cells to alkylating agents or activated toxic substances from the environment, e. g., diol epoxides of PAH, can cause the induction of alkylated DNA bases, chromosome breaks or both. When chromosome breaks of DNA base modifications occur, cell division is delayed until the defect can be repaired. Faulty repair can potentially lead to mutation or cancer.

## Sperm Densities and Ejaculate Volumes

Figure 3 illustrates the sperm density distribution for the group of 132 Florida State University students that were examined. To compare visually the sperm density distribution in this study with data from previous studies the data have been smoothed over 40 million cell/ml increments and replotted with data from previous studies (Figure 4). The plots in Figure 4 suggest that the sperm density distribution has been decreasing with time.

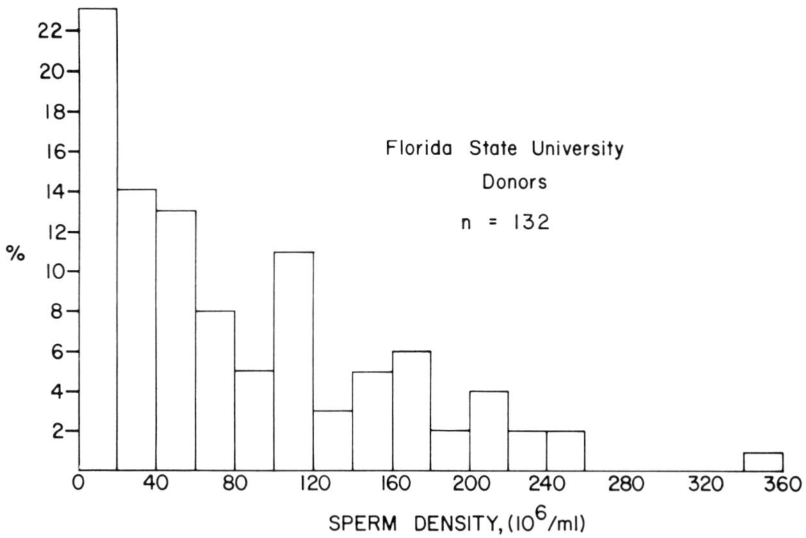


**Figure 3.** Sperm density distribution (increments of 20 million cell/ml) for 132 Florida State University donors.

There are a number of factors which could have contributed to the apparent decrease in the sperm density distribution. It is also true that volunteer donors in a university may not be a group that is representative of the male population as a whole. University students have distinct behavioral and stress parameters. Factors that could have contributed to the decline in median sperm densities include changes in frequency of sexual activity, changes in drug use patterns and changes in the general level of stress within the population.

The ejaculate volume distribution for the group of Florida State University students is plotted along with the similar volume distribution obtained by Rehan et al. [5] in Figure 5. The ejaculate volume distribution for the Florida State University students is shifted to smaller volumes as compared to

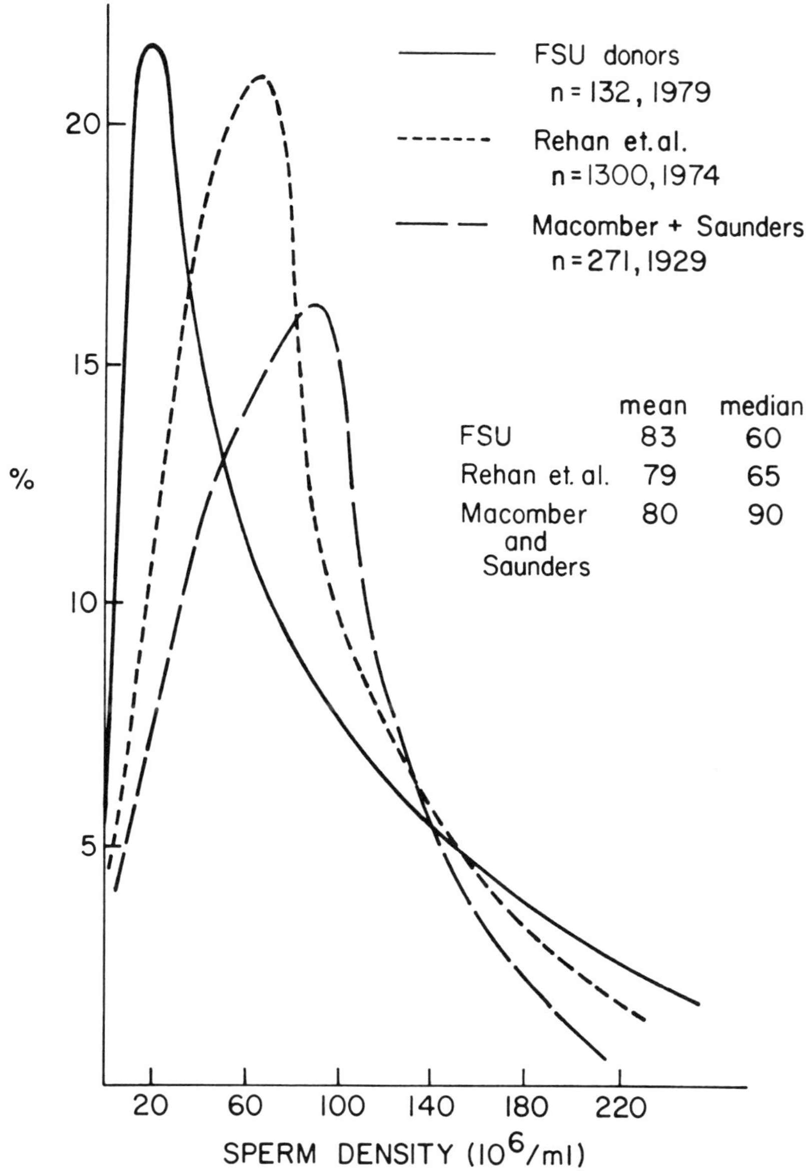


**Figure 4.** Sperm density distributions (smoothed over 40 million-cell/ml increments) for Florida State University donors as compared to the prevasectomy population of Rehan et al. [5] in 1974 and the prenatal clinic population of Macomber and Sanders [7] in 1929.

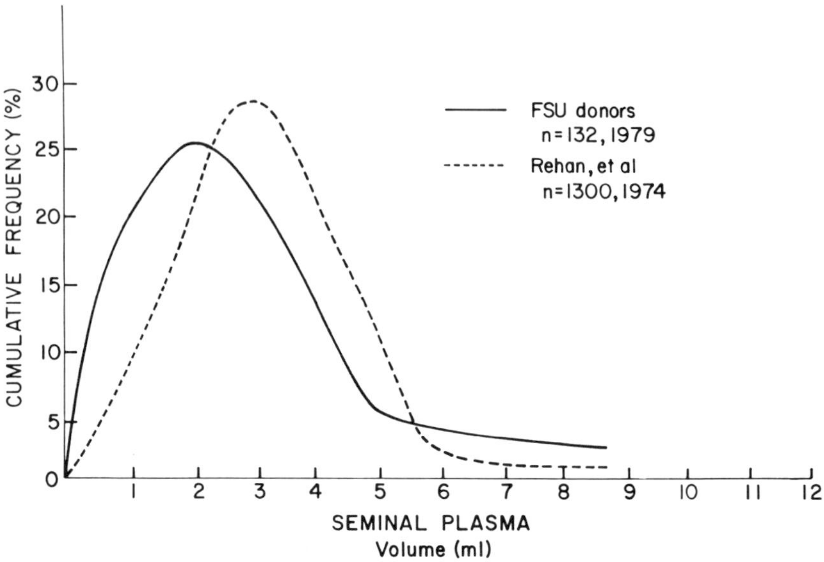


**Figure 5.** Ejaculate volume distribution for Florida State University donors as compared with the prevasectomy population of Rehan et al. [5].

the data of Rehan et al. The differences in the ejaculate volume distributions for the two populations would be consistent with a higher level of sexual activity in the student population.

Macleod and Wang have reviewed reports of male fertility parameters in the United States over the past two decades [20]. During this period median sperm densities have ranged from 60 million to almost 80 million cell/ml, and the number of samples with fewer than 20 million cell/ml varied from 15% to slightly over 20% of the populations examined. These numbers are not distinctly different from the values obtained in this study (median, 60 million cell/ml, proportion with less than 20 million cell/ml, 23%). These values suggest that the student population may reflect the parameters in the general population. The data in Table I indicate very clearly that there has been an apparent decline in male fertility parameters in the general population since 1950. The student population can be used to obtain the data that are needed to determine the relationship, if any exists, between the presence of specific toxic substances and low sperm densities.

## Negative Chemical Ionization Screening For Toxic Substances

In screening applications it is not possible to determine sample recoveries for all compounds because many of the compounds are unknown. Sample recoveries have been determined for hexachlorobenzene, pentachlorophenol, dieldrin, chlordane and octachlorostyrene. Sample recoveries, to some extent, depended on the specific steam distillation head (Figure 2) that was used. Sample recoveries were routinely checked for a representative group of compounds before putting a specific steam distillation head into service. Sample recoveries for all of the compounds mentioned have exceeded 90% in the equipment that was used for this study. Procedural blanks were conducted by taking an equivalent quantity of triple-distilled water that had been subjected to CLLE steam distillation for 1 hr, through the entire sample cleanup procedure, starting with the sample collection vial. To obtain acceptable procedural blanks it was necessary to use high-purity solvents that had been fractionally distilled in glass. Even with extreme precautions, polychlorinated ion clusters would occasionally appear in procedural blank samples. For the data reported here, the ion intensities in the procedural blanks were never larger than one order of magnitude less than the ion intensities for the corresponding ions in the samples examined.

For purposes of statistical evaluation, abundances of given ions were recorded under standard operating conditions. The instrument was not used unless it was possible to detect 1 ng of "ultramark" by direct probe examination. Samples were introduced at 150°C, and recordings were made at constant electron multiplier settings.

A number of compounds appeared in virtually every sample, reflecting the known general contamination of the human population with these substances. Known compounds that appeared in most of the samples include tri-, tetra- and pentachlorophenol, hexachlorobenzene, polychlorobiphenyls (PCB) with 5-8 chlorines, and the DDT metabolites DDE and DDMU. In addition to ions corresponding to these structures, a series of polyhalogenated ions was frequently encountered for which structures cannot be assigned at this time. Ion clusters that contain three chlorines for which there is no reasonable structural assignment included m/z 212, 241, 287 and 318. Frequently encountered unknowns with a four-chlorine isotope cluster included: m/z 229, 231, 239, 317 and 323. Unknown ion clusters with five chlorine atoms included: m/z 230 and 251. Unknown ions with an apparent six-chlorine isotope cluster were observed at m/z 375 and 427. An unknown with seven chlorines was frequently encountered at m/z 463.

In related studies, tissue samples obtained in medical examiner autopsy cases have been screened for the presence of toxic substances. In this screening program, heptachlorepoxide, nonachlor and chlordane have routinely been encountered. It is interesting to note that none of these compounds have appeared in the screening of human seminal plasma. Because the sample sizes were roughly equivalent it must be concluded that the concentration of these three compounds is significantly lower in seminal plasma than it is in fat. The reasons for this difference must be differences in the matrix and the presence of the blood-testicular barrier. Findings of toxic substances in human samples appear to be directly complementary to the findings of the U.S. EPA human monitoring program [21].

## Statistical Analysis

The basic model that we used in this examination of toxic substances in the environment is that of smoking and health. The first indication that tobacco smoking was deleterious to human health was obtained by statistical analysis relating tobacco consumption to the incidence of lung cancer mortality. Sperm density happens to be a quantitative biological parameter that is sensitive to the presence of a number of toxic substances. It is clear that in screening seminal plasma samples of toxic substances, some of the toxic substances will be missed which frequently appear in human populations, such as chlordane, nonachlor and heptachlorepoxide. It is to be hoped that the compounds missed in this study will turn up when further attempts are made to index human body burdens for persistent toxic substances to other quantitative health parameters.

Table II presents the statistical parameters obtained for a simple multiple linear regression analysis of the relationship between these findings for toxic substances and sperm densities. The slope is the particular intensity against sperm density for each item in the multiple regression. The "R square change" parameter reflects the contribution of the individual item to the multiple correlation coefficient R. The significance number is the probability that the individual correlation coefficient for the parameter in question is 0. The smaller the significance number, the more significant the individual parameter is to the overall correlation. The multiple correlation coefficient R for the 20 parameters listed in Table II against sperm density was 0.517. This means that the sum of these parameters accounts for roughly 27% of the variance in sperm density throughout the population. Considering the semiquantitative nature of the intensity data and the very large number of parameters that influence sperm density it is believed that the data in Table II represent a reasonable correlation for the parameters investigated.

Because it is known that smoking appears to have an effect on sperm density [4], donors are asked for information relating to their consumption of tobacco and nontobacco (marijuana) cigarettes. The slopes for tobacco and nontobacco cigarettes against sperm density were 0.07 and -0.06, respectively. The squares of the simple correlation coefficients were 0.005 and 0.009, respectively. The failure to show a negative slope in sperm density as a function of tobacco cigarette smoking is most likely related to the

Table II. Statistical Parameters Relating Sperm Density to Toxic Substances

| Precursor Structure | m/z | Number of Chlorines | Slope (SD/Intensity) | R Square Change | Significance |
|---|---|---|---|---|---|
| | 427 | 6 | 0.22 | 0.048 | 0.040 |
| | 241 | 3 | −0.11 | 0.054 | 0.010 |
| Heptachlorobiphenyl | 373 | 6 | −0.15 | 0.037 | 0.005 |
| | 343 | 4 | −0.16 | 0.021 | 0.005 |
| | 230 | 5 | −0.01 | 0.017 | 0.006 |
| Trichlorophenol | 231 | 4 | 0.08 | 0.012 | 0.007 |
| Hexachloronaphthalene | 313 | 5 | 0.10 | 0.011 | 0.009 |
| Pentachlorophenol | 263 | 5 | 0.00 | 0.013 | 0.010 |
| Hexachlorobiphenyl | 339 | 5 | −0.10 | 0.005 | 0.015 |
| | 463 | 7 | −0.04 | 0.008 | 0.020 |
| | 318 | 3 | −0.09 | 0.015 | 0.021 |
| Tetrachlorodiphenylether (?) | 287 | 3 | −0.09 | 0.008 | 0.026 |
| Hexachlorobenzene | 282 | 6 | 0.04 | 0.005 | 0.035 |
| | 212 | 3 | 0.20 | 0.003 | 0.049 |
| | 239 | 4 | 0.03 | 0.003 | 0.065 |
| | 241 | 3 | 0.02 | 0.002 | 0.087 |
| | 224 | 3 | −0.14 | 0.002 | 0.115 |
| | 251 | 5 | −0.12 | 0.001 | 0.152 |
| Pentachlorobiphenyl | 305 | 4 | −0.09 | 0.001 | 0.198 |
| Octachlorobiphenyl | 407 | 7 | −0.03 | 0.001 | 0.251 |

restricted size of the sample and the relatively small number of smokers within the sample.

It is interesting to note that of the ion clusters, whose identity is known from comparisons with standard NCI mass spectra in Table II, the PCB all have negative slopes against sperm density, and contribute significantly to the overall correlation. PCB basically represent a single parameter, because they may all travel together in the environment and have the same origins. The correlation could probably be improved if these components were added together as a single parameter.

It is not at all likely that the dose-response curve for sperm density as a function of exposure to toxic substances is linear. It is probable that the correlation in Table II could be improved significantly by the use of nonlinear regression.

The partition coefficient for specific toxic substances between the sperm cells and seminal fluid is far from unity. For pentachlorophenol, the concentration in the cells is between 20 and 40 times as high as the concentration in cell-free seminal plasma. Although the cells on average correspond to only 4% of the mass of the ejaculate, the differential in the concentration of toxic substances in the cells means that the presence of the cells is particularly important to the analytical results. As the number of cells in the ejaculate decreases, the ability to detect specific toxic substances in the seminal plasma also decreases. Linear regression models have been examined using concentrations per cell for the independent variables. The correlation was significantly improved. When the correlation was made on an intensity-per-cell basis, all of the entries in Table II had negative slopes against sperm density. The partition ratios are presently being determined for the entries in Table II between cell-free seminal plasma and sperm cells. These data should allow the estimation of the cellular concentration for the materials listed in Table II, and it is anticipated that these data will show a better correlation with sperm densities than simple linear regression.

## SUMMARY

The sperm density distributions obtained for a group of 132 college aged males have been compared with toxic substance burden data as obtained in a NCI screening procedure. The sperm density distribution for this group was similar to the distribution obtained by Zuckerman et al. [6] for a group of more than 4000 prevasectomy patients. NCI screening revealed the presence of a number of unknown polychlorinated substances as well as polychlorophenols, PCB, hexachlorobenzene, DDT metabolites and polychloronaphthalenes. Multiple linear regression was used in an attempt to correlate the presence of specific toxic substances uncovered in the NCI screening with sperm densities. PCB uniformly gave negative slope correlations with sperm densities. For all of the toxic substances that remain in the regression equation (Table II), the multiple correlation coefficient was 0.52, which indicates that these variables account for roughly 27% of the variance in the sperm density distribution.

## ACKNOWLEDGMENTS

It is a pleasure to acknowledge useful discussions with Andrew Wyrobek and Duane Meeter. This work was supported by the National Institute of Environmental Health Sciences (Extramural Program) and the U.S. Environmental Protection Agency.

## REFERENCES

1. Mason, T. J., F. W. McKay, R. Hoover, W. J. Blot and J. F. Fraumeni, Jr. "Atlas of Cancer Mortality for U.S. Counties: 1950–1969," U.S. DHEW Publication No. (NIH) 75-780 (1975).

2. Ames, B. N. "Identifying Environmental Chemicals Causing Mutations and Cancer," *Science* 204:587-593 (1979).
3. Wyrobek, A. J. and W. R. Bruce. "Induction of Sperm-Shape Abnormalities in Mice and Humans," in *Chemical Mutagens, Vol. 5*, A. Hollander and F. J. deSerres, Eds. (New York: Plenum Publishing Corp., 1978), p. 257–285.
4. Viczian, M. "Ergebnisse von Spermauntersuchungen bei Zigarettenrauchen," *Z. Hant Geschlechtskr.* 44:183–187 (1969).
5. Rehan, N. E., A. J. Sobrero and J. W. Fertig. "The Semen of Fertile Men: Statistical Analysis of 1300 Men," *Fertil. Steril.* 26:492–502 (1975).
6. Zukerman, Z., L. J. Rodriquez-Rigan, K. D. Smith and E. Steinberger. "Frequency Distribution of Sperm Counts in Fertile and Infertile Males," *Fertil. Steril.* 28:1310–1313 (1977).
7. Macomber, D., and M. B. Sanders. "The Spermatozoa Count: Its Value in the Diagnosis, Prognosis and Treatment of Sterility," *New England J. Med.* 200:981–984 (1929).
8. Hotchkiss, R. S., K. Brunner and P. G. Grenley. "Semen Analysis of Two Hundred Fertile Men," *Am. J. Med. Sci.* 196:362–365 (1938).
9. Farris, E. J. *J. Urol.* 61:1099 (1949).
10. Falk, H. C., and S. A. Kaufmann. "What Constitutes a Normal Semen?" *Fertil. Steril.* 1:489–503 (1950).
11. MacLeod, J., and R. Z. Gold. "The Male Factor in Fertility and Infertility. II. Spermatozoon Counts in 1000 Men of Known Fertility and in 1000 Cases of Infertile Marriage," *J. Urol.* 66:436–444 (1951).
12. Sobrero, A. J., and N.-E. Rehan. "The Semen of Fertile Men. II. Semen Characteristics of 100 Fertile Men," *Fertil. Steril.* 26:1048–1056 (1975).
13. Glass, R. I., R. N. Lyness, D. C. Mengle, K. E. Powell and E. Kahn. "Sperm Count Depression in Pesticide Applicators Exposed to Dibromochloropropane," *Am. J. Epidemol.* 109(3):346–351 (1979).
14. Tannenbaum, H. P., J. D. Roberts and R. C. Dougherty. "Negative Chemical Ionization Mass Spectrometry: Chloride Attachment Spectra," *Anal. Chem.* 47:49–54 (1975).
15. Dougherty, R. C., J. Dalton and F. J. Biros. "Negative Chemical Ionization Mass Spectra of Polycyclic Chlorinated Pesticides," *Org. Mass. Spectrom.* 6:1171–1181 (1972).
16. Dougherty, R. C., and K. Piotrowska. "Screening by Negative Chemical Ionization Mass Spectrometry for Environmental Contamination with Toxic Residues," *Proc. Nat. Acad. Sci., U.S.* 73:1777–1781 (1976).
17. Hass, J. R., M. D. Friesen, D. J. Harvan and E. C. Parker. "Determination of Polychlorinated Dibenzo-p-dioxins in Biological Samples by Negative Chemical Ionization Mass Spectrometry," *Anal. Chem.* 50: 1474–1480 (1978).
18. Veith, G. D., and L. M. Kiwus. "An Exhaustive Steam-Distillation and Solvent Extraction Unit for Pesticides and Industrial Chemicals," *Bull. Environ. Contam. Toxicol.* 17:631-632 (1977).
19. Kuehl, D. W., M. J. Whitaker and R. C. Dougherty. "Micro-Methods for Toxic Residue Screening," *Anal. Chem.* 52:935-940 (1980).

20. Macleod, J., and Y. Wang. "Male Fertility Potential in Terms of Semen Quality: A Review of The Past and a Study of the Present," *Fertil. Steril.* 31(2):103-116 (1979).
21. Kutz, F. W., A. R. Yobs and S. C. Strassman. "Organochlorine Pesticide Residues in Human Adipose Tissue," *Bull. Soc. Pharm. Environ. Pathol.* IV:17-50 (1976).

# CHAPTER 14

# DEVELOPMENT OF RADIOIMMUNOASSAYS FOR CHLORINATED AROMATIC HYDROCARBONS

**Michael I. Luster, Phillip W. Albro, Kun Chae, Sunil K. Chaudhary and James D. McKinney**

Laboratory of Environmental Chemistry
National Institute of Environmental Health Sciences
Research Triangle Park, North Carolina

## INTRODUCTION

Many of the microconstituents of complex mixtures to which humans are exposed thoughout their lifetimes are chemically uncharacterized and, often, little is known of their toxicologic significance. In regulatory science, detection and quantitation of unidentified hazardous chemicals in complex mixtures are essential to hazard assessment, to exert some measure of regulatory control. Given the complexity of such mixtures, new approaches to identification and control of health hazards need to be developed to encompass both the chemical properties and the biological effects of such components. Highly specific biological systems which reflect toxicologic endpoints may be useful in a bioassay approach to signal the presence of trace amounts of certain industrial or natural contaminants in mixtures which can be subsequently confirmed by chemical methods. Ideally, a suitable bioassay will discriminate between toxic and nontoxic chemical analogs which may be indistinguishable by chemical assay, be sensitive to low concentrations and be qualitative as well as quantitative. The biological endpoint must specifically reflect the presence of only certain chemicals or chemically related compounds.

Although intact animals are often viewed as the preferred system for toxicologic testing in a bioassay approach, methods using the intact animal do not generally lend themselves to rapid and convenient testing of a large number of substances in a screening matrix. Nor do they always or necessarily provide the information sought, which sometimes requires an understanding of the mechanism by which a toxicologic event occurred. Therefore, there is a need for reliable, simple and reproducible indicators such as in vitro methods using specific biochemical endpoints in tissue and cell cultures and protein receptor-type assays. Research in the authors' laboratories has led to the development of radioimmunoassays for certain chlorinated aromatic hydrocarbons.

Polychlorinated aromatic hydrocarbons such as polychlorinated dibenzo-*p*-dioxins (PCDD), biphenyls (PCB) and dibenzofurans (PCDF) are classes of widespread environmental pollutants, of considerable current concern [1]. PCDD occur as contaminants in commercial chlorophenols, and particularly as by-products in the manufacture of chlorophenoxyacids. The primary PCDD found as a contaminant of 2, 4, 5-trichlorophenoxyacetic acid (2, 4, 5-T) is 2, 3, 7, 8-tetra-CDD (TCDD) [2] possibly the most toxic manmade chemical known with an acute oral LD50 of 1 $\mu$g/kg body weight in the guinea pig [3] and approximately 250 $\mu$g/kg in the mouse [4]. TCDD is not the only highly toxic PCDD, and several penta- and hexa- CDD have toxicities comparable to that of TCDD. Aroclors® are commercial preparations of PCB used for the past 50 years in transformers, capacitors, as heat transfer fluids and in other industrial applications. PCB are widely distributed in the environment, have been found in tissues of wildlife and humans [5] and have an acute oral LD50 ranging from 1 to 10 g/kg body weight in rats, rabbits and mice [6]. The toxicities of individual PCB have been studied extensively, and will vary with isomeric composition [7]. Individual Aroclors can consist of up to 100 different chlorobiphenyls; however, the lower chlorinated homologs are less abundant in biological and environmental samples, indicating their more rapid metabolism and degradation to polar compounds [8]. Interest in PCDF resulted from their identification as impurities in various American and European PCB [9] and subsequent identification from PCB-contaminated rice oil in Japan [10]. Like PCDD several PCDF isomers have been found to be highly toxic, with 2, 3, 7, 8-tetra-CDF (TCDF) the most toxic, having an acute oral LD50 between 5 and 10 $\mu$g/kg body weight in the guinea pig [11].

Unitl recently, the only analytical technique with sufficient sensitivity and specificity for determination of chlorinated aromatic hydrocarbons, particularly PCDD, has been high resolution mass spectrometry (MS) [12]. Gas chromatography (GC) combined with low or medium resolution MS in either electron impact or chemical ionization modes [13] has been used recently to estimate levels of PCDD in addition to TCDD itself. The detection limits of these techniques are on the order of a few tens of picograms when the samples are free of interfering contaminants. Further data can be obtained by comparison of retention times employing high resolution GC with authentic standards, but the number of synthetic standards are limited [14].

Because of the cost and complexity of gas chromatography/mass spectrometry (GC/MS) instrumentation and the high degree of skill and experience needed in assays of this type, only a few laboratories are able to perform assays at the present. This situation has resulted in a slow output of analytical data. Additionally, the lack of a confirmatory technique not based on MS has tended to limit the confidence of those not trained in that specialty in the data presently available. For these reasons, development of assays has begun based on the highly sensitive and relatively specific technique of radioimmunoassay (RIA). It is believed that these assays will be applicable both to screening samples to minimize the demand for MS analysis by eliminating "negatives," and for routine monitoring of exposure in environments where specific polychlorinated aromatic hydrocarbons are known to be present.

## DESIGN AND METHODS

### Principle of RIA for Polychlorinated Aromatic Hydrocarbons

RIA are similar to competitive protein-binding assays, except RIA employ specific antibody as the binder rather than a naturally occurring binder protein. In general, RIA are more sensitive and specific than competitive protein-binding assays, and can accurately quantify picograms of test material under optimal conditions. In what follows, the polychlorinated aromatic hydrocarbon is referred to as antigen or hapten (Hap). The hapten is present in two forms in the assay, radiolabeled with $^{125}I$ (Hap*) or unlabeled. During incubation both labeled and unlabeled hapten exist in bound and free forms depending on their interaction with specific antibody (Ab) at any particular time. Yalow and Berson have used the ratios bound:free as the response parameter after equilibrium, based on the treatment of the system in terms of mass equations:

$$(\text{Hap}) + (\text{Ab}) \underset{k_2}{\overset{k_1}{\rightleftarrows}} (\text{Hap Ab})$$

$$K = \frac{k_1}{k_2} = \frac{(\text{Hap Ab})}{(\text{Hap})(\text{Ab})}$$

the molar concentration (molar concentration of antibody x valency of antibody) is Ab°:

$$(\text{Ab}^\circ) = (\text{Ab}) + (\text{Hap Ab})$$

or

$$K(\text{Ab}^\circ) - (\text{Hap Ab}) = \frac{(\text{Hap Ab})}{(\text{Hap})}$$

where Bound (B) = (Ag Hap)

Free (F) = (Hap)

thus, $B/F = K(\text{Ab}^\circ) - B$. When plotting RIA curves from this equation, the plot is neither linear nor log-linear, and the scatter of determinations of the response parameter is markedly different at various points along the curve. A full description of this system has been described [15,16].

The antibody-antigen complex, after equilibration, must be separated from nonbound antigen. Many "separators" have been used, including a second antibody directed against the primary antibody (double antibody assay), dextran-coated charcoal, as well as physical processes such as electrophoresis or dialysis.

Low-molecular-weight molecules, including the polychlorinated aromatic hydrocarbons, are not by themselves capable of inducing an antibody response. Compounds of this type can be covalently coupled to various "carrier" molecules (usually proteins), affording them immunogenicity. The chlorinated aromatic hydrocarbons do not have functional groups in their molecule to bind with carrier proteins to form hapten-carrier complexes. Therefore, it is necessary to derivatize with reactive groups such as amino or carboxy groups. Although a variety of compounds have been derivatized, those compounds used as antigens in the RIA to be described include 1-amino-3, 7, 8-tri-CDD, 4-amino-4-chlorobiphenyl, 2-amino-4, 5, 3′, 4′-tetrachlorobiphenyl (TCBP), 3-amino-2, 6, 2′, 6′-TCBP and 4-amino-2, 7, 8-tri-CDF. The synthesis of the amino-tri-CDD [17] and amino-TCBP [18] have been described. The 4-amino-4-monochlorobiphenyl was purchased from K & K Laboratories, Inc., while the synthesis of the amino-PCDF has recently been described [19].

## Hapten: Protein Conjugation

A series of coupling procedures were evaluated for reproducibility, stability and immunogenicity including azo, acetyl and adipamide linkages. The optimal results occurred by reacting the amino-compounds with the acid chloride of *mono*-methyl adipate followed by converting the adipamide to a mixed anhydride [20]. The protein carriers conjugated to haptens by this mixed anhydride method included various albumins and thyroglobulins, the protein content of the reaction being determined by the biuret method. The number of free amino groups was determined by the ninhydrin assay of Harding and MacLean [21] and was confirmed using trinitrobenzene sulfonate [22]. Free-hydroxy of tyrosyl units was determined using the Folin-Ciocalteu phenol reagent [23]. Tryptophan was measured in the unhydrolyzed protein by the method of Gaitonde and Dovey [24]. The mixed anhydride coupling procedure gave a reproducible degree of conjugation, with 80 ± 2% of the hapten moiety covalently bound to protein over a range of 10–50 mol mixed anhydride/mol of protein. Bound plus adsorbed hapten was measured by ultraviolet (UV) difference spectra, with antigen protein concentration made equal to the corresponding unconjugated protein concentration on the basis of biuret assays. Adsorbed hapten was separated from the protein conjugated hapten by chromatography on Sephadex G-100. Albumin carrier had approximately 12 mol of hapten coupled at the $\epsilon$-amino group of lysine and 3 mol coupled at tyrosine, per mole of albumin. Thyroglobulin bound approximately 80 mol of hapten at lysine and 20 mol at tyrosine, per mole of protein.

## Production of Antiserum

New Zealand White rabbits were immunized on a variety of schedules. The most effective procedure appeared to be weekly administration of 0.5 mg protein-hapten in equal volumes of Tris-buffer and Freund's adjuvant (total of 1.0 ml). The initial immunization was given in complete Freund's adjuvant intradermally into several sites into the back of neck and hind foot pads. Subsequent injections were administered in incomplete Freund's adjuvant intramuscularly into the hind legs. Antibody production was initially monitored by immunodiffusion analysis against a different carrier protein and analogous hapten and later by RIA. Secondary antibody responses were obtained, by a single injection (as described above) after the initial antibody response titer had begun to decay (usually 3-4 months after completing the primary immunization schedule). Serum was stored frozen at -70°C in small portions.

## $^{125}$I-Radiolabeled Hapten

The amino derivatives of the haptens were converted to amides with 5-bromovaleryl chloride as described previously [20]. The bromo compound was reacted with sodium iodide in acetone and the product was extracted with ether. The etheral solution was washed with 10% (aq) sodium metabisulfite, water and was dried over anhydrous sodium sulfate, after which the solvent was evaporated. The crude product was chromatographed on a column containing activated silica gel, eluted with benzene and 10% chloroform in benzene. The product gave a single spot on a silica gel thin-layer chromatography (TLC) plate with benzene as solvent. The unlabeled iodovaleramide derivative was dissolved in acetone (or, preferably, peroxide-free tetrahydrofuran), and injected into a vial containing carrier-free $^{125}$I–sodium iodide. The mixture was held at 50°C for 60 hr in a sand bath. After cooling, the products were taken up in chloroform, washed with 10% sodium metabisulfite and water and dried over anhydrous sodium sulfate. The crude product was passed through silica gel (silicic acid) in chloroform to remove traces of unbound iodine. The final product contained greater than 95% of its radioactivity in a single spot during TLC on silica gel in benzene, and had an estimated specific radioactivity of ~80 Ci/mmol.

## Tissue Extraction and Cleanup

Tissues (liver, adipose and serum) were processed as recommended previously [25] with some slight modifications (Luster et al., in preparation). Soil samples can be extracted with acetone in a Soxhlet extraction apparatus [26] and the extracts purified as for tissue extracts [24]. Small volumes of benzene are added to the final residues and, if desired, are stored frozen.

## Solubility

A central feature of this assay is the use of nonionic detergents to solubilize the extremely hydrophobic polychlorinated aromatic hydrocarbons in a manner permitting their binding to antibodies. Fifteen detergents were compared as to their ability to solubilize $^{14}$C-TCDD (probably the most lipophilic hapten examined) without interfering seriously with the antibody-hapten interaction. Two nonionic detergents, Triton X-305 and Cutscum, provided sufficient micelle formation to negate insolubility, and had minimal effects on inhibiting antibody binding and precipitation in the RIA (Table I). Triton X-45 and X-100 solubilized the TCDD but interfered with antibody

Table I. The Effect of Various Detergents on the TCDD RIA

| Detergents Tested | Result in Assay |
|---|---|
| Triton X-305 | 30 pg–5 ng |
| Cutscum | 100 pg–ng |
| Triton X-45, X-100 | Interference |
| Tergitol TMN, Tween 20, Tween 80 Fluorosurfactants and Ionic Surfactants | Inadequate solubilizer |

binding. Other anionic and ionic surfactants examined did not solubilize TCDD. In general, lower levels of hapten could be measured with Triton X-305 than with Cutscum; however, a wider range of concentrations could be assayed using Cutscum than Triton X-305. Furthermore, although Cutscum alone caused a greater inhibition of the hap-Ab curve than Triton X-305 (approximately 15%), unlike Triton X-305, the resulting inhibition was independent of Cutscum concentration at least up to 5% v/v.

## Preparation of Samples Prior to RIA Analysis

Compounds used as competitive inhibitors, unknowns, working standards or blank controls were appropriately diluted in benzene, added to 12- x 75-mm glass tubes and dried under nitrogen. To each tube was added 0.2 ml of 1% Cutscum or 1% Triton X-305 in methanol and the solvent again evaporated under nitrogen.

## Assay Procedure

Radioimmunoassay of small molecules requires some means of separating free hapten from antibody-bound hapten [27]. The procedure used in these studies was chosen because of its compatibility with detergent-solubilized hapten and involved precipitating the antibody-hap complex with goat antibodies against rabbit gamma-globulin. Haptens from the unknown sample or working standard compete with the $^{125}$I-labeled hapten for binding to the antibody. Thus, the decrease in precipitation of radioactivity is a measure of the amount of unlabeled hapten in the test sample.

The assay buffer (PBS) contained 20 mmol/l of potassium phosphate, 140 mmol/l of NaCl and 200 mg/l of sodium azide. The pH was adjusted to 7.3 with NaOH. Antiserum was diluted with PBS also containing 0.1% bovine gamma globulin (w/v) to prevent nonspecific binding and 0.02% rabbit gamma globulin (w/v) to standardize precipitation of the second antibody. These procedures have been described in detail [17, 28]. Each assay tube as prepared under "Preparation of Samples" received 0.2 ml of PBS, after which the tubes were held in an Ultramet II sonicating cleaner for 40 min and allowed to cool. For RIA analysis, 0.2 ml of one of the antisera diluted in PBS with carrier proteins was added to the tubes. A dilution of antiserum that bound about 40% of the tracer doses was used in all assays. After incubation for 30 min at 37°C, 7000 counts/min (cpm) of the appropriate $^{125}$I-labeled hapten (14,000 dpm) diluted in PBS with 1% detergent (~25 microliter/7000 cpm) was added. This was followed by an additional 30-min incubation at 37°C and a further 65-hr at 4°C. Each tube then received 0.2 ml of cold goat antirabbit gamma-globulin appropriately diluted in PBS which contained 0.05 m*M* ethylenediaminetetraacetate (EDTA). The preparation was then incubated for an additional 6 hr at 4°C. All tubes were centrifuged (4°C, 500 *g*, 30 min) and the radioactivity in the precipitate was measured in a gamma counter.

Standard curves were prepared using sequential twofold dilutions of hapten standard in benzene, evaporating the solvent as described above. Both control (blank) and spiked tissues were extracted and processed as described above to determine general interference and recoveries. All samples were run in duplicate or triplicate.

Incubation times required for maximum reproducible binding were determined from time/temperature studies. General methods for optimizing the conditions for the double-antibody separation system have been described [27]. Nonspecifically bound and precipitated radioactivity was, in these detergent-containing systems, quite minor and reproducible (100–150 cpm), so that radioactivity in pellets of tubes lacking antiserum could simply be subtracted from the radioactivity in assay tubes.

Calibration curves were obtained by plotting (B/Bo) x 100, where B represents counts per minute in tubes containing unlabeled affector (calibration standard, unknown, or inhibitor) and Bo represents counter per minute in the tubes lacking affector, against amount of unlabeled affector on semilog paper as described previously [29].

A complete description of the materials used in these studies and more detailed methodology has been described elsewhere [19,28].

## RESULTS AND DISCUSSION

The final assay conditions (i. e., buffer pH, buffer ionic strength, time and temperature of incubation, etc.) were similar in all assays. Immunization with each of the particular protein-hapten conjugates was performed in a number of rabbits (usually 8-10). Antiserum avidity from individual rabbits to their respective hapten was determined by a series of antibody titration curves as described by Hunter [27]. Avidity is a function of both antibody potency and specificity. The antiserum of highest avidity for each hapten was selected for further experiments. Antisera dilutions that bound about 40% of the tracer dose (without unlabeled hapten present) were used. This resulted in antiserum dilutions which range from 1:1000 to 1:15,000, depending on the hapten tested and antiserum employed, and whether the antisera were obtained after a primary or secondary immunization. In all cases, antiserum reactivity was greater against the amino-derivative than the native compound as would be expected.

## TCDF Assay

The immunizing hapten for the DBF assay was 4-amino-2, 7, 8-tri-CDF, and the standard curves were constructed against unlabeled 2, 3, 7, 8-TCDF. A typical standard curve for inhibition of radioiodinated hapten/antibody binding by TCDF in the presence of Cutscum is shown in Figure 1. Using the equation B/Bo x 100 where B represents the corrected counts per minute in tubes containing unlabeled TCDF and Bo the corrected counts per minute in tubes lacking unlabeled hapten, the theoretical range of this assay is between 20 pg and 4.0 ng if no interference from the test samples is present.

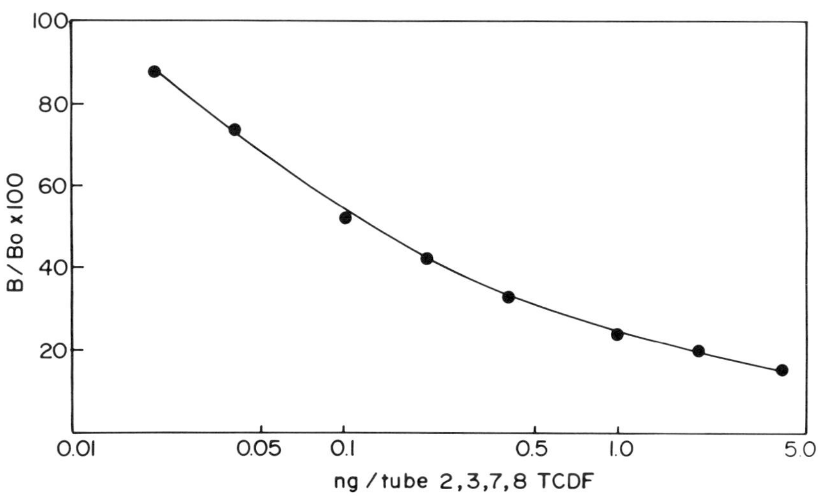


**Figure 1.** Typical standard curve for 2,3,7,8-TCDF with antisera against 4-amino-2,7,8-tri-CDF in the presence of Cutscum.

Table II. Cross Reactivity of 2,3,7,8-TCDF RIA

| Compound | Amount Required for 50% Inhibition of Curve[a] (ng) | Percentage Reactivity[b] |
|---|---|---|
| Dibenzofurans | | |
| Unchlorinated | >100.0 | <0.25 |
| 2,8-$Cl_2$ | 17.0 | 1.5 |
| 3,6-$Cl_2$ | 30.0 | 0.8 |
| 2,3,8-$Cl_3$ | 0.45 | 55.5 |
| 2,3,6,8-$Cl_4$ | 1.25 | 20.0 |
| 2,3,7,8-$Br_4$ | 0.64 | 39.1 |
| 2,3,7,8-$Cl_4$ | 0.25 | 100 |
| 1,3,4,7,8-$Cl_5$ | >100.0 | <0.25 |
| 2,3,4,6,7,8-$Cl_6$ | 12.0 | 2.1 |
| 1,2,3,4,6,7,8,9-$Cl_8$ | >100.0 | <0.25 |
| Biphenyls | | |
| 2,4,2′,4′-$Cl_4$ | 9.9 | 2.5 |
| 2,6,2′,6′-$Cl_4$ | >100.0 | <0.25 |
| 3,4,3′,4′-$Cl_4$ | 12.0 | 2.1 |
| 3,4,3′,4′-$(CH_3)_4$ | >100.0 | <0.25 |
| 3,5,3′,5′-$Cl_4$ | 33.0 | 0.8 |
| 3,4,5,3′,4′,5′-$Cl_6$ | 25.0 | 1.0 |
| Others | | |
| 3,4,3′,4′-$Cl_4$-Biphenyl Ether | >100.0 | <0.25 |
| 3,4,3′,4′-$Cl_4$-Biphenylene | 1.05 | 23.8 |
| 2,3,7,8-Tetrachlorodibenzo-*p*-dioxin | 2.9 | 8.6 |
| 3,4,3′,4′-Tetrachloroazobenzene | 1.4 | 17.9 |
| RIA Working Proteins | >100.0 | <0.25 |

[a]Amounts testable depended on "solubility" in Cutscum.
[b]Amount 2,3,7,8-TCDF required for 50% displacement of RIA curve divided by amount of test compound required for 50% displacement x 100.

Table II summarizes the relative cross reactivity of the antiserum to several PCDF, PCB and other halogenated aromatic hydrocarbons. As would be expected, 2, 3, 7, 8-TCDF is the most cross-reactive compound in the assay assuming that the amino group of the immunizing hapten substitutes for the fourth chlorine. In general, the antisera are fairly specific to 2, 3, 7, 8-TCDF, but have significant cross-reactivity to several compounds with similar halogen substitution (including bromine). Furthermore, some cross-reactivity is caused by the rigid nature of the DBD, DBF, biphenylene and azobenzene, as compared to the less rigid biphenyls, because 3, 4, 3′, 4′-TCBP is not very reactive. Kinetic studies have indicated that abosrption of the antisera with these cross-reacting compounds do not result in a more specific antiserum (unpublished data).

To test the applicability of the TCDF RIA to tissue samples, monkey adipose and rat liver tissues obtained from orally dosed animals were processed as described previously (Table III). A fraction (5%) of the recovered sample was subjected to RIA analysis, while an additional aliquot was used for comparison assay by GC with either negative chemical ionization MS or an electron capture detector as measuring device. In addition, the concentration of TCDF in Aroclors 1242 and 1016 were determined. In almost all instances, good correlation was found. The presence of low-level interfering contaminants that accumulated during sample cleanup will limit the sensitivity of these RIA, however, it should be noted that the interference as reported here is exaggerated because actual values were multiplied by a factor of 20 to determine the TCDF concentration in an entire tissue sample. This interference is represented on a standard curve as approximately 3-5% inhibition, while 250 pg of TCDF causes 50% inhibition.

## PCB Assay

The likelihood that an environmental sample would contain a single PCB congener is relatively remote, because it would probably present itself as a

**Table III. Comparison of RIA with Other Procedures for Determination of TCDF in Various Samples**

| Sample | Amount Processed (g) | Dosage (per kg Body Weight) | Amount Detected (ng) | |
|---|---|---|---|---|
| | | | RIA | EC/GC or GC/MS |
| Monkey Adipose[a] | 0.05 | 0 mg | 0.4 | ND[b](EC/GC) |
| | | 0 mg | 0.4 | ND |
| | | 0.5 mg | 2.3 | Interference |
| | | 0.5 mg | 1.48 | 2.30 |
| | | 1.0 mg | 7.0 | 2.06 |
| | | 1.5 mg | 2.6 | 2.07 |
| Rat Liver | 1.0 | 0 μg | 0.8 | ND (GC/MS) |
| | | 5 μg | 22.0 | 29 |
| | | 50 μg | 82.0 | 152 |
| Aroclor 1242 | 0.1 | | 15.0 | 14.9[c](GC/MS) |
| Aroclor 1016 | 0.1 | | 0.5 | ND |
| Column Control (Background) | | | 0.5 | ND |

[a]Monkey samples were obtained from an earlier study [30].
[b]ND = none detected.
[c]Based on total DBF found (2,3,6-$Cl_3$, 4.7 ng/0.lg; 1,3,6,7-$Cl_4$, 0.7 ng/0.1 g; 2,3,7,8-$Cl_4$, 6.4 ng/0.1 g; 2,3,4,7,8-$Cl_5$, 2.8 ng/0.1 g; 1,2,3,6,7,8-$Cl_6$, $<$ 0.3 ng/0.1 g) [31].

mixture of PCB reflecting their commercial origin. Biological samples, of course, would tend to concentrate the higher-chlorinated biphenyls. Production of antisera against a PCB mixture would not only be technically difficult but would not have any quantitative significance in RIA analysis. Thus, RIA analysis of PCB was approached by producing antisera against specific PCB. Initially, antisera were produced against homologs likely to be found in environmental samples, and included 2-amino-4, 5, 3′, 4′-TCBP and 3-amino-2, 6, 2′, 6′-TCBP. In addition, antisera were produced against 4-amino-4′-MCBP. Cross-reactivity studies with these antisera against compounds either potentially present in Aroclors, biological samples or unique to the laboratory are summarized in Table IV. In all cases, the amino derivative of the hapten was the most reactive compound against the respective antisera. However, antisera to the two TCBP had sufficient cross-reactivity and specificity to their corresponding nonaminated chlorobiphenyls to indicate that the RIA

**Table IV. Percent Cross Reactivity[a] in PCB Assays**

| | Percent Cross Reactivity with Chlorobiphenyl Antisera | | |
|---|---|---|---|
| **Compound Tested** | **2,6,2′,6′** | **3,4,3′,4′** | **4** |
| Biphenyls | | | |
| Biphenyl | –[b] | +/–[c] | 65 |
| 4-Cl | – | +/– | 65 |
| 4-F | – | – | 32 |
| 3,3′-$Cl_2$ | – | – | 5.0 |
| 3,4-$Cl_2$ | – | – | +/– |
| 2,3,2′,3′-$Cl_4$ | +/– | – | 2.4 |
| 2,4,2′,4′-$Cl_4$ | +/– | – | – |
| 2,6,2′,6′-$Cl_4$ | 27 | – | – |
| 3,4,3′,4′-$Cl_4$ | – | 10 | +/– |
| 3,5,3′,5′-$Cl_4$ | – | – | +/– |
| 3,4,3′,4′-$Me_4$ | – | – | – |
| 3,4,2′,4′,5′-$Cl_5$ | – | 12.5 | 1.9 |
| 2,3,6,2′,3′,6′-$Cl_6$ | 43 | – | 3 |
| 3,4,5,3′,4′,5′-$Cl_2$ | – | +/– | 2.4 |
| Decachlorobiphenyl | – | – | +/– |
| 3,4,3′,4′=$Cl_4$-Biphenyl Ether | ND[d] | +/– | ND |
| Various PCDF and PCDD | – | – | – |

[a]Cross reactivity = (ng compound causing 20% displacement of label (values not shown) per ng immunizing ligand causing 20% displacement of label) x 100.
[b] – = compound with less than 0.14% cross reactivity.
[c] +/– = compounds with 0.15-1.49% cross reactivity.
[d]ND = not done.

was sensitive enough to identify qualitatively and semiquantitatively these biphenyls in environmental samples. Antiserum to 4-amino-4-MCBP cross-reacted extensively not only with 4-MCBP but several other low chlorinated biphenyls, indicating a lack of specificity.

At present, these PCB assays would not lend themselves to tissue analysis where PCB mixtures are present, because it is uncertain which PCB homologs are more likely to be present. Before this use, antisera will have to be produced against several of the higher-chlorinated homologs (e. g., 2, 4, 5, 2′, 4′, 5′-HCBP). Nonetheless, the PCB assay has been used to quantify the percentage of several of the PCB congeners present in Aroclors 1242 and 1248 (Table V) and in the case of the TCBP, are in fairly good agreement with GC analysis. These assays have also been adapted to "fingerprint analysis" to determine the probable Aroclor number in a nonbiological sample (immersion oil) as well as the percentage of Aroclor in this sample [28].

**Table V. Comparison of PCB RIA for Determining the Concentration of Their Specific Homolog in Aroclors 1242 and 1248 with Gas Chromatography**

| Biphenyls Analyzed by GC | Antisera Used in RIA | Aroclor 1242 (%) | | Aroclor 1248 (%) | |
|---|---|---|---|---|---|
| | | GC | RIA | GC | RIA |
| 4-MCBP | 4-Amino-4′-MCBP | 0.23 | 4.0 | Trace | 0.6 |
| 3,4,3′,4′-TCBP plus 2,4,5,3′,4′-penta CBP | 2-Amino-4,5,3′,4′-TCBP | 0.34 | 0.24 | ~2.2 | ~3.5 |
| 2,6,2′,6′-TCBP | 3-Amino-2,6,2′,6′-TCBP | 0.17 | 0.24 | Trace | 0.7 |

## PCDD Assay

The sensitivity of the 2, 3, 7, 8-TCDD (immunizing hapten 1-amino-3, 7,8-tri-CDD) was in the order of 100 pg in the presence of Cutscum when no interfering contaminants were present. Table VI gives an indication of the possible interference to be expected from compounds other than PCDD and PCDF. The potential for interference in this assay as well as all the RIA is somewhat self-limiting, because only those amounts of hydrophobic compounds capable of being solubilized by this concentration of Cutscum or Triton X-305 are presented effectively to the antibodies. Thus, while Aroclor 1254 does contain traces of 3, 4, 3′, 4′-TCBP and PCDF [31], only about 5 $\mu$g of Aroclor can be accommodated in 0.2 ml of 0.5% Cutscum. At this level of Aroclor, the cross-reacting components are at concentrations too low to interfere.

**Table VI. Specificity of the Radioimmunoassay with F-12 Antiserum in the Presence of Cutscum**

| Compound | Highest Amount Tested | Percentage Reactivity[a] |
|---|---|---|
| 3,4,3′,4′-TCBP | 5 ng | 6 |
| 2,6,2′,6′-TCBP | 200 ng | 0 |
| 3,5,3′,5′-TCBP | 100 ng | 0 |
| 3,4,5,3′,4′,5′-HCBP | 100 ng | 0 |
| 2,4,5,2′,4′,5′-HCBP | 100 ng | 0 |
| Aroclor 1254 | 1 μg | 0 |
| 3,4,3′,4′-Tetrachlorobiphenyl Ether | 200 ng | 0.1 |
| DEHP [di (2-Ethylhexyl) phthalate] | 100 μg | 0 |
| Tetrachloro DEHP | 200 ng | 0.1 |
| Anthracene | 100 ng | 0 |
| α-Tocopherol Acetate | 200 ng | 0 |
| DDE | 400 ng | 0 |
| 9-Fluorenone | 100 ng | 0 |
| 2,7-Dichlorofluorescein | 200 ng | 0 |
| Pentachlorophenol | 10 μg | 0 |
| 2,4,5-T (Commercial) | 10 μg | 37 |
| Cholesterol Oleate | 100 μg | 0 |

[a]Percentage inhibition of $^{125}$I-binding by maximum amount of test substance relative to percentage inhibition by 5 ng of 2,3,7,8-TCDD.

Table VII depicts the relative cross reactivity of several PCDD and PCDF using two of the antisera. In the case of F-12, some generalization can be made on the antigenic determinants responsible for antibody binding. The ring system must contain halogen, but the presence of two or more chlorine atoms in *peri* positions greatly interfers with binding. Either the 1 and 9 or 4 and 6 positions or both sets must lack substitution for effective binding to occur. Thus, 1, 2, 3, 7, 8, 9-hexa-CDD should, if available for testing, be an effective competitor. In the case of F-12, only one of the two oxygen atoms is recognized by the antiserum, because TCDD and TCDF show approximately the same binding. However, TCDD and TCDF show different reactivities with GC-5 antiserum, indicating the second oxygen interferes with binding. This would suggest that this antiserum can be used to distinguish TCDD and TCDF.

The PCDD RIA was able to detect 0.7 pmol of 2, 3, 7, 8-TCDD using Cutscum and as little as 0.08 pmol with Triton X-305. These limits were based on nonoverlapping ranges of blank and test replicates. The applicability of this assay to tissue samples was examined with liver and adipose samples from monkeys that had been used in a toxicity study involving 2, 3, 7, 8-

Table VII. Cross Reactivity in Chlorinated DBD Assay

| | Cross Reactivity[a] | |
|---|---|---|
| | Antiserum GC-5 | Antiserum F-12 |
| Dibenzo-*p*-Dioxin | | |
| Unchlorinated | 4 | $<1$ |
| 2,3-$Cl_2$ | 44 | 16 |
| 2,7-$Cl_2$ | 56 | 20 |
| 2,8-$Cl_2$ | 52 | 17 |
| 2,3,7-$Cl_3$ | 73 | 77 |
| 1,2,3,4-$Cl_4$ | 20 | $<1$ |
| 2,3,7,8-$Cl_4$ | 100 | 100 |
| 1,2,3,7,8-$Cl_5$ | 99 | 97 |
| 1,2,4,7,8-$Cl_5$ | 76 | 36 |
| 1,2,3,4,7,8-$Cl_6$ | 99 | 9 |
| 1,2,3,6,7,8-$Cl_6$ | 99 | 9 |
| Octachloro | 100 | 8 |
| Dibenzofuran | | |
| Unchlorinated | 2.5 | $<1$ |
| 2,8-$Cl_2$ | 12 | ND[b] |
| 2,3,8-$Cl_3$ | 2 | ND |
| 2,3,6,8-$Cl_4$ | 6 | 40 |
| 2,3,7,8-$Cl_4$ | 25 | 92 |
| Octachloro | 14 | 8 |
| 2,3,7,8-$Br_4$ | ND | 46 |

[a]100 x (inhibition of $^{125}$I-binding by 4 pmol of test compound)/(inhibition by 4pmol of 2,3,7,8-TCDD).
[b]ND = not done.

TCDD [32]. Sample size ranged from 3 to 50 mg of tissue for the radioimmunoassay, while 200 mg samples were used for comparison assays by GC with either negative chemical ionization MS [13] or an electron-capture detector as measuring device. The results are summarized in Table VIII. Of the three techniques, GC with an electron capture detector has the greatest potential for interference, and thus can only suggest an upper limit for the amount of TCDD in a sample. In the absence of a suitable internal standard (e. g., $^{37}$Cl-TCDD), the mass spectral technique gives results, the accuracy of which depends on how soon the unknown sample was run after preparing the standard curve. In contrast, the unknown and standard curve are run simultaneously in the immunoassay procedure. Considering the many differences in the principles involved in the three assay methods, the agreement of results in Table VIII was very acceptable.

**Table VIII. Comparison of Three Assay Methods for Determination of 2,3,7,8-TCDD in Monkey Tissue**

| Animal No.[a] | Tissue | TCDD (ppb) | | |
|---|---|---|---|---|
| | | RIA | GC/MS | EC/GC |
| 373 | Adipose | ND[b] | ND | ND |
| 373 | Liver | ND | – | ND |
| 374 | Adipose | ND | ND | ND |
| 374 | Liver | ND | – | ND |
| 380 | Adipose | 41 | 28 | 87 |
| 380 | Liver | 20 | – | 17 |
| 391 | Adipose | 1800 | 1740 | 1810 |
| 391 | Liver | 94 | – | 30 |

[a]Monkeys 373 and 374 were controls and dosed orally with corn oil alone. Monkeys 380 and 391 were experimental and received a single oral dose of 70 μg/kg or 350 μg/kg TCDD in corn oil, respectively.
[b]ND = none detected.
[c]– = not done.

## CONCLUSIONS

Double-antibody radioimmunoassays have been developed for quantifying a number of chlorinated aromatic hydrocarbons of current concern from environmental samples, including animal tissues. Antisera against amino-derivatives of 3, 7, 8-tri-CDD, 2, 7, 8-tri-CDF, 3, 4, 3′, 4′-TCBP, 2, 6, 2′, 6′-TCBP and 4-MCBP were produced in rabbits by conjugating these compounds to proteins using the mixed anhydride method. Extensive characterization studies indicated the antisera were, in general, fairly specific to their non-aminated analogs. Values for these isomers in various samples including biological tissues correlated well between RIA and analytical instrumentation.

The RIA described in this chapter have by no means been brought to their maximum limits of specificity or sensitivity. Further improvements should be obtained by increasing the specific activity of the radioiodinated haptens and improving sample cleanup procedures with respect to sample recovery and removal of interfering contaminants and production of antisera with increased avidity. The importance of antisera quality in these assays is exemplified by the different reactivity of the two TCDD antisera (GC-5 and F-12) to TCDF, as well as the greater sensitivity obtained with a TCDF antiserum (~ 20 pg) compared to the TCDD antisera (~ 100 pg). This is probably primarily caused by animal variation, because immunization schedules, assay conditions and specific activity of the radiolabeled haptens were similar in both cases. The importance of sample cleanup cannot be overemphasized. The low-level interference obtained following cleanup of adipose and, particularly, liver samples at present is a primary factor in limiting the sensitivity potential.

At present, the assays should be applicable both to screening samples to minimize the demand for MS analysis by eliminating "negative" samples, and routine monitoring of exposure in environments where specific polychlorinated aromatic hydrocarbons are known to be present. Positive tissue samples should be confirmed with analytic instrumentation, at least until the assay has been exhaustively scrutinized. Although RIA quantification of contaminated tissue samples correlates with analytic instrumentation, the full potential of these assays must await further validation, including examination of other environmental samples, particularly human tissue samples, and determination of the feasibility of performing these assays routinely in clinical laboratories without the need for specialized personnel.

Sensitive biochemical and immunological targets in cells are potentially effective as screens for specific toxicants found in environmental matrices because of the multiplicity of structures and molecules available. Although there are many possible biological targets for any given toxicant, they are not infinite, and it is conceivable that a panel of several different cell or cell component systems may provide nearly all of such targets. However, a need exists for the continued development and validation of these methods. The use of newer techniques of molecular biology for screening the specific detection of biologically active trace components will provide additional tools for making better-informed decisions concerning environmental health hazards.

## REFERENCES


1. Nicholson, W. J., and J. A. Moore, Eds. *Health Effects of Halogenated Aromatic Hydrocarbons*, 320:1–730 (1979).
2. Courtney, K. D., D. W. Gaylor, M. D. Hogan, H. C. Falk, R. R. Bates and I. Mitchell. "Teratogenic Evaluation of 2,4,5-T," *Science* 168: 864-866 (1970).
3. Schewtz, B. W., P. J. Gehring and R. J. Kociba. "Toxicological Properties of Pentachlorophenol Relative to Its Content of Chlorinated Dibenzo-*p*-dioxins," *Pharmacologist* 15:395-403 (1973).
4. McConnell, E. E., J. A. Moore, J. K. Haseman and M. W. Harris. "The Comparative Toxicity of Chlorinated Dibenzo-*p*-dioxins in Mice and Guinea Pigs," *Toxicol. Appl. Pharmacol.* 44:335-356 (1978).
5. Risebrough, R. W., P. Rieche, D. B. Peakall, S. G. Herman and M. W. Kirven. "Polychlorinated Biphenyls in the Global Ecosystem," *Nature* 220:1098-1099 (1968).

6. Kimbrough, R. D. "Toxicity of Chlorinated Hydrocarbons and Related Compounds: A Review Including Chlorinated Dibenzodioxins and Chlorinated Dibenzofurans," *Arch. Environ. Health* 25:125-131 (1972).
7. McKinney, J. D., K. Chae, B. N. Gupta, J. A. Moore and J. A. Goldstein. "Toxicological Assessment of Hexachlorobiphenyl Isomers and 2,3,7,8-Tetrachlorodibenzofuran in Chicks. I. Relationship of Chemical Parameters," *Toxicol. Appl. Pharmacol.* 36:65-80 (1976).
8. Grant, D. L., W. E. J. Phillips and D. C. Villeneuve. "Metabolism of a PCB (Aroclor 1254) Mixture in the Rat," *Bull. Environ. Contam. Toxicol.* 6:102-112 (1971).
9. Vos, J. G., J. H. Koeman, H. L. van der Maas, M. C. ten Noever de Brauw and R. H. de Vos. "Identification and Toxicological Evaluation of Chlorinated Dibenzofuran and Chlorinated Naphthalene in Two Commercial Polychlorinated Biphenyls," *Cosmet. Toxicol.* 8:625-673 (1970).
10. Kuratsune, M., Y. Masuda and J. Nagayama. "Some of the Recent Findings Concerning Yusho," paper presented at the National Conference on PCBs, Chicago, IL, November 19-21, 1975.
11. Moore, J. A., B. N. Gupta and J. G. Vos. "Toxicity of 2,3,7,8-Tetrachlorodibenzofuran–Preliminary Results," U.S. EPA, EPA-560-6-75-004 (1976), pp. 77-80.
12. Baughman, R., and M. Meselson. "An Analytical Method for Detecting TCDD (Dioxin) Levels of TCDD in Samples from Vietnam," *Environ. Health Persp.* 5:27-36 (1973).
13. Hass, J. R., M. D. Friesen, D. J. Harvan and C. E. Parker. "Determination of Polychlorinated Dibenzo-*p*-dioxins in Biological Samples by Negative Chemical Ionization Mass Spectrometry," *Anal. Chem.* 50(11):1474-1479 (1978).
14. Rappe, C., H. R. Buser and H. P. Bosshardt. "Dioxins, Dibenzofurans and Other Polyhalogenated Aromatics: Production, Use, Formation and Distribution," *Ann. N.Y. Acad. Sci.* 320:1-18 (1979).
15. Yalow, R. S., and S. A. Berson. "Immunoassay of Endogenous Plasma Insulin in Man," *J. Clin. Invest.* 39:1157-1175 (1960).
16. Yalow, R. S., and S. A. Berson. "Introduction and General Considerations," in *Principles of Competitive Protein Binding Assay*, W. Odell and W. H. Daughaday, Eds. (Philadelphia: Lippincott, 1971), p. 1.
17. Chae, K., L. K. Cho and J. D. McKinney. "Synthesis of 1-Amino-3,7,8-trichlorodibenzo-*p*-dioxin and 1-Amino-2,3,7,8-tetrachlorodiobenzo-*p*-dioxin as Haptenic Compounds," *Agric. Food Chem.* 25(5):1207-1209 (1977).
18. Chaudhary, S. K., and P. W. Albro. "A Convenient Method for the Preparation of 2-Amino-4,5,3′,4′-tetrachlorobiphenyl," *Org. Prep. Proc. Int.* 10:46-55 (1978).
19. Norstrom, A., S. K. Chaudhary, P. W. Albro and J. D. McKinney. "Synthesis of Chlorinated Dibenzofurans and Chlorinated Aminodibenzofurans from the Corresponding Diphenyl Ethers and Nitrodiphenylethers," *Chemosphere* 6:331-343 (1979).
20. Albro, P. W., M. I. Luster, K. Chae, S. K. Chaudhary, G. Clark, L. D. Lawson, J. T. Corbett and J. D. McKinney. "A Radioimmunoassay for Chlorinated Dibenzo-*p*-dioxins," *Toxicol. Appl. Pharmacol.* 50:137-146 (1979).

21. Harding, V. J., and R. M. MacLean. "Estimation of Amino Groups with Ninhydrin," *J. Biol. Chem.* 24:503-517 (1976).
22. Mokrasch, L. D. "Use of 2,4,6-Trinitrobenzene-Sulfonic Acid for the Coestimation of Amines, Amino Acids, and Proteins in Mixtures," *Anal. Chem.* 18(1):64-71 (1967).
23. Kabat, A. E., and M. M. Mayer. *Experimental Immunochemistry* (Springfield, IL: Charles C. Thomas, 1968), p. 556.
24. Gaitonde, M. K., and T. Dovey. "A Rapid and Direct Method for the Quantitative Determination of Tryptophan in the Intact Protein," *Biochem. J.* 117(5):907-911 (1970).
25. Albro, P. W., and B. Corbett."Extraction and Clean-Up of Animal Tissues for Subsequent Determination of Mixtures of Chlorinated Dibenzo-*p*-Dioxins and Dibenzofurans," *Chemosphere* 7:381-385 (1977).
26. Seidl, G., and K. Ballschmiter. "Isolation of PCB's from Soil, Recovery Rates Using Different Solvent Systems," *Chemosphere* 5:373-376 (1976).
27. Hunter, W. M. "Radioimmunoassay," in *Handbook of Experimental Immunology*, D. M. Weir, Ed. (Oxford, England: Blackwell Scientific Publ. (1973), p. 17.1.
28. Luster, M. I., P. W. Albro, G. Clark, K. Chae, S. K. Chaudhary, L. D. Lawson, J. T. Corbett and J. D. McKinney. "Production and Characterization of Antisera Specific for Chlorinated Biphenyl Species: Initiation of a Radioimmunoassay for Aroclors," *Toxicol. Appl. Pharmacol.* 50:147-155 (1979).
29. Luster, M. I., P. W. Albro, K. Chae, G. Clark and J. D. McKinney. "Radioimmunoassays for Mono-(2-ethylhexyl) phthalate in Unextracted Plasma," *Clin. Chem.* 24(3):429-432 (1978).
30. Moore, J. A., E. E. McConnell, D. W. Dalgard and M. W. Harris. "Comparative Toxicity of Three Halogenated Dibenzofurans in Guinea Pigs, Mice and Rhesus Monkeys," *Ann. N.Y. Acad. Sci.* 320:151-163 (1979).
31. Albro, P. W., and C. E. Parker. "Comparison of the Composition of Aroclor 1242 and Aroclor 1016," *J. Chromatog.* 169:161-166 (1979).
32. McConnell, E. E., J. A. Moore and D. W. Dalgard. "Toxicity of 2,3,7,8-tetrachlorodibenzo-*p*-dioxin in Rhesus Monkeys (*Macaca mulatta*) Following a Single Oral Dose," *Toxicol. Appl. Pharmacol.* 43(1):175-187 (1978).

# SECTION 3

# STRUCTURE-ACTIVITY AND TOXICITY PREDICTION

# CHAPTER 15

# DEVISING DESCRIPTORS FOR TOXIC STRUCTURE-ACTIVITY STUDIES

**A. J. Hopfinger,* R. Pearlstein, R. Potenzone, Jr.† and O. Kikuchi‡**

Department of Macromolecular Science

**G. Klopman**

Department of Chemistry
Case Western Reserve University
Cleveland, Ohio

## INTRODUCTION

Every molecule possesses a distinct propensity to be a toxicant. The source(s) of this propensity resides somewhere in the chemical makeup of the molecule. If these "sources" can be identified, the hope exists of computing the toxic properties of a compound before it is made or released to the environment. The question is, "what level of investigation into the chemical integrity of a molecule must be achieved to uncover the toxic promoting sources?" An approach to answer this question is to measure, or calculate, features of a molecule and to compare (correlate) the magnitude of these molecular descriptors to the magnitudes of an observed biological response (toxic potency) of a living species "exposed" to the

*Author to whom correspondence should be addressed.
†Present address: Office of Toxic Substances, Environmental Protection Agency, Washington, DC.
‡Present address: Department of Chemistry, The University of Tsukuba, Sakura-Mura, Ibaraki, Japan.

molecule. This clearly requires the existence of reliable and accurate biological measures of toxicity.

As one might guess, there exists a direct relationship between the sophistication of the molecular descriptor measured and the effort required to make the measurement. One optimistically hopes that the depth of the probe into the chemical architecture needed to understand the toxicity of a molecule is not so great as to invalidate, from practical considerations, the determination of the requisite molecular features.

The purpose of this chapter is to discuss the types of molecular descriptors which can be generated for usage in toxic quantitative structure-activity relationship (QSAR) studies. A necessary part of this discussion will include comparing and contrasting different formalisms or approaches to performing structure-activity investigations and how they can be used on toxic data bases.

## NONROUTE OF ACTION TOXIC CORRELATION QSAR

A first level for a toxic QSAR study might be to treat the data in the same manner as has become popular in medicinal chemistry QSAR studies. That is, one uses a set of descriptors, dependent directly and only on the chemical connectivity structure of a molecule, as the independent correlation features. In addition, although multiple action steps, and/or metabolic pathways are recognized as possibly influencing activity, one form of each compound, usually the parent species, is assumed to be the dominant factor in controlling biological potency.

A constraint which enhances the reasonableness of this latter assumption is that the compound data base be structurally congeneric. If not, more than one toxic mechanism may be at play, and there may not be a consistent means of selecting equivalent physicochemical forms for all of the compounds. The congeneric constraint further manifests itself when linear regression methods are used to establish a quantitative relationship between biological activity and the set of descriptors. If a structurally noncongeneric data base is used, it is possible that equivalent descriptor terms in respective correlation equations cannot be identified statistically. That is, one will be comparing physicochemical features of compounds which may "look alike" but are actually "apples" and " oranges" with respect to one another.

Descriptors which can be included in toxic QSAR studies of this form are given in Table I.

Most of the descriptors in Table I are probably familiar to workers in QSAR except perhaps for $F_{H_2O}$, $F_{oct}$ and the (B,C,D) descriptors. $F_{H_2O}$,

**Table I. Molecular Descriptors Used in Toxic QSAR Studies Analogous to Popular Medicinal Structure-Activity Studies**

| | Descriptor | Reference | Explanation |
|---|---|---|---|
| 1. | Log P ($\pi$, f) | 2 | Water/1-octanol partition coefficient |
| 2. | MR | 3 | Molecular refractivity |
| 3. | $\sigma$ | 4 | Hammett's electronic factor |
| 4. | Q | 5 | Del Re charge density |
| 5. | $E_s$, V | 6 | Taft's steric parameter and volume parameters |
| 6. | $R_v$ | 7 | Van der Waal radius |
| 7. | $\chi_\mu^\nu$ | 8 | Molecular connectivity indices |
| 8. | $F_{H_2O}$ | 9, 10 | Aqueous free energy |
| 9. | $F_{oct}$ | 9, 10 | 1-octanol free energy |
| 10. | B, C, D | 11, 12 | Principal component physicochemical descriptors |
| 11. | $I_x$ | 13 | Indicator variable for property x |
| 12. | $S_x$ | 14 | Structure fragments |

the aqueous free energy, and $F_{oct}$, the 1-octanol free energy, are group substituent constants used in the same way as are $\pi$ constants [1]. They are defined and determined from the two relationships:

$$\pi(x) = 0.735[F_{H_2O}(x) - F_{oct}(x)] \tag{1}$$

$$F_{H_2O}(x) = 1.36 \, ln \, A_{H_2O}(x) \tag{2}$$

where x = the group
$A_{H_2O}(x)$ = the aqueous activity of x

Since $\pi(x)$ is known, one need only measure $A_{H_2O}(x)$ as done by Hine and Mookerjee [15] to determine both $F_{H_2O}(x)$ and $F_{oct}(x)$. From equation 1 it is seen that $F_{H_2O}(x)$ and $F_{oct}(x)$ are the two components of the partition coefficient substituent constant $\pi(x)$.

The (B,C,D) parameters are a universal set of empirical descriptors derived from a principal component analysis of 18 different physicochemical properties of some 139 structurally diverse molecules [11,12]. As such they represent the absolute and unique minimal number of measures (three) needed to account for the 18 different physicochemical features considered in the analysis. Unique correlation equations have been determined to compute the 11 physicochemical features of any molecule in terms of the (B,C,D) descriptors.

The three descriptors can be applied to any molecule, which is a significant advantage. However, the (B,C,D) descriptors are empirical and do not distinctly correspond to any observable physicochemical property. Hence, correlations established with these features are difficult to identify with reality, e.g., model of toxic action.

More generally, it is to be emphasized that structure-activity investigations directly using descriptors listed in Table I cannot elucidate specific factors that might relate to cause-and-effect, because no mode of action is postulated. If one goes the normal route of using linear regression analysis to establish the QSAR, an arbitrary mathematical relationship between descriptor value(s) and some measure of toxicological activity is generated which only has limited statistical significance over the range of descriptor space to which it was fit.

Fujita and Hansch [16] generated such a toxic QSAR for a set of 32 polycyclic hydrocarbons and benzacridines for which rough carcinogenic activity data were available. The QSAR is:

$$\log(A) = 28.07Q_k + 0.32 \log(P-5) - 0.14(\log(P-5))^2 - 35.26 \quad (3)$$

where $A$ = the carcinogenic activity

$Q_k$ = the residual charge density in the k-regions of the molecules.

The correlation coefficient is 0.865 and the standard deviation ± 0.4.

## STATISTICAL ROUTE OF ACTION TOXIC CORRELATION QSAR

The next level of a toxic QSAR study begins to explicitly seek out features responsible for toxicity. For example, it is generally believed that the sustained bioaccumulation in an animal of an intrinsically nontoxic agent can lead to acute toxicity through long-term exposure. Since toxic agents are "flushed" through an animal via an aqueous medium, highly lipid-soluble, poorly aqueous-soluble compounds have an immediate strike against them as possible toxic agents. Therefore, compounds possessing high log P and/or $F_{oct}$ values, e.g., very hydrophobic, should be flagged as potentially dangerous materials.

Unfortunately, as we have already seen, both log P and $F_{oct}$ are descriptors which are used in the nonmode of action toxic QSAR described above. Put another way, log P and $F_{oct}$ may correlate with some measure of toxic potency not entirely because of bioaccumulation. These descriptors may also reflect, for example, the in vivo transport properties necessary to sustain a high level of toxicity. Therefore, to generate a QSAR which contains more information than the nonroute of action toxic QSAR, one of two options needs to be taken. Firstly one can assume an explicit route of action in which log P and/or $F_{oct}$ appear in two or more action steps. "Tuning" such a model, with respect to choice and mathematical form of the descriptors so as to optimize the statistical significance, leads to a "best" route of action model. The nonrigorous and sometimes inconsistent means of arriving at the QSAR retains itself as a necessary evil of the whole methodology.

The availability of additional biological and/or physicochemical measures provides a preferable second alternative. If, for example, some measure(s) of bioaccumulation in a lipid medium were available, a distinct correlation could be established between the molecular descriptors and bioaccumulation. A second correlative relationship could be established between the toxic measures and the descriptors plus the bioaccumulation data. The substitution of the bioaccumulation-descriptor correlation relationship into the toxic-(descriptor plus bioaccumulation) correlation would again yield a relationship only involving toxicity and molecular descriptors. However, this relationship contains the set of molecular descriptors in two weighted terms which allows one to see how much each molecular descriptor distinctly contributes to toxicity from: (1) bioaccumulation and (2) other sources.

The point to be made is that the availability of multiple physicochemical and toxic measures and/or, less preferably, assumed routes of action allows toxicity mechanisms to be dissected. The dissection, in turn, allows insight into which factors, steps and/or terms are most crucial to toxicity. When different measures of toxicity are available for a compound data base, or a single measure of toxicity is available for two or more compound data bases, the dissection can allow common action features to be identified. Such common action features may lay a foundation for a generalized theory of toxicity for the included compounds or toxic measures.

## SIMULATION AND MODELING OF TOXIC MECHANISMS

The toxic QSAR methods described above are not always satisfactory to chemical and biological scientists. The ultimate reliability of even the route of action toxic correlation QSAR rests on a statistical premise which relates isolated molecular descriptors to a toxic measure. In addition, the set of descriptors used in such QSAR, as reported in Table I, do not explicitly include the effects of three-dimensional shape on chemical activity and reactivity. The preferable alternative to the types of QSAR presented above would be to model or simulate chemical and physicochemical behavior of toxic compounds using detailed three-dimensional structural and electronic descriptors derived from molecular mechanics [7,17,18] and quantum mechanics [19]. The simulation/modeling approach appears to be particularly well suited for toxicity investigations because a specific metabolic species of an applied compound is often the actual toxic agent. Chemical modeling offers a means of predicting probable metabolites, whereas in correlation-type QSAR methods one must *assume* a chemical form (route of action) for each compound. Unfortunately, workers currently using correlation methods usually limit themselves to including only the parent chemical structure of a compound in their toxic QSAR. For example, some workers have included benzo[a]pyrene (B[a]P]) in nonroutes of action toxic correlation QSAR, which is not directly carcinogenic, rather than its 7,8-diol-9,10-epoxide metabolite, which is strongly suspected of being responsible for carcinogenic activity [20].

## SOME EXAMPLES OF TOXIC SIMULATION/MODELING STUDIES AND CORRESPONDING DESCRIPTORS

The 7,8-diol-9,10-epoxide of benzo[a]pyrene, BPDE, can exist in four isomers (Figure 1). The benzyl 7-hydroxyl group can be *cis* or *trans* with respect to the epoxy oxygen atom. The *cis* isomers are experimentally found to be more reactive with DNA [21,22], but less carcinogenic [23] than the *trans* isomers. The high reactivity of the *cis* isomer has been explained in terms of a postulated hydrogen bond between the 7-hydroxyl group and the epoxy oxygen atom [21,22]. BPDE, like many known carcinogens, binds to DNA [24-27]. The observed site of alkylation of BPDE to DNA involves the $C_{10}$ and nitrogen of the 2-$NH_2$ group of guanine [25]. This is a relatively unusual site of alkylation. Most often alkylation occurs at the N-7 position of guanine [28]. Other minor alkylation sites include 0-6 of guanine, N-1, N-3, and N-7 of adenine, and N-3 of cytosine [28].

The CNDO/2L molecular orbital method [29] was used to examine the ring-opening reaction of the epoxide ring induced by the back-side attack of a nucleophile at the $C_{10}$ atom [30]. The interaction energies calculated for the BPDE-nucleophile systems indicate that the *cis*(ax,ax′) isomer is the most reactive with a nucleophile, and that the *trans*(eq,eq′) isomer is more reactive than the other conformer, *trans*(ax,ax′). In the *cis*(eq,eq′) and *trans*(ax,ax′) isomers, the angle between the plane of the epoxide ring and that of the conjugated subsystem is smaller than that in the *cis*(ax,ax′) and *trans*(eq,eq′) isomers. Consequently, the back-side attack of a nucleophile against the $C_{10}$ atom is sterically restricted to greater extent in the *cis*(eq,eq′) and *trans*(ax,ax′) isomers than in the *cis*(ax,ax′) and *trans*(eq,eq′) isomers.

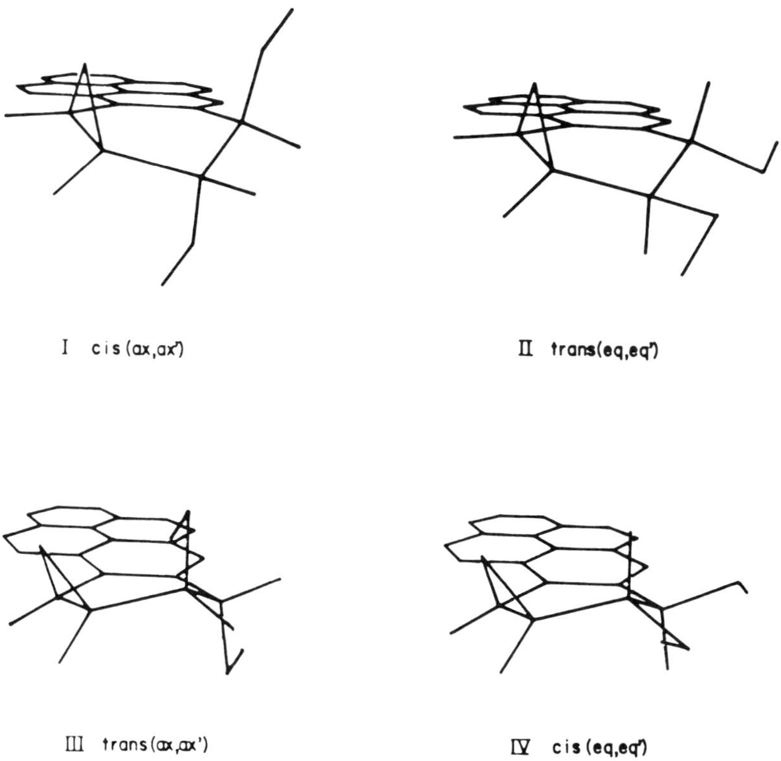


**Figure 1.** Schematic models for four isomers of benzo[a] pyrene 7,8-diol-9,10-epoxide.

Intramolecular hydrogen bonding between the 7-hydroxyl group and the epoxide oxygen atom (structure Ih) is predicted to not only stabilize the *cis*(ax,ax′) isomer, but also increase its reactivity toward nucleophiles. Reactivity calculations also suggest a different mechanism for stabilization of a carbonium ion during ring-opening of the epoxy group than that proposed in the literature [31]. Overall, the experimentally observed high reactivity of the *cis*(ax,ax′) and *trans*(eq,eq′) isomers can be explained in terms of the predicted conformational properties of the four isomers of BPDE.

The molecular descriptors used to model the structural and reactive properties of BPDE are given in Table II. These descriptors are much more specific to particular parts of a molecule than those given in Table I. This reflects the relative structural detail inherent to each of the two sets of descriptors.

There is considerable evidence that the onset of carcinogenisis involves the interaction of the active form of a carcinogen with cellular macromolec-

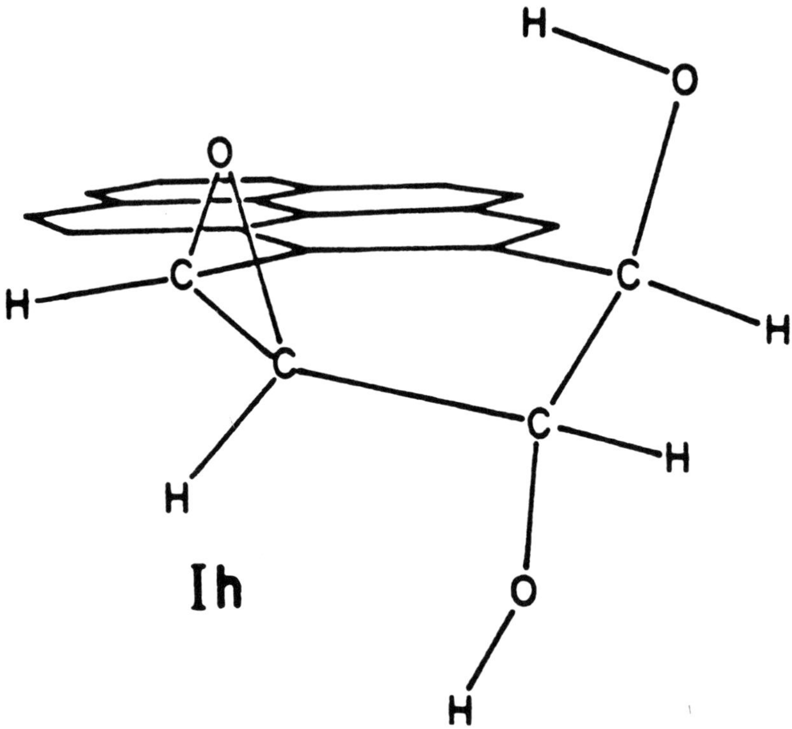

Ih

Table II. Electronic Descriptors Used in the Modeling of the Four Isomers of BPDE with $NH_3$ (a Model Nucleophile)[a]

| Descriptor | Explanation |
|---|---|
| Intramolecular | |
| 1. $E_T$ and $\Delta E_T$ | Total molecular conformer energy and differences in conformer energies |
| 2. $E_o(X)$ | Orbital energy |
| X = HOMO | Highest occupied molecular orbital |
| X = LUMO | Lowest unoccupied molecular orbital |
| 3. LCAO coefficient of $\phi_i$ | Linear combination of atomic orbital coefficient of orbital $\phi_i$ |
| 4. $P(\phi_i)$ | Electron population of $\phi_i$ |
| 5. $Q^a$ | Atomic charge densities |
| Intermolecular | |
| 1. $E(BPDE \ldots NH_3)$ | Interaction energy of BPDE and $NH_3$ |
| 2. $T_e(BPDE \ldots NH_3)$ | Electron transfer property (percent) |
| 3. $H_2(X_1, X_2)$ | Two center energies of $X_1$ and $X_2$ |
| $X_1$ = BP diol epoxide | |
| $X_2$ = N atom of $NH_3$ | |

[a] These atomic charge densities are computed from three-dimensional molecular orbital methods as opposed to bonding topology empirical formalisms like that of Del Re in Table I.

ules and the alkylation of DNA in particular. Thus, it is of interest to model the alkylation specificity of carcinogens with DNA. Specificity can be realized through both physical and chemical interactions between the DNA and the alkylating agent. Chemical interactions include the destruction and formation of covalent chemical bonds. These interactions, best characterized in terms of electronic molecular properties, can be calculated using molecular orbital methods like those employed in the analysis of BPDE. The physical association is characterized in terms of nonbonded interactions as can be calculated from molecular mechanics [7,17].

The nonbonded potential interactions between an alkylating agent and DNA reflect the respective conformations of the two molecules and their competitive interactions with the solvent medium. The result of these physical interactions may be that the site of chemical modification and the relative orientations of the two molecules near that site are not random events. In fact, well before the molecules are within range for chemical reaction, the physical forces may have significantly influenced the trajectory and orientation of the alkylating agent, and possibly the conformations of the molecules as well.

An initial investigation has been completed [32] of a computer simulation model, using molecular mechanics of the physical interaction between two simple known alkylating species ($CH_3^+$ and the dimethyl aziridinium ion, $Az^+$) and four tetrameric sequences of B-form DNA [33]. The goal of these intermolecular structure calculations is to identify preferred physical association sites on DNA as a function of alkylating agent, DNA sequence and DNA conformation. As far as this goal can be achieved, we may begin to understand how the physical association process is related to experimentally observed DNA alkylation products.

The DNA · · · alkylator intermolecular geometry is shown in Figure 2. These modeling calculations simply consist of "driving" the alkylator about the DNA and seeking the physical association energy minima. This leads to energy surfaces of the type shown in Figure 3 for $(G\text{-}C)_4$ interacting with $CH_3^+$. Electrostatic interactions are most important in determining these preferential physical association sites. In turn, the intermolecular energy minima depend on the charge distribution assigned to the DNA sequence. However, for three reported DNA charge distributions, only two distinct sets of energy minima were obtained for the $CH_3^+$-like ion interacting with $(G\text{-}C)_4$, $(A\text{-}T)_4$ and $[(G\text{-}C) \cdot (A\text{-}T)]_2$ deoxyribonucleic acids. These minima correspond to physical association geometries in which the $CH_3^+$-like ion is near known alkylation sites. The results of the $Az^+ \cdots [(G\text{-}C) \cdot (A\text{-}T)]_2$ interaction are virtually identical to those found for the $CH_3^+$-like ion. Aqueous solvation energies have little effect on the physical association of $Az^+$ with $[(G\text{-}C) \cdot (A\text{-}T)]_2$.

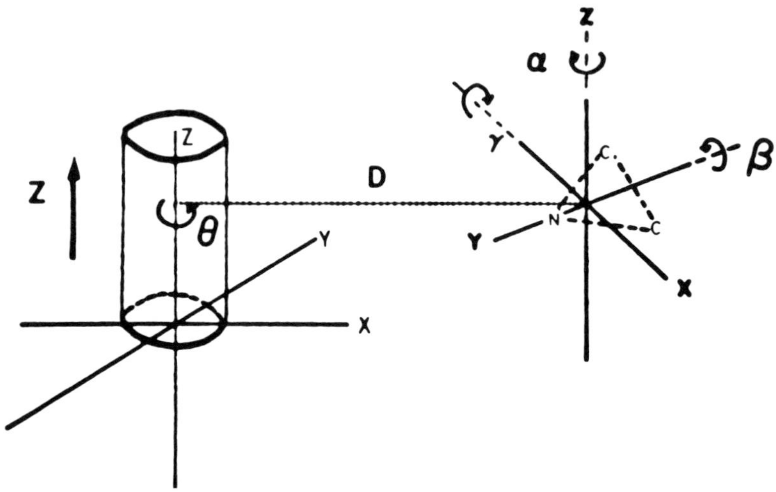


**Figure 2.** Intermolecular geometry of the DNA double-helix (cylinder) and alkylating agent (triangle). D,$\theta$,Z,$\alpha$ and $\beta$ are defined.

The molecular descriptors which specify physical association specificity of alkylators with DNA are given in Table III. These descriptors might be considered as information concerning the elusive drug-receptor interaction of pharmacology. Clearly, the descriptors in Table III primarily reflect the importance of intermolecular stereochemistry on biological activity.

## MERGING OF TOXIC QSAR METHODS AND DESCRIPTORS

The various classes of toxic descriptors given in Tables I to III and, to some degree, the different QSAR formalisms can be merged by proposing a model of action which requires descriptors from each table. Such a model has been formulated for a set of carcinogenic cyclic nitrosamines. In constructing this model it was found necessary to employ nonlinear regression analysis to establish a correlation equation. This is a mathematical consequence of allowing multiple metabolic species.

Lijinsky and co-workers [34] have developed a data base containing two quantitative measures of carcinogenic potency for a set of cyclic nitrosamines. The first carcinogenic measure, TD50, is the average time, in weeks, for 50% of a set of Sprague-Dawley rats to die relative to a control set of equal population. An upper limit of 100 weeks has been placed on each experiment. The second measure is an overall assessment of relative carcinogenicity (RC) based on observations made over the course of the experiments.

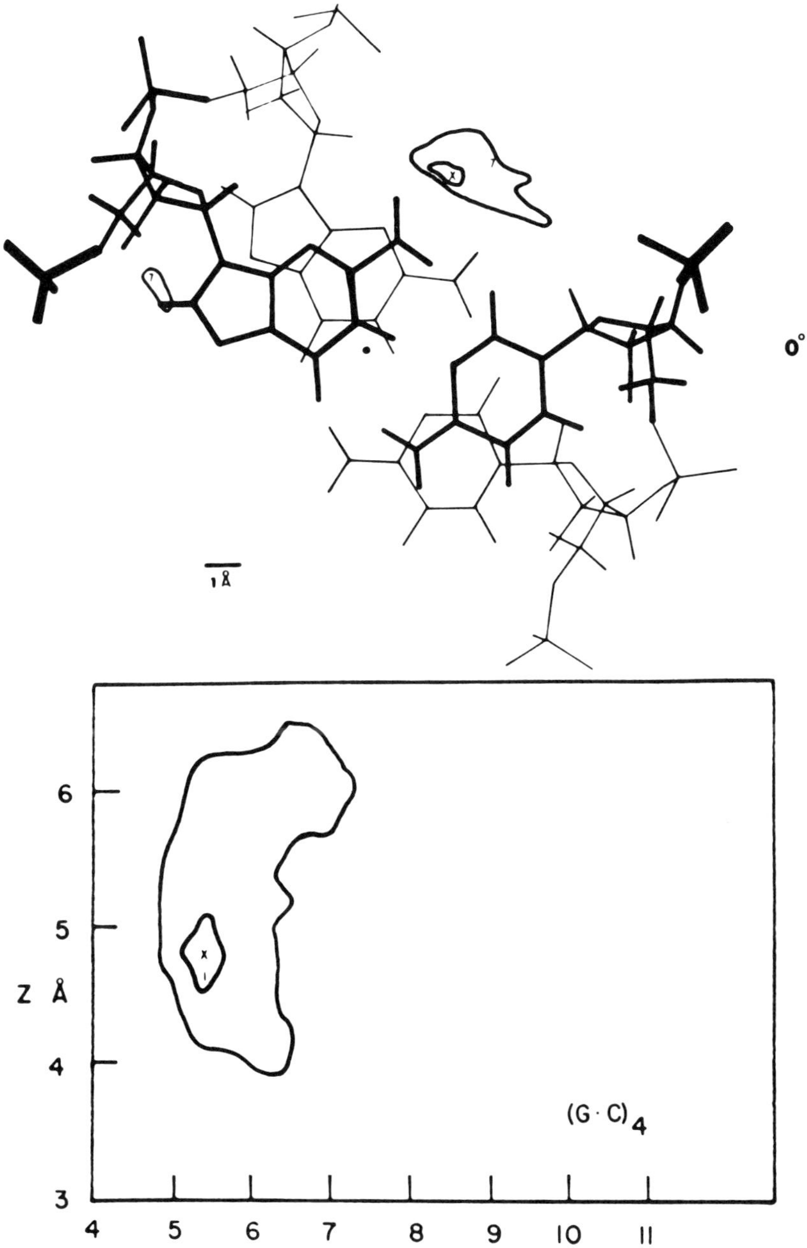


**Figure 3.** Intermolecular energy maps for $CH_3^+$ interacting with $(G\text{-}C)_4$ with isoenergy contours plotted (kcal/mol) (a) The spatial variables are D and $\theta$; (b) the spatial variables are D and Z. x = global minimum; o = secondary minima; solvent contributions not included.

**Table III. Physical Association Descriptors Used in DNA . . . Alkylation Modeling**

| | Descriptor | Explanation |
|---|---|---|
| 1. | $\Delta E_p\,(DNA[X_1]\ldots[X_2])$ | Relative physical association energy minima of DNA sequence $X_1$ with alkylator $X_2$ |
| 2. | $\vec{S}^a$ | Spatial location of physical association energy minima |
| 3. | $\vec{O}^a$ | Spatial orientation of physical association minima |

[a]These are each three component vectors. A vector exists for each unique energy minimum.

RC is recorded on a discrete scale from 0 to 4, with zero being "noncarcinogenic" and four being "extremely carcinogenic."

Exposure to the nitrosamine was achieved by placing a fixed dosage in the animal's drinking water. The sites of tumor formation were recorded for each compound tested. For specific testing details see Lijinsky and Taylor [35-37]. It is to be emphasized that this data base was not constructed from biological experiments designed for QSAR studies. The experiments were developed only to ascertain whether or not a compound is "carcinogenic." Consequently, relatively high doses have been used, which lead to a narrow range of responses.

The QSAR study was begun by considering the classification model used by Hansch [38] to develop his linear-free energy relationships and making some generalizations:

$$\frac{d(\text{response})}{dt} = ACFK \tag{4}$$

where
A = the probability of a molecule to reach the critical site in a given time interval
C = the applied concentration
$\frac{d(\text{response})}{dt}$ = the biological effect
F = the fraction of molecules reaching the critical site which have been transformed into an active metabolite
K = the activity of the metabolite, i.e., its reactivity toward the target molecule

Usually, the generalization F has been set equal to one, that is, explicit metabolic considerations have been neglected. K accounts for drug-target interactions.

It is further noted that several metabolites are allowed in the postulated metabolic pathway of Figure 4. Therefore, Equation 4 becomes:

$$\frac{d(\text{response})}{dt} = AC \sum_i F_i K_i \qquad (5)$$

where i refers to the $i^{th}$ metabolite and the constraint $\Sigma F_i = 1$ is present. Equation 5 can be solved under three different biological boundary conditions:

1. concentration and time are constant;
2. concentration and response are constant; and
3. response and time are constant.

The $TD_{50}$ and RC measures fall into the second classification. Consequently, the final form of the drug action equation becomes

$$\frac{1}{t} = A \sum_i F_i K_i \qquad (6)$$

An expression for $K_i$ was formulated in terms of a product of structural switches:

$$K_i = \prod_u S_{ui} \qquad (7)$$

$$S_{ui} = (1 - V_{ui} X_{ui}) \qquad (8)$$

where $X_{ui}$ = 1 or 0 depending on the presence or absence of descriptor u in metabolite i

$V_{ui}$ = a measure of the importance of descriptor u in metabolite i in the production of the observed response

The descriptors employed include those given in Tables I to III. A in Equation 6 was separately considered as represented by a Gaussian function in log P multiplied by the population of the boat conformer. The parent compound was used to determine the values of log P in A. The program MULFIT, which is a form of nonlinear regression analysis, was used to determine the coefficients for the A term, the $V_{ui}$ and the $F_i$. The values of the $F_i$, in turn, provide the information to determine which metabolic species are most important in the action model. The $V_{ui}$ indicate which

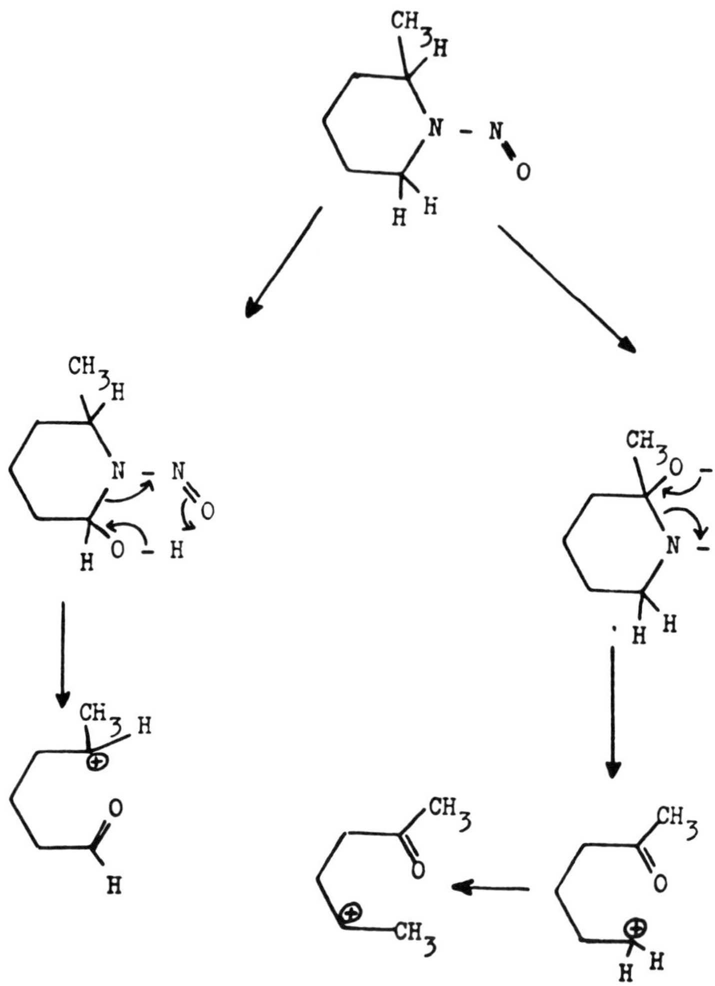

Figure 4. Possible mechanism of metabolic activation of 2-methyl nitrosopiperidine to carbonium ion metabolites.

molecular descriptors are most important in the action of a particular metabolite.

The set of equations (6-8) employing some of the molecular descriptors from Tables I to III were used to describe the action model. The optimum action model achieved to date for the cyclic nitrosamines listed in Table IV is,

$$\frac{100}{TD_{50}} = A(F_1P_1 + F_2P_2) \tag{9}$$

**Table IV. Cyclic Nitrosamines Used in the Mechanism of Action Model QSAR**

| Molecule | Exp. TD59 [34] (Weeks) |
|---|---|
| Nitrosopiperidine | 38.0 |
| 2-Methyl- | 80.0 |
| 3-Methyl- | 55.0 |
| 4-Methyl- | 40.0 |
| 2,6-Dimethyl | 125.0 |
| 3,5-Dimethyl | 100.0 |
| 2,2,6,6-Tetramethyl- | 125.0 |
| 4-t-Butyl- | 125.0 |
| 3-Hydroxy- | 43.0 |
| 4-Hydroxy- | 44.0 |
| 4-Keto | 45.0 |
| 2-Carboxy- | 125.0 |
| 4-Carboxy- | 125.0 |
| 4-Chloro- | 41.0 |
| 3,4-Dichloro | 20.0 |
| 3,4-Dibromo | 36.0 |
| 1,2,3,6-Tetrahydropyridine | 28.0 |
| N-Nitroso-3-pyrroline | 80.0 |
| N-Nitroso-hexamethyleneimine | 28.0 |
| N-Nitroso-heptamethyleneimine | 25.0 |
| Dimethyl-nitrosamine | 25.0 |
| Diethyl-nitrosamine | 30.0 |
| *Bis*-(2-Chloro)- | 84.0 |
| *Bis* (2-Cyano)- | 125.0 |
| *Bis* (2-Methoxy)- | 63.0 |

where 100 is an arbitrary scaling constant chosen equal to the maximum time duration of the experiments, and

$$A = (8.34 \exp [0.05(\log P - 1.32)^2]) (1 + \exp(-0.26\, \Delta E_T))^{-1}$$

where $\Delta E_T$ = the difference in energy between the chair and boat ring conformers shown in Figure 5 for nitrosopiperidine

The fraction of each metabolite reaching the target site is chosen to be uniform, e.g., $F_1$ = (set) = $F_2$ = (set) = 0.5. That is, a nonselective oxidizing agent (P-450?) has been assumed in setting equal weights to the two metabolic pathways (see Figure 4). $P_1$ and $P_2$ are the switch variable products defined as:

$$P_1 = \prod_{j=1}^{6} (1 - V_{j1} X_{j1})$$

$$P_2 = \prod_{j=1}^{6} (1 - V_{j2} X_{j2})$$

where $X_{11}$ or $X_{12}$ = 1 if $C\text{-}C^{\oplus}$ is formed, else = 0

$X_{21}$ or $X_{22}$ = 1 if $(C)_n\text{-}C\text{-}C^{\oplus}$, for $n \geqslant 1$, is formed, else = 0

$X_{31}$ or $X_{32}$ = 1 if $(C)_2{>}C\text{-}C^{\oplus}$ is formed, else = 0

$X_{41}$ or $X_{42}$ = 1 if $C\text{-}C\text{-}C^{\oplus}\text{-}C$ is formed, else = 0

$X_{51}$ or $X_{52}$ = 1 if $X\text{-}C({-})\text{-}C^{\oplus}$ (X=halogen) is formed, else = 0

$X_{61}$ or $X_{62}$ = 1 if $C{=}C\text{-}C^{\oplus}$ is formed, else = 0

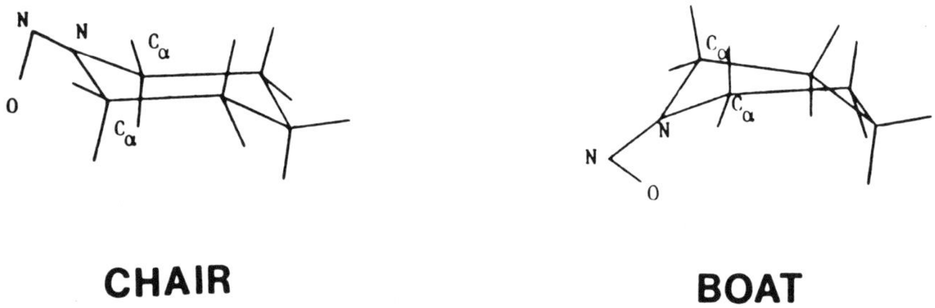


**Figure 5.** Molecular stick models of the chair and boat conformer states of nitrosopiperidine.

The assignment of the $X_{ji}$ were made from an analysis of the $E_T$ values for each of the model metabolites.

The resulting nonlinear regression fit of the $V_{j1}$ are $V_{11} = 0.50$; $V_{21} = 0.438$; $V_{31} = 0.484$; $V_{41} = 1.000$; $V_{51} = 0.021$; and $V_{61} = -0.007$.

Figure 6 is a plot of predicted TD50, using Equation 9, vs the observed TD50. The major outlyer is 4-keto-nitrosopiperidine. It is not possible to compute a correlation coefficient for this fitting procedure because nonlinear regression methods have been employed.

Equation 9 indicates that log P is of only marginal significance in specifying activity. The optimum value for log P is 1.32. This finding is consistent with the cluster and regression QSAR where log P was not found to be an important descriptor [39]. Overall, this suggests that transport processes may not be important in the carcinogenic potency of these cyclic nitrosa-

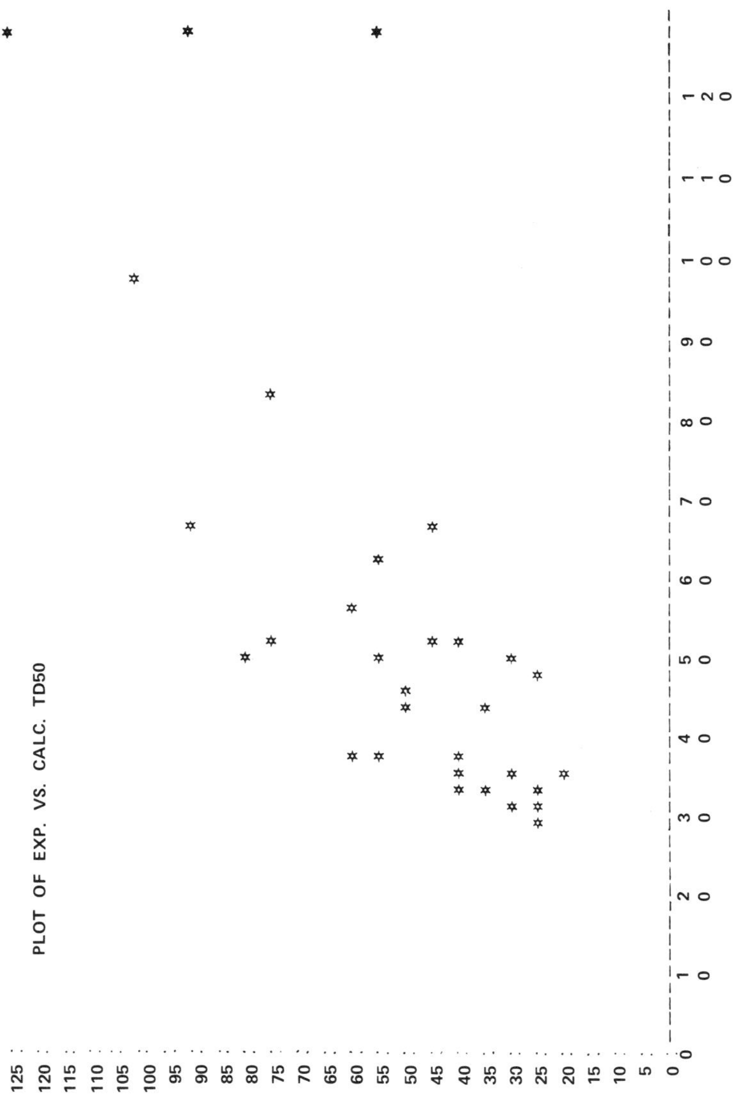


**Figure 6.** A plot of experimental TD50 using the mechanism of action QSAR. TD50 > 100 are assigned a value of 125.

mines. $\Delta E_T$ appears in Equation 9 as a minor descriptor whose increasing value increases carcinogenicity (TD50 decreases). The physicochemical role of $\Delta E_T$ in this QSAR has not yet been explained.

The role of the carbonium ion metabolites of the cyclic nitrosamines in specifying carcinogenic potency can be estimated from an analysis of $V_{ji}$. The following conclusions have been made:

1. $V_{41} = 1.0$ implies that secondary carbonium ions are not carcinogenic.
2. $V_{11} \cong V_{21} \cong V_{31} \cong 0.5$ suggests that the nature of the side-chain of the carbonium ion is not important to specifying carcinogenic potency. Further, the common default option to each of these cases ($X_{1i} = X_{2i} = X_{3i} = 0$, $i = 1,2$) corresponds to the formation of $-CH_3^{\oplus}$. Thus $-CH_3^{\oplus}$ is estimated to be twice as carcinogenic as each of the three alternative classes.
3. $V_{51} \cong V_{61} \cong 0$ implies that halogen substitution or formation of a double bond at an adjacent carbon to the carbonium ion enhances carcinogenic potency to about the same level as $-CH_3^+$ carcinogenic potency.
4. Qualitatively, carcinogenic potency can be ranked as,

$$\overset{\text{Hal}}{\diagdown}\!\!\!\diagup C{-}C^{\oplus} \cong C{=}C{-}C^{\oplus} \cong CH_3^{\oplus} > R{-}C^{\oplus} \gg R{-}C{-}C^{\oplus}{-}C{-}R'.$$

This in turn has led to the conclusion that the alkylation mechanism of N-nitrosamines may not involve carbocation intermediates, because the most active carbocation predicted from the model is a primary form. This species is too unstable to exist any reasonable length of time necessary for specific DNA alkylation. A very recent paper [40] suggests that the formation of alkyldiazonium ions from cyclic nitrosamines are probably the crucial metabolites with respect to carcinogenicity.

## CONCLUSIONS

Obviously, the modeling approach is much more detailed with regard to chemical structure than the statistical correlation methods mentioned earlier. One pays for this additional structural information in terms of the computational time and cost required. Perhaps the best current way to compare and contrast the correlation and modeling approaches to studying toxicity is in terms of practicality. If one takes a very pragmatic position and only wishes to develop a relationship between some measure of toxicity and some simple molecular descriptors, without regard to a physicochemical or mechanistic basis, and without regard to generality or reliability, then the nonroute of action correlation QSAR are appropriate. On the other hand, as soon as one wishes to gain information about possible routes of action, multiple measures of physicochemical and/or biological data and/or postulated reactions are required. These latter investigations, which focus specifically on mechanistic aspects, take the form of computer simulation and/or modeling of chemical processes. The descriptors determined from modeling are more specific and detailed, with respect to molecular structure, than the directly dependent molecular connectivity descriptors used in classic correlation QSAR studies.

## ACKNOWLEDGMENTS

We gratefully acknowledge the financial support of the National Cancer Institute (Contract No. NO1-CP-76927), the National Science Foundation (Grant No. ENV 77-74061) and the National Institutes of Health (Contract No. 217041).

## REFERENCES

1. Hansch, C., A. Leo, S. H. Unger, K. H. Kim, D. Nikaitami and E. J. Lien. "Aromatic Substituent Constants for Structure-Activity Correlations," *J. Med. Chem.* 16:1207 (1973).
2. Rekker, R. *The Hydrophobic Fragment Constant* (New York: Elsevier, 1977).
3. Hansch, C., S. H. Unger and A. B. Forsythe. "Strategy in Drug Design. Cluster Analysis as an Aid in the Selection of Substituents," *J. Med. Chem.* 16:1217 (1973).
4. Ariëns, E. J. *Drug Design, Vols. 1-6* (New York: Academic Press, Inc., 1971-1976).
5. Del Re, G., B. Pullman and T. Yonezawa. "Electronic Structure of the α-Amino Acids of Proteins. I. Charge Distributions and Proton Chemical Shifts," *Biochem. Biophys. Acta* 75:153 (1963).
6. Verloop, A. J. "The Use of Linear Free Energy Parameters and Other Experimental Constants in Structure-Activity Studies," in *Drug Design, Vol. 3*, E. J. Ariëns, Ed. (New York: Academic Press, Inc., 1972), p. 133.
7. Hopfinger, A. J. *Conformational Properties of Macromolecules* (New York: Academic Press, Inc., 1973).
8. Kier, L. B., and L. Hall. *Molecular Connectivity in Chemical Research* (New York: Academic Press, Inc., 1976).
9. Hopfinger, A. J., and R. D. Battershell. "Application of SCAP to Drug Design. I. Prediction of Octanol-Water Partition Coefficients Using Solvent-Dependent Conformational Analysis," *J. Med. Chem.* 19: 569 (1976).
10. Forsythe, K. H., and A. J. Hopfinger. "A Quantitative Model of Biomolecular Solvation," in *Biomolecular Structure, Conformation, Function and Evolution, Vol. 2*, R. Srinivasan, Ed. (Oxford: Pergamon Press, 1980), p. 563.

11. Cramer, R. D., III. "BC(DEF) Parameters. 1. The Intrinsic Dimensionality of Intermolecular Interactions in the Liquid State," *J. Am. Chem. Soc.* 102(6):1837 (1980).
12. Cramer, R. D., III. "BC(DEF) Parameters. 2. An Empirical Structure-Based Scheme for the Prediction of Some Physical Properties," *J. Am. Chem. Soc.* 102(6):1849 (1980).
13. Hansch, C., C. Silipo and E. E. Steller. "Formulation of *De Novo* Substituent Constants in Correlation Analysis: Inhibition of Dihydofolate Reductase by 2,4-Diamino-5-(3,4-dichlorophenyl)-6-Substituted Pyrimidines," *J. Pharm. Sci.* 64:1186 (1975).
14. Cramer, R. D., III. "Quantitative Drug Design," in *Annual Reports in Medical Chemistry, Vol. 11,* F. H. Clarke, Ed. (New York: Academic Press, Inc., 1976), p. 301.
15. Hine, J., and P. D. Mookerjee. "The Intrinsic Hydrophilic Character of Organic Compounds. Correlations in Terms of Structural Contributions," *J. Org. Chem.* 40:292 (1975).
16. Hansch, C., and T. Fujita. "$\rho$-$\sigma$-$\pi$ Analysis. A Method for the Correlation of Biological Activity and Chemical Structure," *J. Am. Chem. Soc.* 86:1616 (1964).
17. Allinger, N. L., J. T. Sprague and T. Kiljefors. "Conformational Analysis. CIV. Structures, Energies, and Electronic Absorption Spectra of the [$\eta$] Paracyclophanes," *J. Am. Chem. Soc.* 96:5100 (1974).
18. Potenzone, R., Jr., E. Cavicchi, H. J. R. Weintraub and A. J. Hopfinger. "Molecular Mechanics and the CAMSEQ Processor," *Computers Chem.* 1:187 (1977).
19. Kier, L. B. *Molecular Orbital Theory in Drug Research* (New York: Academic Press, Inc., 1971).
20. Depierre, J. W., and L. Ernster. "The Metabolism of Polycyclic Hydrocarbons and Its Relationship to Cancer," *Biochem. Biophys. Acta* 473:149 (1977).
21. Hulbert, P. B. "Carbonium Ion as Ultimate Carcinogen of Polycyclic Aromatic Hydrocarbons," *Nature* 256:146 (1975).
22. Yagi, H., O. Hernandez and D. M. Jerina. "Synthesis of (±)-7,$\beta$,8$\alpha$-Dihydroxy-9$\beta$,10$\beta$-epoxy-7,8,9,10-tetrahydrobenzo(a)pyrene, a Potential Metabolite of the Carcinogen Benzo(a)pyrene with Stereochemistry Related to the Antileukemic Tripolides," *J. Am. Chem. Soc.* 97:6881 (1975).
23. Kapitulnik, J., W. Levin, A. H. Conney, H. Yagi and D. M. Jerina. "Benzo[a]pyrene and Newborn Mice," *Nature* 266:378 (1977).
24. Sims, P., P. L. Grover, A. Swaisland, K. Pal and A. Hewer. "Metabolic Activation of Benzo(a)pyrene Proceeds by a Diol-Epoxide," *Nature* 252:326 (1974).
25. Weinstein, I. B., A. M. Jeffrey, K. W. Jennette, S. H. Blobstin, R. G. Harvey, G. Harris, H. Autrup, H. Kasai and K. Nakanishi. "Benzo(a)-pyrene Diol Epoxides as Intermediates in Nucleic Acid Binding *in vitro* and *in vivo*," *Science* 193:592 (1976).
26. King, H. W. S., M. R. Osborne, F. A. Beland, R. C. Harvey and P. Brooks. "(±)-7$\alpha$,8$\beta$-Dihydroxy-9$\beta$,10$\beta$-epoxy-7,8,9,10-tetrahydrobenzo(a)pyrene as an Intermediate in the Metabolism and Binding to DNA of Benzo(a)pyrene," *Proc. Nat. Acad. Sci. U. S.* 73:2679 (1976).

27. Koreeda, M., P. D. Moore, H. Yagi, H. J. C. Yeh and D. M. Jerina. "Alkylation of Polyguanylic Acid at the 2-Amino Group and Phosphate by the Potent Mutagen (±)-7,8α-Dihydroxy-9β,10β-epoxy-7,8,9,10-tetrahydrobenzo(a)pyrene," *J. Am. Chem. Soc.* 98:6720 (1976).
28. Lawley, P. D. "Carcinogenesis by Alkylating Agents," in *Chemical Carcinogens,* ACS Monograph 173, C. E. Searle, Ed. (Washington, DC: American Chemical Society, 1976), p. 83.
29. Kikuchi, O., A. J. Hopfinger and G. Klopman. "A New Type of Semi-empirical Molecular Orbital Method for Large Molecules," *J. Theor. Biol.* 77:129 (1979).
30. Kikuchi, O., A. J. Hopfinger and G. Klopman. "Electronic Structure and Reactivity of Four Stereo Isomers of Benzo(a)pyrene 7,8-Diol-9,10-epoxide," *Cancer Biochem. Biophys.* 4:1 (1979).
31. Whalen, D. L., A. M. Ross, H. Yagi, J. M. Karle and D. M. Jerina. "Stereoelectronic Factors in the Solvolysis of Bay Region Diol Epoxides of Polycyclic Aromatic Hydrocarbons," *J. Am. Chem. Soc.* 100: 5218 (1978).
32. Pearlstein, R., S. Tripathy, R. Potenzone, Jr., D. Malhotra, A. J. Hopfinger, G. Klopman and N. Max. "Physical Association of Two Simple Alkylators to Some DNA Sequences," *Biopolymers* 19:311 (1980).
33. Adams, R. K. P., R. H. Burdon, A. M. Campbell and R. M. S. Smellie. *Davidson's–The Biochemistry of Nucleic Acids* (New York: Academic Press, Inc., 1976), p. 94.
34. Lijinsky, W., Chemical Carcinogenesis Program, Frederick Cancer Research Center, Frederick, MD. Personal communication.
35. Lijinsky, W., and H. W. Taylor. "Carcinogenicity Tests of N-Nitroso Derivatives of Two Drugs, Phenmetrazine and Methylphenidate," *Cancer Lett.* 1:359 (1976).
36. Lijinsky, W., and H. W. Taylor. "Carcinogenicity of Methylated Dinitrosopiperazines in Rats," *Cancer Res.* 35:1270 (1975).
37. Lijinsky, W., and H. W. Taylor. "The Effect of Substituents on the Carcinogenicity of N-Nitrosopyrrodines in Sprague-Dawley Rats," *Cancer Res.* 36:1988 (1976).
38. Tute, M. S. "Principles and Practice of Hansch Analysis: A Guide to Structure-Activity Correlation for the Medicinal Chemist," in *Advances in Drug Research, Vol. 6,* N. J. Harper and A. B Simmons, Eds. (New York: Academic Press, Inc., 1971), p. 1.
39. Petit, B., R. Potenzone, Jr., A. J. Hopfinger, G. Klopman and M. Shapiro. "A Hierarchal QSAR Molecular Structure Calculator Applied to a Carcinogenic Nitrosamine Data Base," *Computer Assisted Drug Design,* E. C. Olson and R. E. Christoffersen, Eds., ACS Symp. Series 112 (Washington, DC: American Chemical Society, 1979), p. 553.
40. Andreozzi, P., G. Klopman and A. J. Hopfinger. "Theoretical Study of the Carcinogenic Metabolism of N-Nitrosamines," *Cancer Biochem. Biophys.* (submitted).

# CHAPTER 16

# HYDROPHOBICITY, THE UNDERLYING PROPERTY IN MOST BIOCHEMICAL EVENTS

**Albert J. Leo**
Chemistry Department
Pomona College
Claremont, California

## INTRODUCTION

In considering how the word "environment" is commonly used today–the environment being whatever surrounds, encircles or envelops–one realizes that some sort of *barrier* is implied which must separate the "interior" (which is us, or some other organism that concerns us) from the "exterior," which is the rest of the world. Since it is obvious that no organism can exist in isolation, the interior must communicate with the exterior through the barrier or set of barriers. Currently popular scenarios for biogenesis see these early barriers as effective ways of keeping chemical reactions from quickly reaching equilibrium conditions–nonequilibrium chemistry being characteristic of life (Figure 1).

The vast time interval which separates us from these events makes it difficult or impossible to convert this sort of speculation into an empirically supported theory, but since it is useful to order ideas, it was proposed that hydrophobic forces [1, 2] were primarily, if not solely, responsible for the creation of the interior region of the first protocells. On this event, then, the further development of the biosphere depended. Everyone appreciates that life processes have evolved to be remarkably efficient, specific and responsive to delicate control mechanisms. Therefore it is unlikely that these properties, which distinguish biochemistry from ordinary organic chemistry, would

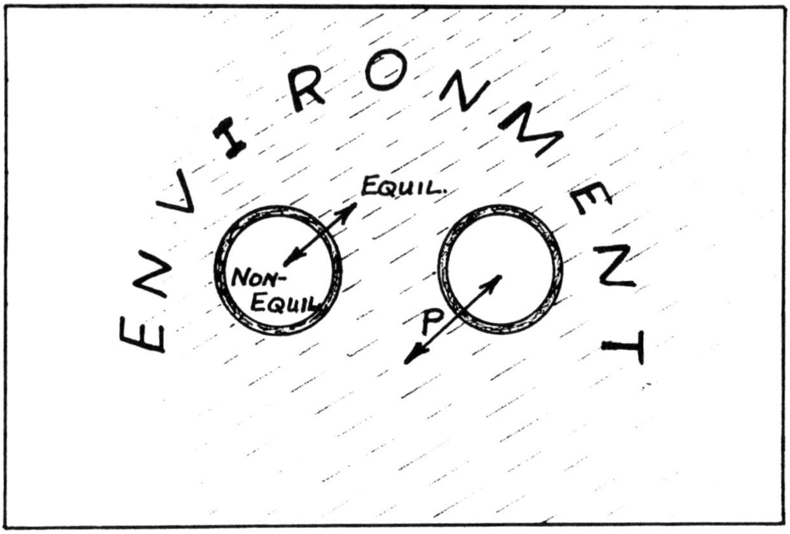


**Figure 1.** "Protocells" facing the first environmental challenge.

have developed unless, under selective pressure operating over billions of years, forces other than those of a simply hydrophobic nature were called on to regulate environmental effects.

Although it is highly speculative, this hypothesis provides an overview from which we can better judge the usefulness and limitations of the hydrophobic parameter. The correlations which follow support the view that hydrophobic forces provide the underlying "substrata" for biological interactions, but these forces are often supplemented by more specific and selective "active transport" processes (Figure 2). A simple but useful corollary with environmental implications is this: In the study of the potential hazard of a truly "xenobiotic" class of chemicals, the specific and selective forces, which are much more difficult to find parameters for are much less likely to turn up in rate-controlling transport steps, but can, of course, result in higher activity with a key enzyme than the natural substrate.

After a considerable amount of study of biological systems of varying degrees of complexity, it is the conclusion of Hansch and co-workers that the partitioning of a solute between octanol and water provides a practical model system for quantitatively predicting how that solute will interact through nonspecific hydrophobic forces with nonpolar portions of biosystems. In the first series of regression equations which follow, hydrophobicity is the only parameter needed to explain a particular physicochemical or biological response, but that does not mean that it is always just a "fossil"

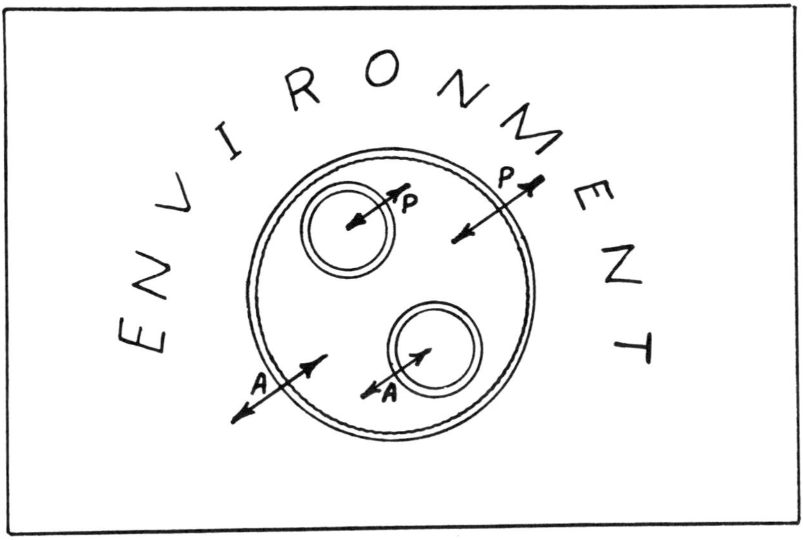


**Figure 2.** Active transport produces selective nonequilibrium.

carryover from an earlier epoch. From the later equations it will be apparent that not only do hydrophobic forces play an important role in the "random walk" of a toxicant as it enters an organism and migrates to an active site, but when the toxicant happens to be a specific enzyme inhibitor, these forces can also aid in the required orientation step. As one might expect, an equation which purports to "explain" a more complex response requires additional parameters before the various roles can be separated.

## LINEAR HYDROPHOBIC DEPENDENCE

### Model Systems

The equations in Table I have been selected from among hundreds developed by Hansch and co-workers which illustrate some actions of model systems where the logarithm of the octanol-water partition coefficient is linearly related to a measure of binding. Note that the logarithm of the partition coefficient is used to put the parameter on the same scale as other free-energy based parameters [3]. In Equation 1, the macromolecule is nonbiological, and it can be seen that the partition coefficient of a series of acetanilides is also a good measure of how they will bind to a polyamide. By "a good measure," it can be understood that the correlation coefficient of

**Table I. Solute Binding**

| | n | r | s | Equation Number |
|---|---|---|---|---|
| Model Systems | | | | |
| Nylon (by acetanilides) [4] | | | | |
| $\log K = 0.69 \log P - 1.16$ | 7 | 0.961 | 0.20 | 1 |
| Activated carbon (by phenoxyacetic acids from 20% solution) [5] | | | | |
| $\log \%\ \text{ads.} = 0.81 \log P - 2.13$ | 16 | 0.952 | 0.21 | 2 |
| Biological Material | | | | |
| Bovine hemoglobin (phenols, amines and hydrocarbons ) [6] | | | | |
| $\log 1/C = 0.67 \log P + 1.96$ | 17 | 0.941 | 0.16 | 3 |

0.961 indicates that the single parameter, log P, explains over 92% of the variance in the binding data. The standard deviation of 0.2 is acceptable for the reproducibility of this type of measurement. The number of data points (7) is not large, but it need not be if only one parameter is employed.

What the equation does not say is also important to keep in mind. Before reaching the conclusion that hydrophobic forces are paramount in the binding of acetanilides to nylon, one must first examine how other parameters vary with the structural changes in the solute set. If there were a high degree of collinearity between log P and, for example, molar refractivity among the seven structures in the study, other structures which separate these two parameters would have to be tested and included in the regression. Without taking this obvious precaution it would be foolhardy to assign a "causative" role to a term in any regression equation regardless of the favorable correlation coefficient.

Equation 2 shows the relationship between the octanol-water log P and the binding of phenoxyacetic acids to activated carbon. Again, the result is consistent with the belief that the manner in which octanol solvates the lipid portion of the phenoxyacetic acids is analogous to the mutual nonpolar contact of these acids to the carbon surface. Furthermore, the coefficient of the log P term leads one to infer that the process of aqueous desolvation is more complete when the solute is enveloped by octanol than when it adsorbs onto a carbon surface.

Equation 3 relates the hydrophobic parameter to the way a variety of small solute molecules (phenols, amines and hydrocarbons) bind to a real biochemical macromolecule, bovine hemoglobin, in vitro. In equation 3, C is the concentration needed to get a binding ratio of 0.5 to 1. A very similar equation can be derived for a 1:1 binding ratio of miscellaneous solutes to bovine serum albumin [6].

When one considers that these three binding equations are just examples of hundreds which have been derived, it does not take a great deal of imagination to assign a significant role to hydrophobic forces in the environmental transport of hazardous chemicals, whether environmental transport refers to the migration of chemicals from spills or improperly barricaded landfills or whether it refers to their transport and storage within animal organisms. (Figure 3) [7].

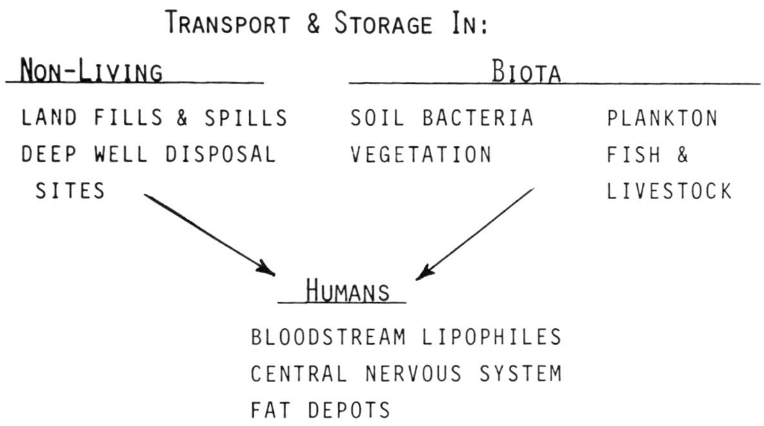


**Figure 3.** Environmental importance of binding.

Hydrophobic forces, acting in a presumed nonspecific manner, can have some directly measurable biological effects which can be seen as toxic in character. Perhaps the effect most frequently encountered is membrane perturbation or even disaggregation. Again it makes sense to examine simple model systems from the realm of physical organic chemistry: the disaggregation by alcohols of silinized glass beads and the change in resistance across a black lipid membrane (BLM). The relationships with log P are shown as Equations 4 and 5 (Table II). In the experiment "explained" by Equation 4, the 0.2-mm glass beads were given a lipid-like surface, but the forces which clump the beads in a pure aqueous environment are undoubtedly less complex than those responsible, for example, for the integrity of an erythrocyte membrane.

**Table II. Membrane Effects**

| | n | r | s | Equation Number |
|---|---|---|---|---|
| Model Systems | | | | |
| Glass beads, silinized (by alcohols) [8] | | | | |
| $\log 1/C = 0.98 \log P - 0.80$ | 4 | 0.995 | 0.77 | 4 |
| BLM (by alcohols) [8] | | | | |
| $\log 1/C = 1.16 \log P - 0.51$ | 7 | 0.985 | 0.26 | 5 |
| Biosystems | | | | |
| Red cell rupture [9] | | | | |
| $\log 1/C = 0.96 \log P - 0.30$ | 6 | 0.999 | 0.06 | 6 |
| Nerve depolarization (by alcohols) [8] | | | | |
| $\log 1/C = 0.84 \log P + 3.31$ | 30 | 0.979 | 0.18 | 7 |

## Biosystems

It is, perhaps, not surprising that one can quantitatively relate hydrophobicity, as measured by the octanol-water partition coefficient, to some other physico-chemical process which appears likely to respond to the lipophilic nature of one of its components. Therefore, because there are many honest skeptics who distrust octanol because it bears little chemical resemblance to biological membrane material, it is important to extend the equations using log P from model systems to real biological phenomena. Red cell hemolysis can serve as a first example, as seen in Equation 6 of Table II.

The coefficients of the log P terms in Equations 4 and 6 can be considered equal, so it appears safe to conclude that the response to changes in hydrophobicity of the alcohols used is the same in the model system as in the biological one. The only difference is in the intercept, and this indicates that the red cells will rupture at a lower concentration of any given alcohol than that needed to disaggregate silinized beads.

Of course, membranes (especially those on nerve cells) can indicate some response to an adsorbed solute before an actual rupture occurs. Using a model BLM system, the concentration of added alcohol necessary to lower the resistance across one square centimeter by a constant amount ($10^8$-$10^6$ ohms) can be taken as a measure of how a nerve membrane might react in an intact animal. In the BLM this potential lowering is related to the hydrophobicity of the alcohols by Equation 5. If an actual nerve, such as a mollusc ganglion, is observed, and the endpoint taken as the amount of alcohol needed to change the rest potential by 20 mV, a very similar dependence on log P can be seen as shown in Equation 7 [10].

**Table III. Intact Animals**

| | n | r | s | Equation Number |
|---|---|---|---|---|
| Narcosis in Tadpoles [8] | | | | |
| $\log 1/C = 0.90 \log P + 0.91$ | 57 | 0.962 | 0.31 | 8 |
| Bioaccumulation in Trout [11] | | | | |
| $\log k_1/k_2 = 0.54 \log P + 0.12$ | 8 | 0.984 | 0.34 | 9 |

Moving up in complexity of the responding biosystem and taking an intact animal, such as a tadpole, barnacle or goldfish, the same type of linear relationship can be developed between log P and narcotic action. Overton's famous early work with tadpoles narcotized by a miscellaneous assortment of organic solutes results in Equation 8 (Table III).

In all probability most of the hazardous chemicals we should be worrying about in our environment act through more specific and unique mechanisms than those which have been presented so far. Rationalizing these more complex biointeractions not only requires additional parameters, but the hydrophobic dependence is often nonlinear. Before discussing the implications of these more complex relationships, there is an important phenomenon which, although undoubtedly a combination of complex events, appears on an overall basis and for several important chemical classes to be a simple linear function of log P. This is bioaccumulation.

It is becoming obvious that one cannot deal adequately with the problem of chronic toxicity until he or she has addressed that of bioaccumulation. Regardless of whether one considers chronic toxicity a greater problem than acute toxicity, most people agree that the former is more difficult because it is harder to pinpoint and document. Of course, persistence or chemical half-life, is of primary importance in the estimation of chronic toxicity hazard. Bioaccumulation, however, is almost on a par with it, for it is a process which assures both long-term and intimate exposure. A relatively unpublicized danger of the storage of lipophilic chemicals in fat deposits within the human body is the possibility of their sudden release when the fat is called upon for energy reserves. This may not be as important for an American housewife on a "crash diet," but it can still mean higher blood concentrations of the chemical than existed during initial exposure. Not so fortunate would be a nursing mother in a third-world country beset with famine where mother and baby might be in a seriously weakened condition to begin with.

Several relationships between bioaccumulation and hydrophobicity have been published to date, but one of the earliest to gain widespread attention used the ratio of uptake rate to clearance rate for a variety of hydrocarbons and their halogen derivatives in small trout [11]. This appears as Equation 9 (Table III). As mentioned above, the simplicity of Equation 9 is probably fortuitous. In summing several biological processes involved, the higher terms in hydrophobicity and any dependence on electronic or steric factors just happen to cancel each other.

## NONLINEAR HYDROPHOBIC DEPENDENCE

If the majority of toxic behavior followed the same pattern as shown in the first nine equations, the task of the U.S. Environmental Protection Agency would be simplified a great deal. Because nature is not so accommodating, the dependence of toxicity on hydrophobicity can be expected to be nonlinear whenever the biological response reflects, not simple protein binding or membrane penetration, but rather the rate of multicompartment transport or the oriented binding at an enzymic site. Thus far Hansch's co-workers have characterized three nonlinear types: parabolic, bilinear and position-dependent hydrophobic relationships.

### Model Systems

When one considers a solute moving through successive compartments alternating between water and a lipid substance, a similar parabolic curve can be obtained using either a mathematical nonsteady-state model or using a physical model of interconnected water-octanol cells. These are depicted graphically in Figure 4 [12]. In the mathematical model, the rate at which a drug reaches the 20th compartment corresponds very closely with a true parabola, whereas for the fourth compartment in the physical model, the observed curve approximates a parabola more closely as time goes on. While the present data are insufficient to know for sure, it would appear that a bilinear expression would produce an even better fit for all three time intervals: 4, 7 and 30 hr.

### Biosystems

A parabola very nicely describes the rate of appearance of benzeneboronic acids in mouse brain after intraperitoneal injection. The dependence on hydrophobicity is given by:

$$\log 1/C = -0.54 (\log P)^2 + 2.47 \log P - 1.05 \quad n=14; r=0.915; s=0.214 \qquad (10)$$

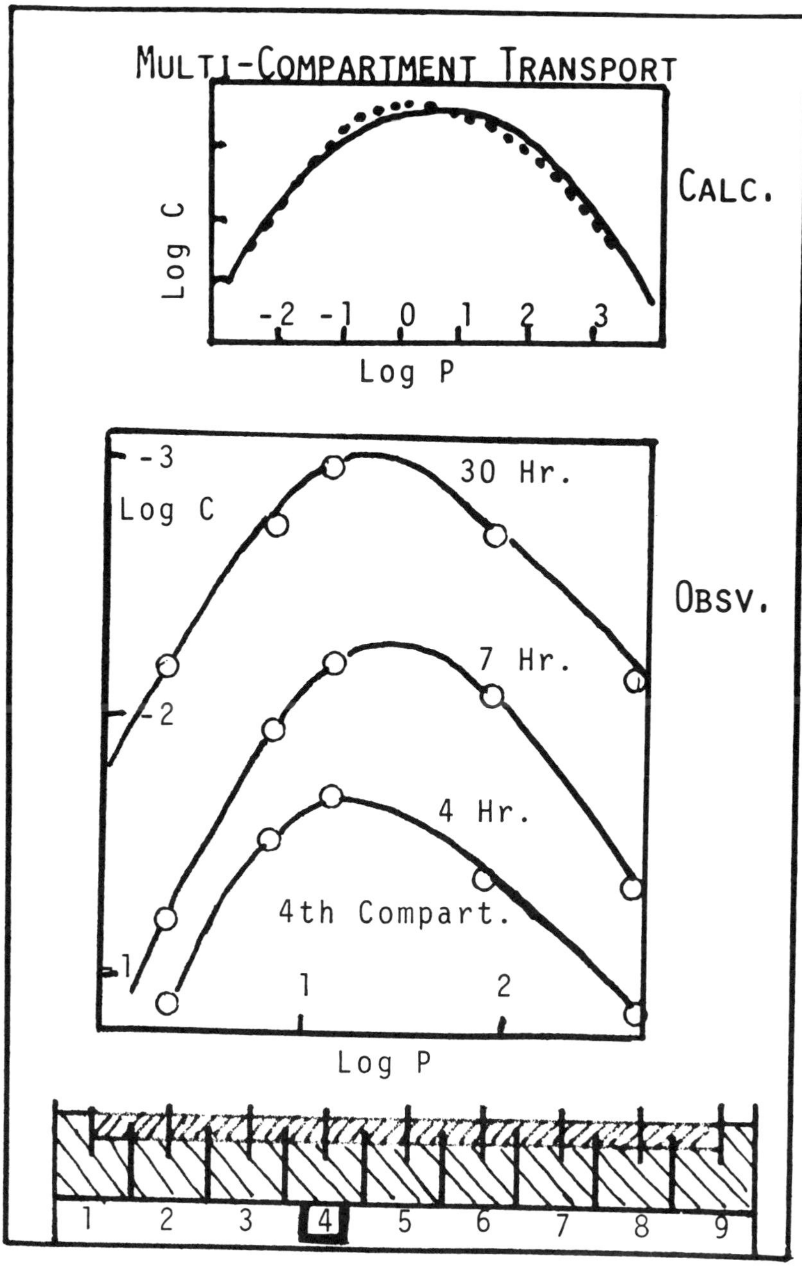


Figure 4. Mathematical and experimental modeling of transport.

Under certain conditions, the two "limbs" of the parabola may differ significantly in slope, and a bilinear relation gives a more precise fit of the data. Diffusion-controlled rate of membrane penetration appears to be one of these conditions. Another apparently exists when the structural variation in a series of substrate analogs allows extension out of the cleft containing the active site and into "free" solvent space. At any rate, a number of relationships which were once considered adequately fit by a parabola are better fit by a bilinear expression of the type:

$$\log BR = a\log P - b\log(\beta P+1) + c$$

where $a$ and $b$ = the slopes of the "up" and "down" legs
$\beta$ = the distance of optimal log P from the Y axis
$c$ = the distance of the intercept on the X axis

Bacterial inhibition by N-alkylpyridines is a type of toxic response for which the data corresponds well to a bilinear expression of the type given in Equation 12 (Figure 5) [13].

Reactions involving enzyme or complement inhibition can often be carried out sufficiently free of obscuring side reactions so that position-dependent hydrophobic character is seen to be important. The rather complex Equation 13 was developed to rationalize the action of 67 inhibitors of bacterial dihydrofolate reductase [14]:

$$\log 1/C = 1.13\pi_5 - 1.10\ MR_5 - 2.39\ I_1 - 4.09\ I_2 - 2.37\ I_3 + 8.26 \qquad (13)$$

$$n=67;\ r=0.926;\ s=0.672$$

From Equation 13 it is seen that enzyme inhibition by the 2,4-diaminoquinazolines does not depend significantly upon overall hydrophobicity, but hydrophobic substituents in the 5-position do enhance activity (Figure 6). It should be noted, however, that the in vivo action of these quinazolines as antimalarials is best fit with a similar equation, except that a negative $(\log P)^2$ becomes significant. It appears likely that this reflects optimization of the transport through the animal body and through the parasite to the enzyme site.

Of course, inhibiting bacterial or plasmodial dihydrofolate reductase is a desired toxicity, but it would be surprising if many chemical pollutants were not toxic to humans through some similar enzyme inhibition step which was strongly position-dependent. If the position effect were strong enough, it could effectively mask the usual transport role for hydrophobicity.

There is no questioning the fact that potential carcinogenicity is a menacing specter when chronic toxicity from environmental sources is being con-

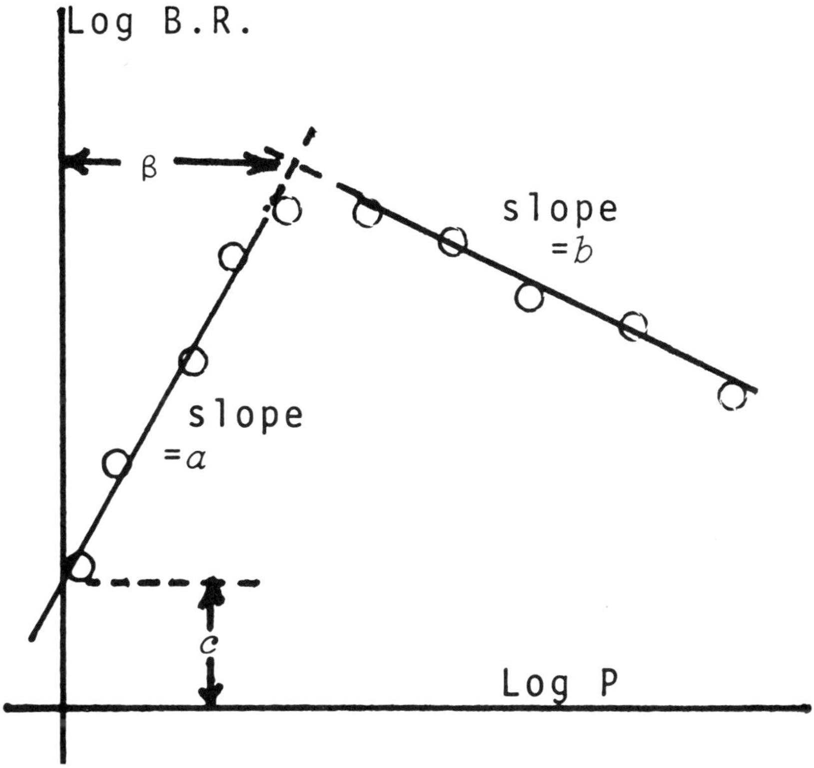


**Figure 5.** Bilinear relationships; log BR = *a*log P – *b*(*β*log P + 1) + *c*; log 1/C = 1.03 log P –1.32 log (*β*P + 1) + 2.56; n = 9, 4= 0.998, s= 0.07, log $P_0$ = 3.05; C = bacterial inhibition of N-alkylpyridines.

sidered. One promising avenue to the acquisition of pertinent data quickly and cheaply enough is the Ames test and its numerous modifications. But even the bacterial mutagenicity step itself is not a simple response, and extrapolation to untested compounds on the basis of structural similarities is not going to be as satisfactory as had first been hoped.

For solutes needing no microsomal (S-9) activation, there may be no dependence upon hydrophobic character. This is seen in Equation 14 (Table IV), which correlates the concentration of phenylenediamine platinum derivatives needed to produce a fixed number of revertants in *Salmonella* TA-92 [15]. For the relatively hydrophilic triazines, which do need microsomal activation to mutate TA-92, there is a positive relationship with log P as seen in Equation 15 (Table IV) [16]. A hydrophobic parameter is significant for the very lipophilic anilinoacridines acting as mutants, but, as

IN VITRO:

$$\text{Log } 1/C = 1.13\ \pi\text{-}5 - 1.10\ MR\text{-}5 - 2.39\ I_1 - 4.09\ I_2 - 2.37\ I_3 + 8.26$$

16-6 n=67; r=.926; s=.67

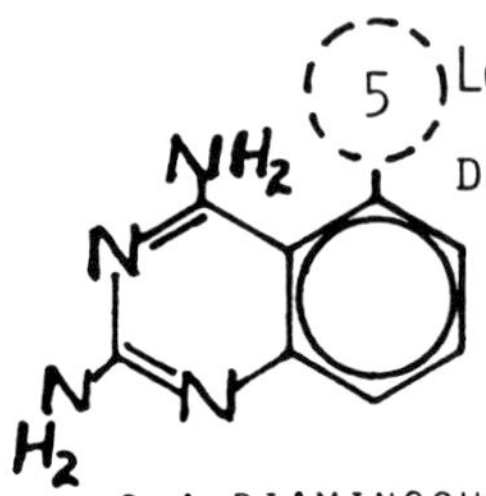


IN VIVO (as Anti-Malarial):

NEEDS $-(\text{Log P})^2$ TERM

2,4-DIAMINOQUINAZOLINES

**Figure 6.** Enzyme inhibition: bacterial dihydrofolate reductase.

**Table IV. Bacterial Mutation**[a]

| | n | r | s | Equation Number |
|---|---|---|---|---|
| *o*-Phenylenediamine Platinums (TA-92; no S-9 [15] | | | | |
| $\log 1/C = 0.0$ lob $P + 2.80\ \sigma$ | 11 | 0.98 | 0.27 | 14 |
| Triazines (TA-92 + S-9) [16] | | | | |
| $\log 1/C = 1.09 \log P - 1.63\ \sigma^+ + 5.58$ | 17 | 0.97 | 0.32 | 15 |
| 9-Anilinoacridines (TA-1537; no. S-9) [17] | | | | |
| $\log M_{50} = -2.57\ R_m + 2.60$ | 11 | 0.81 | 0.60 | 16 |
| Aniline Mustards (TA-100 + S-9) [18] | | | | |
| $\log 1/C = 0.35\pi - 0.09\pi^2 + 1.65$ | 13 | 0.94 | 0.23 | 17 |

[a]The substituent parameters $\sigma$, $\sigma^+$ and $\pi$ are defined in Reference 3.

can be seen in Equation 16, the relationship is now **inverse** [17], (In this case hydrophobicity was measured as $R_m$.). Finally, with the aniline mustards, which are direct alkylating agents, but which nevertheless require microsomal activation to mutate TA-100 or TA-1535, a parabolic hydrophobic dependence is seen in Equation 17 of (Table IV) [18].

These four classes of mutagens give an indication of the problems which must be faced in predicting, through structural comparison, the other chemical classes which have not been studied in such great detail. Even the fundamental hydrophobic parameter is no sure guide, because nonlinear responses must be anticipated, and one must know beforehand on which segment of the curve a particular class of chemicals lies. Of course, with the four classes for which these quantitative structure-activity relationships have been derived, one would be justified in predicting that untested triazine analogs would be more mutagenic as they were made more hydrophobic (holding electronic properties constant, of course). The reverse would be true for the anilinoacridines. And, although hydrophobicity is immaterial in the mutagenic potency of the platinums, it is ambivalent in the aniline mustards.

The aniline mustard analogs, reported in Equation 17 as mutagens, have also been tested for lung tumorgenesis in strain A mice by Leo et al. [18]. The inverse relationship between these two activities (mutagenicity and carcinogenicity) is not really so strange if one postulates a pair of competing reactions, one or the other of which can be favored by a change in test conditions. This final possibility must not be overlooked, and it waves a large yellow caution flag in the race to use our rapidly expanding banks of structural and parametric information to predict environmental hazards.

## ACKNOWLEDGEMENTS

This work was supported by Contract NO1-CM-67062 from the National Cancer Institute and by the Pomona College Medicinal Chemistry Project.

## REFERENCES

1. Hildebrand, J. H. "A criticism of the Term 'Hydrophobic Bond'," *J. Phys. Chem.* 72:1841 (1969).
2. Hildebrand, J. H. "Is There a 'Hydrophobic Effect'?" *Proc. Natl. Acad. Sci., U.S.A.* 76:194 (1979).
3. Hansch, C., and A. Leo. *Substituent Constants for Correlation Analysis in Chemistry and Biology* (New York: Wiley Interscience, 1979), p. 1.
4. Hansch, C., and F. Helmer. "An Extrathermodynamic Approach to the Study of the Adsorption of Organic Molecules by Membranes," *J. Polymer Sci.* (A-1):3295-3302 (1968).
5. Dunn, W., III, and C. Hansch. "Chemicobiological Interactions and the Use of Partition Coefficients in their Correlation," *Chem.-Biol. Interact.* 9:75-95 (1974).
6. Helmer, F., K. Kiehs and C. Hansch. "The Linear Free Energy Relationship Between Partition Coefficients and the Binding and Conformational Perturbation of Macromolecules by Small Organic Compounds," *Biochemistry* 7:2858-2863 (1968).
7. Leo, A. "Structural Correlates of Carcinogenesis and Mutagenesis," FDA/OS Symposium (1977), pp. 55-62.
8. Hansch, C., and W. Dunn, III. "Linear Relationships Between Lipophilic Character and Biological Activity of Drugs," *J. Pharmaceut. Sci.* 61:1-19 (1972).
9. Hansch, C., and W. Glave. "Structure-Activity Relationships in Membrane Perturbing Agents," *Mol. Pharmacol.* 7:337-354 (1971).

10. Hansch, C. "Bioisosterism," *Intra Sci. Chem. Repts.* 8:17-25 (1974).
11. Neeley, W., D. Branson and G. Blau. "Partition Coefficients to Measure Bioconcentration Potential of Organic Chemicals in Fish," *Environ. Sci. Technol.* 8:1113-1115 (1974).
12. Hansch, C., Q. Steward and J. Iwasa. "The Correlation of Localization Rates of Benzeneboronic Acids in Brain and Tumor Tissue with Substituent Constants," *Mol. Pharmacol.* 1:87-92 (1965).
13. Kubinyi, H. Personal communication.
14. Hansch, C., J., Fukanaga, P. Jow and J. Hynes. "Quantitative Structure Activity Relationships of Antimalarial and Dihydrofolate Reductase Inhibition by Quinazolines and 5-Substituted Benzyl-2,4-diaminopyrimidines," *J. Med. Chem.* 20:96-102 (1977).
15. Venger, B., and C. Hansch. "Mutagenicity of X-O-Phenylenediamine Platinum Dichlorides in the Ames Test: A Quantitative Structure Activity Analysis," Mutat. Res. (submitted).
16. Venger, B., C. Hansch, G. Hathway and Y. Amrein. "Ames Test of 1-(X-Phenyl)-3,3-Dialkyltriazines: A Quantitative Structure Activity Study," *J. Med. Chem.* 22:473-476 (1979).
17. Ferguson, L., and W. Denny. "Potential Antitumor Agents 30. Mutagenic Activity of Some 9-Anilino-acridines: Relationships Between Structure, Mutagenic Potential and Antileukemic Activity," *J. Med. Chem.* 22:251-255 (1979).
18. Leo, A., A. Panthananickal, C. Hansch, J. Theiss, M. Shimkin and A. Andrews. "Comparison of Mutagenic and Carcinogenic Activities of Aniline Mustards," *Cancer Res.* (submitted).

# CHAPTER 17

# COFACTORS IN ENVIRONMENTAL HEALTH AND DISEASE: COCARCINOGENS AND TUMOR PROMOTERS

**Benjamin L. Van Duuren and Susan Melchionne**

Laboratory of Organic Chemistry and Carcinogenesis
Institute of Environmental Medicine
New York University Medical Center
New York, New York

## INTRODUCTION

In recent years a great deal of effort has been spent on uncovering new carcinogens and studying the mode of action of well known carcinogens such as nitroso compounds, aromatic hydrocarbons and aromatic amines and their occurrence in air, water, foods and other environmental sources. With advances in levels of detection of carcinogens by sophisticated modern instrumentation, these endeavors have led to governmental controls, improved safety measures in industry and, at times, confusion in the minds of the public.

On the other hand, it has been known for almost 30 years that some materials are noncarcinogenic, but can enhance by several orders of magnitude the potency of low-level known environmental carcinogens.

The first material of this nature to be discovered was the tumor promoter, croton oil, which is derived from the seeds of a rare tropical plant, *Croton tiglium* L., indigenous to India and Sri Lanka. For more than two decades, biologists interested in chemical carcinogenesis have examined the unusual behavior of this material. It was not until the mid-1960s that the active principles of croton oil, the phorbol esters, were isolated and chemically characterized. The history of the early biological and chemical characterization studies have been well documented [1-4] and will not be repeated in this review.

During recent years these phorbol esters have become widely available; hence, their effects have been examined in a wide array of biochemical and biological studies. These studies will be summarized in this chapter.

The phorbol esters, however, are not environmental factors in cancer causation. Although croton oil was used in earlier years as a purgative in veterinary medicine [5], it is no longer used for this purpose. Other known tumor promoters are much less active, e.g., anthralin (1,8-dihydroxy-9-anthrone) and phenol [1]. Thus, the phorbol esters, although valuable tools in studies on chemical carcinogenesis, are less relevant to environmental health and disease than another group of compounds known as cocarcinogens.

Many cocarcinogens are ubiquitous environmental agents. It is only within recent years that these compounds have been given more attention. Indeed, it is expected that as more of these agents become known and their mode of action becomes understood, great advances in cancer cause and prevention will be made. The paucity of information in the area of cocarcinogens—endogenous and exogenous—is clear from scanning a recent monograph on the subject of tumor promoters and cocarcinogens. Pitifully few reviews in this monograph ventured to touch on the subject of cocarcinogens [4].

This review will focus on the biological distinction between tumor promoters and cocarcinogens, their structure-activity relationships and mode of action. The subject matter will deal mostly with mouse skin experiments but other in vivo and in vitro systems will be referred to.

A brief discussion of tumor inhibition in mouse skin cocarcinogenesis studies will emerge as a part of this review, but because of the wide scope of the subject of tumor inhibition, it will not be covered in detail.

## DEFINITION OF INITIATORS, PROMOTERS AND COCARCINOGENS

The terms "tumor promoter" and "cocarcinogen" were used in the introduction, and it is now necessary to define them. These terms are used interchangeably at times. This is unfortunate, because they clearly differ in operational terms in animal experimentation. Furthermore, because of the wide range in chemical structures of these agents, they are not all expected to exert their effects by the same mode of action; this will become clear in later sections of this review. The confusion about terminology arose because the mode of action of these compounds cannot presently be described, despite a great deal of information, particularly about promoters. It is clear, however, that promoters and cocarcinogens can be classed together as *co-factors*, regardless of mode of action. For discussion purposes, they are defined here in operational terms in animal experiments. Most of these animal experiments have dealt with mouse skin bioassays, but test systems in other organs have recently become available and will be discussed briefly.

**Initiators and Promoters**

A typical experiment involving initiators and promoters is used in what has become known as two-stage carcinogenesis in mouse skin. In this type of experiment a single dose of an initiator is applied to mouse skin. The initiator is usually a mouse skin carcinogen, such as the aromatic hydrocarbons, benzo[a]pyrene (B[a]P), 7,12-dimethylbenz[a]anthracene (DMBA) or 3-methylcholanthrene (3-MC). The initiator, if carcinogenic, is applied at such a dose that it does not cause tumors on mouse skin during the lifespan of the animals, i.e., a subcarcinogenic dose. Some initiators result in tumors in other organs, but not in the skin, e.g., urethane [6], others have been shown not to be carcinogenic at all [7]. The application of the initiator is followed by repeated applications of the promoter for six months to a year or, in more extensive experiments, for the lifespan of the group of animals on test, i.e., until there are no survivors. In the case of the very potent phorbol ester promoters from croton oil such as phorbol myristate acetate (PMA), this treatment results in the rapid (30 days) appearance of multiple benign tumors, i.e., papillomas, which progress in about six months to squamous carcinomas of the skin. These malignant tumors invade the connective tissue below the skin and, if allowed to grow, will kill the animal. The dose of a potent promoter, such as PMA, is remarkably low, 2.5-5.0 $\mu$g per application. This has been determined from extensive dose-response studies with PMA [8]. The frequency of application of the promoter is important; if the frequency of application is decreased from thrice to twice or once weekly, the tumor response decreases (as is also observed with repeated application of a carcinogen). This decreased frequency of application results in regression and disappearance of what was clinically defined earlier in the experiment as a papilloma [9].

The outstanding features of the phorbol ester promoters are the rapid rate of appearance and the large number of papillomas per animal, sometimes 12-15. These compounds are much more potent than other promoters such as anthralin, phenol and others [1]. In fact, the two-stage model for tumor induction using DMBA as initiator and PMA as promoter is the most rapid way of tumor induction on mouse skin by any chemical or combination of chemicals.

### Cocarcinogens

In cocarcinogenesis experiments, a low dose of a carcinogen, such as B[a]P, is applied simultaneously and repeatedly with the cocarcinogen. Tumors appear later than in initiation-promotion experiments, but the end result is that the carcinogenicity of B[a]P is enhanced three- or fourfold. Not all cocarcinogens are promoters and vice versa, which further complicates definitions. This aspect will be discussed in another section of this review dealing with the mode of action of these compounds.

## TYPES OF TUMOR PROMOTERS AND STRUCTURE-ACTIVITY RELATIONSHIPS

By far the most extensively studied tumor promoters and in fact the first ones discovered are the phorbol esters from croton oil. The phorbol esters are fatty acid esters of the tetracyclic diterpene alcohol phorbol. This compound was first discovered, isolated and its structure was already partially described between 1930 and 1942 by Flaschenträger and co-workers [10-12]. Its detailed structure was determined in 1967 by independent research in two laboratories [13,14], by X-ray analysis of appropriate bromine-containing phorbol esters. Phorbol has yet to be synthesized because of its complex structure. Since then a variety of esters of phorbol and those of one of its epimers has been made semisynthetically and tested for tumor-promoting activity [15]. Some of the esters synthesized are shown in Figures 1 and 2. The biological data obtained with some of these compounds are summarized in Table I [1,8,15-22].

It is clear from these findings that in this series a high degree of structural specificity is required for tumor-promoting activity. The most remarkable result was that epimerization of the 4a$\beta$-hydroxyl of PMA, structure 1b, to the 4a$\alpha$-conformation, structure 2b, resulted in complete loss of tumor-promoting activity. The same applies when comparing the biological results of structures 1c and 2c. Structures 1b and 2b were examined using Dreiding molecular models; 1a has a rigid structure in which ring D is *trans*-connected with ring C. Because ring C is fixed in an envelope conformation with the fold between C-4a and C-1b, it imposes strain, and ring D, therefore, is not planar. In structure 2a, 4a$\alpha$-phorbol, ring D is *cis*-connected with ring C. This ring then has more flexibility with the fold through C-4 and C-7b. As a result, ring D is coplanar. These Dreiding molecular model studies agree with ultraviolet (UV), nuclear magnetic resonant (NMR) and X-ray studies [13,14,20,23]. Structures 3 and 5, which represent minor changes in the PMA structure, still retain some promoting activity but are much less active

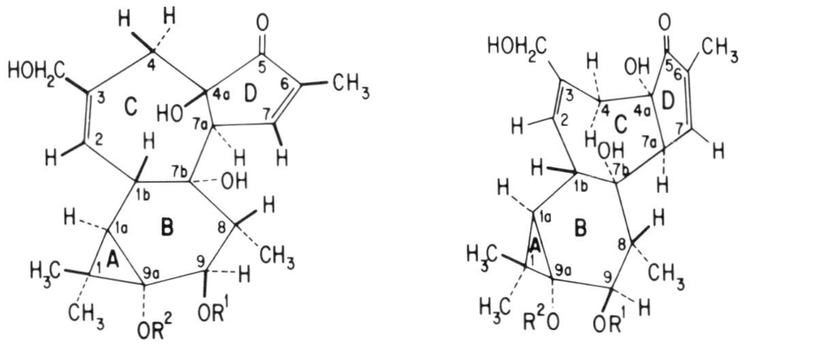

4aβ CONFORMATION

1a. $R^1 = R^2 = H$
1b. $R^1 = CO(CH_2)_{12}CH_3$; $R^2 = COCH_3$
1c. $R^1 = R^2 = CO(CH_2)_8CH_3$
1d. $R^1 = R^2 = COCH_3$
1e. $R^1 = R^2 = COC_6H_5$

4aα CONFORMATION

2a. $R^1 = R^2 = H$
2b. $R^1 = CO(CH_2)_{12}CH_3$; $R^2 = COCH_3$
2c. $R^1 = R^2 = CO(CH_2)_8CH_3$

**Figure 1.** Structures for 4aβ-phorbol and 4aα-phorbol and some of their esters discussed in text (see Table I). Structure 1a, phorbol; 1b, phorbol myristate acetate; 1c, phorbol-9,9a-didecanoate; 1d, phorbol-9,9a-diacetate; 1e, phorbol-9,9a-dibenzoate; 2a, 4aα-phorbol; 2b, 4aα-phorbol myristate acetate; 2c, 4aα-phorbol didecanoate.

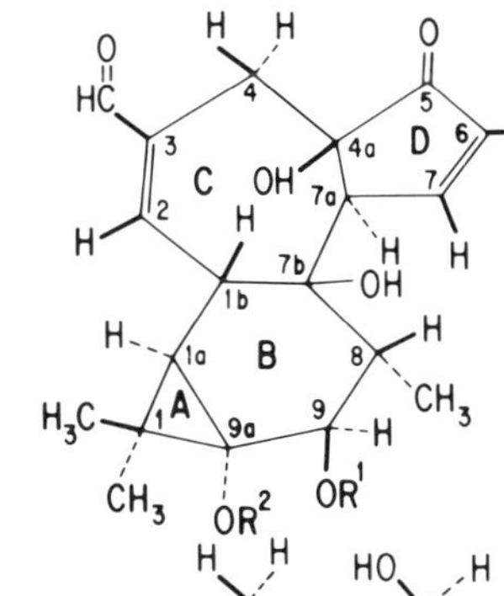

3

5

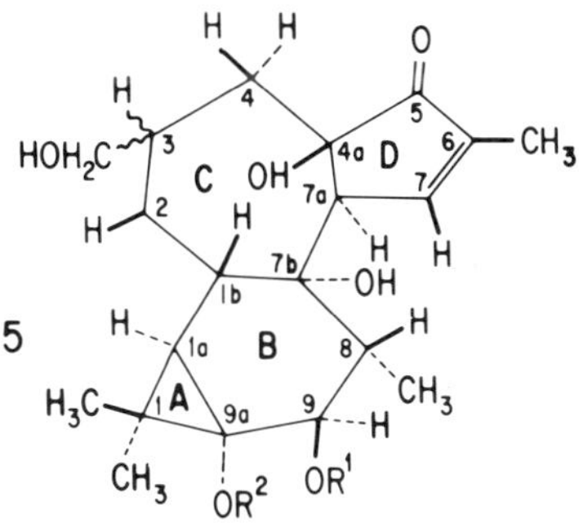

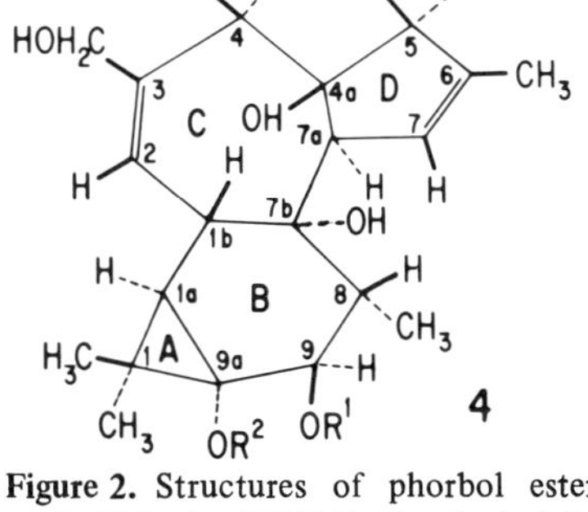

4

3. PAMA
4. PHMA
5. DPMA
$R^1 = CO(CH_2)_{12}CH_3$; $R^2 = COCH_3$

**Figure 2.** Structures of phorbol esters. Structure 3, phorbol-9-myristate-9a-acetate-3-aldehyde (PAMA); 4, phorbolol-9-myristate-9a-acetate (PHMA); 5, 2,3-dihydrophorbol-9-myristate-9a-acetate (DPMA).

Table I. Tumor-Promoting Activity of Phorbol Derivatives on Mouse Skin

| Compound[a] | Structure Number | Days on Test/Median Survival Time (days) | Days to First Tumor | Mice with Papillomas/ Total Papillomas |
|---|---|---|---|---|
| Phorbol [1] | 1a | 196/>196 | | 0[b] |
| Phorbol-9,9a-diacetate [17] | 1d | 182/>182 | | 0[c] |
| Phorbol-9,9a-dibenzoate [19] | 1e | 196/>196 | 112 | 7/-[b] |
| Phorbol-9,9a-didecanoate [16] | 1c | 196/>196 | 42 | 16/-[b] |
| 4aα-PDD [20] | 2c | 434/>434 | | 0[d] |
| 4aα-PMA [20] | 2b | 443/>443 | | 0[d] |
| PAMA [22] | 3 | 461/>461 | 188 | 10/25[d] [2][e] |
| PHMA [22] | 4 | 380/>380 | 54 | 29/181[d] [10][e] |
| DPMA [21] | 5 | 433/>433 | 220 | 9/16[d] [4][e] |
| PMA [8] | 1b | 435/352 | 49 | 30/617[d] [15][e] |

[a] References are to papers describing preparation and/or partial synthesis of test compounds.

[b] Female CD-1 mice (28 to 32/group) were initiated with 51.2 μg 7,12-dimethylbenz[a]anthracene and promoted beginning two weeks later, two times weekly for the duration of the test, with 11.4 μg phorbol-9,9a-didecanoate, 97 μg phorbol-9,9a-dibenzoate, and 62 μg phorbol. All three compounds were applied in 0.15 ml acetone per application. The number of mice with papillomas is approximated from percentages; total papillomas were not given [16].

[c] Female CD-1 mice, exact number not specified, were initiated with 51.2 μg 7,12-dimethylbenz[a]anthracene and promoted beginning two weeks later, two times weekly for the duration of the test, with 7.6 μg phorbol-9,9a-diacetate per application [18].

[d] Female ICR/Ha Swiss mice (30/group) were initiated with 20 μg 7,12-dimethylbenz[a]anthracene and promoted beginning two weeks later, three times weekly for the duration of the test, with 10 μg each of 4aα-PDD, 4aα-PMA, PAMA, PHMA, DPMA and PMA. All promoting treatments were in 0.1 ml acetone per application [15,21].

[e] Number in brackets = number of mice in which papillomas progressed to squamous cell carcinomas.

than PMA itself. PHMA, structure 4, is the most active of the modified phorbol esters. The removal of the long-chain moiety (decanoate or myristate) from the phorbol ring results in complete loss of biological activity [16]. The relevance of this structural specificity of PMA with regard to mode of action will be discussed in a later section of this review.

In recent years a wide variety of compounds obtained from plants, mainly from the *Euphorbiaceae* species have been isolated and some of them have been characterized [24,25]. Some of these compounds have ring systems and ester functions similar to that of the phorbol esters. However, detailed structure-promoting activity studies have yet to be carried out on these compounds.

An intriguing tumor-promoting agent is anthralin [26,27], 1,8-dihydroxy-9-anthrone, which has been used in the treatment of psoriasis [28]. Studies on structure-promoting activity of this compound and a series of analogs showed again that minor changes cause a decrease or loss of activity. Of the 18 compounds shown in Figure 3, only compounds 1,4,5,7 and 16 have noteworthy tumor-promoting activity as shown in Table II. Three other compounds 2,12 and 17, showed marginal activity, whereas the others were all inactive. All 18 compounds were inactive as whole carcinogens when applied to mouse skin for the duration of the test (370 days) [27].

Some observations on structure and tumor-promoting activity can be made. In comparing compounds 1, 4 and 5, it is noteworthy that the 1, 8 and 9 substituents are the same and intact. Esterification of the 1 or 9 positions (compounds 2 and 3) results in loss of tumor-promoting activity. Also, where the three groups are intact, but the middle ring is opened, as in 10, activity is lost. The addition of an acetyl, structure 4, or myristoyl group, structure 5, on the 10 position of anthralin does not markedly affect tumor-promoting activity compared with anthralin. Compounds 11-15 were all inactive. It was also found in an earlier study that anthrone and 1,8-dihydroxynaphthalene are inactive as tumor promoters [26]. It was concluded from these studies that the structural features of anthralin necessary for tumor-promoting activity are at least one phenolic hydroxyl group hydrogen-bonded to the C-9 carbonyl oxygen and one benzylic proton at the C-10 position.

These findings suggested that metal chelation may play a role in the tumor-promoting activity of anthralin. Metal chelation studies carried out using Cu, Zn, Mn, Mg and Ca as metal ions, however, did not show any direct correlation between chelation and tumor-promoting activity [27].

Another interesting feature was that molecular rigidity is necessary for tumor-promoting activity; this is seen by comparing structure 10 with structures 1, 4 and 5.

In the early phases of studies on chemical carcinogens in tobacco smoke condensate (TSC) it became apparent that the known aromatic hydrocarbon

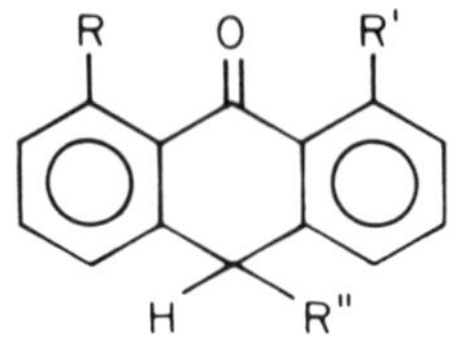

**1,** R, R′ = OH; R″ = H
**2,** R, R′ = $OCOCH_3$; R″ = H
**3,** R, R′ = OCO-$(CH_2)_{12}CH_3$; R″ = H
**4,** R, R′ = OH; R″ = $COCH_3$
**5,** R, R′ = OH; R″ = $CO(CH_2)_{12}CH_3$
**6,** R, R′, R″ = OH

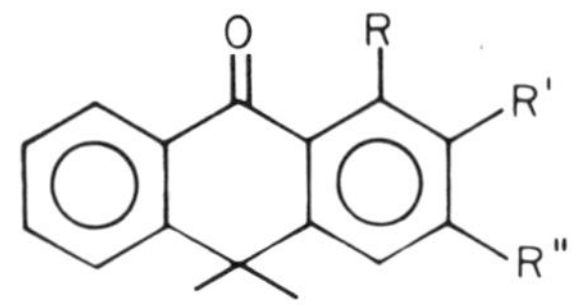

**7,** R = OH; R′, R″ = H
**8,** R, R′ = OH; R″ = H
**9,** R = H; R′, R″ = OH

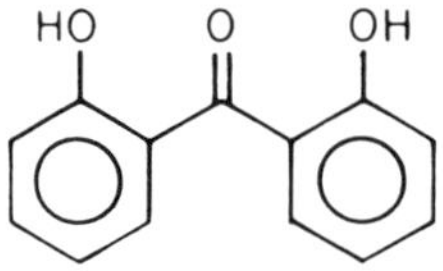

**10**

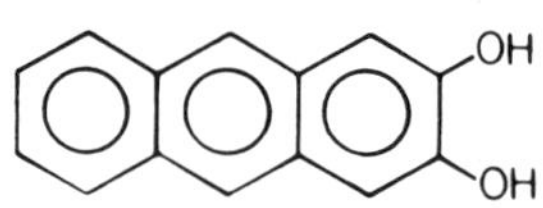

**11**

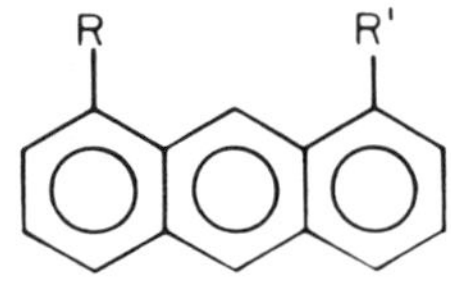

**12,** R = OH; R′ = H
**13,** R, R′ = OH

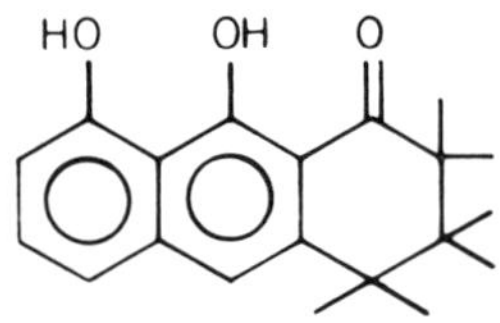

**14**

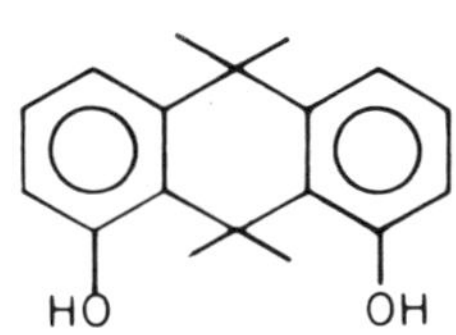

**15**

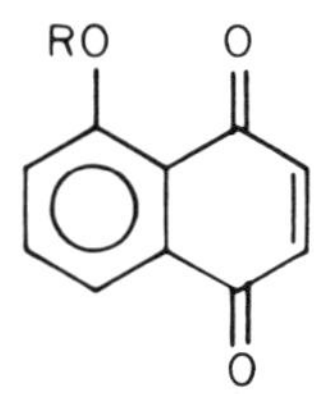

**16,** R = H
**17,** R = $COCH_3$
**18,** R = $CO(CH_2)_{12}CH_3$

**Figure 3.** Structures of anthralin (structure 1) and some of its analogs. Analogs 2,4,5,7, 12,16 and 17 are named in Table II. Structure 3, 1,8-dimyristoyl-9-anthrone; 6, 1,8, 10-trihydroxy-9-anthrone; 8, 1,2-dihydroxy-9-anthrone; 9, 2,3-dihydroxy-9-anthrone; 10, 2,2′-dihydroxybenzophenone; 11, 2,3-dihydroxyanthracene; 13, 1,8-dihydroxy-anthracene; 14, 3,4-dihydro-8,9-dihydroxy-1(2H)-anthracenone; 15, 1,8-dihydroxy-9,10-dihydroanthracene; 18, myristoyljuglone.

Table II. Tumor-Promoting Activity of Anthralin and Related Compounds in Mouse Skin [27]

| Figure 3 Compound No. | Test Compound | Dose (μg)[a] | Days to First Papilloma | Mice with Papillomas/Total Papillomas[b] |
|---|---|---|---|---|
| 1 | 1,8-Dihydroxy-9-anthrone (anthralin) | 80 | 68 | 12/22 (0) |
| 2 | 1,8-Diacetoxy-9-anthrone | 124 | 322 | 2/3 (0) |
| 4 | 1,8-Dihydroxy-10-acetyl-9-anthrone | 15 | 89 | 6/10 (1) |
| 5 | 1,8-Dihydroxy-10-myristoyl-9-anthrone | 300[c] | 55 | 12/15 (2)[d] |
| 7 | 1-Hydroxy-9-anthrone | 80[e] | 154 | 10/12 (4)[d] |
| 12 | 1-Hydroxyanthracene | 80[f] | 486 | 1/1 (0) |
| 16 | Juglone | 62 | 148 | 3/4 (2) |
| 17 | Acetyljuglone | 76 | 370 | 1/1 (0) |

[a] 30 female ICR/Ha Swiss mice per group except where noted. A single treatment with 20 μg of 7,12-dimethylbenz[a]anthracene in 0.1 ml of acetone was followed two weeks later by thrice weekly application of the test compounds in 0.1 ml of acetone. Duration of test was 370 days except where noted. Not shown in this table are those tests in which the compounds were applied without pretreatment with initiator or with initiator alone. No skin tumors were observed with any of these tests. Skin tumors were also not observed in the no-treatment groups, and the incidences of spontaneous tumors at other sites were identical with those observed in the many earlier experiments in which female ICR/Ha Swiss mice were used as controls.

[b] Number of mice with squamous carcinoma of skin in parentheses.

[c] 20 mice; duration of test was 521 days; median survival time = 423 days.

[d] One mouse with metastatic squamous carcinoma of lung.

[e] 20 mice; duration of test = 521 days; median survival time = 391 days.

[f] 20 mice; duration of test = 521 days; median survival time = 474 days.

and heterocyclic carcinogens isolated from TSC could not account for its observed carcinogenicity on mouse skin. It was recognized as early as 1958 that tumor promoters and/or other cofactors must be involved [29,30].

This led to an intensive study on the promoting activity of a series of phenols which are known or suspected components of TSC using single applications of B[a]P or DMBA as initiators followed by maximum tolerated doses of the phenols applied repeatedly to mouse skin for a year or more. Of the 16 compounds tested only 1, phenol itself, showed notable, but weak promoting activity [31]. This led to the conclusion that other cofactors must be involved in tobacco carcinogenesis. These are the cocarcinogens discussed below.

Other miscellaneous compounds earlier considered of interest as promoters were the "Tweens and Spans" which are surface-active agents; they are long-chain fatty acid esters of hexitol anhydride derived from sorbitol and related materials [5]. The massive doses of these materials used in two-stage carcinogenesis studies [32,33] and the possibility of impurities discouraged further research on the Tweens and Spans [1].

## BIOLOGICAL AND BIOCHEMICAL PROPERTIES OF INITIATORS AND PROMOTERS AND MODE OF ACTION OF PROMOTERS

There are several features of two-stage carcinogenesis which are quite remarkable. One is that the dose of initiator, e.g., DMBA, is several orders of magnitude lower than that required for DMBA alone, even when applied repeatedly, to elicit a tumor response comparable to the two-stage experiment using PMA as promoter. It has also been calculated that the dose of PMA required for a high yield of tumors is about two orders of magnitude less than the quantity of DMBA required when DMBA is tested as a carcinogen by itself on mouse skin [9]. Considering the low dosages of DMBA and PMA used [8], the tumor response in terms of both total papillomas and carcinomas of the skin, is astoundingly higher and tumors appear dramatically earlier than by any known mouse skin carcinogen, including such potent mouse skin carcinogens as DMBA, B[a]P or 3-MC.

Other features of the two-stage model that are important are the reversibility of promotion, discussed above, the persistence of the initiating effect and the effect of aging. The permanence of the initiating effect was discovered over 30 years ago [34] and it was more recently examined in detail [35]. The procedure used and carcinoma incidences observed are shown schematically in Figure 4. The complete experiment involved six other groups which were controls and received initiator or promoter only at the

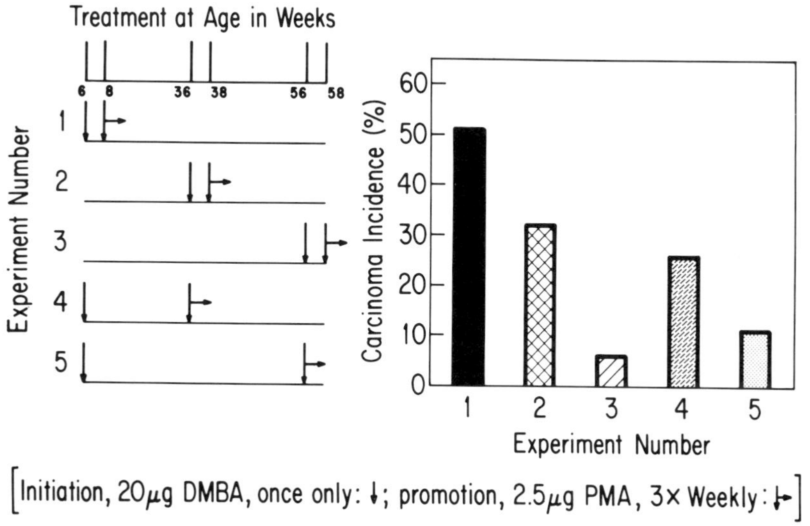


**Figure 4.** Diagrammatic protocol for effect of aging and interval between initiation and promotion on two-stage tumorigenesis in mouse skin and the carcinoma incidence in percent.

various time intervals shown in Figure 4, plus a solvent control. The results of this experiment are relevant not only to the matter of persistence of the initiating effect, but also to the effect of aging in two-stage carcinogenesis.

These experiments showed that there is a decrease in tumor yield when there is a prolonged time interval between initiation and promotion (group 5) or when old animals are initiated followed by promotion (group 3). Thus, the age of the animals at the beginning of the secondary treatment is important in determining the final tumor yields. The experiments also clearly show the permanence of the effect of the initiator, i.e., comparing groups 1 and 5.

Using the same experiments referred to above, the effect of aging on tumor induction in two-stage carcinogenesis was further analyzed [36]. The results of the pertinent experiments are illustrated in Figures 5 and 6. These figures show life table analyses, probably not familiar to many chemists. It uses a formula which takes into account the tumor incidences together with the number of surviving animals at any point during the course of the experiment [37]. The conclusion from these experiments was that the percentage of tumor-bearers decreases as the age of the animals at the onset of promotion increases, or when initiation and promotion occur in older animals, i.e., comparing groups 1 and 3. The average number of tumors per tumor bearer similarly decreases with increasing age at the onset of the experiment [35].

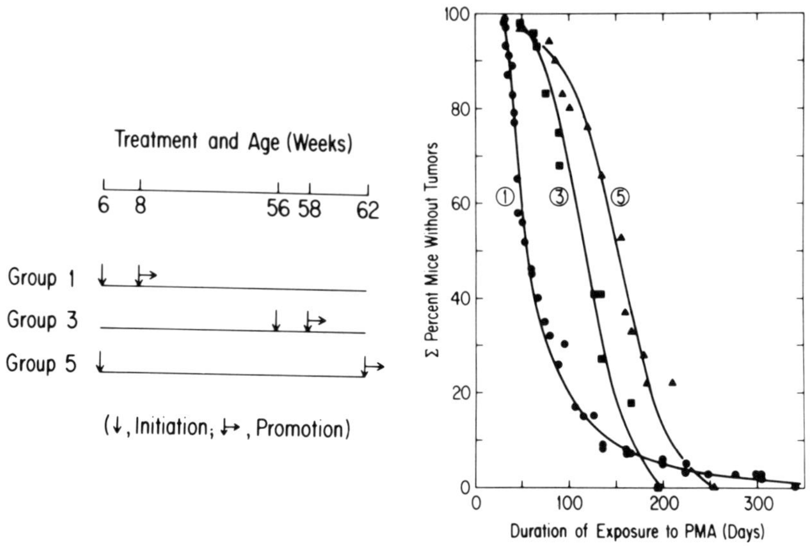


**Figure 5.** Life table analysis; percentage of animals without tumors compared with duration of exposure.

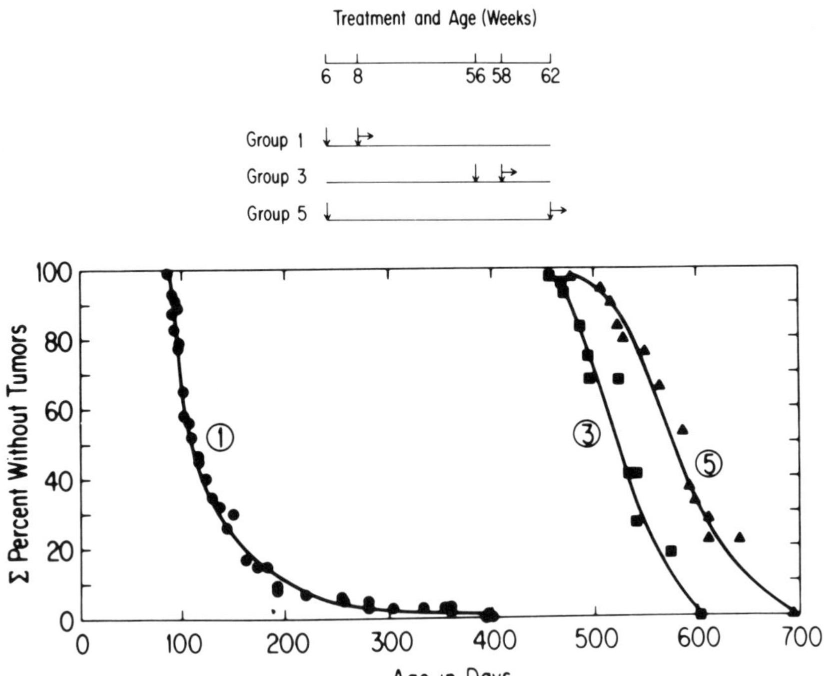


**Figure 6.** Life table analysis; percentage of animals without tumors compared with age.

A biological feature of PMA and other promoters which has elicited a great deal of discussion is the fact that they cause in the mouse hyperplasia, (thickening of the epidermis) and inflammation of the skin. To some researchers this property is not relevant in tumor-promotion. Many materials do not possess promoting activity, yet cause these same effects [38]. In addition, there is no clear-cut correlation between potency of promoting activity and inflammatory response [39], and the dose-response curve for PMA as a promoter does not parallel its hyperplastic activity [8,40]; others believe that hyperplasia is a relevant part of the process of tumor promotion [41]. In any event, the phenomenon is not of much aid in elucidating the mechanism of action of promoters.

PMA has only recently been shown to be a promoter in sites other than skin by the demonstration that two-stage carcinogenesis occurs in the forestomach of the mouse using DMBA as initiator [42]. PMA and related promoters have been shown to have a variety of biological effects in cell culture and other in vitro systems. The biologic effects of PMA in vivo and in vitro are summarized in Table III [1,8,42-59]. Related biochemical effects in vivo and in vitro are summarized in Table IV [39,45,48,60-71]. Some of the observed effects are clearly related to the mitogenic effect of PMA and do not reveal much or anything about its mode of action.

One of the early observations concerning the possible mode of action of the phorbol esters was that the active compounds are lipophilic-hydrophilic in nature [1]. This observation, taken together with the high structural specificity required for promoting activity of PMA and its analogs, suggests

**Table III. Biological Effects of Phorbol Myristate Acetate**

| In Vivo | In Vitro |
|---|---|
| Tumor promoter in mouse skin [1] | Inducer of cell division in BalbC/3T3 cells and in thymic lymphoblasts [47-49] |
| Tumor promoter in mouse forestomach [42] | Causes aggregation of human blood platelets [50] |
| Cocarcinogen in mouse skin [43] | Tumor promoter in C3H/10T1/2 cells [51] |
| Inducer of mitosis (mitogenic), hyperplasia inflammation [8,44,45] | Inhibits terminal differentiation of cells in culture [52,53] |
| Interferes with epidermal differentiation in mouse skin [46] | Alters membrane permeability [54] and increases membrane fluidity [55] |
| | Interferes with differentiation in cell culture [53,56] |
| | Inhibits epidermal growth factor in several cell types [57-59] |

**Table IV. Biochemical Effects of Phorbol Myristate Acetate**

| |
|---|
| Stimulates DNA, RNA and protein synthesis in cell culture and in mouse skin [44,45,48,60] |
| Induces ornithine decarboxylase in epidermal cell culture and in mouse skin [39,61,62] |
| Releases lysosomal enzymes (rabbit liver) in vitro [63,64] |
| Induces cell membrane enzymes ($Na^+K^+$ ATPase and 5′-nucleotidase) in microsomal preparations from cell cultures [65] |
| Inhibits DNA repair in human lymphocytes and HeLa cells [66-68] |
| Stimulates histone synthesis and phosphorylation in mouse skin [69,70] |
| Binds to rat liver plasma membranes in vitro [71] |

that binding of the phorbol ester to the plasma membrane of the cell is a primary step in tumor promotion [1,47,72]. This concept has now become widely accepted and is supported from several biochemical and biological studies listed in Tables III and IV. Thus, it has been shown that PMA alters membrane permeability [54] and increases membrane fluidity [55,73]. In addition, it has been shown by spectrofluorimetry that PMA binds to rat liver plasma membranes [71,72].

Although a large number of biochemical effects have been observed, as shown in Table IV, it is not clear which of these effects are relevant to the mechanism of tumor promotion. Thus, one of the observed effects, induction of ornithine decarboxylase, can also be accomplished by mechanical abrasion of mouse skin [39]. However, the importance of binding of PMA to the plasma membrane as a primary step in promotion is now clear. The nature of the receptor sites in the membrane is unknown. However, the high structural specificity required for promoting activity using the phorbol ester and anthralin compounds indicates that the receptor sites are also highly specific. It is likely that the long-chain ester moiety becomes inserted or intercalated in some way in the lipid-rich layer of the plasma membrane and that the phorbol moiety binds to an external protein site.

## USE OF TWO-STAGE CARCINOGENESIS FOR SCREENING POTENTIAL CARCINOGENS

The two-stage mouse skin model for screening potential carcinogens has emerged from several studies using halogenated hydrocarbons as initiators with PMA as promoter [74,75]. Tests with four of these halogenated compounds are listed in Table V. None of these compounds are carcinogenic by repeated application on mouse skin. Nevertheless, they are all carcinogenic by other routes of administration [75-80] in mice and/or rats as shown in

Table V. Initiation-Promotion for Screening Potential Carcinogens

| Initiation-Promotion[a] | | | Other Bioassays | | |
|---|---|---|---|---|---|
| Compound[b] | Days to First Tumor | Mice with Papillomas/ Total Papillomas | Species | Route of Administration | Tumors |
| Allyl chloride | 197 | 7/10 ($p<0.025$) | Mouse [76] | Feeding | Cancer, forestomach |
| 1,2-Dibromo-3-chloropropane | 257 | 6/6 ($p<0.05$) | Mouse | Skin | Cancer, forestomach |
| | | | Mouse, rat [77] | Feeding | Cancer, forestomach |
| Vinylidene Chloride | 271 | 8/9<br>1 cancer ($p<0.005$) | Mouse [78] | Inhalation | Adenocarcinoma, kidney |
| Epichlorohydrin [79] | 92 | 9/12<br>1 cancer ($p<0.005$) | Mouse [79]<br>Rat [80] | Subcutaneous<br>Inhalation | Sarcomas<br>Cancer, nasal passages |

[a] 30 female ICR/Ha Swiss mice per group; duration of test 400–500 days. Reference 75 except where other reference numbers are indicated.
[b] All compounds inactive when applied repeatedly on mouse skin.

Table V. Also included in this table is epichlorohydrin from earlier studies [79]. These routes of administration include feeding, inhalation and subcutaneous injection, which result in tumors at sites other than skin. Although this represents a limited series, it suggests that this assay be further explored.

## COCARCINOGENIC AGENTS

### Biological Aspects

In Berenblum's classical experiments, croton oil and B[a]P, when applied simultaneously to mouse skin, resulted in a remarkable enhancement of tumor induction compared to either agent applied alone [81]. This type of test is thus operationally different from the two-stage carcinogenesis experiments described above and, moreover, is the way in which humans are exposed to cigarette smoke, air pollutants and other environmental cofactors. A series of experiments using the cocarcinogenesis protocol was used to examine various structural types [43].

Five major compound types were tested for cocarcinogenicity on mouse skin. There were di- and triphenols, noncarcinogenic aromatic hydrocarbons, long-chain aliphatic hydrocarbons, long-chain fatty acids and alcohols. A summary of some of these findings are given in Table VI [43].

**Table VI. Cocarcinogenesis on Mouse Skin[a]**

| Compound | Dose (mg) | Days on Test | Days to First Tumor | Tumor Bearers[b]/ Total No. of Tumors |
|---|---|---|---|---|
| Catechol | 2 | 368 | 299 | 36/90 (31) |
| Pyrogallol | 5 | 440 | 253 | 40/95 (33) |
| Decane | 25 | 440 | 230 | 38/73 (34) |
| Undecane | 25 | 440 | 195 | 44/105 (41) |
| Pyrene | 0.012 | 368 | 186 | 26/42 (20) |
| Benzo[e]pyrene | 0.015 | 368 | 246 | 33/79 (27) |
| Fluoranthene | 0.040 | 440 | 99 | 39/126 (37) |
| Controls | | | | |
| Benzo[a]pyrene | 0.005 | 368 | 251 | 14/16 (10) |
| Benzo[a]pyrene | 0.005 | 440 | 210 | 16/26 (12) |

[a] 50 female ICR/Ha Swiss mice per group; cocarcinogens applied simultaneously with 0.005 mg benzo[a]pyrene, thrice weekly for 368 or 440 days [43].

[b] Papillomas of skin; number of animals with squamous carcinoma of skin given in parentheses.

In these experiments, 21 pure chemicals and related compounds were tested for cocarcinogenicity. The compounds were applied to mouse skin, 50 female ICR/Ha Swiss mice per group, thrice weekly, together with 5 μg per application of B[a]P. The duration of these tests was 440 days. The compounds listed in Table VI all enhance significantly the carcinogenicity of B[a]P, but did not notably reduce the days to first tumors, except in the case of fluoranthene. The results with the other compounds are given in the original papers and the carcinoma incidences for some of these compounds are shown in Figure 7. The rate of tumor appearance for representative cocarcinogens and tumor inhibitors are illustrated in Figures 8 and 9.

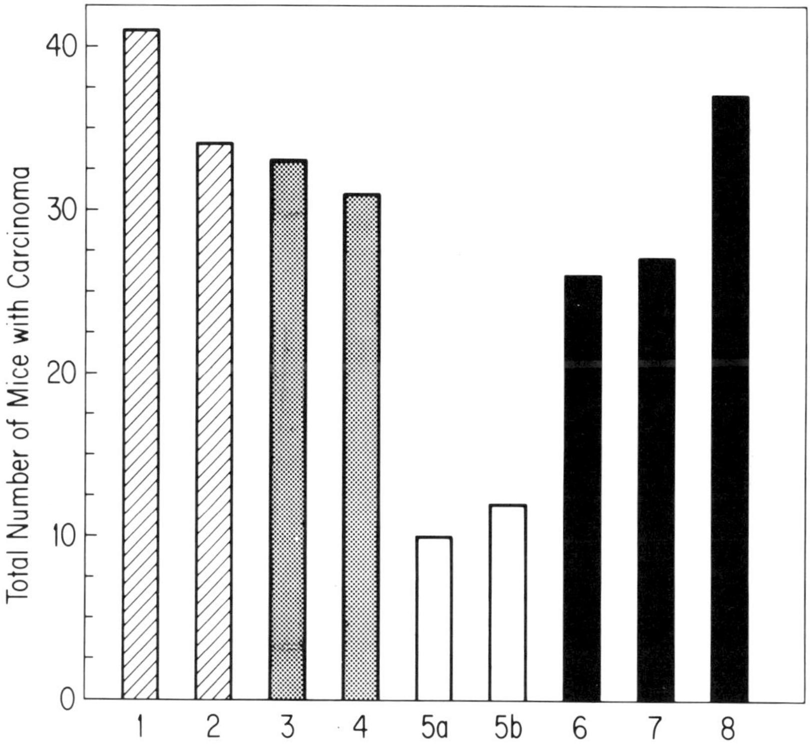


**Figure 7.** Carcinoma incidences in cocarcinogenesis experiments using 50 female ICR/Ha mice per group. 1, Undecane, 25 mg per application, + B[a]P, 5 μg per application at 440 days; 2, decane, 25 mg per application + B[a]P, 5 μg per application at 440 days; 3, pyrogallol, 5 mg per application + B[a]P, 5 μg per application at 440 days; 4, catechol, 2 mg per application + B[a]P, 5 μg per application at 368 days; 5a, B[a]P, 5 μg per application, control at 368 days; 5b, B[a]P, 5 μg per application, control at 440 days; 6, pyrene, 40 μg per application, + B[a]P, 5 μg per application at 440 days; 7, benzo[e]pyrene, 15 μg per application + B[a]P, 5 μg per application, at 368 days; 8, fluoranthene, 40 μg per application + B[a]P, 5 μg per application at 440 days.

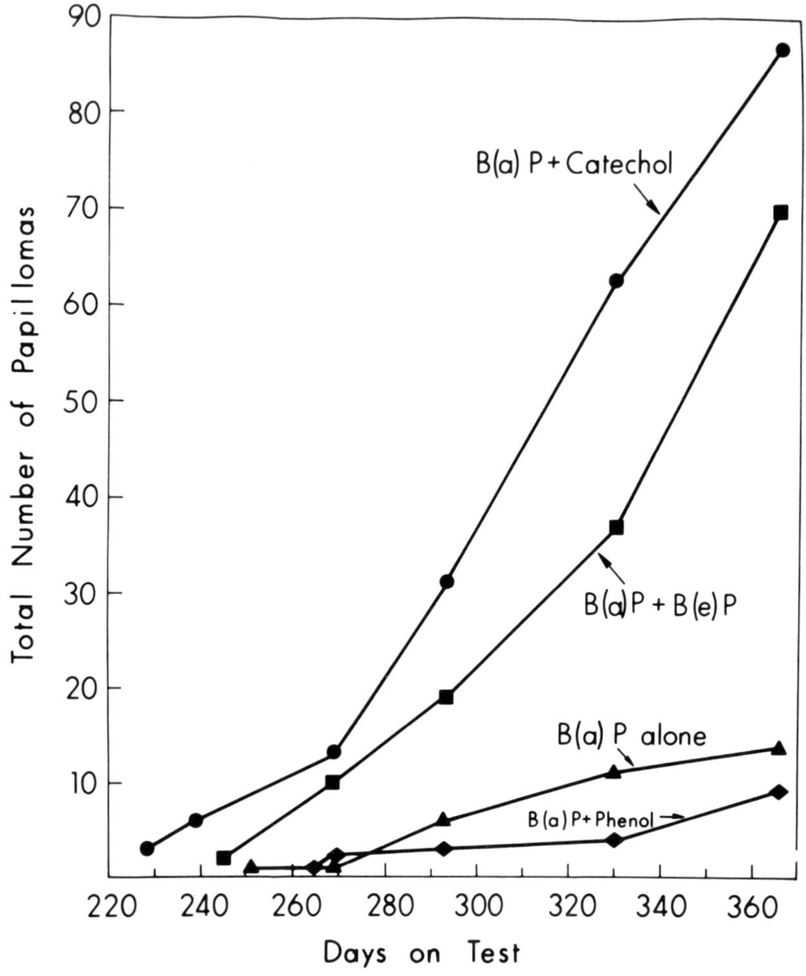


**Figure 8.** Rate of appearance of papillomas in cocarcinogenesis experiments. B[a]P applied at 5 μg per application; catechol, 2 mg per application; B[e]P, 15 μg per application; phenol, 3 mg per application in 0.1 ml acetone three times weekly for 368 days. Fifty female ICR/Ha mice per group.

None of the cocarcinogens in Table VI are tumor promoters or carcinogens on mouse skin. Instead, it is a series of compounds which appears innocuous but is, indeed, harmful in the presence of minute amounts of a carcinogen. It is also important to note that these compounds are not mutagenic in bacterial systems.

Recently, the same type of experiment was carried out with catechol as cocarcinogen using a tumor-susceptible strain of mice called SENCAR mice

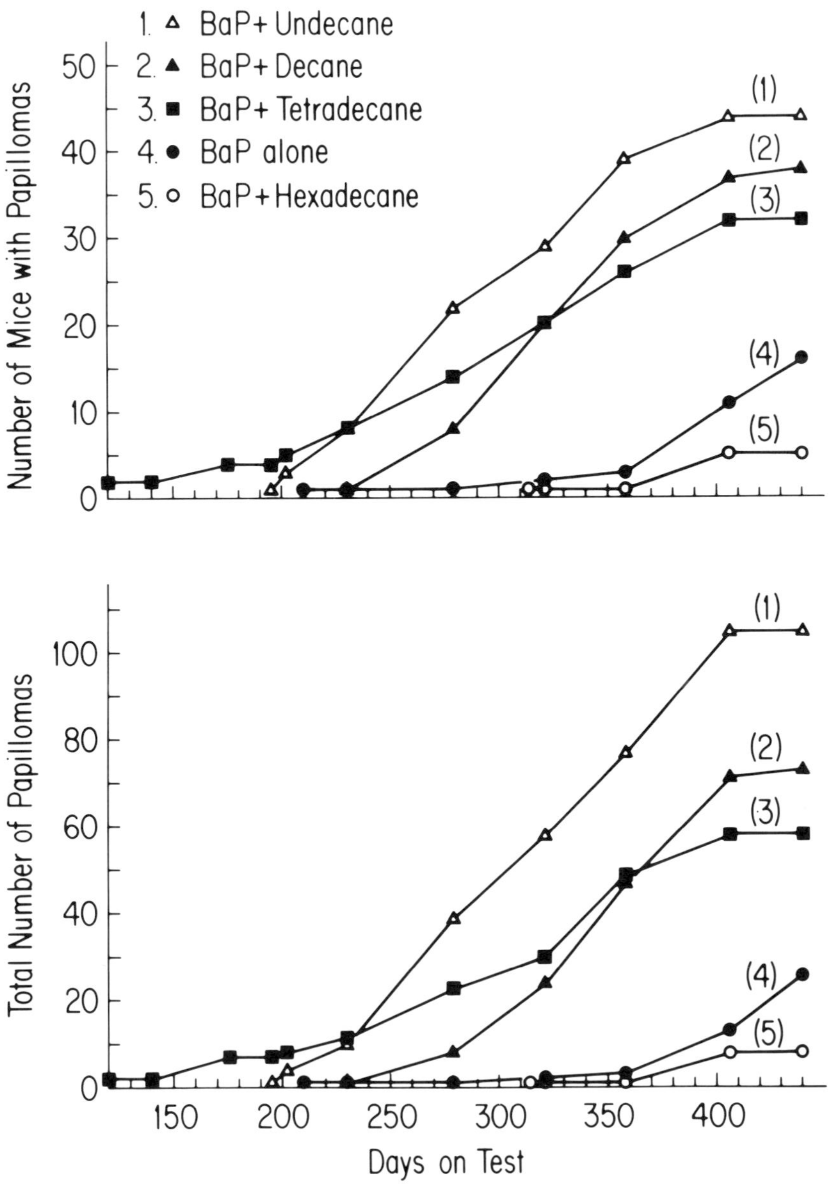


**Figure 9.** Papilloma incidence in cocarcinogenesis experiments expressed as total papillomas and as number of mice with papillomas at 440 days. Dose per application: B[a]P, 5 μg; undecane, 25 mg; decane, 25 mg; tetradecane, 25 mg; hexadecane, 25 mg.

[82]. These results are summarized in Table VII. It is of interest to compare the results given for catechol in Table VI, i.e., with ICR/Ha mice, with the results in SENCAR mice (Table VII). Although the group sizes were different, the dosages were the same in the two experiments. The SENCAR mice are sensitive for cocarcinogenesis on mouse skin, particularly in terms of days to first tumor. There was no significant difference in tumor response in male and female SENCAR mice.

**Table VII. Cocarcinogenesis in SENCAR Mice Using Benzo[a]pyrene and Catechol[a]**

| Sex | Compund | Dose (mg) | Days to First Tumor | Tumor Bearers[b]/ Total No. Tumors |
|---|---|---|---|---|
| Female | Catechol | 2 | | 0 (0) |
| Male | Catechol | 2 | | 0 (0) |
| Female | B[a]P | 0.005 | 266 | 5/5 (2) |
| Male | B[a]P | 0.005 | 230 | 5/6 (2) |
| Female | B[a]P | 0.005 | 147 | 17/78 (8) |
| | + catechol | 2 | | |
| Male | B[a]P | 0.005 | 107 | 13/44 (8) |
| | + catechol | 2 | | |

[a] 20 mice/group; solutions applied simultaneously three times weekly to the dorsal skin in 0.1 ml acetone for 323 days [82].

[b] Papillomas of skin; number of animals with squamous carcinoma of skin given in parentheses.

## Structure-Activity Relationships of Cocarcinogens and Possible Modes of Action

It is noteworthy that, although catechol is a potent cocarcinogen, its position isomers, resorcinol and hydroquinone, are not only inactive, but partially inhibit the tumorigenicity of B[a]P [43]. The cocarcinogenicities of these various phenols are compared in Figure 10. In the aliphatic hydrocarbon series, decane ($C_{10}H_{22}$), undecane ($C_{11}H_{24}$) and tetradecane ($C_{14}H_{30}$) are potent cocarcinogens. Their longer-chain analogs, hexadecane ($C_{16}H_{34}$), eicosane ($C_{20}H_{42}$) and octacosane ($C_{28}H_{58}$) are inactive as cocarcinogens, and some of these longer-chain hydrocarbons also partially inhibit B[a]P carcinogenicity. In other recent studies similar structural specificities for tumor promoters, both in the anthralin series [27] and in the phorbol ester series [15], have been observed.

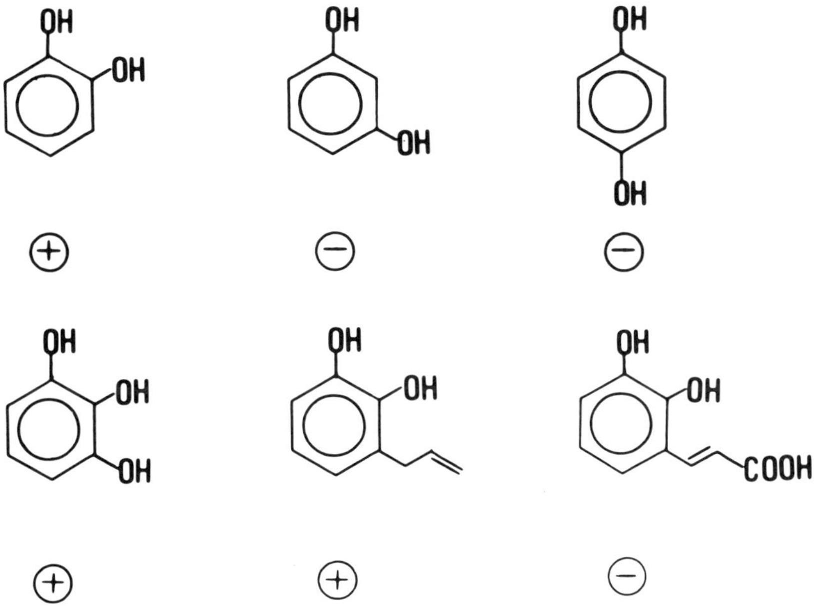


**Figure 10.** Cocarcinogenicity ⊕ or tumor inhibition ⊖ with B[a]P on mouse skin for catechol and five related phenols.

Because the compound types which were cocarcinogenic in these tests vary so widely in their chemical structures, it is unlikely that they all have the same mode of action. Several possible mechanisms come to mind to account for the cocarcinogenicity or tumor-inhibitory activity of these compounds. They include: (1) induction of carcinogen-activating enzymes: (2) other alterations of metabolic pathways, e.g., activation or deactivation of detoxifying enzymes; (3) physical effects, i.e., increased or decreased rate of carcinogenic absorption; and (4) effects on DNA repair mechanisms. These possible modes of action are in need of further studies.

## COMPARISON OF PROMOTERS AND COCARCINOGENS

In the course of the work on cocarcinogens cited above, the cocarcinogenic activities of a series of compounds with their tumor-promoting activities were compared. Phenol, for example, is a weak promoter [31], while in the cocarcinogenesis experiments referred to above, it is a tumor inhibitor. Only the two most powerful known tumor promoters, PMA and anthralin, showed both types of activity. These comparisons for representative compounds are

**Table VIII. Comparison of Tumor-Promoting and Cocarcinogenic Agents [43]**

| Compound | Tumor-Promoting Activity | Cocarcinogenic Activity |
|---|---|---|
| PMA | + | + |
| Anthralin | + | + |
| Phenol | + | - |
| Catechol | - | + |
| Pyrogallol | - | + |
| Pyrene | - | + |
| Fluoranthene | - | + |

shown in Table VIII. A detailed list comparing tumor-promoting and cocarcinogenic activities has been reported [43].

## SUMMARY AND CONCLUSIONS

From the studies described in this review, dealing primarily with mouse skin as the in vivo test system, it is clear that three types of cofactors exert effects in chemical carcinogenesis: promoters, cocarcinogens and inhibitors of tumorigenesis. The most extensively studied cofactors in terms of mode of action are the tumor promoters.

Tumor promoters of two major groups of chemicals are known; the phorbol esters which are of plant origin and the anthralin series of compounds which are all related to anthralin, a medicinal agent. Miscellaneous other weak promoters are known. A wide variety of biochemical effects of the phorbol esters have been observed in vivo and in vitro; only a few of these effects are expected to be relevant to tumor promotion. The primary site of interaction of PMA is at the plasma membrane, and this is a highly specific binding. The binding results in transmembrane signaling, which triggers this series of intracellular biochemical effects.

Cocarcinogens come in a wide variety of compound types, including long-chain aliphatic and aromatic hydrocarbons, phenols and others. These compounds are probably of great importance in environmental cancer and their mode(s) of action need further study.

The relationship between promoters and cocarcinogens has been studied to a limited extent. It is clear that not all promoters are cocarcinogens and vice versa. The wide variety of compound types involved suggests different mechanisms of action for the various structural types.

The tumor inhibitory agents offer new opportunities to study the mechanism of action of chemical carcinogens, such as the aromatic hydrocarbons and in addition, future research on tumor inhibition should lead to new approaches in cancer prevention.

## REFERENCES


1. Van Duuren, B. L. "Tumor-Promoting Agents in Two-Stage Carcinogenesis," *Prog. Exp. Tumor Res.* 11:31-68 (1969).
2. Hecker, E. "Isolation and Characterization of the Cocarcinogenic Principles from Croton Oil," *Meth. Canc. Res.* 6:439-484 (1971).
3. Van Duuren, B. L. "Tumor-Promoting and Cocarcinogenic Agents," in *Chemical Carcinogenesis,* C. E. Searle, Ed. (Washington, DC: American Chemical Society, 1976), p. 24.
4. Slaga, T. J., A. Sivak and R. K. Boutwell, Eds. *Carcinogenesis, Vol. 2: Mechanisms of Tumor Promotion and Cocarcinogenesis* (New York: Raven Press, 1978).
5. Stecher, P. G., Ed. *The Merck Index,* 8th ed. (Rahway, NJ: Merck & Co., 1968).
6. Haran, N., and I. Berenblum. "The Induction of the Initiating Phase of Skin Carcinogenesis in the Mouse by Oral Administration of Urethane (Ethyl Carbamate)," *Brit. J. Cancer* 10:57-60 (1956).
7. Van Duuren, B. L., A. Sivak, B. M. Goldschmidt, C. Katz and S. Melchionne. "Initiating Activity of Aromatic Hydrocarbons in Two-Stage Carcinogenesis," *J. Nat. Cancer Inst.* 44:1167-1173 (1970).
8. Van Duuren, B. L., A. Sivak, A. Segal, I. Seidman and C. Katz. "Dose-Response Studies with a Pure Tumor-Promoting Agent, Phorbol Myristate Acetate," *Cancer Res.* 33:2166-2172 (1973).
9. Boutwell, R. K. "The Function and Mechanism of Promoters of Carcinogenesis," *CRC Crit. Rev. Toxicol.* 2:419-443 (1974).
10. Flaschenträger, B. "Über den Giftstoff im Crotonöl, Versammlungsberichte," *Z. angew. Chem.* 43:1011-1012 (1930).
11. Flaschenträger, B., and F. V. Falkenhausen. "The Poisons in Croton Oil. II. The Constitution of Krotophorbolone," *Ann. Chem.* 514:252-260 (1934).
12. Flashcenträger, B., and G. Wigner. "The Poisons in Croton Oil. V. The Isolation of Croton Resin, Thin Oil and Phorbol from Croton Oil by Alcoholysis," *Helv. Chim. Acta* 25:569-581 (1942).
13. Pettersen, R. C., G. Ferguson, L. Crombie, M. L. Games and D. J. Pointer. "The Structure and Stereochemistry of Phorbol, Diterpene Parent of Co-carcinogens of Croton Oil," *Chem. Commun.* pp. 716-717 (1967).
14. Hoppe, W., F. Brandl, I. Strell, M. Röhrl, J. Gassmann, E. Hecker, H. Bartsch, G. Kreibich and C. V. Szczepanski. "Röntgenstrukturanalyse des Neophorbols," *Angew. Chem.* 79:824 (1967).
15. Van Duuren, B. L., S. -S. Tseng, A. Segal, A. C. Smith, S. Melchionne and I. Seidman. "Effects of Structural Changes on the Tumor-

Promoting Activity of Phorbol Myristate Acetate on Mouse Skin," *Cancer Res.* 39:2644-2646 (1979).

16. Baird, W. M., and R. K. Boutwell. "Tumor-Promoting Activity of Phorbol and Four Diesters of Phorbol in Mouse Skin," *Cancer Res.* 31:1074-1079 (1971).
17. Szczepanski, C. V., H. -U. Schairer, M. Gschwendt and E. Hecker. "Zur Chemie des Phorbols. III. Mono- und Diacetate des Phorbols," *Ann. Chem.* 705:199-210 (1967).
18. Baird, W. M., P. W. Melera and R. K. Boutwell. "Acrylamide Gel Electrophoresis Studies of the Incorporation of Cytidine-$^3$H into Mouse Skin RNA at Early Times After Treatment with Phorbol Esters," *Cancer Res.* 32:781-788 (1972).
19. Schairer, H. U., H. W. Thielmann, M. Gschwendt, G. Kreibich, R. Schmidt and E. Hecker. "Polybenzoate und -acetate des Phorbols und Phorbol-3-ols und funktionelle Derivate der Allygruppierung des Phorbols," *Z. Naturforsch. B.* 23:1430-1433 (1968).
20. Tseng, S. -S., B. L. Van Duuren and J. J. Solomon. "Synthesis of 4aα-Phorbol-9-myristate 9a-Acetate and Related Esters," *J. Org. Chem.* 42:3645-3649 (1977).
21. Segal, A., B. L. Van Duuren, U. Maté, J. J. Solomon, I. Seidman, A. Smith and S. Melchionne. "Tumor-Promoting Activity of 2,3-Dihydrophorbol Myristate Acetate and Phorbolol Myristate Acetate in Mouse Skin," *Cancer Res.* 38:921-925 (1978).
22. Segal, A., B. L. Van Duuren and U. Maté. "The Identification of Phorbolol Myristate Acetate as a New Metabolite of Phorbol Myristate Acetate in Mouse Skin," *Cancer Res.* 35:2154-2159 (1975).
23. Thielmann, H. W., and E. Hecker. "Beziehungen zwischen der Struktur von Phorbolderivaten und ihren entzündlichen und tumorpromovierenden Eigenschaften," in *Fortschritte der Krebsforschung. Molekularbiologie, Wachstum, Klinik* (Stuttgart: F. K. Schattauer Verlag, 1969) p. 171.
24. Hecker, E. "Co-carcinogene oder bedingt Krebsauslösende Faktoren," *Naturwissen.* 65:640-648 (1978).
25. Kinghorn, A. D. "Characterization of an Irritant 4-Deoxyphorbol Diester from *Euphorbia tirucalli*," *J. Nat. Prod.* 42:112-115 (1979).
26. Segal, A., C. Katz and B. L. Van Duuren. "Structure and Tumor-Promoting Activity of Anthralin (1,8-Dihydroxy-9-anthrone) and Related Compounds," *J. Med. Chem.* 14:1152-1154 (1971).
27. Van Duuren, B. L., A. Segal, S. -S. Tseng, G. M. Rusch, G. Loewengart, U. Maté, D. Roth, A. Smith, S. Melchionne and I. Seidman. "Structure and Tumor-Promoting Activity of Analogues of Anthralin (1,8-Dihydroxy-9-anthrone)," *J. Med. Chem.* 21:26-31 (1978).
28. Perutz, A. *Handbuch der Haut und Geschlechts Krankheiten. Vol. 5*, X. Jadassohn, Ed. (Berlin: Springer-Verlag, 1930), p. 155.
29. Van Duuren, B. L. "The Polynuclear Aromatic Hydrocarbons in Cigarette-Smoke Condensate," *J. Nat. Cancer Inst.* 21:623-630 (1958).
30. Orris, L., B. L. Van Duuren and A. I. Kosak. "The Carcinogenicity for Mouse Skin and the Aromatic Hydrocarbon Content of Cigarette-Smoke Condensates," *J. Nat. Cancer Inst.* 21:557-561 (1958).

31. Van Duuren, B. L., A. Sivak, L. Langseth, B. M. Goldschmidt and A. Segal. "Initiators and Promoters in Tobacco Carcinogenesis," *Nat. Cancer Inst. Monog.* No. 28, pp. 173-180 (1968).
32. Setälä, H. "Tumor-Promoting and Cocarcinogenic Effects of Some Non-ionic Lipophilic-Hydrophilic (Surface Active) Agents. An Experimental Study on Skin Tumors in Mice," *Acta Path. Microbiol. Scand. Suppl.* 115:7-91 (1956).
33. Saffiotti, U., and P. Shubik. "Studies on Promoting Action in Skin Carcinogenesis," *Nat. Cancer Inst. Monog.* No. 10, pp. 489-507 (1963).
34. Berenblum, I., and P. Shubik. "The Persistence of Latent Tumour Cells Induced in the Mouse's Skin by a Single Application of 9:10-Dimethyl-1:2-benzanthracene," *Brit. J. Cancer* 3:384-386 (1949).
35. Van Duuren, B. L., A. Sivak, C. Katz, I. Seidman and S. Melchionne. "The Effect of Aging and Interval Between Primary and Secondary Treatment in Two-Stage Carcinogenesis on Mouse Skin," *Cancer Res.* 35:502-505 (1975).
36. Van Duuren, B. L., A. C. Smith and S. M. Melchionne. "Effect of Aging in Two-Stage Carcinogenesis on Mouse Skin with Phorbol Myristate Acetate as Promoting Agent," *Cancer Res.* 38:865-866 (1978).
37. Palmes, E. D., L. Orris and N. Nelson. "Skin Irritation and Skin Tumour Production by Beta Propiolactone (BPL)," *Am. Ind. Hyg. Assoc. J.* 23:257-264 (1962).
38. Boutwell, R. K., and D. K. Bosch. "The Tumor-Promoting Action of Phenol and Related Compounds for Mouse Skin," *Cancer Res.* 19:413-424 (1959).
39. Marks, F., S. Bertsch and G. Fürstenberger. "Ornithine Decarboxylase Activity, Cell Proliferation, and Tumor Promotion in Mouse Epidermis *in Vivo*," *Cancer Res.* 39:4183-4188 (1979).
40. Raick, A. N., K. Thumm and B. R. Chivers. "Early Effects of 12-o-Tetradecanoyl-phorbol-13-acetate on the Incorporation of Tritiated Precursors into DNA and the Thickness of the Interfollicular Epidermis, and Their Relation to Tumor Promotion in Mouse Skin," *Cancer Res.* 32:1562-1568 (1972).
41. Frei, J. V., and P. Stephens. "The Correlation of Promotion of Tumour Growth and of Induction of Hyperplasia in Epidermal Two-Stage Carcinogenesis," *Brit. J. Cancer* 22:83-92 (1968).
42. Goerttler, K., H. Loehrke, J. Schweizer and B. Hesse. "Systemic Two-Stage Carcinogenesis in the Epithelium of the Forestomach of Mice Using 7,12-Dimethylbenz(a)anthracene as Initiator and the Phorbol Ester 12-o-Tetradecanoylphorbol-13-acetate as Promoter," *Cancer Res.* 39:1293-1297 (1979).
43. Van Duuren, B. L., and B. M. Goldschmidt. "Cocarcinogenic and Tumor-Promoting Agents in Tobacco Carcinogenesis," *J. Nat. Cancer Inst.* 56:1237-1242 (1976).
44. Baird, W. M., J. A. Sedgwick and R. K. Boutwell. "Effects of Phorbol and Four Diesters of Phorbol on the Incorporation of Tritiated Precursors into DNA, RNA, and Protein in Mouse Epidermis," *Cancer Res.* 31:1434-1439 (1971).

45. Raick, A. N. "Ultrastructural, Histological, and Biochemical Alterations Produced by 12-o-Tetradecanoyl-phorbol-13-acetate on Mouse Epidermis and Their Relevance to Skin Tumor Promotion," *Cancer Res.* 33:269-286 (1973).
46. Raick, A. N. "Cell Differentiation and Tumor-Promoting Action in Skin Carcinogenesis," *Cancer Res.* 34:2915-2925 (1974).
47. Sivak, A., and B. L. Van Duuren. "Phenotypic Expression of Transformation: Induction in a Cell Culture by a Phorbol Ester," *Science* 157:1443-1444 (1967).
48. Sivak, A., and B. L. Van Duuren. "RNA Synthesis Induction in Cell Culture by a Tumor Promoter," *Cancer Res.* 30:1203-1205 (1970).
49. Whitfield, J. F., J. P. MacManus and D. J. Gillan. "Calcium-Dependent Stimulation by a Phorbol Ester (PMA) of Thymic Lymphoblast DNA Synthesis and Proliferation," *J. Cell. Physiol.* 82:151-156 (1973).
50. Zucker, M. B., W. Troll and S. Belman. "The Tumor-Promoter Phorbol Ester (12-o-Tetradecanoyl-phorbol-13-acetate), a Potent Aggregating Agent for Blood Platelets," *J. Cell Biol.* 60:325-336 (1974).
51. Mondal, S., D. W. Brankow and C. Heidelberger. "Two-Stage Chemical Oncogenesis in Cultures of C3H/10T½ Cells," *Cancer Res.* 36:2254-2260 (1976).
52. Yamasaki, H., E. Fibach, U. Nudel, I. B. Weinstein, R. A. Rifkind and P. A. Marks. "Tumor Promoters Inhibit Spontaneous and Induced Differentiation of Murine Erythroleukemia Cells in Culture," *Proc. Nat. Acad. Sci., U.S.* 74:3451:3455 (1977).
53. Ishii, D. N., E. Fibach, H. Yamasaki and I. B. Weinstein. "Tumor Promoters Inhibit Morphological Differentiation in Cultured Mouse Neuroblastoma Cells," *Science* 200:556-559 (1979).
54. Sivak, A., F. Ray and B. L. Van Duuren. "Phorbol Ester Tumor-Promoting Agents and Membrane Stability," *Cancer Res.* 29:624-630 (1969).
55. Fisher, P. B., M. Flamm, D. Schachter and I. B. Weinstein. "Tumor Promoters Induce Membrane Changes Detected by Fluorescence Polarization," *Biochem. Biophys. Res. Commun.* 86:1063-1068 (1979).
56. Mufson, R. A., P. B. Fisher and I. B. Weinstein. "Effects of Phorbol Ester Tumor Promoters on the Expression of Melanogenesis in B-16 Melanoma Cells," *Cancer Res.* 39:3915-3919 (1979).
57. Lee, L. -S., and I. B. Weinstein. "Tumor-Promoting Phorbol Esters Inhibit Binding of Epidermal Growth Factor to Cellular Receptors," *Science* 202:313-315 (1978).
58. Lee, L. -S., and I. B. Weinstein. "Mechanism of Tumor Promoter Inhibition of Cellular Binding of Epidermal Growth Factor," *Proc. Nat. Acad. Sci., U.S.* 76:5168-5172 (1979).
59. Brown, K. D., P. Dicker and E. Rozengurt. "Inhibition of Epidermal Growth Factor Binding to Surface Receptors by Tumor Promoters," *Biochem. Biophys. Res. Commun.* 86:1037-1043 (1979).
60. Yuspa, S. H., T. Ben., E. Patterson, D. Michael, K. Elgjo and H. Hennings. "Stimulated DNA Synthesis in Mouse Epidermal Cell Cultures Treated with 12-O-Tetradecanoylphorbol-13-acetate," *Cancer Res.* 36:4062-4068 (1976).

61. O'Brien, T. G., R. C. Simsiman and R. K. Boutwell. "Induction of Polyamine Biosynthetic Enzymes in Mouse Epidermis by Tumor Promoting Agents," *Cancer Res.* 35:1662-1670 (1975).
62. Yuspa, S. H., U. Lichti, T. Ben, E. Patterson, H. Hennings, T. Slaga, N. Colburn and W. Kelsey. "Phorbol Esters Stimulate DNA Synthesis and Ornithine Decarboxylase Activity in Mouse Epidermal Cell Cultures," *Nature* 262:402-404 (1976).
63. Weissman, G., W. Troll, B. L. Van Duuren and G. Sessa. "A New Action of Tumor-Promoting Agents: Lysis of Cell and Intracellular Membranes," *J. Clin. Invest.* 46:1131 (1967).
64. Weissmann, G., W. Troll, B. L. Van Duuren and G. Sessa. "Studies on Lysosomes. X. Effects of Tumor-Promoting Agents Upon Biological and Artificial Membrane Systems," *Biochem. Pharmacol.* 17:2421-2434 (1968).
65. Sivak, A., B. T. Mossman and B. L. Van Duuren. "Activation of Cell Membrane Enzymes in the Stimulation of Cell Division," *Biochem. Biophys. Res. Comm.* 46:605-609 (1972).
66. Gaudin, D., R. S. Gregg and K. L. Yielding. "DNA Repair Inhibition: A Possible Mechanism of Action of Cocarcinogens," *Biochem. Biophys. Res. Commun.* 45:630-636 (1971).
67. Gaudin, D., R. S. Gregg and K. L. Yielding. "Inhibition of DNA Repair by Carcinogens," *Biochem. Biophys. Res. Commun.* 48:945-949 (1972).
68. Teebor, G. W., N. J. Duker, S. A. Ruacan and K. T. Zachary. "Inhibition of Thymine Dimer Excision by the Phorbol Ester, Phorbol Myristate Acetate," *Biochem. Biophys. Res. Commun.* 50:66-70 (1973).
69. Raineri, R., R. C. Simsiman and R. K. Boutwell. "Stimulation of the Phosphorylation of Mouse Epidermal Histones by Tumor-Promoting Agents," *Cancer Res.* 33:134-139 (1973).
70. Raineri, R., R. C. Simsiman and R. K. Boutwell. "Stimulation of the Synthesis of Mouse Epidermal Histones by Tumor-Promoting Agents," *Cancer Res.* 37:4584-4589 (1977).
71. Van Duuren, B. L., S. Banerjee and G. Witz. "Fluorescence Studies on the Interaction of the Tumor Promoter Phorbol Myristate Acetate and Related Compounds with Rat Liver Plasma Membranes," *Chem.-Biol. Interact.* 15:233-246 (1976).
72. Van Duuren, B. L., G. Witz and B. M. Goldschmidt. "Structure-Activity Relationships of Tumor Promoters and Cocarcinogens and Interaction of Phorbol Myristate Acetate and Related Esters with Plasma Membranes," in *Carcinogenesis, Vol. 2: Mechanisms of Tumor Promotion and Cocarcinogenesis,* T. J. Slaga, A. Sivak, and R. K. Boutwell, Eds. (New York: Raven Press, 1978), p. 491.
73. Weinstein, I. B., H. Yamasaki, M. Wigler, L. -S. Lee, P. B. Fisher, A. Jeffrey and D. Grunberger. "Molecular and Cellular Events Associated with the Action of Initiating Carcinogens and Tumor Promoters," in *Carcinogens: Identification and Mechanisms of Action,* A. C. Griffin and C. R. Shaw, Eds. (New York: Raven Press, 1979), p. 399.
74. Van Duuren, B. L. "Carcinogenicity and Metabolism of Some Halogenated Olefinic and Aliphatic Hydrocarbons," in *Banbury Report 5: Ethylene Dichloride, A Potential Health Risk?* B. Ames, P. Infante

and R. Reitz, Eds. (Cold Spring Harbor, NY: Banbury Center, Cold Spring Harbor Laboratory, 1980), p. 185.

75. Van Duuren, B. L., B. M. Goldschmidt, G. Loewengart, A. C. Smith, S. Melchionne, I. Seidman and D. Roth. "Carcinogenicity of Halogenated Olefinic and Aliphatic Hydrocarbons in Mice," *J. Nat. Cancer Inst.* 63:1433-1439 (1979).

76. U.S. Public Health Service. "Bioassay of Allyl Chloride for Possible Carcinogenicity," NCI-CG-TR-73. DHEW Publication No. (NIH) 78-1323, U.S. Government Printing Office (1978).

77. U.S. Public Health Service. "Bioassay of Dibromochloropropane for Possible Carcinogenicity," NCI-CG-TR-28. DHEW Publication No. (NIH) 78-828, U.S. Government Printing Office (1978).

78. Maltoni, C. "Recent Findings on the Carcinogenicity of Chlorinated Olefins," *Environ. Health Persp.* 21:1-5 (1977).

79. Van Duuren, B. L., B. M. Goldschmidt, C. Katz, I. Seidman and J. S. Paul. "Carcinogenic Activity of Alkylating Agents," *J. Nat. Cancer Inst.* 53:695-700 (1974).

80. U.S. Public Health Service. "Epichlorohydrin Nasal Cancer by Inhalation in Rats. Memorandum from Center for Disease Control," U.S. Government Printing Office (1977).

81. Berenblum, I. "The Cocarcinogenic Action of Croton Resin," *Cancer Res.* 1:44-47 (1941).

82. Van Duuren, B. L., and W. Troll. Unpublished data.

# CHAPTER 18

# THE IMPORTANCE OF METABOLISM IN CARCINOGENESIS

**David B. Clayson**

Eppley Institute for Research in Cancer
University of Nebraska Medical Center
Omaha, Nebraska

## INTRODUCTION: DEFINITION OF A CARCINOGEN

There is a growing body of opinion that perhaps as much as 90% of human cancer is associated with environmental factors [1, 2]. However, there is firm evidence for only a relatively small proportion of human cancer being caused by specific synthetic or naturally occurring chemicals as a result of occupation, medical treatment or environmental exposure (Table I) [3]. An agent which leads to an increase in cancer incidence in a human or animal population is known as a carcinogen [4, 5]. Such definitions as are presently available do not recognize that different carcinogens may work through different mechanisms of action and, therefore, the term "carcinogen" is an umbrella term for all agents having this effect. This lack of specificity about how cancer is induced is a major reason for many present difficulties with carcinogens and carcinogen regulation.

This chapter will mainly be concerned with chemicals that induce cancer, and also interact with and alter the cell genome leading to the production of microbial or mammalian cell mutation, DNA repair, sister chromatid exchanges and other genotoxic effects. At this time, it is imprudent to assume that carcinogenesis is necessarily a mutagenic process, although evidence suggesting that carcinogenesis has a large genetic component is becoming more convincing because (1) patients with DNA repair deficiency, that is, *Xero-*

**Table I. Examples of Agents Shown to Induce Cancer in Humans**

| | Site |
|---|---|
| Habit | |
| Cigarette Smoking | Lung, etc. |
| Occupation | |
| Soots, Tars, Pitches | Skin, Lung |
| 2-Naphthylamine, 4-Aminobiphenyl | Bladder |
| Asbestos | Lung, Pleura |
| Vinyl Chloride Monomer | Liver |
| Drugs | |
| Immunosuppressants | Reticulum Cell Sarcoma |
| Analgesics (Phenacetin) | Renal Pelvis |
| Chlornaphazin | Bladder |
| Diethylstilbestrol | Vagina |
| Food Contaminants | |
| Aflatoxin $B_1$ | Liver |

*derma pigmentosum*, have a high rate of cancer, (2) of the close parallel between chemicals that, after any necessary metabolism, induce mutation and those that induce cancer, and (3) a genetic change is a plausible way of explaining the apparently irreversible nature of the change from normal to cancer cells.

## MECHANISMS OF GENOTOXIC CARCINOGENIC ACTION

The mode of action of genotoxic carcinogens can very simplistically be divided into three broad phases: metabolic activation, tissue interaction and tumor development (Figure 1). In the first phase, the genotoxic carcinogen is converted either spontaneously, as in the case of the biological alkylating agents (e. g., oxirans, nitrogen mustards, or alkylalkanesulfonates) or enzymatically to an electron deficient, highly reactive species, or electrophile [8,9]. Such an electrophile, in the second phase, interacts avidly with electron-rich groups in the tissues. Electrophiles, therefore, react with cellular macromolecules, such as DNA, RNA or protein, as well as with small molecules [8, 9]. The consequences of such an interaction have been studied most closely with DNA, which may either undergo repair processes to remove the chemically induced lesions, or may replicate before repair is complete to "lock in" genetic damage (Figure 2). In the latter case, populations of altered cells may ensue, among which are the tumor progenitor cells. The third phase of carcinogenesis is the development of the tumor progenitor cells to frank clinical neoplasia.

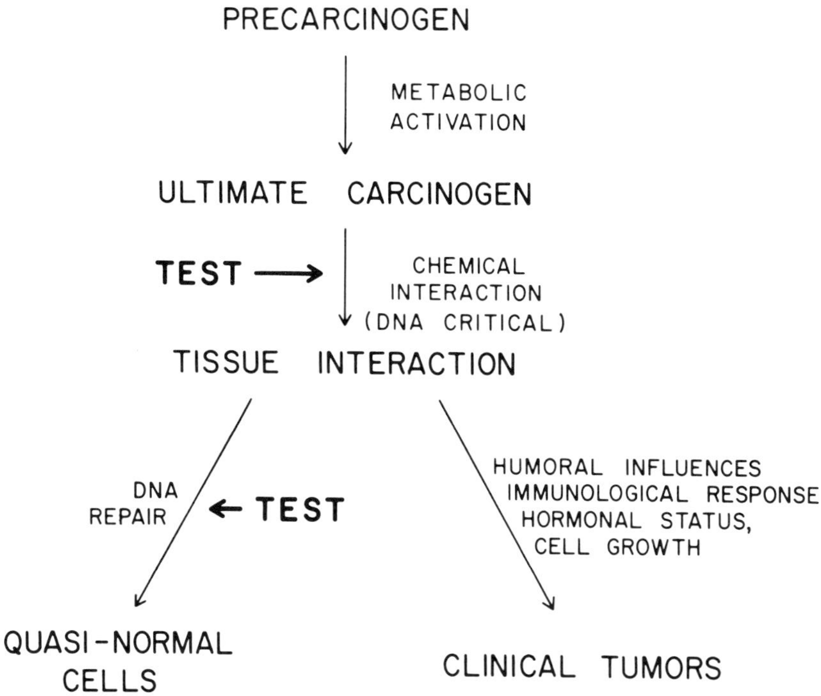


**Figure 1.** The mechanism of chemical carcinogenesis. TEST shows critical events in chemical carcinogenesis which have led to short-term prescreening tests for carcinogens.

This model for carcinogenesis permits the understanding of the need to define a variety of modes of action for chemical carcinogens. Each of us is exposed from before birth to death to low levels of a variety of naturally occurring carcinogens, such as sunlight and aflatoxin. It would, therefore, be surprising if our tissues did not contain some tumor progenitor cells. Agents which favor the development of tumor progenitor cells to frank clinical cancer, will, therefore, appear to induce cancer and be classified as carcinogens. Estrogens, for example, may stimulate the growth of mammary tumors induced by viruses [10] or chemicals [11, 12] and, therefore, be classified as carcinogens. Such tumor-enhancing agents may or may not require metabolism to their active form or to detoxified products, but will not be considered further here.

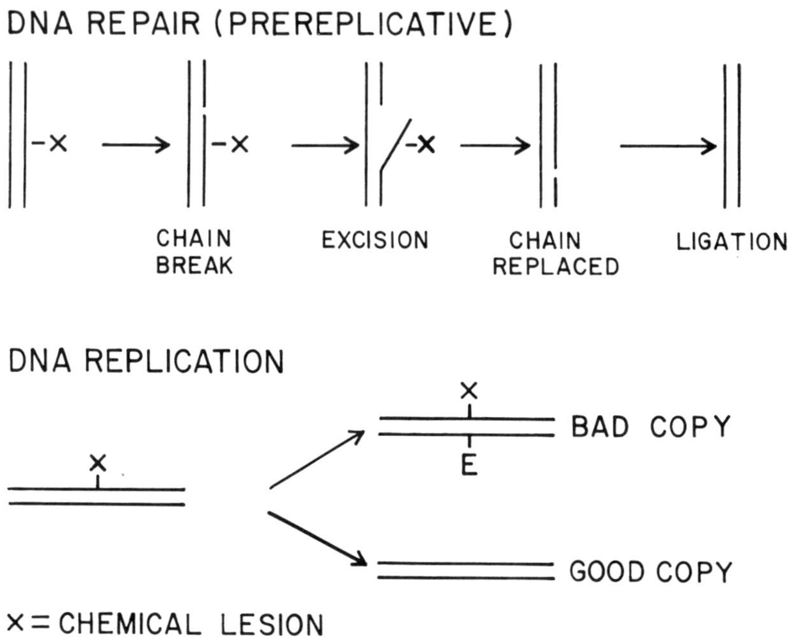


**Figure 2.** Effect of chemical lesion in DNA (X) in DNA repair and replication. E indicates that an error has been induced in one DNA strand.

## EVIDENCE FOR THE METABOLIC ACTIVATION OF GENOTOXIC CARCINOGENS

Consideration of earlier data on tumors induced by aromatic amines, such as 2-N-fluorenylacetamide (2-FAA), 2-naphthylamine, or 4-aminobiphenyl (Table II) suggested that tumors were often located on the routes of excretion from the body, such as the liver, urinary tract, intestine, rat ear duct or mammary gland [13]. With aromatic amines, tumors are not commonly induced in the oral cavity or stomach after feeding, nor at the injection site after injection (Figure 3). This possibly indicates that a derivative of the carcinogen formed in the body, a metabolite, was the ultimate carcinogen. The first studies to adduce firm evidence in support of this concept were those of the Millers and their co-workers [14,15]. A new metabolite of 2-FAA was isolated and shown to be N-hydroxy-2-FAA (Figure 4). This metabolite proved to be somewhat more carcinogenic than 2-FAA, especially in weanling rats; it was not found in guinea pits, which are apparently not susceptible to 2-FAA carcinogenicity, although this species is

**Table II. Species Response to Aromatic Amine Carcinogens**

| Species | 2-Naphthylamine | 4-Aminobiphenyl | 2-AAF |
|---|---|---|---|
| Humans | Bladder | Bladder | ? |
| Dog | Bladder | Bladder | Liver, Bladder |
| Monkey | Bladder | ? | None |
| Rabbit | None | Bladder | Bladder, Ureter |
| Hamster | Bladder | None | Liver |
| Rat | Bladder | Breast | Liver, Breast, etc. |
| Mouse | Liver | Liver | Liver, etc. |

affected by N-hydroxy-2-FAA. This, and other evidence, led the Millers to regard it as the first stage in the metabolic activation of 2-FAA. It could not, however, be regarded as the ultimate carcinogen, because 2-FAA interacts with nucleic acids and proteins in the living animal, whereas in the test tube, there was no significant level of reaction between N-hydroxy-2-FAA and DNA or RNA. An observation that *O*-acylated derivatives of N-OH-FAA were highly reactive and carcinogenic led this group to study the *O*-sulfate of N-hydroxy-2-FAA as the possible ultimate carcinogen. The enzyme sulfotransferase, in rat liver cytosol, was shown to be able to transfer sulfate from an activated source, phosphoadenosine phosphosulfate, to N-hydroxy-2-FAA in the presence of the necessary cofactors. This enzyme had a greater activity in male than in female rate liver, corresponding to the greater susceptibility of the former to 2-FAA-induced hepatocarcinogenesis. There was also a parallelism between the activities of this enzyme in the liver of various species and their susceptibility to 2-FAA-induced hepatocarcinogenesis [16] (Table III). The sulfate ester of 2-FAA is extremely unstable; the sulfate ion acts as a leaving group, thus forming a nitrenium ion that is a potent electrophile. The instability of the sulfate ester makes it extremely difficult to isolate it from animal tissues; it also makes it very difficult to prove satisfactorily that it is a carcinogen. Evidence that it or a related entity is, in fact, produced, is supplied by chemical studies that show DNA or RNA from 2-FAA or N-hydroxy-2-FAA-treated rat liver contain the product of interaction of the nitrenium ion at the 8-position of guanine [17,18]. Additional indirect evidence in support of sulfate ester formation was obtained by Weisburger et al. who demonstrated that the reason why acetanilide, in a large excess, inhibited N-hydroxy-2-FAA carcinogenesis in the rat liver was that *p*-hydroxyacetanilide conjugated with sulfate and reduced the effective concentration of active sulfate ions sufficiently to inhibit N-hydroxy-2-FAA activation. This inhibition was reversed by feeding a higher level of sulfate in the diet [19].

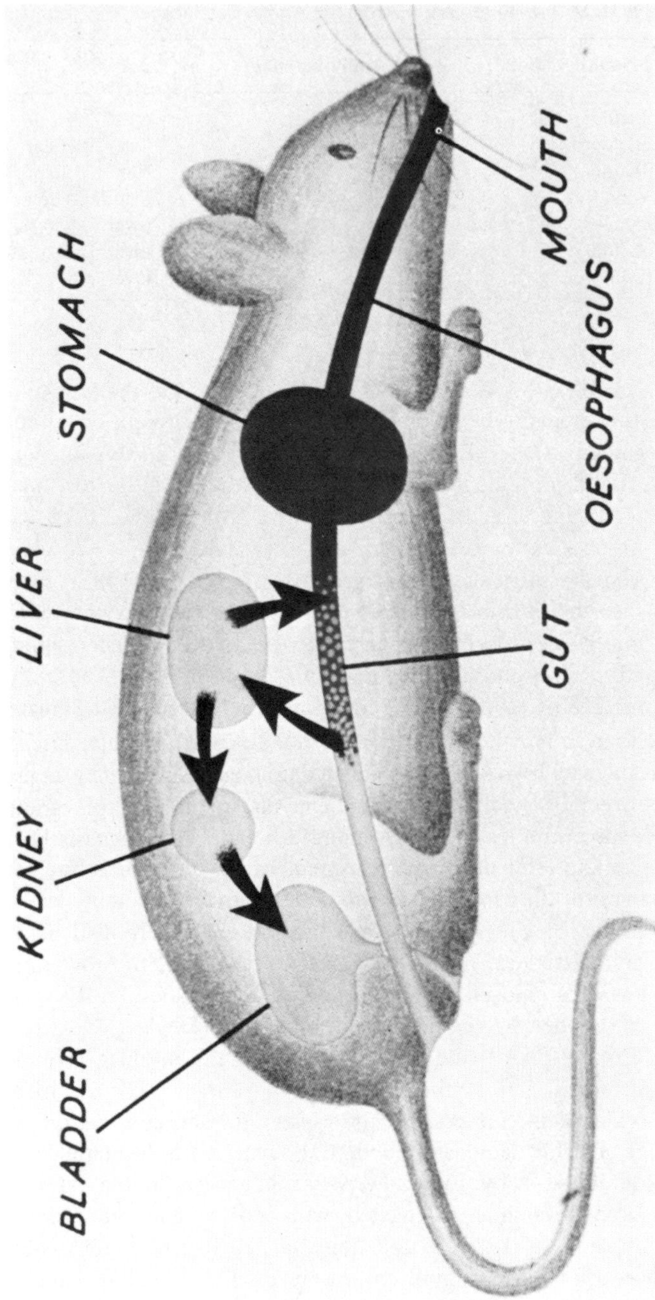


**Figure 3.** After administration of aromatic amines, tumors are often located on routes of excretion rather than at the site of administration. Dark areas (mouth, esophagus) are exposed to highest levels of carcinogen. Light areas (liver, kidney, guts, bladder) are exposed to metabolites and develop tumors.

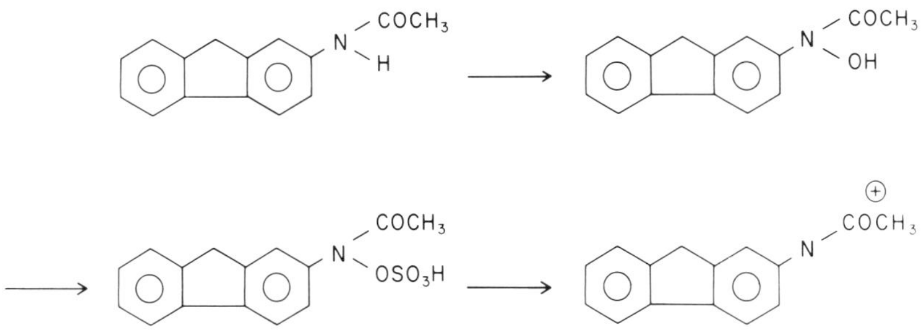

**Figure 4.** Metabolic activation of 2-fluorenylacetamide.

**Table III. Sulfotransferase Levels in Liver of Various Species [16]**

| Species | Sex | Enzyme Level | Hepatocarcinogenicity |
|---|---|---|---|
| Rat | M | 23 | +++ |
| Rat | F | 4 | + |
| Mouse | M | $<0.5$ | + |
| Hamster | M | $<0.5$ | + |
| Guinea Pig | M | $<0.3$ | - |

Thus in rat liver, it appears that 2-FAA is activated by N-hydroxylation followed by sulfate formation and the production of a nitrenium ion. Such a model does not apply to all tissues in which 2-FAA induces tumors. Thus, the rat ear duct and the rat mammary gland do not contain detectable levels of sulfotransferase, although 2-FAA induces tumors at these sites [20]. It now appears that although N-hydroxylation is the key to the metabolic activation of 2-FAA and other carcinogenic aromatic amines, intermediates other than the sulfate ester are involved. These intermediates are each capable of decomposing to a nitrenium ion [21, 22].

Other relatively stable carcinogens are likewise activated in the animal to produce ultimate carcinogens that lead to strongly electrophilic intermediates (Figure 5). Thus, for example, carcinogenic polycyclic aromatic hydrocarbons lead to bay-region diolepoxides by a three-stage process of epoxidation, hydrolysis to the dihydrodiol and epoxidation of the isolated double bond [23, 24]. Aflatoxin $B_1$ is converted to the 2, 3-oxiran [25, 26], nitrosamines are hydroxylated at the alpha position to the nitroso group [27, 28], while vinyl chloride is converted to the oxiran, which may act

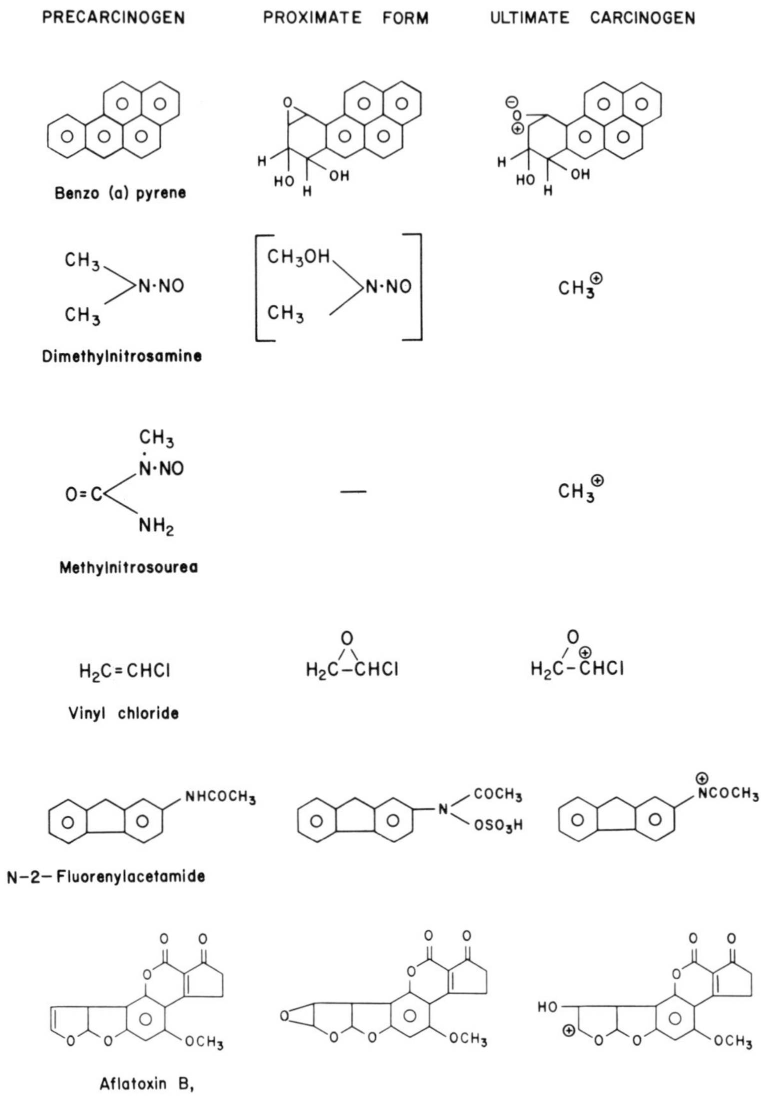


**Figure 5.** Active metabolites of selected carcinogens.

directly or as the derived aldehyde [29, 30]. Thus, metabolic activation has provided a unifying concept to link together many of the diverse structures that behave as genotoxic chemical carcinogens (Figure 5).

## SHORT-TERM PRESCREENING TESTS

The practical importance of these concepts of metabolic activation is clearly illustrated in the development of the short-term prescreening tests for carcinogens. It may be argued that if the critical events in the chemical induction of cancer can be identified, it may be possible to design quicker and less expensive tests for carcinogenicity. If, for example, interaction with specific regions in DNA is critical, mutation might be linked with carcinogenesis. In 1955, Burdette [31] wrote a review clearly demonstrating that mutagenicity and carcinogenicity were seldom the property of the same chemical agents; only the directly acting biological alkylating agents shared these properties. Ames and co-workers [32, 33] developed histidine-requiring mutants of *Salmonella typhimurium* as prescreening tools for carcinogens. His success depended almost entirely on the fact that a metabolizing system was introduced [34]. The strains of *S typhimurium* he developed do not contain the capability to activate metabolically many classes of carcinogens; the addition of the 9000-g supernatant from rat liver cells and the necessary cofactors enabled Ames to claim an 80–90% correlation between mutagenesis and carcinogenesis.

Getting the answer wrong in 1 of 5 or 1 of 10 cases is not particularly satisfactory. One difficulty may well be that preparation of the liver homogenate leads to changes in metabolic capability. Thus, enzymes in the endoplasmic reticulum may be dissociated from each other, and the cellular mechanisms that control the level of cofactors available in each cellular compartment may be destroyed. The technique introduced by Huberman and co-workers [35, 36] involves the growth of mutatable mammalian cells (V79 cells) on a feeder layer of primary explants of mammalian cells from a chosen tissue. Primary explants are used to preserve normal in vivo metabolism. With liver cells [36] as the feeder layer, it has been possible to differentiate between liver carcinogens and nonliver carcinogens. Benzo[a]pyrene gives a positive result when connective tissue cells (fibroblasts) are used as a feeder cell layer [37], but not when liver cells are used. Aflatoxin B1 shows the opposite activities. Thus, these results agree with the tissue specificity of the two carcinogens. This approach clearly has great potential. Langenbach [36] is exploiting it to study the capability of cells from a variety of other tissues, such as lung and bladder, to activate carcinogens. This approach promises a method for determining the capability of human cells to metabolically activate carcinogens, using a relatively small sample of cells. This approach may enable us to determine whether man, like the guinea pig, is deficient in the capability to metabolize specific classes of carcinogens to their ultimate carcinogenic forms.

## ENZYME INDUCTION, COFACTORS AND POISONS

The metabolism of a foreign compound involves activating and detoxifying reactions occurring simultaneously. Therefore, a change in the activity of a particular enzyme or enzymes may affect the proportion of a carcinogen that is converted to an electrophile and the resulting amount of the electrophile that reaches the critical target. Enzyme cofactors, enzyme poisons and enzyme induction may each alter the proportion of a carinogen that is activated.

Riboflavin in the diet is inhibitory to the hepatocarcinogenic action of 4-dimethylaminoazobenzene [38]. This was shown to be caused by riboflavin being an essential cofactor for the enzyme, N-demethylase, which converts the dye into an inactive form, aminoazobenzene [39]. This is but one example of the profound influence that nutritional variables have on carcinogenic activity, a field which has recently been reviewed [40-43].

Enzyme poisons have not been so intensively studied. Berry et al. [44] demonstrated that the ability of 3-methylcholanthrene (3-MC) to initiate skin tumors was considerably enhanced by 1,1,1-trichloropropene oxide (TCPO), an agent that inhibits epoxide hydratase. TCPO may prevent epoxide derivatives of 3-MC from being detoxified by hydrolysis to the dihydrodiol and may, therefore, increase its carcinogenic potential. However, oxirans are often carcinogens in their own right [45], so it is not possible to be convinced completely that enhancement of tumor yield occurs by metabolic rather than direct cocarcinogenic interaction of these two chemicals (Table IV).

**Table IV. Initiation-Promotion Studies: Effect of TCPO on 3-MC Initiation of Mouse Skin [44]**

| | No. Skin Tumors[a] (%) | Papilloma[b] Mouse |
|---|---|---|
| 3-MC + croton oil | 60 | 1.6 |
| 3-MC + TCPO + croton oil | 70 | 2.6 |

[a]At 28 weeks.
[b]Figures estimated from charts.

The discovery of enzyme induction is one of the most important contributions of carcinogenesis research to biochemistry. In 1952, Richardson et al. [45] reported that cofeeding 3-MC and 3′-methyl-4-dimethylaminoazobenzene to rats strongly inhibited liver cell carcinomas induced by the latter compound alone (Table V). Conney et al. [46] showed that feeding 3-MC greatly increased the levels of the detoxifying enzymes azoreductase and N-demethylase, thus explaining the inhibition of carcinogenicity. They went on to demonstrate that this induction of specific enzymes was not limited to these detoxifying enzymes and that a wide range of chemicals, carcinogens and noncarcinogens had this property [47]. Such agents included polycyclic hydrocarbons, their quinones, chlorocarbons, polychlorinated aromatics and barbituates. 3-MC, Aroclor® and phenobarbital are now in common use to stimulate the metabolizing enzymes in laboratory rodents. So far as carcinogenesis is concerned, enzyme induction during tumor initiation generally appears to have a protective effect on the host [48, 49], but as Wattenberg [50] has recently commented, knowledge of the mechanisms of carcinogen activation and cellular interaction are still so incomplete as to make their immediate application to the prevention of human cancer imprudent.

**Table V. - Inhibition of Liver Tumor Induction by 3′-Methyl-4-Dimethylamino Azobenzene by Dietary 3-MC [45]**

| Treatment | No. of Rats | % of Liver Tumors (Malignant) |
|---|---|---|
| 3′-MeDAB (0.6%) | 54 | 98 |
| 3′-MeDAB + 3-MC (0.0067%) | 20 | 0 |

An example from another area will perhaps make some of the difficulties clearer. A very low ("zero") protein diet inhibits the toxic effects of dimethylnitrosamine in liver. The overall effect of this diet is to permit administration of a higher dose of the carcinogen and thus, to enhance the yield of tumors of the kidney, which is not protected by this regimen [51-53]. At this stage, we are painfully ignorant of the metabolic capabilities of most tissues other than the liver, lung and kidney.

Another difficulty is that single chemicals may not only be enzyme inducers. Commercially important antioxidants (e.g., BHT and BHA) exhibit more protective action than their power of enzyme induction would indicate. It has been suggested that they also act as free radical scavengers and may, therefore, lower the effective levels of electrophiles at critical sites in the tissues. However, the two highly beneficial properties must be counter balanced by the fact that recent reports suggest that certain of these agents may enhance the yield of lung tumors in mice [54].

## AGE OF ANIMAL AND METABOLIC ACTIVATION

It is well established that the stage of development and the age of an animal may have a profound effect on its capability to metabolize carcinogens. In the rat, for example, the fetal liver is largely a hemopoietic organ responsible for furnishing the animal with blood cells. In the first five or so days after birth, the hemopoietic element regresses and normal parenchymal cells are formed. This is reflected by the fact that the fetal liver is deficient in metabolic capability, which builds up in early independent life.

Such changes affect the response of the fetus to different types of carcinogens. Thus, as shown by Ivankovic and Druckrey [55], the biological alkylating agent ethylnitrosourea, which requires no metabolic activation, affects the rat fetus about 50 times as strongly as it does the adult animal. That is, the developing nervous system is more responsive to the carcinogenic stimulus than is the fully developed adult tissue. This particular experiment has led to the belief that the fetus is exquisitely sensitive to carcinogens. Yet, Althoff and co-workers failed to demonstrate any marked fetal sensitivity in hamsters to a series of nitrosamines which were administered to their mothers during gestation [56-58]. The nitrosamines penetrate the fetus, but the necessary enzymes for metabolic activation are probably absent, so tumors do not develop.

One aspect of this problem does not yet appear to have received the prominence it deserves. It has been known for many years that if a neonatal female rodent is given a large dose of testosterone at about the time of birth, she behaves biologically and biochemically as if she were a male for the remainder of her life [59]. That is to say, the genetically female animal is "imprinted" with male characteristics. Lucier has shown that similarly treating a rodent with a suitable chemical, such as a tetrachlorobiphenyl or a polycyclic aromatic hydrocarbon, also leads to imprinting. Enzyme levels in the treated animal are permanently different from those in untreated animals [60-62] (Table VI).

A number of important questions are raised by this work. First, is such a phenomenon confined to rodents, which seems unlikely, or is it shared by other species, such as man? Second, if imprinting occurs in man, how much of the differences that are habitually assigned to heterozygosity are, in fact, caused by imprinting by unsuspected toxic agents during early life. Third, is protection of the human race possible; that is, do such exposures obey normal dose-response relationships and are there thresholds? Fourth,

**Table VI. Effect of TCDD (3 μg/kg Given on Day 5 of Gestation) on Benzo[a]pyrene Hydrolase Activity in Fetal Liver [60]**

| Day Relative to Birth | Untreated | TCDD-Treated |
|---|---|---|
| -16 | | TCDD given |
| -1 | 0.073 | 1.131 |
| +1 | 0.075 | 0.859 |
| +8 | 0.184 | 1.324 |

how does such imprinting affect carcinogenesis and other forms of toxicity later in life? These are major questions and deserve intensive study.

## METABOLIC THRESHOLDS

One of the greatest difficulties in the regulation of carcinogens is the problem of demonstrating experimentally whether or not there is a threshold dose value for any carcinogen, below which cancer will not be induced. Experimentation to decide this point directly is impractical because of the huge number of animals needed to establish that a specific dose of carcinogen induces a very low tumor incidence. The National Center for Toxicological Research has recently established the dose of 2-FAA that induces liver and bladder tumors in 1% of a mouse population. Even this relatively substantial tumor incidence required over 20,000 animals for its evaluation [63].

Gehring et al. [64] suggested that dose-response curves for carcinogens may show discontinuities, because there are such discontinuities in the dose response curve for critical events in carcinogenesis. This interesting concept may be illustrated in the case of metabolic activation. Metabolizing enzymes may become saturated with substrate and, as a result, the plasma concentration of the substrate will remain longer at an elevated level. In consequence, other enzymes capable of metabolizing the substrate, which do not have as high an affinity for it, become more prominent and the overall metabolic pattern will change. If the lower-affinity enzyme produces a carcinogenically active metabolite, the result will be that at low substrate levels, little, if any, active metabolite will be produced; at high levels, a disproportionate amount will occur, which, as metabolic activation is critical in carcinogenesis, will lead to a real or apparent threshold in the carcinogenesis dose-response curve. Great caution should, however, be exercised in using this concept in carcinogen regulation. The balance of enzymes, and possibly their relative affinity for a given substrate, may vary even from tissue to tissue as well as from species to species. At our present level of knowledge, this makes difficult transspecies extrapolation of such potential threshold values to man. Furthermore, if the lower-affinity enzyme is activating, the carcinogen will become proportionally less effective at high dose levels.

## CONCLUSION

The metabolic activation of genotoxic carcinogens other than the direct biological alkylating agents is a critical and necessary event in carcinogenesis. It is at this time perhaps the best understood aspect of chemical carcinogensis. An understanding of metabolic activation is critical to the successful development of our present generation of short-term prescreening tests for carcinogens. Metabolic activation helps the understanding of why specific chemicals and other factors, such as enzyme inducers, affect the rate of tumor formation. It also partly explains why the sensitivity of the mammalian organism to specific carcinogens differs at different stages of development. In the future, it may be demonstrated that "imprinted" changes in the pattern of metabolizing enzymes explain some of the immense variation in susceptibility of the human population to carcinogens and other toxic agents. Finally, if true, the concept of metabolic thresholds may lead to scientifically sensible regulation of specific environmental carcinogens.

## REFERENCES

1. Higginson, J. "Geographical Pathology in Environmental Carcinogenesis," Proceedings of the Eleventh Canadian Cancer Research Conference, Toronto, Canada (1976), pp. 48-57.
2. Wynder, E. L., and G. B. Gori. "Guest Editorial: Contributions of the Environment to Cancer Incidence: An Epidemiologic Exercise," *J. Nat. Cancer Inst.* 58:825-831 (1977).
3. Fraumeni, J. F., Ed. *Persons at High Risk of Cancer: An Approach to Cancer Epidemiology and Control.* (New York: Academic Press, Inc., 1975), pp. xvii, 544.
4. Clayson, D. B. *Chemical Carcinogenesis* (London: J&A Churchill, 1962).
5. "General Criteria for Assessing the Evidence for Carcinogenicity of Chemical Substances: Report of the Subcommittee on Environmental Carcinogenesis, National Cancer Advisory Board," *J. Nat. Cancer Institute* 58:461-463 (1977).
6. Reed, W. H., E. Boder and M. Gardner. "Congenital and Genetic Skin Disorders with Tumor Formation," *Birth Defects* 10:265-284 (1974).

7. Ames, B. N. "Environmental Chemicals Causing Cancer and Genetic Birth Defects: Developing a Strategy for Minimizing Human Exposure," California Policy Seminar (1977) pp. 1-37.
8. Miller, J. A. "Carcinogenesis by Chemicals: An Overview," *Cancer Res.* 30:559-576 (1970).
9. Miller, E. C., and J. A. Miller "The Metabolism of Chemical Carcinogens to Reactive Electrophiles and Their Possible Mechanisms of Action in Carcinogenesis," in *Chemical Carcinogens,* C. E. Searle, Ed. ACS Monograph No. 173, (Washington, DC: American Chemical Society, 1976), pp. 737-762.
10. Gardner, W. U., T. P. Dougherty and W. L. Williams. "Lymphoid Tumors in Mice Receiving Steroid Hormones," *Cancer Res.* 4:73-87 (1944).
11. Strong, L. C., and G. M. Smith. "The Local Induction of Carcinoma of the Mammary Gland by Methylcholanthrene," *Yale J. Biol. Med.* 11: 589-592 (1939).
12. Bonser, G. M., and J. W. Orr. "The Morphology of 160 Tumors Induced by Carcinogenic Hydrocarbons on the Subcutaneous Tissues of Mice," *J. Pathol. Bacteriol.* 49:171-183 (1939).
13. Clayson, D. B. "A Working Hypothesis for the Mode of Carcinogenesis of Aromatic Amines," *Brit. J. Cancer* 7:40-61 (1953).
14. Cramer, J. W., J. A. Miller and E. C. Miller. "N-Hydroxylation: A New Metabolic Reaction Observed in the Rat with the Carcinogen, 2-Acetylaminofluorene," *J. Biol. Chem.* 235:885-888 (1960).
15. Miller, J. A., J. W. Cramer and E. C. Miller. "The N- and Ring-Hydroxylation of 2-Acetylaminofluorene During Carcinogenesis in the Rat," *Cancer Res.* 20:950-962 (1960).
16. DeBaun, J. R., E. C. Miller and J. A. Miller. "N-Hydroxy-2-acetylaminofluorene Sulfotransferase: Its Probable Role in Carcinogenesis and in Protein-(Methion-S-yl) Binding in Rat Liver," *Cancer Res.* 30:577-595 (1970).
17. Kriek, E. "On the Mechanism of Action of Carcinogenic Aromatic Amines. I. Binding of 2-Acetylaminofluorene and N-Hydroxy-2-acetylaminofluorene to Rat Liver Nucleic Acids *In Vivo*," *Chem.-Biol. Interact.* 1:3-17 (1969).
18. Kriek, E., J. A. Miller, V. Juhl and E. C. Miller. "8-(N-2-Fluorenylacetamide) Guanosine, An Arylamidation Reaction Product of Guanosine and the Carcinogen, N-Acetoxy-N-2-fluorenylacetamide in Neutral Solution," *Biochemistry* 6:177-182 (1967).
19. Weisburger, J. H., R. S. Yamamoto, G. M. Williams, P. H. Grantham, T. Matsushima and E. K. Weisburger. "On the Sulfate Ester of N-Hydroxy-N-2-fluorenylacetamide as a Key Ultimate Hepatocarcinogen in the Rat," *Cancer Res.* 32:491-500 (1972).
20. Irving, C. C., D. H. Janss, and L. T. Russell. "Lack of N-Hydroxy-2-acetylaminofluorene Sulfotransferase Activity in the Mammary Gland and Zymbal's Gland of the Rat," *Cancer Res.* 31:387-391 (1971).
21. Bartsch, H., J. A. Miller and E. C. Miller. "N-Acetoxy-N-Acetylaminoarenes and Nitrosoarenes: One-Electron Non-Enzymatic and Enzymatic Oxidation Products of Various Carcinogenic Aromatic Acethydroxamic Acids," *Biochem. Biophys. Acta* 273:40-51 (1972).
22. Bartsch, H., M. Dworkin, J. A. Miller and E. C. Miller. "Electrophilic

N-Acetoxyaminoarenes Derived from N-Acetylaminoarenes by Enzymatic Deacetylation and Transacetylation in Liver," *Biochem. Biophys. Acta* 286: 272-298 (1972).

23. Chouroulinkov, I., A. Gentil, P. L. Grover and P. Sims. "Tumour Initiating Activities on Mouse Skin of Dihydrodiols Derived from Benzo(a)-Pyrene," *Brit. J. Cancer* 34:523-532 (1976).
24. Jerina, D. M., and J. W. Daly. "Oxidation of Carbon," in *Drug Metabolism*, D. V. Parkes and R. L. Smith, Eds. (London: Taylor and Francis, 1977), pp. 15-35.
25. Lin, J.-K., K. A. Kennan, E. C. Miller and J. A. Miller, "Reduced Nicotinamide Adenine Dinucleotide Phosphate-Dependent Formation of 2,3-Dihydro-2,3-Dihydroxyaflatoxin $B_1$ from Aflatoxin $B_1$ by Hepatic Microsomes," *Cancer Res.* 38:2424-2428 (1978).
26. Croy, R. G., J. M. Essigmann, V. N. Reinhold and G. N. Wogan. "Identification of the Principle Aflatoxin-$B_1$-DNA Adduct Formed *In Vivo* in Rat Liver," *Proc. Nat. Acad. Sci., U.S.* 75:1745-1749 (1978).
27. Ward, J. M., J. M. Rice, P. R. Roller and M. L. Wenk. "Natural History of Intestinal Neoplasms Induced in Rats by a Single Injection of Methylacetoxymethylnitrosamine," *Cancer Res.* 37:3046-3052 (1977).
28. Joshi, S. R., J. M. Rice, M. L. Wenk, P. P. Roller and L. K. Keefer. "Brief Communication–Selective Induction of Intestinal Tumors in Rats by Methyl(acetoxymethyl)nitrosamine, an Ester of the Presumed Reactive Metabolite of Dimethylnitrosamine," *J. Nat. Cancer Inst.* 58:1531-1535 (1977).
29. Maltoni, C. "Recent Findings on the Carcinogenicity of Chlorinated Olefins," *Environ. Health Persp.* 21:1-5 (1977).
30. "Vinyl Chloride, Polyvinyl Chloride and Vinyl Chloride - Vinyl Acetate Co-polymers," IARC Monographs on the Evaluation of the Carcinogenic Risk of Chemicals to Humans. International Agency for Research on Cancer, Lyon, France, Vol. 19 (1979), pp. 377-438.
31. Burdette, W. J. "The Significance of Mutation in Relation to the Origin of Tumors: A review," *Cancer Res.* 15:201-226 (1955).
32. Ames, B. N., W. E. Durston, E. Yamasaki, and F. D. Lee. "Carcinogens are Mutagens–A Simple Test System Combining Liver Homogenates for Activation and Bacteria for Detection," *Proc. Nat. Acad. Sci., U.S.* 70:2281-2285 (1973).
33. Ames, B. N., F. D. Lee and W. E. Durston. "An Improved Bacterial Test System for the Detection and Classification of Mutagens and Carcinogens," *Proc. Nat. Acad. Sci., U.S.* 70:782-786 (1973).
34. Garner, R. C., E. C. Miller and J. A. Miller. "Liver Microsomal Metabolism of Aflatoxin $B_1$ to a Reactive Derivative Toxic to *Salmonella typhimurium* TA 1530," *Cancer Res.* 32:2058-2066 (1972).
35. Huberman, E., and L. Sachs. "Mutability of Different Genetic Loci in Mammalian Cells by Metabolically Activated Carcinogenic Polycyclic Hydrocarbons," *Proc. Nat. Acad. Sci., U.S.* 73:188-192 (1976).
36. Langenbach, R., H. J. Freed and E. Huberman. "Liver Cell-Mediated Mutagenesis of Mammalian Cells by Liver Carcinogens," *Proc. Nat. Acad. Sci., U.S.* 75:2864-2867 (1978).
37. Langenbach, R., H. J. Freed, D. Raveh and E. Huberman. "Cell Speci-

ficity in Metabolic Activation of Aflatoxin $B_1$ and Benzo(a)Pyrene to Mutagens for Mammalian Cells," *Nature* 276:277-279 (1978).
38. Kensler, C. J., K. Sugiura, N. F. Young, C. R. Halter and C. P. Rhoads. "Partial Protection of Rats by Riboflavin with Casein Against Liver Cancer Caused by Dimethylnitrosamine," *Science* 93:308-310 (1941).
39. Miller, J. A., and E. C. Miller. "The Carcinogenic Amino-Azo Dyes," *Adv. Cancer Res.* 1:339-396 (1953).
40. Clayson, D. B. "Nutrition and Experimental Carcinogenesis: A Review," *Cancer Res.* 35:3292-3300 (1975).
41. de Waard, F. "Breast Cancer Incidence and Nutritional Status with Particular Reference to Body Weight and Height," *Cancer Res.* 35:3351-3356 (1975).
42. Lipsett, M. B. "Hormones, Nutrition and Cancer," *Cancer Res.* 35:3359-3361 (1975).
43. Rogers, A., and P. M. Newberne. "Dietary Effects on Chemical Carcinogenesis in Animal Models for Colon and Liver Tumors," *Cancer Res.* 35:3421-3426 (1975).
44. Berry, D. L., T. J. Slaga, A. Viaje, N. M. Wilson, J. DiGiovanni, M. R. Juchau and J. K. Selkirk. "Effect of Trichloropropene Oxide on the Ability of Polyaromatic Hydrocarbons and Their K-Region Oxides to Initiate Skin Tumors in Mice and to Bind to DNA *In Vitro*," *J. Nat. Cancer Inst.* 58:1051-1055 (1977).
45. Richardson, H. L., A. R. Stier and E. Borsos-Nactnebel. "Liver Tumor Inhibition and Adrenal Histologic Responses in Rats to Which 3′-Methyl-4-Dimethylaminoazobenzene and 20-Methylcholanthrene were Simultaneously Administered," *Cancer Res.* 12:356-361 (1952).
46. Conney, A. H., E. C. Miller and J. A. Miller. "The Metabolism of Methylated Aminoazodyes. V. Evidence for Induction of Enzymic Synthesis in the Rat by 3-Methylcholanthrene," *Cancer Res.* 16:450-459 (1956).
47. Arcos, J. C., A. H. Conney and N. G. Buu-Hoi. "Induction of Microsomal Enzyme Synthesis by Polycyclic Aromatic Hydrocarbons of Different Molecular Sizes," *J. Biol. Chem.* 236:1291-1296 (1961).
48. Wattenberg, L. W. "Inhibition of Carcinogenic and Toxic Effects of Polycyclic Hydrocarbons by Phenolic Antioxidants and Ethoxyquin," *J. Nat. Cancer Inst.* 48:1425-1430 (1972).
49. Wattenberg, L. W. "Effects of Dietary Constituents on the Metabolism of Chemical Carcinogens," *Cancer Res.* 35:3326-3331 (1975).
50. Wattenberg, L. W. "Guest Editorial–Inhibition of Chemical Carcinogenesis," *J. Nat. Cancer Inst.* 60:11-18 (1978).
51. Swann, P. F., and A. E. McLean. "Cellular Injury and Carcinogenesis. The Effect of a Protein-Free High Carbohydrate Diet on the Metabolism of Dimethylnitrosamine," *Biochem. J.* 124:283-288 (1971).
52. Hard, G. C., and W. H. Butler. "Cellular Analysis of Renal Neoplasm, Light Microscopic Study of Interstitial Lesions Induced in the Rat Kidney by a Single Carcinogenic Dose of Dimethylnitrosamine," *Cancer Res.* 30:3806-3815 (1970).
53. McLean, A. E. M., and P. N. Magee. "Increased Renal Carcinogenesis by Dimethylnitrosamine in Protein Deficient Rats," *Brit. J. Exp. Pathol.* 51:587-590 (1970).

54. Witschi, H., D. Williamson and S. Lick. "Enhancement of Urethan Tumorigenesis by Butylated Hydroxytoluene," *J. Nat. Cancer Inst.* 58:300-305 (1977).
55. Ivankovic, S., and H. Druckrey. "Transplacentare Erzeugung maligner Tumoren des Nervensystem. I. Ethylnitrosoharnstoff (ANH) an BD-IX Ratten," *Z. Krebsforsch.* 71:320-360 (1968).
56. Althoff, J., C. Grandjean, S. Marsh, P. Pour and H. Takahashi. "Transplacental Effects of Nitrosamines in Syrian Hamsters. II. Nitrosopiperidine," *Z. Krebsforsch.* 90:71-77 (1977).
57. Althoff, J., P. Pour, C. Grandjean and S. Marsh. "Transplacental Effects of Nitrosamines in Syrian Hamsters. III. Dimethyl- and Dipropylnitrosamine," *Z. Krebsforsch.* 90:79-86 (1977).
58. Althoff, J., C. Grandjean and P. Pour. "Transplacental Effect of Nitrosamines in Syrian Hamsters. IV. Metabolites of Dipropyl- and Dibutylnitrosamine," *Z. Krebsforsch.* 90:119-126 (1977).
59. Kirkman, H. "Estrogen-Induced Tumors of the Kidney. IV. Incidence in Female Syrian Hamsters," *Nat. Cancer Inst. Monog. Series* 1:59-91 (1959).
60. Lucier, G. W., B. R. Sonawanes, O. S. Modaniel and G. E. R. Hook. "Perinatal Stimulation of Hepatic Microsomal Enzymes Following Administration of TCDD to Pregnant Rats," *Chem.-Biol. Interact.* 11:15-26 (1975).
61. Dieringer, C. S., C. A. Lamartinier and G. W. Lucier. "Effects of DES on Perinatal Development of Hepatic Steroid Metabolizing Enzymes," *Environ. Health Persp.* 20:201-242 (1977).
62. Davies, G. J. W. A. Mclachan, and G. W. Lucier. "Effect of 7,12-Dimethylbenz(a)anthracene (DMBA) on the Perinatal Development of Gonads in Mice," *Teratology* 17:33 (1978).
63. Staffa, J. A., and M. A. Mehlman. "Innovations in Cancer Risk Assesment ($ED_{01}$ Study," in proceedings of a symposium sponsored by the National Center for Toxicological Research, U.S. Food and Drug Administration and the American College of Toxicology (Park Forest South, IL: Pathotox Publishers, 1979), pp. 1-246.
64. Gehring, P. J., P. G. Watanabe, J. D. Young and J. E. LeBeau. "Metabolic Thresholds Must be Considered in Assessing the Carcinogenic Hazard of Chemicals," *Collection of Dow Scientific Papers* 2:56-70 (1976).

CHAPTER 19

# METABOLIC FORMATION AND REACTIONS OF BAY-REGION DIOL EPOXIDES: ULTIMATE CARCINOGENIC METABOLITES OF POLYCYCLIC AROMATIC HYDROCARBONS

**D. R. Thakker and H. Yagi**

Section on Oxidation Mechanisms
Laboratory of Bioorganic Chemistry
National Institute of Arthritis, Metabolism and Digestive Diseases
National Institutes of Health
Bethesda, Maryland

**D. L. Whalen**

Laboratory of Chemical Dynamics
Department of Chemistry
University of Maryland
Catansville, Maryland

**W. Levin, A. W. Wood and A. H. Conney**

Department of Biochemistry and Drug Metabolism
Hoffmann-La Roche Inc.
Nutley, New Jersey

**D. M. Jerina**

Section on Oxidation Mechanisms
Laboratory of Bioorganic Chemistry
National Institute of Arthritis, Metabolism and Digestive Diseases
National Institutes of Health
Bethesda, Maryland

## INTRODUCTION

Polycyclic aromatic hydrocarbons (PAH), formed by incomplete combustion of organic matter, occur widely as environmental pollutants. Automobile exhaust, cigarette smoke and chimney soot are a few of the common sources of PAH, some of which are highly carcinogenic, mutagenic and toxic. A few examples of PAH are shown in Figure 1. Biological activity of the carcinogenic PAH is a consequence of their metabolic activation to one or more chemically reactive intermediates. In the case of benzo[a]pyrene (B[a]P), the most thoroughly examined PAH, the metabolic activation pathway for the formation of an ultimate carcinogen consists of the following enzymatic steps:

$$\text{B[a]P} \xrightarrow[\text{P-450}]{\text{cytochrome}} \text{B[a]P 7,8-oxide} \xrightarrow[\text{hydrolase}]{\text{epoxide}} \text{B[a]P 7,8-dihydrodiol}$$

$$\xrightarrow[\text{P-450}]{\text{cytochrome}} \text{B[a]P 7,8-diol-9,10-epoxides}$$

There are four possible isomers of B[a]P 7,8-diol-9,10-epoxides: (+)- and (-)- B[a]P diol epoxides-*1** and their diastereomers (+)- and (-)-B[a]P diol epoxides-*2* (Figure 2). Of these four isomeric bay-region diol epoxides, only (+)-B[a]P diol epoxide-*2* has been shown to be a highly carcinogenic metabolite of B[a]P [1]. The experimental evidence which has led to the identification of B[a]P 7,8-diol-9,10-epoxide as an ultimate carcinogen of B[a]P has been reviewed recently [2-4]. The epoxide groups of the highly mutagenic and/or carcinogenic 7,8-diol-9,10-epoxides of B[a]P form part of the sterically hindered region between C-10 and C-11 of B[a]P (Figures 1 and 2). The use of the term "bay-region" has been introduced to describe such hindered regions in PAH [5]. The high biological activity of the 7,8-diol-9,10-epoxides of B[a]P has been explained by the bay-region theory. The theory postulates that bay-region epoxides of PAH, present on a saturated angular benzo-ring, should be highly chemically reactive and presumably biologically active [5-8]. The degree of chemical reactivity should be predictable from electronic considerations. Thus, perturbational molecular orbital calculations by the method of Dewar [9] have indicated that forma-

---

*Isomer-*1* always denotes that diastereomer of the diol epoxide in which the benzylic hydroxyl group and oxirane oxygen are *cis* to each other. Isomer-*2* denotes the other isomer, in which these two groups are *trans* to each other; for example, B[a]P diol epoxide-*1* denotes (±)-7β,8α-dihydroxy-9β,10β-epoxy-7,8,9,10-tetrahydro B[a]P. Unless otherwise specified, racemic mixtures of diol epoxides are implied.

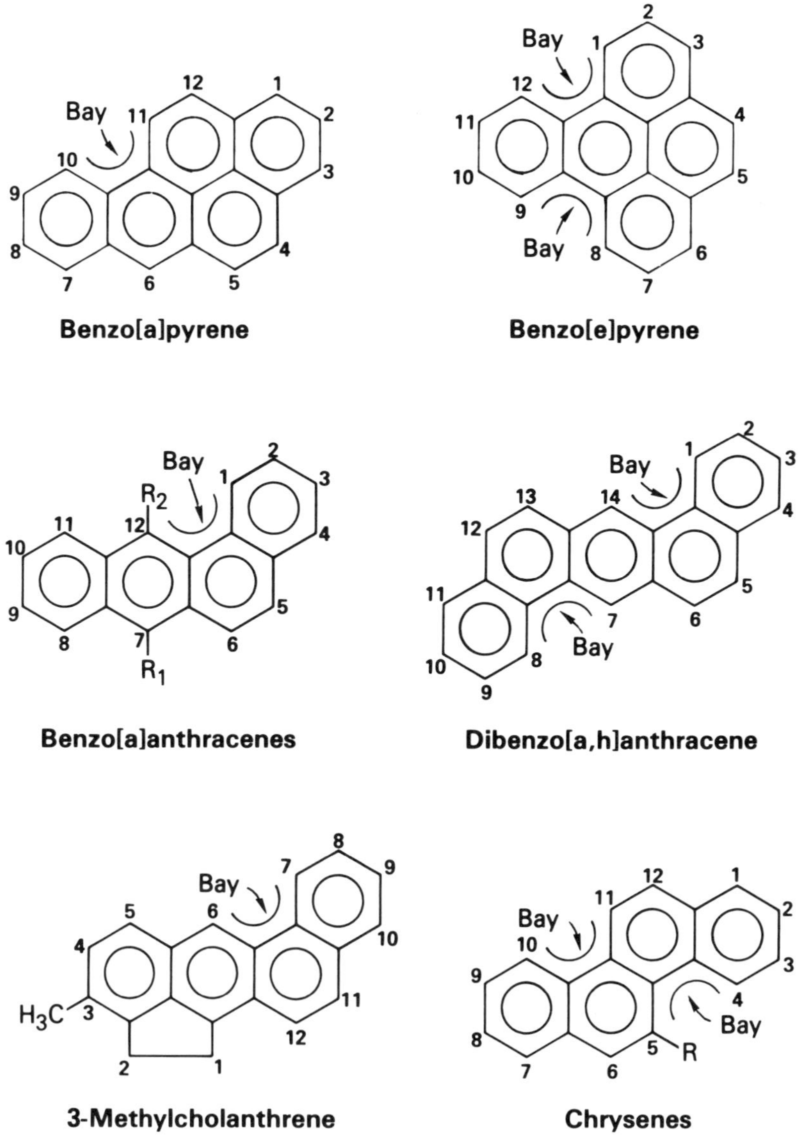


**Figure 1.** Structures of several PAH. The substituents R can represent either hydrogen or methyl groups.

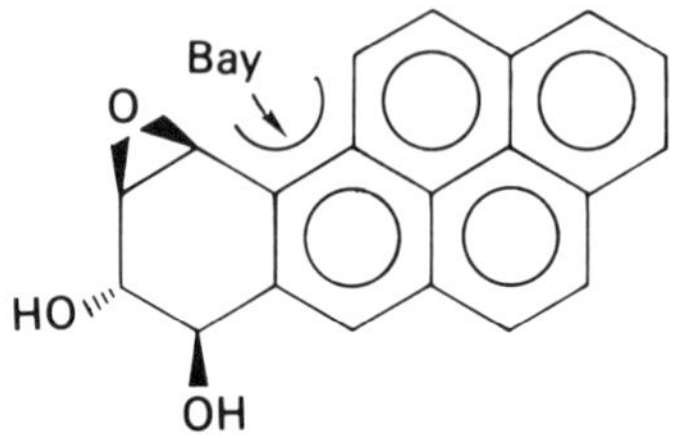


(−)-B[a]P DIOL EPOXIDE-*1*

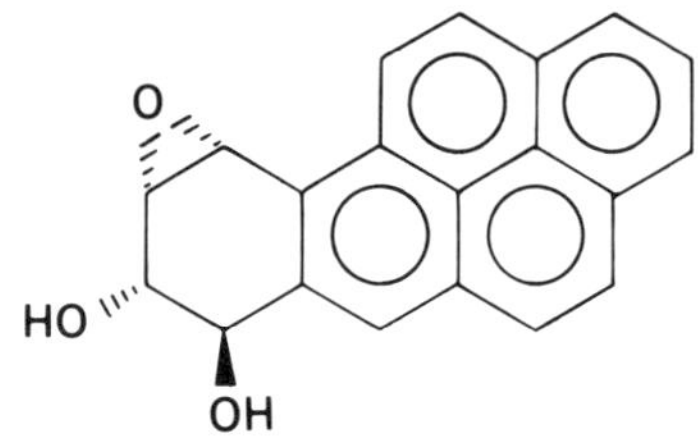


(+)-B[a]P DIOL EPOXIDE-*2*

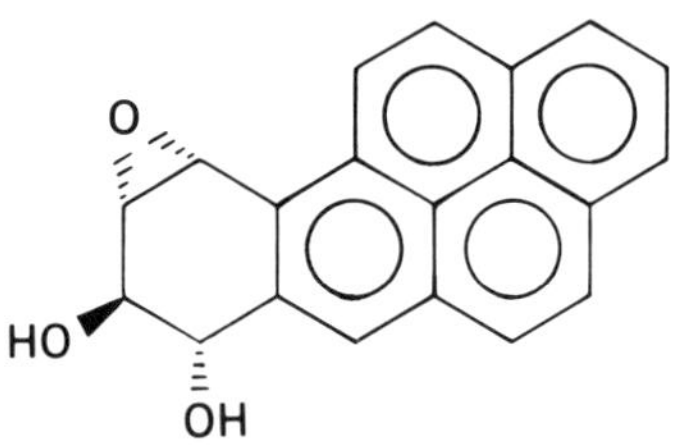


(+)-B[a]P DIOL EPOXIDE-*1*

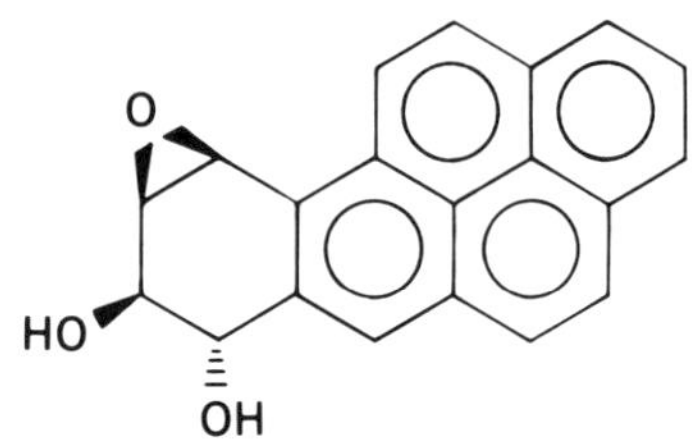


(−)-B[a]P DIOL EPOXIDE-*2*

**Figure 2.** Structures of the isomeric B[a]P 7,8-diol-9,10-epoxides. (+)- and (–)-B[a]P diol epoxides-*1* as well as (+)- and (–)-B[a]P diol epoxides-*2* are enantiomeric pairs.

tion of carbonium ions at benzylic positions on a saturated benzo-ring of a given hydrocarbon is easiest (highest value of $\Delta E_{deloc}$), when that carbonium ion forms part of a bay-region [5-8]. A fundamental assumption of the bay-region theory is that higher reactivity, which can be estimated by predicted ease of carbonium ion formation, is paralleled by greater biological activity. Since the initial predictions of the bay-region theory, bay-region diol epoxides have been shown to be or have been implicated as ultimate carcinogenic forms of eight PAH in addition to B[a]P. These are benzo[a]anthracene (BA), dibenzo[a,h]anthracene (DBA), 7-methyl BA, 7,12-dimethyl BA, 3-methylcholanthrene (3-MC), chrysene, 5-methylchrysene [2,3] and 15,16-dihydro-11-methylcyclopenta[a]phenanthrene-17-one [10]. Synthesis, chemical reactivity, metabolic formation and biological activity of bay-region diol epoxides is the subject of the present chapter.

## SYNTHESIS

Bay-region diol epoxides of PAH have been synthesized from the corresponding *trans*-dihydrodiols with a bay-region double bond [11-15]. Conformation of the hydroxyl groups of dihydrodiols plays an important role in the synthesis of diol epoxides. For benzo-ring dihydrodiols, four stereochemical possibilities exist with respect to the relative positions of the diol group and the olefinic double bond: (1) no bay-region is present, e.g., BA 8,9-dihydrodiol; (2) only the double bond forms part of a bay-region, e.g., B[a]P 7,8-dihydrodiol;* (3) both the diol group and the double bond form part of bay-regions, e.g., benzo[e]pyrene (B[e]P) 9,10-dihydrodiol; or (4) only the diol group forms part of a bay-region, e.g., B[a]P 9,10-dihydrodiol. In the first two cases, the hydroxyl groups of the nonbay-region dihydrodiols exist predominantly in a quasiequatorial conformation. In the latter two cases, the hydroxyl groups of the bay-region dihydrodiols exist predominantly in a quasiaxial conformation because of steric crowding in the bay region [16]. In the case where the hydroxyl groups are quasi-equatorial, such as those of B[a]P 7,8-dihydrodiol, direct epoxidation by peroxy acid results in the selective formation of the diol epoxide-*2* (compare Figure 2 and Scheme 1), due to the directing effects of the equatorial allylic hydroxyl group of the dihydrodiol [17]. For synthesis of B[a]P diol epox-

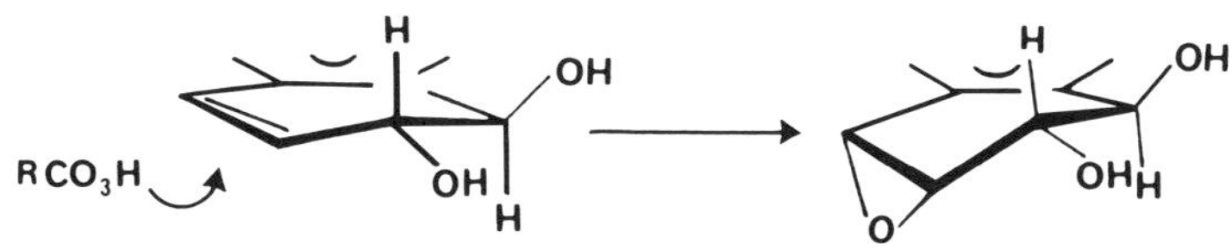


Scheme 1

ide-*1* (Figure 2), B[a]P 7,8-dihydrodiol is allowed to react with N-bromo-acetamide in the presence of water to form a bromotriol stereoselectively by attack of bromine from the same face of the molecule as was attacked by peroxy acid. The bromotriol, on treatment with base, produces diol epoxide-*1* (Scheme 2). Synthesis of diol epoxides of B[e]P (Figure 3) [11] emphasizes the importance of the conformation of the hydroxyl groups to the stereoselectivity of these reactions. B[e]P 9,10-dihydrodiol has its bay-region hydroxyl groups in a quasiaxial conformation because of steric constraints by the proximate bay-region [16]. Consequently, the stereo-selectivity of the epoxidation reaction with peroxy acid is lost, and both B[e]P diol epoxides-*1* and *-2* are formed in approximately equal amounts

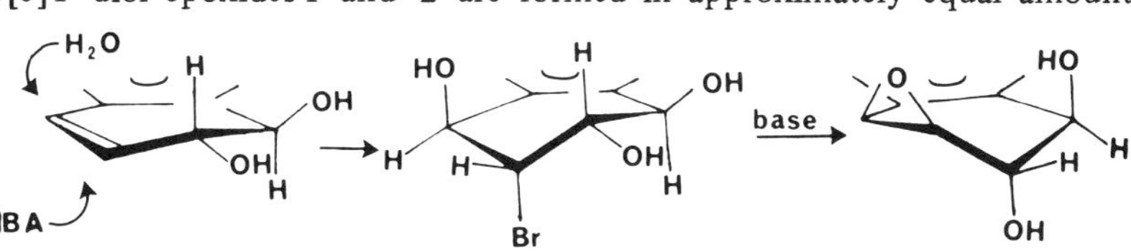


Scheme 2

---

*BA 8,9-dihydrodiol, (±)-*trans*-8,9-dihydroxy-8,9-dihydro BA. All the other dihydro-diols mentioned in this chapter are also *trans* dihydrodiols and are similarly abbreviated.

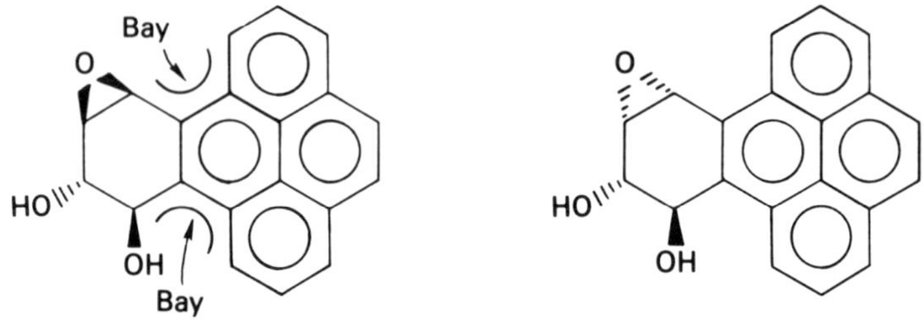


B[e]P 9,10-DIOL-11,12-EPOXIDE-*1* B[e]P 9,10-DIOL-11,12-EPOXIDE-*2*

**Figure 3.** Bay-region diol epoxides of B[e]P.

under a wide variety of epoxidation conditions [11]. Separation of the two diol epoxides is possible by high-performance liquid chromatography (HPLC) on a silica gel column with tetrahydrofuran in hexane as mobile phase [11]. High stereoselectivity is also lost for the reaction of N-bromoacetamide with B[e]P 9,10-dihydrodiol because of the quasiaxial conformation of its hydroxyl groups. These general considerations have been applied to the synthesis of diastereomeric bay-region diol epoxides of BA [13], phenanthrene and chrysene [14], triphenylene [11], and dibenzo [a,h]- and [a,i] pyrene [15].

## REACTIONS

Both B[a]P diol epoxides-*1* and -*2* are highly reactive compounds. In aqueous solutions each diol epoxide is hydrolyzed rapidly to a pair of tetraols (Scheme 3). In addition, diol epoxide-*1* also isomerizes to form a keto-diol in neutral and alkaline solutions [11,14,18] (Scheme 3). Similar hydrolysis and isomerization products have been detected for bay-region diol epoxides of other PAH. A pH-rate profile for hydrolysis of the B[a]P diol epoxides-*1* and -*2* is shown in Figure 4. Plots of log $k_{obsd.}$ vs pH for both diol epoxides have a slope of −1 at low pH values, indicative of an acid-catalyzed solvolysis mechanism. However, at pH values greater than 4.5 for B[a]P diol epoxide-*1* and 6.5 for B[a]P diol epoxide-*2*, the reaction rates become independent of pH. Thus, both of the bay-region diol epoxides of B[a]P undergo spontaneous hydrolysis above pH 7 in water. The rate constants for acid catalyzed and spontaneous hydrolysis reactions were obtained from the equation:

$$k_{obsd} = k_H a_{H^+} + k_o$$

where $k_{obsd}$ = the pseudofirst-order rate constant
$k_H$ = the rate constant for acid-catalyzed hydrolysis
$k_o$ = the rate constant for spontaneous hydrolysis

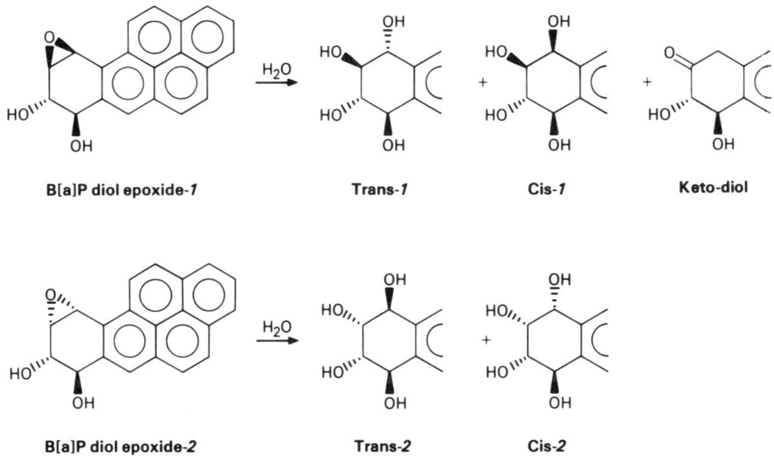


Scheme 3

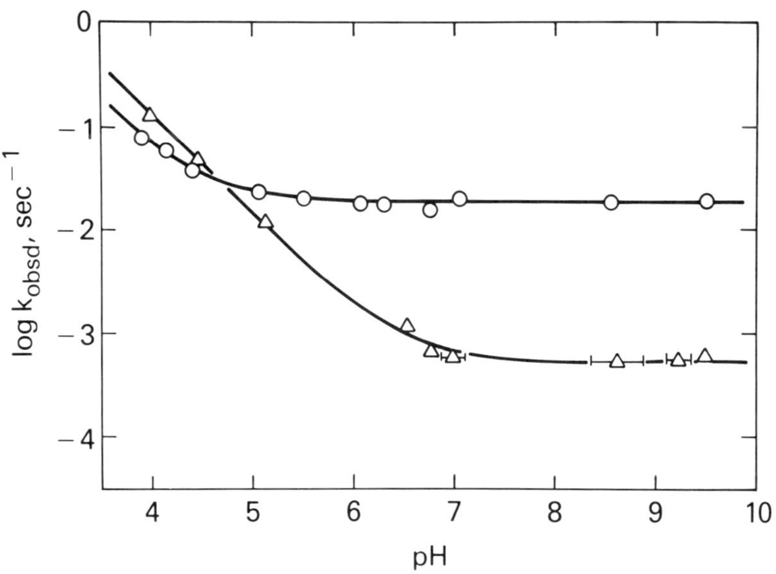


**Figure 4.** Plots of log $k_{obsd.}$ vs pH for hydrolysis of B[a]P diol epoxides-*1* (–o–) and -*2* (–△–) in water (0.1 *M* $NaClO_4$, $10^{-4}$ *M* EDTA) at 25°C. Rates were measured by monitoring absorbance change at 278–279 nm. The pH generally did not change by more than 0.05 during each rate determination with the exception of some measurements for B[a]P diol epoxide-*2* in the spontaneous region where a greater change of pH was observed. The ranges of pH observed during these rate measurements are shown by horizontal error bars. The data are taken from Reference 18.

The various rate constants for hydrolysis of B[a]P diol epoxides in water as well as in 10 and 25% dioxane-water are summarized in Table I [18]. Although B[a]P diol epoxide-*2* is slightly more than twice as reactive as its diastereomeric diol epoxide-*1* toward acid-catalyzed hydrolysis, diol epoxide-*1* is as much as 33-fold more reactive than B[a]P diol epoxide-*2* toward spontaneous hydrolysis. The spontaneous hydrolysis proceeds at a much slower rate in dioxane-water than in water. For example, spontaneous hydrolysis of B[a]P diol epoxide-*1* is 25-fold slower in 25% dioxane-water than in water.

**Table I. Rate Constants for Hydrolysis of B[a]P Diol Epoxides-*1* and -*2* in Water and Dioxane-Water Mixtures at 25°C[a] [14]**

| Compound | Solvent | $k_H$ ($m^{-1}$ $sec^{-1}$) | $k_o$ ($sec^{-1}$) |
|---|---|---|---|
| B[a]P diol epoxide-*1* | Water | $5.8 \pm 0.9 \times 10^2$ | $1.8 \pm 0.1 \times 10^{-2}$ |
| B[a]P diol epoxide-*2* | | $1.4 \pm 0.2 \times 10^3$ | $5.4 \pm 0.8 \times 10^{-4}$ |
| B[a]P diol epoxide-*1* | 10% dioxane-water (v/v) | $5.1 \pm 0.4 \times 10^2$ | $4.2 \pm 0.3 \times 10^{-3}$ |
| B[a]P diol epoxide-*2* | | $1.4 \pm 0.2 \times 10^3$ | $1.3 \pm 0.5 \times 10^{-4}$ |
| B[a]P diol epoxide-*1* | 25% dioxane-water (v/v) | $4.1 \pm 0.1 \times 10^2$ | $7.2 \pm 0.3 \times 10^{-4}$ |
| B[a]P diol epoxide-*2* | | $7.9 \pm 0.2 \times 10^2$ | b |

[a]All solutions contained $10^{-4}$ *M* EDTA. Ionic strength was adjusted to 0.1 with $NaClO_4$ in all cases. Rate constants were calculated from weighted least-squares plots of $k_{obsd.}$ vs $a_{H^+}$.

[b]No spontaneous hydrolysis of B[a]P diol epoxide-*2* was detected in 25% dioxane-water at pH ~ 7.

The distribution of tetraol products formed from B[a]P diol epoxides-*1* and -*2* as a function of pH are shown in Figure 5. B[a]P diol epoxide-*1* gives predominantly the tetraol formed by *cis*-opening of the oxirane ring by water at C-10 to produce *cis-1* (Scheme 3) over the entire pH range studies, along with the formation of small amounts of a keto diol (Scheme 3) at neutral to alkaline pH. In contrast, isomer-*2* gives predominantly the tetraol formed by *trans*-opening of the oxirane ring by water at C-10 to product *trans-2* (Scheme 3) in the acidic pH-range, whereas 1:1 mixture of *trans-2* and *cis-2* tetraols is formed at neutral to alkaline pH. The change in product distribution with pH signifies a change in solvolysis mechanism for B[a]P diol epoxide-*2*.

Interestingly, when hydrolysis of B[a]P diol epoxides-*1* and -*2* is carried out in 10% dioxane-water solutions containing phosphate buffer, the rates

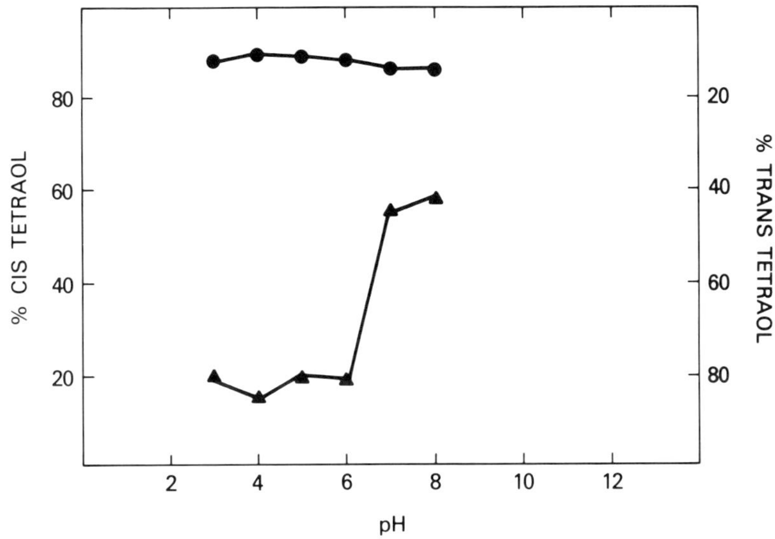


**Figure 5.** Distribution of tetraol products from B[a]P diol epoxides-*1* (–●–) and -*2* (–▲–) as a function of pH. For solvolysis conditions see the legend for Figure 4. The tetraols were separated by HPLC. For chromatographic conditions see Reference 18.

of hydrolysis show a first-order dependence on the buffer concentrations [19]. A mechanism in which dihydrogen phosphate ion ($H_2PO_4^{-2}$) acts as a general acid, and transfers a proton to diol epoxides in the rate-limiting step to form a triol carbonium ion (Scheme 4) has been suggested [19]. The triol carbonium ion can either react with water to give tetraols or with $H_2PO_4^{-2}$ to form phosphate esters. Such general acid catalysis has also been observed [19] with acetic acid (pH 4.8-5.1), Tris-$H^+$ (pH 7.9-8.5), HO-$CH_2CH_2$-$NH_3^+$ (pH 8.5-9.0) and phenol (pH 9.2-9.6). This general acid catalysis by weak acids has considerable biological importance since it suggests an important detoxification mechanism for diol epoxides in vivo.

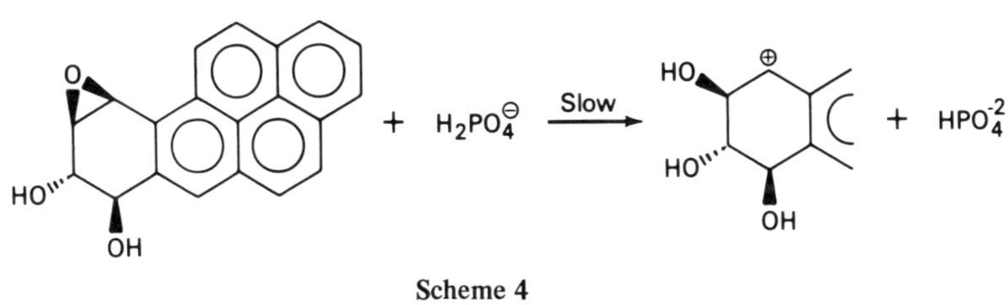


Scheme 4

When B[a]P diol epoxides are allowed to react with nucleophiles under $SN_2$ conditions, i.e., reactions of B[a]P diol epoxides with *p*-nitrothiophenolate in *t*-butanol, B[a]P diol epoxide-*1* is as much as 150-fold more reactive than B[a]P diol epoxide-*2* [17]. Anchimeric assistance by the benzylic hydroxyl group to opening of the epoxide ring appears to be responsible for the much higher reactivity of isomer-*1* over isomer-*2* under such conditions.

The highly reactive bay-region diol epoxides of B[a]P react covalently with nucleic acid bases [20-28] as well as with the phosphate backbone of nucleic acids [21,25]. When B[a]P is applied on the skin of mice or is metabolized by cells in culture, its principal covalent adduct is formed by attack of the exocyclic amino group of guanine in RNA or DNA at C-10 of the B[a]P diol epoxides (Figure 6) [21,22,24,27]. Such covalent interactions of B[a]P diol epoxides are believed to be responsible for some of the mutagenicity of B[a]P on metabolic activation and for its carcinogenicity in animals.

## METABOLIC FORMATION

### Bay-Region Diol Epoxides of B[a]P

Bay-region diol epoxides of B[a]P are formed from the parent hydrocarbon by a three-step enzymatic pathway which involves initial oxidation of B[a]P by cytochrome P-450 to B[a]P 7,8-oxide, hydrolysis of the oxide

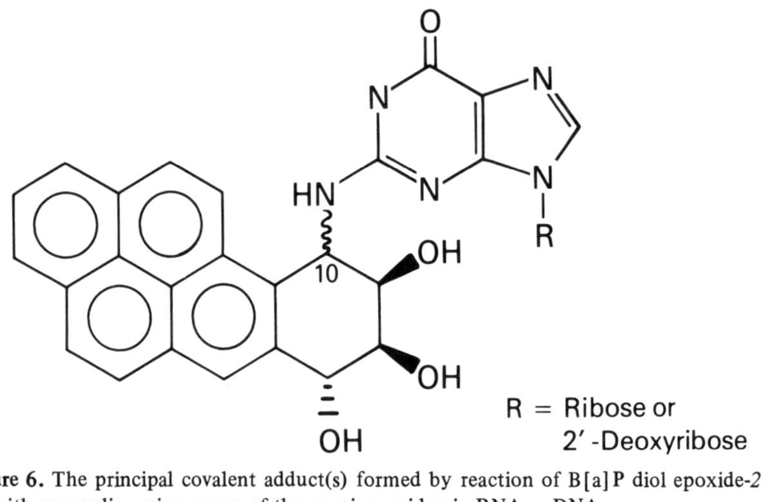


**Figure 6.** The principal covalent adduct(s) formed by reaction of B[a]P diol epoxide-*2* with exocyclic amino group of the guanine residue in RNA or DNA.

by epoxide hydrolase to form B[a]P 7,8-dihydrodiol and subsequent cytochrome P-450 catalyzed oxidation to the bay-region diol epoxides. The metabolism of B[a]P 7,8-dihydrodiol is a highly regio- and stereoselective process. For example, 83-92% of the total metabolites from (±)-B[a]P 7,8-dihydrodiol with hepatic microsomes from 3-MC-treated rats are the bay-region diol epoxides; whereas, 60-70% of the total metabolites are bay-region diol epoxides when microsomes from untreated or phenobarbital-treated rats are used as the enzyme sources [29]. The bay-region diol epoxides of B[a]P are formed with a high degree of stereoselectivity when (+)- and (-)-enantiomers of B[a]P 7,8-dihydrodiol are used as substrates [30]. (-)-B[a]P [7R,8R]-dihydrodiol is metabolized by hepatic microsomes from 3-MC-treated rats to form B[a]P diol epoxides-*2* and -*1* in the ratio of 6 to 1, whereas these two diol epoxides are formed in the ratio of 1:22 when (+)-B[a]P [7S,8S]-dihydrodiol is used as a substrate [30]. Metabolic formation of predominantly (+)-diol epoxide-*2* (Figure 2) from the (-)-[7R,8R]-enantiomer of B[a]P 7,8-dihydrodiol and of predominantly (+)-diol epoxide-*1* (Figure 2) from the (+)-[7S,8S]-enantiomer of B[a]P 7,8-dihydrodiol indicates that oxygen is inserted at the 9,10-position from the same face of the hydrocarbon for both enantiomers (Scheme 5). The metabolically formed B[a]P 7,8-dihydrodiol, which contains (-)-[7R,8R]-enantiomer to the extent of 96%, is metabolized by hepatic microsomes from 3-MC-treated rats predominantly to (+)-diol epoxide-*2* (88% of total metabolites) [30,31]. High stereoselectivity was also observed in the metabolism of (-)-B[a]P 7,8-dihydrodiol by various forms of cytochrome P-450 purified from rabbit liver microsomes [32]. The ratio of the two diastereo-

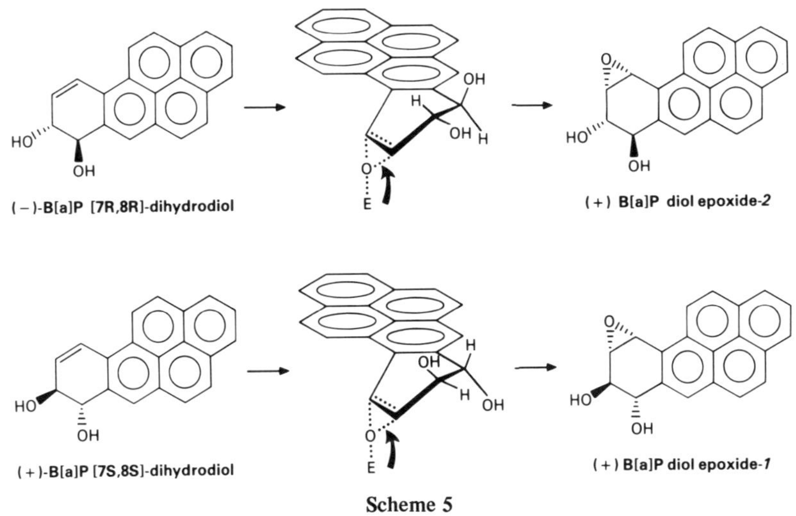


Scheme 5

meric diol epoxides formed by various forms of cytochrome P-450 varied over approximately 40-fold range [32].

## Bay-Region Diol Epoxides of BA, Phenanthrene, Chrysene and B[e]P

Bay-region diol epoxides are formed from dihydrodiols of these four PAH with different degrees of regiospecificity. For example, less than 10% of the total metabolites of racemic BA 3,4-dihydrodiol are bay-region diol epoxides [33], whereas approximately 60-70% of total metabolites formed from metabolically formed and highly enantiomerically enriched phenanthrene 1,2-dihydrodiol and chrysene 1,2-dihydrodiol can be accounted for as bay-region diol epoxides. In analogy to the metabolism of (-)-B[a]P [7R,8R]-dihydrodiol, the (-)-[R,R]-enantiomer of BA 3,4-dihydrodiol is also metabolized by rat liver microsomes to predominantly (+)-BA 3,4-diol-1,2-epoxide-*2*. However, the metabolism of (+)-BA [3S,4S]-dihydrodiol differed from that of (+)-B[a]P [7S,8S] dihydrodiol in that very little, if any, bay-region diol epoxides were formed from this substrate [33]. Racemic B[e]P 9,10-dihydrodiol is metabolized to only trace quantities, if any, of the bay-region 9,10-diol-11,12-epoxides [33,34].

## BIOLOGICAL ACTIVITY

### Bay-Region Diol Epoxides of B[a]P

#### *Mutagenicity*

The diastereomeric B[a]P diol epoxides-*1* and -*2* are two of the most mutagenic derivatives of B[a]P known in bacterial [35-37] and mammalian cells [36-39]. B[a]P diol epoxide-*1* is 4.8- and 1.6-fold more active than B[a]P diol epoxide-*2* toward *Salmonella typhimurium* strains TA-98 and TA-100, respectively; whereas B[a]P diol epoxide-*2* is approximately 2.5-fold more mutagenic than B[a]P diol epoxide-*1* toward Chinese hamster V79 cells [36]. Since each of the diastereomeric B[a]P diol epoxides can exist as a pair of enantiomers, mutagenic activities of the four isomeric B[a]P 7,8-diol-9,10-epoxides were measured. In Chinese hamster V-79 cells, (+)-diol epoxide-*2* is 6- to 18-fold more mutagenic than the other three isomers [40]. (-)-Diol epoxide-*1* is 1.3- to 9.5-fold more mutagenic in *S. typhimurium* strains TA-98 and TA-100 than the other three isomers [4,40].

*Carcinogenicity*

(+)-B[a]P diol epoxides-*1* and -*2* showed very weak or no tumorigenic activity on mouse skin in chronic studies [41]. However, B[a]P diol epoxide-*2* did show moderate tumorigenicity in initiation-promotion studies on mouse skin [42]. B[a]P diol epoxide-*2* was found, however, to be highly tumorigenic to newborn mice when injected intraperitoneally [43]. At a total dose of 28 nmol, (±) B[a]P diol epoxide-*2* was ∿2.5-fold more tumorigenic than its metabolic precursor B[a]P 7,8-dihydrodiol in newborn mice (Table II) [43]. When the four possible isomers of B[a]P 7,8-diol-9,10-epoxides were tested as carcinogens in the newborn mouse model, (+)-B[a]P diol epoxide-*2* was found to be highly tumorigenic. The other three isomers

**Table II. Tumorigenicity of B[a]P, B[a]P 7,8-dihydrodiol and B[a]P Diol Epoxides in Newborn Mice[a]**

| Compound | Lung Adenomas per Mouse |
|---|---|
| Solvent | 0.13 |
| B[a]P | 0.24 |
| B[a]P 7,8-dihydrodiol | 1.77 |
| B[a]P diol epoxide-*1* | 0.14 |
| B[a]P diol epoxide-*2* | 4.42 |

[a]Swiss-Webster mice were injected intraperitoneally within 24 hr of birth and on the 8th and 15th day after birth with 4, 8 and 16 nmol, respectively, of compounds. The mice were killed at 6–7 months of age (data taken from Reference 43).

**Table III. Tumorigenicity of the Isomeric B[a]P Diol Epoxides in Newborn Mice[a]**

| Compound | Lung Adenomas per Mouse |
|---|---|
| Solvent | 0.12 |
| B[a]P | 0.15 |
| (–)-B[a]P diol epoxide-*1* | 0.25 |
| (+)-B[a]P diol epoxide-*1* | 0.33 |
| (–)-B[a]P diol epoxide-*2* | 0.12 |
| (+)-B[a]P diol epoxide-*2* | 7.67 |

[a]Swiss-Webster mice were injected intraperitoneally within 24 hr of birth and on the 8th and 15th day after birth with 2, 4 and 8 nmol, respectively, of the isomeric diol epoxides. The mice were killed at 6–7 months of age (data taken from Reference 1). See Figure 2 for structures of isomeric B[a]P diol epoxides.

of B[a]P 7,8-diol-9,10-epoxide and B[a]P were essentially inactive at the same dose (Table III) [1]. Hence, (+)-B[a]P diol-epoxide-*2* has been established as an ultimate carcinogenic metabolite of B[a]P.

### Bay-Region Diol Epoxides of BA, Phenanthrene and Chrysene

As predicted by the bay-region theory, the 3,4-diol-1,2-epoxides of BA were found to be highly mutagenic compounds relative to the non-bay-region diol epoxides of BA [44,45]. Furthermore, in an initiation-promotion experiment on mouse skin, the diastereomeric BA 3,4-diol-1,2-epoxides caused 10- to 40-fold more papillomas/mouse than did BA. Isomer-*2* was two- to threefold more active than isomer-*1* [46]. (±)-BA 3,4-diol-1,2-epoxide-*2* was at least sevenfold more tumorigenic than (+)- or (−)-BA 3,4-dihydrodiol when tested in the newborn mouse model [47], whereas (±)-BA 3,4-diol-1,2-epoxide-*1* was very weakly tumorigenic in this tumor model [47].

Mutagenicity studies with bacterial and mammalian cells which show relatively high mutagenicity for bay-region diol epoxides of chrysene are consistent with the predictions of the bay-region theory [48]. Bay-region diol epoxides of phenanthrene have relatively lower mutagenic activity than those of chrysene, although values of $\Delta E_{deloc}$ for the formation of bay-region benzylic carbonium ions are comparable for these two hydrocarbons. The small size and high polarity of the phenanthrene diol epoxides may be determining factors in the lower mutagenic activities of the bay-region diol epoxides of phenanthrene compared to those of chrysene. Consistent with these conclusions is the observation that 3,4-epoxy-1,2,3,4-tetrahydrophenanthrene, which lacks the polar hydroxyl groups, is quite mutagenic toward bacterial and mammalian cells [48].

## CONCLUSIONS

There are now numerous examples of bay-region diol epoxides as ultimate carcinogenic forms of PAH. Mutagenicity and/or carcinogenicity studies with bay-region diol epoxides of B[a]P, BA and chrysene have provided the most direct evidence for high biological activities of bay-region diol epoxides. Furthermore, mutagenicity studies in the presence of metabolic activation systems and tumor studies with precursor dihydrodiols of bay-region diol epoxides in the case of DBA, 7-methyl BA, 7,12-dimethyl BA, 3-MC, 5-methylchrysene and 15,16-dihydro-11-methylcyclopenta[a]phenanthrene-

17-one have provided strong circumstantial evidence for the involvement of bay-region diol epoxides in the mutagenicity and carcinogenicity of these PAH (see references cited in References 2, 3 and 10). The bay-region theory of PAH carcinogenesis has provided a rationale for the high chemical reactivity and hence, high biological activity of bay-region diol epoxides.

In addition to the high chemical reactivity, other factors, such as relative and absolute stereochemistry of the bay-region diol epoxides and the precursor dihydrodiols, the conformation of their hydroxyl groups, and size of the parent hydrocarbon, play very significant roles in the carcinogenicity of PAH. The role of absolute and relative stereochemistry as a determinant of carcinogenicity has been well illustrated by tumor studies in the newborn mouse model. Although (+)-B[a]P-7,8-diol-9,10-epoxide-*2* is highly tumorigenic, its (-)-enantiomer as well as the other two diastereomeric diol epoxides are almost completely inactive at equivalent doses. The extent to which a PAH is transformed to its dihydrodiol with a bay-region double bond and the extent to which the dihydrodiol is transformed to bay-region diol epoxides can also play an important role in the carcinogenicity of PAH. For example, despite the moderately high carcinogenicity of the BA 3,4-diol-1,2-epoxides, the very low metabolic conversion of BA to its 3,4-dihydrodiol and of the dihydrodiol to bay-region diol epoxides can account for the very weak carcinogenicity of BA. Another factor important for the high carcinogenicity of bay-region diol epoxides is the refractory nature of these diol epoxides toward enzymatic hydrolysis catalyzed by epoxide hydrolase [29,36,44,48]. This may enable the diol epoxides to survive for sufficient time to reach target molecules such as nucleic acids. Studies are in progress to explore the role of these and other factors as determinants of the carcinogenicity of PAH.

## REFERENCES


1. Buening, M. K., P. G. Wislocki, W. Levin, H. Yagi, D. R. Thakker, H. Akagi, M. Koreeda, D. M. Jerina and A. H. Conney. "Tumorigenicity of the Optical Enantiomers of the Diastereomeric Benzo[a]pyrene 7,8-diol-9,10-Epoxides in Newborn Mice: Exceptional Activity of (+)-7$\beta$-8$\alpha$-dihydroxy-9$\alpha$,10$\alpha$-epoxy-7,8,9,10-tetrahydrobenzo[a]-pyrene," *Proc. Nat. Acad. Sci., U.S.* 75:5358-5361 (1978).
2. Nordqvist, M., D. R Thakker, H. Yagi, R. E. Lehr, A. W. Wood, W. Levin, A. H. Conney and D. M. Jerina. "Evidence in Support of the Bay Region Theory as a Basis for the Carcinogenic Activity of Polycyclic Aromatic Hydrocarbons," in *Molecular Basis of Environmental Toxicity*, R. S. Bhatnagar, Ed. (Ann Arbor, MI: Ann Arbor Science Publishers, Inc., 1980), p. 329.

3. Conney, A. H., W. Levin, A. W. Wood, H. Yagi, R. E. Lehr and D. M. Jerina. "Biological Activity of Polycyclic Hydrocarbon Metabolites and the Bay Region Theory," in *Advances in Pharmacology and Therapeutics, Vol. 9, Toxicology*, Y. Cohen, Ed. (Oxford: Pergamon Press, 1978), p. 43.
4. Jerina, D. M., H. Yagi, D. R. Thakker, J. M. Karle, H. D. Mah, D. R. Boyd, G. Gadaginamath, A. W. Wood, M. Buening, R. L. Chang, W. Levin and A. H. Conney. "Stereoselective Metabolic Activation of Polycyclic Aromatic Hydrocarbons," in *Advances in Pharmacology and Therapeutics, Vol. 9, Toxicology*, Y. Cohen, Ed. (Oxford: Pergamon Press, 1978), p. 53.
5. Jerina, D. M., R. E. Lehr, H. Yagi, O. Hernandez, P. M. Dansette, P. G. Wislocki, A. W. Wood, R. L. Chang, W. Levin and A. H. Conney. "Mutagenicity of Benzo[a]pyrene and the Description of a Quantum Mechanical Model which Predicts the Ease of Carbonium Ion Formation from Diol Epoxides," in *In Vitro Metabolic Activation in Mutagenesis Testing*, F. J. de Serres, J. R. Fouts, J. R. Bend and R. M. Philpot, Eds., (Amsterdam: Elsevier/North-Holland Biomedical Press, 1976), p. 159.
6. Jerina, D. M., and J. W. Daly, "Oxidation at Carbon," in *Drug Metabolism–From Microbe to Man*, D. V. Parke and R. L. Smith, Eds. (London: Taylor and Francis, Ltd., 1976), p. 13.
7. Jerina, D. M., R. E. Lehr, M. Schaefer-Ridder, H. Yagi, J. M. Karle, D. R. Thakker, A. W. Wood, A. Y. H. Lu, D. Ryan, S. West, W. Levin and A. H. Conney. "Bay Region Epoxides of Dihydrodiols: A Concept which Explains the Mutagenic and Carcinogenic Activity of Benzo[a]-pyrene and Benzo[a]anthracene," in *Origins of Human Cancer*, H. Hiatt, J. D. Watson and I. Winsten, Eds. (Cold Spring Harbor, NY: Cold Spring Harbor Laboratory, 1977), p. 369.
8. Jerina, D. M., and R. E. Lehr. "The Bay-Region Theory. A Quantum Mechanical Approach to Aromatic Hydrocarbon-Induced Carcinogenicity," in *Microsomes and Drug Oxidations*, V. Ullrich, I. Roots, A. Hildebrandt and R. W. Estabrook, Eds. (Elmsford, NY: Pergamon Press, 1978), p. 709.
9. Dewar, M. J. S. *The Molecular Orbital Theory of Organic Chemistry* (New York: McGraw-Hill Book Company, 1969), pp. 214, 304.
10. Coombs, M. M., A. M. Kissonerghis, A. A. Jeffrey and C. Vase. "Identification of Proximate and Ultimate Forms of the Carcinogen 15,16-Dihydro-11-methylcyclopenta[3]phenanthrene-17-one," *Cancer Res.* 39:4160-4165 (1978).
11. Yagi, H., D. R. Thakker, O. Hernandez, M. Koreeda and D. M. Jerina. "Synthesis and Reactions of the Highly Mutagenic 7,8-diol-9,10-Epoxides of the Carcinogen Benzo[a]pyrene," *J. Am. Chem. Soc.* 99:1604-1611 (1977).
12. Yagi, H., D. R. Thakker, R. E. Lehr and D. M. Jerina. "Benzo-Ring Diol Epoxides of Benzo[e]pyrene and Triphenylene," *J. Org. Chem.* 44:3439-3442 (1979).
13. Lehr, R. E., M. Schaeffer-Ridder and D. M. Jerina. "Synthesis and Reactivity of Diol Epoxides Derived from non-K-Region *trans*-Dihydrodiols of Benzo[a]anthracene," *Tetrahedron Lett.* (1976) pp. 539-542.

14. Whalen, D. L., A. M. Ross, H. Yagi, J. M. Karle and D. M. Jerina. "Stereoelectronic Factors in the Solvolysis of Bay Region Diol Epoxides of Polycyclic Aromatic Hydrocarbons," *J. Am. Chem. Soc.* 100:5218-5221 (1978).
15. Lehr, R. E., S. Kumar, P. T. Cohenour and D. M. Jerina. "Dihydrodiols and Diol Epoxides of Dibenzo[a,i]- and [a,h]pyrene," *Tetrahedron Lett.* (1979) pp. 3819-3821.
16. Jerina, D. M., H. Selander, H. Yagi, M. C. Wells, J. F. Davey, V. Mehadevan and D. T. Gibson. "Dihydrodiols from Anthracene and Phenanthrene," *J. Am. Chem. Soc.* 98:5988-5996 (1976).
17. Yagi, H., O. Hernandez and D. M. Jerina. "Synthesis of (±)7β,8α-Dihdyroxy-9β,10β-epoxy-7,8,9,10-tetrahydrobenzo[a]pyrene, a Potential Metabolite of the Carcinogen Benzo[a]pyrene with Stereochemistry Related to the Antileukemic Triptolide," *J. Am. Chem. Soc.* 97:6881-6883 (1975).
18. Whalen, D. L., J. A. Montemarano, D. R. Thakker, H. Yagi and D. M. Jerina. "Changes in Mechanisms and Product Distributions in the Hydrolysis of Benzo[a]pyrene 7,8-Diol 9,10-Epoxide Metabolites Induced by Changes in pH," *J. Am. Chem. Soc.* 99:5522-5524 (1977).
19. Whalen, D. L., A. M. Ross, J. A. Montemarano, D. R. Thakker, H. Yagi and D. M. Jerina. "General Acid Catalysis in the Hydrolysis of Benzo[a]pyrene 7,8-Diol 9,10-Epoxides," *J. Am. Chem. Soc.* 101:5086-5088 (1979).
20. Daudel, P., M. Duquesue, P. Vigny, P. L. Grover and P. Sims. "Fluorescence Spectral Evidence that Benzo[a]pyrene-DNA Products in Mouse Skin Arise from Diol-Epoxides," *FEBS Lett.* 57:520-525 (1975).
21. Koreeda, M., P. D. Moore, H. Yagi, H. J. C. Yeh and D. M. Jerina. "Alkylation of Polyguanylic Acid at the 2-Amino Group and Phosphate by the Potent Mutagen (±)-7β,8α-Dihydroxy-9β,10β-epoxy-7,8,9,10-tetrahydrobenzo[a]pyrene," *J. Am. Chem. Soc.* 98:6720-6722 (1976).
22. Jeffrey, A. M., K. W. Jennete, S. H. Blobstein, I. B. Weinstein, F. A. Belend, R. G. Harvey, H. Kasai, I. Miura and K. Nakanishi. "Structure of Guanosine Adducts Formed by Reactions with a Tetrahydrodiol Epoxide of Benzo[a]pyrene," *J. Am. Chem. Soc.* 98:5714-5715 (1976).
23. King. H. W. S., M. R. Osborne, F. A. Belend, R. G. Harvey and P. Brookes. "(±)-7α,8β-Dihydroxy-9β,10β-epoxy-7,8,9,10-tetrahydrobenzo[a]pyrene Is an Intermediate in the Metabolism and Binding to DNA of Benzo[a]pyrene," *Proc. Nat. Acad. Sci., U.S.* 73:2679-2681 (1976).
24. Weinstein, I. B., A. M. Jeffrey, K. W. Jennette, S. H. Blobstein, R. G. Harvey, H. Kasai and M. Nakanishi. "Benzo[a]pyrene Diol Epoxides as Intermediates in Nucleic Acid Binding *In Vitro* and *In Vivo*," *Science* 193:592-595 (1976).
25. Gamper, H. B., A. S.-C. Tung, K. Straus, J. C. Bartholomew and M. Calvin. "DNA Strand Scission by Benzo[a]pyrene Diol Epoxides," *Science* 197:671-674 (1977).
26. Moore, P. D., M. Koreeda, P. G. Wislocki, W. Levin, A. H. Conney, H. Yagi and D. M. Jerina. "*In Vitro* Reactions of the Diastereomeric 9,10-Epoxides of (+) and (-)-*trans*-7,8-Dihydroxy-7,8-dihydrobenzo[a]pyrene with Polyguanylic Acid and Evidence for Formation of an

Enantiomer of Each Diastereomeric 9,10-Epoxide from Benzo[a]-pyrene in Mouse Skin," in *Drug Metabolism Concepts, ACS Symposium Series No. 44*, D. M. Jerina, Ed. (Washington, DC.: American Chemical Society, 1977), p. 127.

27. Koreeda, M., P. D. Moore, P. G. Wislocki, W. Levin, A. H. Conney, H. Yagi and D. M. Jerina. "Binding of Benzo[a]pyrene 7,8-Diol-9,10-epoxides to DNA, RNA, and Protein of Mouse Skin Occurs with High Stereo-selectivity," *Science* 199:778-781 (1978).
28. Meehan, T., and K. Straub. "Double Standed DNA Stereoselectivity Binds Benzo[a]pyrene Diol Epoxides," *Nature* 277:410-412 (1979).
29. Thakker, D. R., H. Yagi, A. Y. H. Lu, W. Levin, A. H. Conney and D. M. Jerina. "Metabolism of Benzo[a]pyrene: Conversion of (±)-*trans*-7,8-Dihydroxy-7,8-dihydrobenzo[a]pyrene to Highly Mutagenic 7,8-Diol-9,10-epoxides," *Proc. Nat. Acad. Sci., U.S.* 73:3381-3385 (1976).
30. Thakker, D. R., H. Yagi, H. Akagi, M. Koreeda, A. Y. H. Lu, W. Levin, A. W. Wood, A. H. Conney and D. M. Jerina. "Metabolism of Benzo[a]-pyrene: VI Stereoselective Metabolism of Benzo[a]pyrene and Benzo-[a]pyrene 7,8-dihydrodiol to Diol Epoxides," *Chem.-Biol. Interact.* 16:281-300 (1977).
31. Yang, S. K., D. W. McCourt, P. P. Roller and H. V. Gelboin. "Enzy-matic Conversion of Benzo[a]pyrene Leading Predominantly to the Diol-Epoxide r-7, 5t-8-Dihydroxy-5-9,10-oxy-7,8,9,10-tetrahydrobenzo-[a]pyrene Through a Single Enantiomer of r-7, t-8-Dihydroxy-7,8-dihydrobenzo[a]pyrene," *Proc. Nat. Acad. Sci., U.S.* 73:2594-2598 (1976).
32. Deutsch, J., J. C. Leutz, S. K. Yang, H. V. Gelboin, Y. L. Chiang, K. P. Vatsis and M. J. Coon. "Regio- and Stereoselectivity of Various Forms of Purified Cytochrome P-450 in the Metabolism of Benzo[a]pyrene and (–)-*trans*-7,8-Dihydroxy-7,8-dihydrobenzo[a]pyrene as Shown by Product Formation and Binding to DNA," *Proc. Nat. Acad. Sci., U.S.* 75:3123-3127 (1978).
33. Thakker, D. R., W. Levin, H. Yagi, M. Tada, A. H. Conney and D. M. Jerina. "Comparative Metabolism of Dihydrodiols of Polycyclic Aro-matic Hydrocarbons to Bay Region Diol Epoxides," in *The Fourth International Symposium on Polynuclear Aromatic Hydrocarbons*, A. Bjorseth and A. J. Dennis, Eds. (Columbus, OH: Battelle Labora-tories, 1980), p. 267.
34. Wood, A. W., W. Levin, D. R. Thakker, H. Yagi, R. L. Chang, D. E. Ryan, P. E. Thomas, P. M. Dansette, N. Whittaker, S. Turujman, R. E. Lehr, S. Kumar, D. M. Jerina and A. H. Conney. "Biological Activity of Benzo[e]pyrene: An Assessment Based on Mutagenic Activity and Metabolic Profiles of the Polycyclic Hydrocarbon and Its Derivatives," *J. Biol. Chem.* 254:4408-4415 (1979).
35. Wislocki, P. G., A. W. Wood, R.L. Chang, W. Levin, H. Yagi, O. Hernandez, D. M. Jerina and A. H. Conney. "High Mutagenicity and Toxicity of a Diol Epoxide Derived from Benzo[a]pyrene," *Biochem. Biophys. Res. Commun.* 68:1006-1012 (1976).
36. Wood, A. W., P. G. Wislocki, R. L. Chang, W. Levin, A. Y. H. Lu, H. Yagi, O. Hernandez, D. M. Jerina and A. H. Conney. "Mutagenicity

and Cytotoxicity of Benzo[a]pyrene Benzo-Ring Epoxides," *Cancer Res.* 36:3358-3366 (1976).

37. Malaveille, C., T. Kuroki, P. Sims, P. L. Grover and H. Bartsch. "Mutagenicity of Isomeric Diol Epoxides of Benzo[a]pyrene and Benz[a]-anthracene in S. typhimurium TA 98 and TA 100 and V79 Chinese Hamster Cells," *Mutation Res.* 44:313-318 (1977).
38. Huberman, E., L. Sachs, S. K. Yang and H. V. Gelboin. "Identification of Mutagenic Metabolites of Benzo[a]pyrene in Mammalian Cells," *Proc. Nat. Acad. Sci., U.S.* 73:607-611 (1976).
39. Newbold, R. F., and P. Brookes. "Exceptional Mutagenicity of a Benzo[a]pyrene Diol Epoxide in Cultured Mammalian Cells," *Nature (New Biol.)* 261:52-54 (1976).
40. Wood, A. W., R. L. Chang, W. Levin, H. Yagi, D. R. Thakker, D. M. Jerina and A. H. Conney. "Differences in Mutagenicity of the Optical Enantiomers of the Diastereomeric Benzo[a]pyrene 7,8-diol-9,10-epoxides," *Biochem. Biophys. Res. Commun.* 77:1389-1396 (1977).
41. Levin, W., A. W. Wood, P. G. Wislocki, J. Kapitulnik, H. Yagi, D. M. Jerina and A. H. Conney. "Carcinogenicity of Benzo-Ring Derivatives of Benzo[a]pyrene on Mouse Skin," *Cancer Res.* 37:3356-3361 (1977).
42. Slaga, T. J., W. M. Bracken, A. Viaje, W. Levin, H. Yagi, D. M. Jerina and A. H. Conney. "Comparisons of the Tumor-Initiating Activities of Benzo[a]pyrene Arene Oxides and Diol Epoxides," *Cancer Res.* 37: 4130-4133 (1977).
43. Kapitulnik, J., P. G. Wislocki, W. Levin, H. Yagi, D. M. Jerina and A. H. Conney. "Tumorigenicity Studies with Diol-Epoxides of Benzo-[a]pyrene Which Indicate That (±)-*trans*-7β,8α-Dihydroxy-9α,10α-epoxy-7,8,9,10-tetrahydrobenzo[a]pyrene Is an Ultimate Carcinogen in Newborn Mice," *Cancer Res.* 38:354-358 (1978).
44. Wood, A. W., R. L. Chang, W. Levin, R. E. Lehr, M. Schaefer-Ridder, J. M. Karle, D. M. Jerina and A. H. Conney. "Mutagenicity and Cytotoxicity of Benzo[a]anthracene Diol Epoxides and Tetrahydro-epoxides: Exceptional Activity of the Bay Region 1,2-Epoxides," *Proc. Nat. Acad. Sci., U.S.* 74:2746-2750 (1977).
45. Slaga, T. J., E. Huberman, J. K. Selkirk, R. G. Harvey and W. M. Bracken. "Carcinogenicity and Mutagenicity of Benz[a]anthracene Diols and Diol-Epoxides," *Cancer Res.* 38:1699-1704 (1978).
46. Levin, W., D. R. Thakker, A. W. Wood, R. L. Chang, R. E. Lehr, D. M. Jerina and A. H. Conney. "Evidence That Benzo[a]anthracene 3,4-diol-1,2-epoxide Is an Ultimate Carciogen on Mouse Skin," *Cancer Res.* 38:1705-1710 (1978).
47. Wislocki, P. G., M. K. Buening, W. Levin, R. E. Lehr, D. R. Thakker, D. M. Jerina and A. H. Conney. "Tumorigenicity of the Diastereomeric Benz[a]anthracene 3,4-Diol-1,2-epoxides and the (+)- and (–)-Enantiomers of Benz[a]anthracene 3,4-Dihydrodiol in Newborn Mice," *J. Nat. Cancer Inst.* 63:201-204 (1979).
48. Wood, A. W., R. L. Chang, W. Levin, D. G. Ryan, P. E. Thomas, H. Mah, J. M. Karle, H. Yagi, D. M. Jerina and A. H. Conney. "Mutagenicity and Tumorigenicity of Phenanthrene and Chrysene Epoxides and Diol Epoxides," *Cancer Res.* 39:4069-4077 (1979).

# CHAPTER 20

# $^{13}C$ NUCLEAR MAGNETIC RESONANCE STUDIES OF THE STRUCTURE AND STEREOCHEMISTRY OF PRODUCTS DERIVED FROM THE CONJUGATION OF GLUTATHIONE WITH ALKENE AND ARENE OXIDES

**R. H. Cox, O. Hernandez, B. Yagen, B. Smith,**
**J. D. McKinney and J. R. Bend**

Laboratory of Environmental Chemistry and
Laboratory of Pharmacology
National Institute of Environmental
Health Sciences
Research Triangle Park, North Carolina

## INTRODUCTION

It is now widely accepted that the metabolism of chemicals in the body can lead to the formation of both more (metabolic activation) and less toxic compounds (detoxication). There has been increasing evidence presented over the past several years that metabolic activation may be required in the toxic effects produced by many alkenes and aromatic hydrocarbons including the benzenes, naphthalenes and polynuclear aromatics (PAH) such as benzo[a]-pyrene [1-3]. The arene oxides arising by metabolic activation of aromatic hydrocarbons have been implicated as causative agents in mutagenesis, carcinogenesis and tissue necrosis [1,4-7]. These toxic effects are thought to result from the covalent binding of the arene oxides with cellular constituents such as nucleic acids and proteins. [6,7].

The alkene and arene oxides are thought to arise from the action of the cytochrome P-450 monooxygenase system on alkenes and aromatic hydrocarbons, respectively. Once the oxide is formed, it may undergo nonenzymatic rearrangement [3] (to produce phenols in the case of arene oxides), react with epoxide hydrase to form dihydrodiols [7] or react with the glutathione S-transferase enzyme system to produce glutathione derivatives which are further biotransformed to various sulfur-containing conjugates [8]. Although the formation of dihydrodiols may be a detoxication process for certain arene oxides, there is accumulating evidence that further oxidation of selected dihydrodiols to produce diol epoxides may lead to substances more toxic than the original arene oxides [9-13].

The detoxication of alkene and arene oxides by the glutathione S-transferases results in the initial formation of a glutathione (GSH) conjugate (Figure 1). The GSH conjugate may be metabolized further by loss of the glutamic acid residue via a γ-glutamyltransferase (cysteinylglycine conjugate) removal of the glycine (cysteine conjugate) and N-acetylation of the S-substituted cysteine (mercapturic acid [8]. These conjugates may be excreted via the bile, feces and/or as urinary metabolites. Although there has been con-

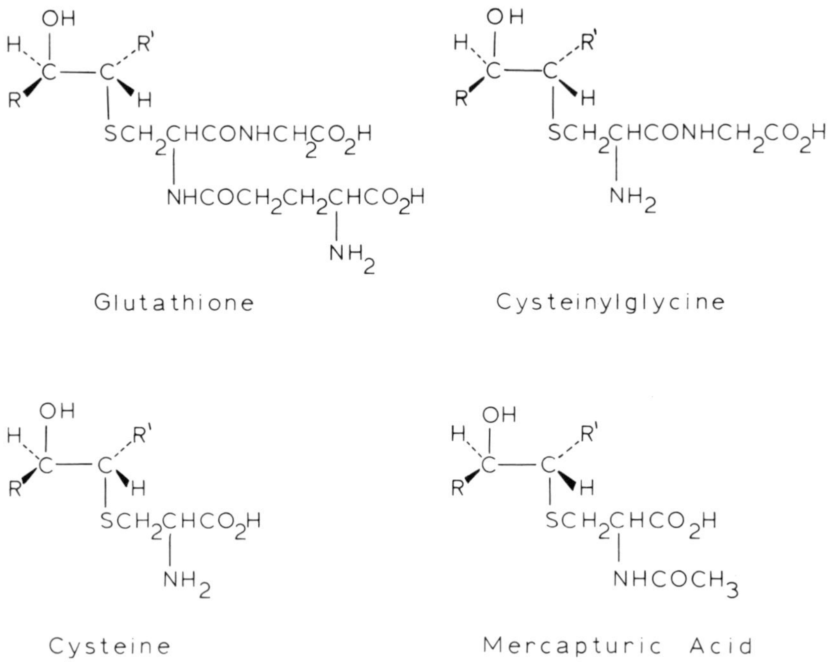


**Figure 1.** Structures of the glutathione conjugate of an epoxide and its possible metabolic products.

siderable effort devoted to investigating the metabolism and excretion of mercapturic acid conjugates of epoxides and the reactions of oxides with model nucleophiles, there has been surprisingly little work on the structure of the GSH conjugates derived from alkene and arene oxides.

In theory, for an unsymmetrical oxide, the addition of the thiol of GSH to an oxide can produce eight possible isomers (Figure 2). Addition can occur at either of the two carbons of the oxide (positional isomers) and the resulting hydroxy and thioether groups may be either *cis* or *trans*. (Studies involving the reaction of arene oxides with model nucleophiles show that the predominant product results from *trans* addition [14-16].) Furthermore because GSH is optically active, each of the possible adducts may exist as a mixture of diastereomers. Studies of the mercapturic acid metabolites isolated from the urine of rats treated with styrene [17] show two major metabolites identified as N-acetyl-S-(1-phenyl-2-hydroxyethyl) cysteine (65%) and N-acetyl-S-(2-phenyl-2-hydroxyethyl) cysteine (34%) and a minor metabolite, N-acetyl-S-(phenacyl) cysteine (1%). The two major metabolites occur as a mixture of diastereoisomers. The excretion of S-(1-phenyl-2-hydroxyethyl) glutathione in the bile from isolated perfused rat liver after infusing with styrene oxide has recently been described [18]. When either 1,2-epoxy-1,2,3,4-tetrahydronaphthalene or 1,2-dihydronaphthalene is administered to rabbits [19], the mecapturic acid N-acetyl-S-(2-hydroxy-1,2,3,4-tetrahydro-1-

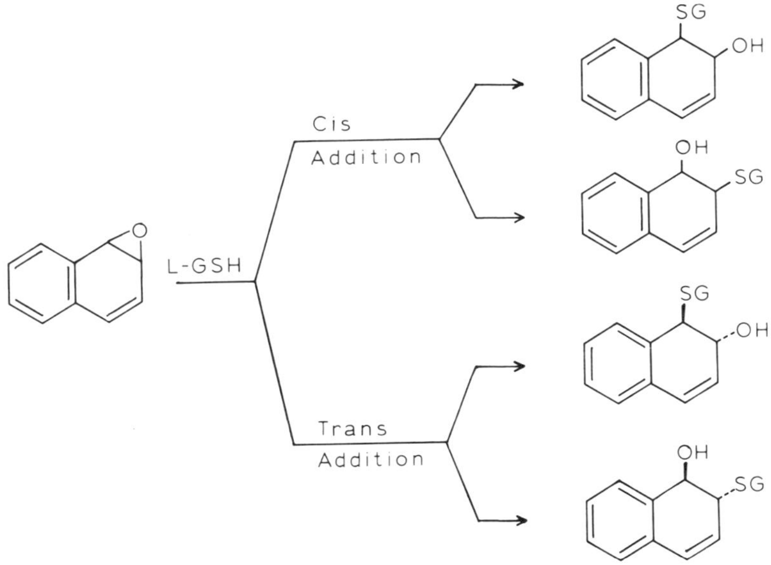


**Figure 2.** Possible products from the conjugation of glutathione (GSH) with an arene oxide. Each of the products can be a mixture of diastereoisomers.

naphthyl) cysteine was excreted in the urine. Rat liver slices have been shown to convert 1,2-dihydronaphthalene into S-(2-hydroxy-1,2,3,4-tetrahydro-1-naphthyl) glutathione [20]. This conjugate was converted into the cysteine conjugate by rat kidney homogenates and into the mercapturic acid by kidney slices. The chemically formed conjugate between naphthalene-1,2-oxide and GSH has been shown recently [21] to result from attack by the thiol at carbon 2, and not at carbon 1 as suggested previously [22]. Because of the lack of data on the structures of the GSH conjugates of epoxides and their metabolites and the prominent role that formation of these conjugates can play in the detoxication of electrophiles, the structures of the GSH conjugates of selected alkene and arene oxides have been investigated with the goal of establishing the ratio of positional isomers and their relative stereochemistry, and of comparing the ratio of products obtained from chemical vs enzymatic conjugation.

Of the various methods available for structural determinations, it appeared that nuclear magnetic resonance (NMR) spectroscopy would yield the most useful information. After several attempts at determining the ratio of positional isomers of the styrene oxide-GSH conjugates using $^{1}$H NMR (these attempts were unsuccessful because of the complexity of the spectra at 100 MHz), the use of $^{13}$C NMR was begun, and it has subsequently been used extensively for this purpose. At first glance, $^{13}$C NMR might not appear to be a suitable method for structural work with metabolites because of its lack of sensitivity. However, recent advances in instrumentation and in the reduction of sample size required have made $^{13}$C NMR on milligram sample sizes relatively routine. Furthermore, $^{13}$C NMR offers several advantages over $^{1}$H NMR that were ideally suited for the needs of this study. First, individual peaks are usually observed for each carbon in the molecule, allowing one to determine if a mixture of positional isomers is present. Second, the "doubling" of peaks from carbon atoms near asymmetric centers allows one to detect the presence of mixtures of diastereoisomers. Finally, the peaks caused by individual isomers are "well-separated" in many cases such that integration of the peak areas is possible, thereby allowing one to quantify the isomers present.

Reported here are $^{13}$C NMR studies of the structure and stereochemistry of both chemically and enzymatically derived GSH conjugates of some alkene and arene oxides.

## EXPERIMENTAL

The methods used to obtain the compounds used in this investigation have been described elsewhere [23]. Samples for NMR analysis were prepared in 5-mm sample tubes using a minimum amount of $D_2O$ as solvent. A small amount of *p*-dioxane was added as an internal reference and chemical shifts were converted to the TMS scale using the relationship $\delta$TMS = $\delta$dioxane + 67.4 ppm. The $^{13}C$ NMR spectra were obtained on a Varian Associates XL-100-12 spectrometer equipped with the 620-L disk data system operating in the Fourier transform mode. Typical parameters used in obtaining the spectra were as follows:

1. spectral width = 5000 Hz;
2. pulse angle = 30°;
3. repetition rate = 2 sec;
4. data points = 8 K;
5. exponential broadening = −0.5;
6. probe temperature = 30°; and
7. 100-Hz square-wave, modulated proton decoupling at 10 W power.

Single-frequency, off-resonance, proton decoupled (SFORD) spectra were obtained by offsetting the decoupler frequency 500 Hz upfield from TMS. Chemical shifts were assigned on the basis of shifts of model compounds, the SFORD spectra and comparison among the compounds examined here.

## RESULTS AND DISCUSSION

### Styrene Oxide

Styrene oxide was chosen for initial study because (1) of the large production of styrene by the chemical industry [24]; (2) styrene is metabolized initially to styrene oxide [25]; (3) styrene has been found as a contaminant in drinking water [26] and cigarette smoke [27]; (4) styrene oxide is used to assay for glutathione S-transferase activity [28,29], and (5) styrene has been shown to be mutagenic in the presence of a microsomal activating system [30]. The 25-MHz natural abundance $^{13}C$ NMR spectrum of the styrene oxide-GSH conjugates derived from chemical synthesis is given in Figure 3A. From the number of peaks present in the spectrum it is obvious that there is more than one compound present. Inspection of the region between 140 and 150 ppm (characteristic of substituted aromatic carbons) reveals at least three peaks, indicating the presence of at least three compounds. The region between 60 and 80 ppm (characteristic of aliphatic carbons attached to one oxygen) also reveals at least three peaks. The SFORD spectrum shows that the peak at ~67 ppm is a methylene ($CH_2$) carbon whereas the peaks at ~75 ppm are caused by a methine (CH) carbon. These results verify the presence of both the possible positional isomers (attachment

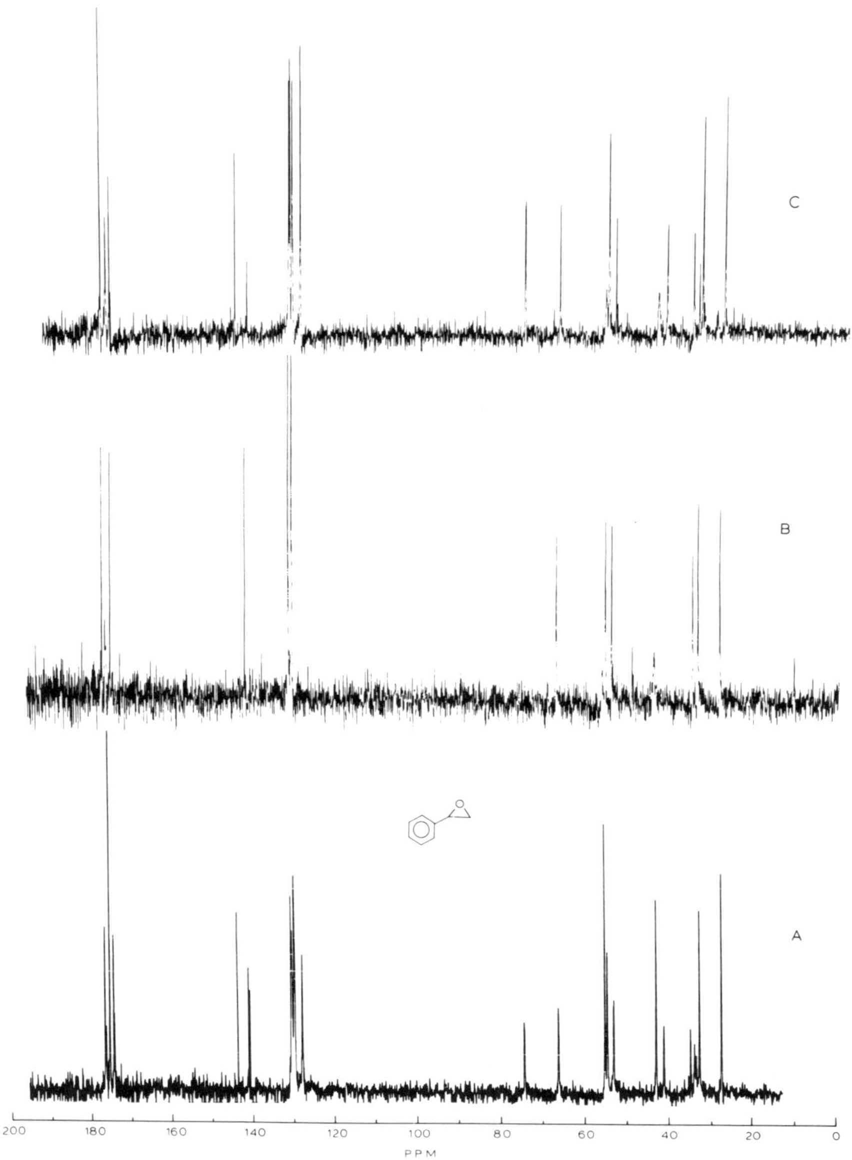


**Figure 3.** $^{13}C$ NMR spectra of the glutathione conjugates derived chemically from styrene oxide: (A) conjugates derived from racemic styrene oxide; (B) one of the benzylic thioether conjugates, peak one from the HPLC separation (see text); and (C) one of the benzylic thioether conjugates and the two primary thioether conjugates, peak two from the HPLC separation.

of sulfur to the carbons of the oxide). The apparent doubling of certain peaks in the spectrum also indicates that each of the positional isomers is present as a mixture of diastereoisomers (Figure 4).

Further experiments were performed to identify the isomers present. Reverse phase, high-pressure liquid chromatography (HPLC) of the above sample separates the components into two peaks. These peaks were collected and their $^{13}$C NMR spectra were examined. The first eluting peak gives a $^{13}$C NMR spectrum (Figure 3B) that indicates the presence of only one isomer. From the SFORD spectrum and chemical shift considerations, it is clear that the first eluting peak in the HPLC separation is one of the diastereoisomers of the benzylic thioether conjugates (Figure 4). The $^{13}$C NMR spectrum of the second eluting peak is given in Figure 3C. Comparison of this spectrum with that from the first eluting peak and with that from the original mixture shows that the second eluting peak contains the other benzylic thioether diastereoisomer and the two diastereoisomers (two peaks at ~75ppm) of the primary thioether (Figure 4).

At this point it was possible to assign the $^{13}$C chemical shifts of the two benzylic thioether conjugates; however, it was not clear as to the assignment of the stereochemistry of these benzylic thioether conjugates. Furthermore,

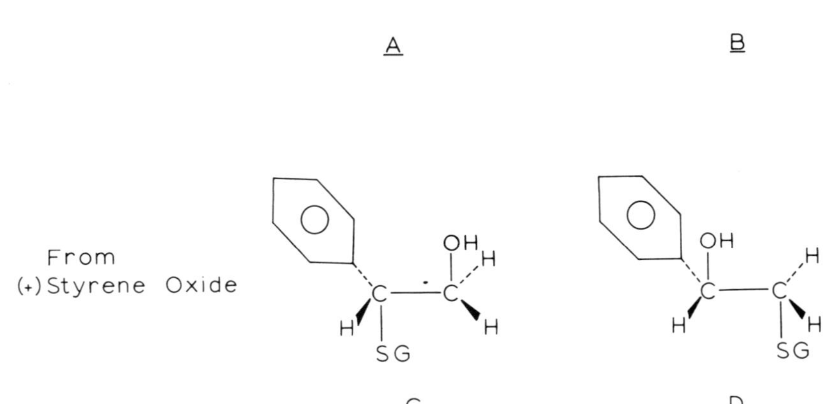


**Figure 4.** Structures of the glutathione conjugates derived from styrene oxide.

the assignment of the primary thioether conjugates was not possible because of the similarity between the chemical shifts of the glutathione part of the conjugates and because the two primary thioether diastereoisomers were present as an equal mixture.

To resolve the above questions, the optically pure isomers of styrene oxide were prepared, and the $^{13}C$ NMR spectra of the GSH conjugates of each of the optically pure isomers of styrene oxide were obtained. The $^{13}C$ spectrum of the GSH conjugates derived from (-) styrene oxide shows the presence of both positional isomers. These isomers separate by HPLC, giving rise to two peaks with identical retention volumes to those observed for the original synthetic mixture (± styrene oxide conjugates). The spectrum of the conjugates derived from (+) styrene oxide also indicates the presence of two positional isomers. These isomers are not separated by HPLC, and give rise to a peak with identical retention volume to the second eluting peak observed for the original mixture.

Thus, the above results demonstrate clearly that both of the possible positional isomers are produced as a mixture of diastereoisomers by the chemical conjugation of styrene oxide with GSH. Chemical shifts for these four isomers are given in Table I. The chemical shifts were assigned using model compounds [31] (*t*-butylthiol derivatives, mercapturic acid conjugates and glutathione), the SFORD spectra and comparison of the spectra obtained from the conjugates derived from the optically pure isomers and the isomers obtained from HPLC separation. With these results in hand, it becomes clear that $^{13}C$ NMR could be used to assay for glutathione S-transferase activity with styrene oxide as a substrate. Either the substituted aromatic carbon peaks (~141 and 144 ppm) or the hydroxyl-bearing aliphatic carbons (~67 and 74 ppm) could be used to determine the presence of positional isomers. The peaks caused by the substituted aromatic carbon of the benzylic thioether (~141 ppm) could be used to determine the relative amounts of the diastereoisomers, whereas the hydroxyl-bearing carbon peaks (~74 ppm) could be used to determine the relative amounts of the diastereoisomers of the primary thioether conjugates.

The GSH conjugates of styrene oxide derived enzymatically using rat liver cytosol were also examined for comparison with those produced synthetically. The $^{13}C$ spectrum shows the presence of both positional isomers as a mixture of diastereoisomers. However, the relative amounts of the positional isomers differ. Integration of either the peaks caused by the substituted aromatic carbons, the protonated aromatic carbons, or the hydroxyl-bearing aliphatic carbons shows that the chemical conjugation results in ~60% relative yield of the benzylic thioether (structure A and C, Fig. 4). Similar integration of the spectrum of the enzymatically produced conjugates shows that the benzylic thioether conjugates are produced in ~90% relative

Table I. $^{13}$C NMR Chemical Shifts of the GSH Conjugates of Styrene Oxide[a]

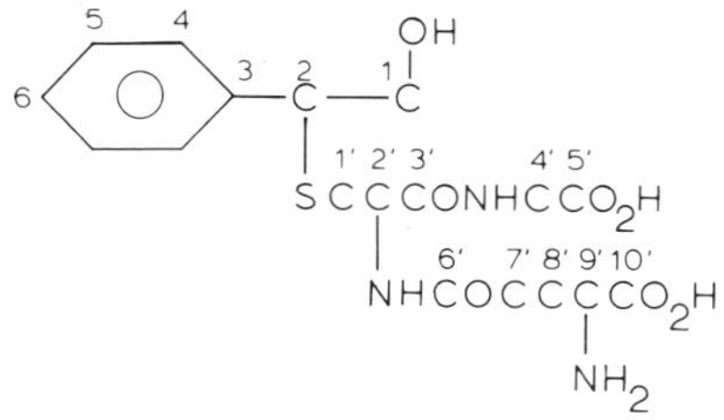

| Carbon/Isomer[b] | A | B | C | D |
|---|---|---|---|---|
| 1 | 67.25 | 42.10 | 66.42 | 41.96 |
| 2 | 54.20 | 74.79 | 53.34 | 74.95 |
| 3 | 141.95 | 144.41 | 140.92 | 144.38 |
| 4 | 131.44 | 128.48 | 130.75 | 128.43 |
| 5 | 130.61 | 131.14 | 129.92 | 130.90 |
| 6 | 130.61 | 130.61 | 129.92 | 129.92 |
| 1′ | 35.08 | 34.98 | 34.11 | 34.59 |
| 2′ | 55.67 | 55.67 | 54.99 | 54.99 |
| 3′ | 174.85 | 174.85 | 173.19 | 173.19 |
| 4′ | 44.24 | 44.24 | 45.29 | 45.29 |
| 5′ | 176.09 | 176.09 | 176.53 | 176.53 |
| 6′ | 176.84 | 176.84 | 177.74 | 177.74 |
| 7′ | 33.82 | 33.83 | 33.43 | 33.43 |
| 8′ | 28.68 | 28.68 | 28.68 | 28.68 |
| 9′ | 56.39 | 56.39 | 56.05 | 56.05 |
| 10′ | 175.92 | 175.92 | 176.53 | 176.53 |

[a]In ppm downfield from TMS.
[b]Structures refer to Figure 4.

yield. Thus, these results show that the enzyme system has a greater preference for attachment of the sulfur at the benzylic carbon. These results are in qualitative agreement with the results of a study where styrene was administered to rats and the mercapturic acids were isolated from the urine [17]. The benzylic thioether mercapturic acid conjugate was produced in 65% relative yield.

The results with styrene oxide suggest that, during the opeining of the epoxide ring, the sulfur of GSH will preferentially become attached to the carbon, resulting in the more stable carbonium ion. To check this observation further and to investigate other structural effects on the conjugation reaction, the conjugation of GSH with *trans*-β-methylstyrene oxide and α-methylstyrene oxide has been studied.

The $^{13}$C NMR spectrum of the chemically derived GSH conjugates of *trans*-β-methylstyrene oxide is given in Figure 5. It is clear from the number

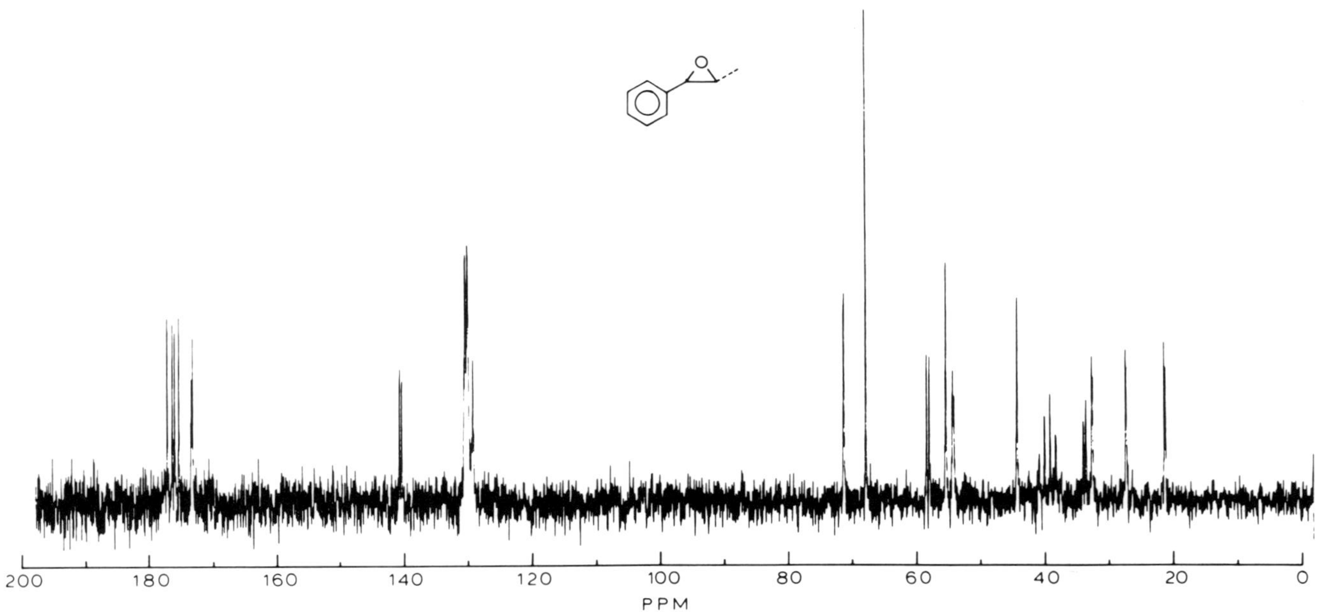


**Figure 5.** $^{13}C$ NMR spectrum of the glutathione conjugates derived chemically from *trans*-β-methylstyrene oxide. The peak at 67.4 ppm is caused by dioxane added as an internal reference.

of peaks present in the spectrum that there are at least two or more isomers present. Closer inspection of the spectrum shows that the two peaks observed for the substituted aromatic carbon (∿140 ppm) are similar to the peaks observed for the benzylic thioether conjugates of styrene oxide. No evidence for peaks similar to those observed for the primary thioether conjugates of styrene oxide (~144 ppm) is observed. Furthermore, the peaks observed for the hydroxyl-bearing carbon (~70 ppm) also indicate the presence of only one of the two possible positional isomers. Thus, the results with *trans*-β-methylstyrene oxide show that only the benzylic thioether GSH conjugates (Figure 6) are produced as a mixture of diastereoisomers. Chemical shift assignments are given in Figure 6. The $^{13}$C NMR spectrum of the GSH conjugates of *trans*-β-methylstyrene oxide derived enzymatically (rat liver

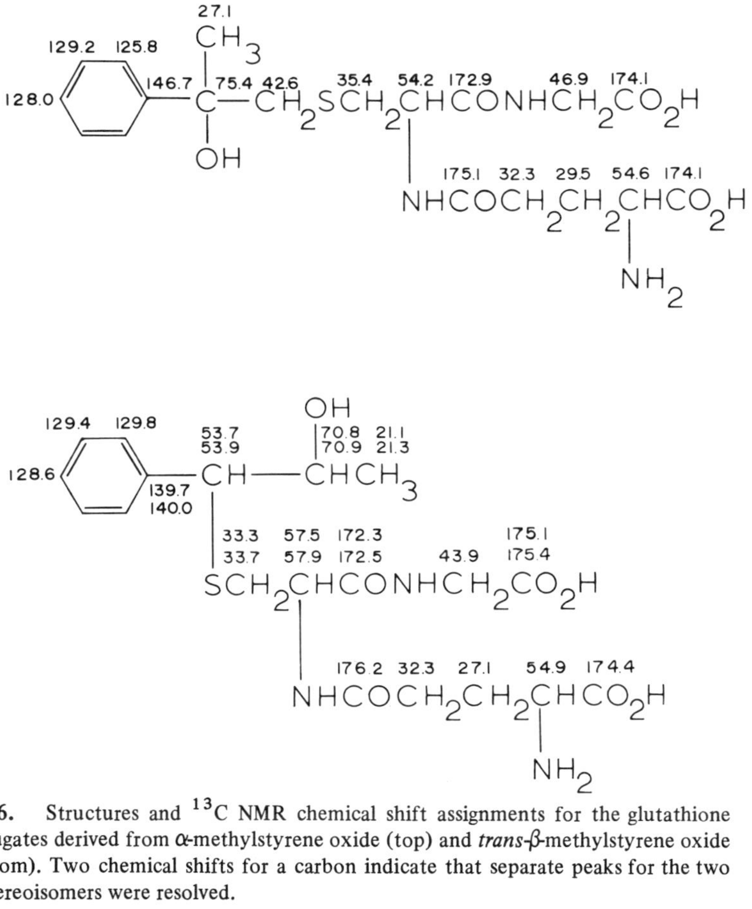

**Figure 6.** Structures and $^{13}$C NMR chemical shift assignments for the glutathione conjugates derived from α-methylstyrene oxide (top) and *trans*-β-methylstyrene oxide (bottom). Two chemical shifts for a carbon indicate that separate peaks for the two diastereoisomers were resolved.

cytosol) is identical to that given by the chemically produced conjugates (Figure 6).

The $^{13}C$ NMR spectrum of the GSH conjugates produced chemically from α-methylstyrene oxide is given in Figure 7. Again, there is only one peak (~146 ppm) for the substituted aromatic carbon. However, in this case, it is in the region where this carbon atom in the primary thioether conjugates of styrene oxide (Figure 1) absorbs. Only one peak is observed for the hydroxyl-bearing aliphatic carbon. These results suggest that only the primary thioether conjugates are formed with α-methylstyrene oxide (Figure 6). This was confirmed by the SFORD spectrum, which shows that the hydroxyl-bearing carbon peak at 75.4 ppm is a quaternary carbon. The spectrum of the enzymatically (rat liver cytosol) produced α-methylstyrene oxide -GSH conjugates is identical to that given in Figure 7 for the conjugates from chemical synthesis. Thus, for α-methylstyrene oxide, both chemical and enzymatic conjugation produces the primary thioether GSH conjugates as a mixture of diastereoisomers.

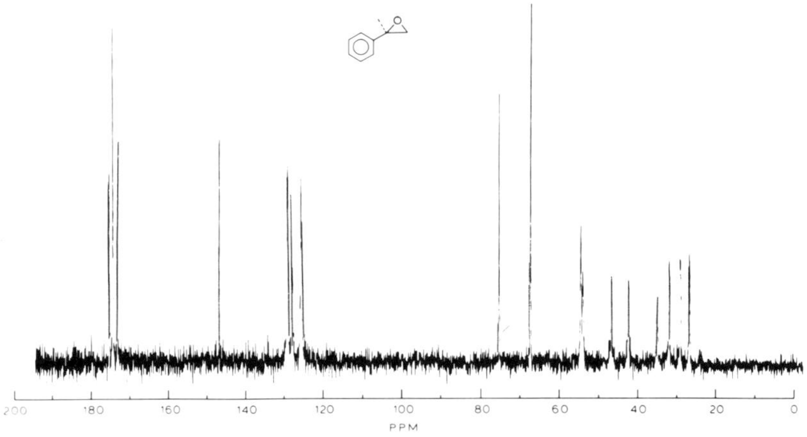


**Figure 7.** $^{13}C$ NMR spectrum of the glutathione conjugates derived chemically from α-methylstyrene oxide. The peak at 67.4 ppm is caused by dioxane added as an internal reference.

The results with the styrene oxides suggest that, all other factors being equal, the enzymatic conjugation will result in products in which the sulfur of GSH becomes attached to the carbon in the epoxide that is capable of forming the more stable carbonium ion on ring opening. It is equally clear that steric factors can reverse this trend. Of the two epoxide carbons in styrene oxide, the benzylic carbon forms the more stable carbonium ion and is also slightly more sterically hindered than the primary carbon. Enzymatic conversion produces ~90% of the benzylic thioether GSH conjugates. For *trans*-β-methylstyrene oxide, the benzylic carbon forms the more stable carbonium ion. In this case the steric hindrance about each of the epoxide carbons is approximately equal. Enzymatic conversion produces only the benzylic thioether conjugates. In the case of α-methylstyrene oxide, again, the benzylic carbon forms the more stable carbonium ion. However, for this epoxide it is clear that the steric hinderance about the benzylic carbon is much greater than that about the primary carbon. Enzymatic conversions produces only the primary thioether conjugates. Therefore, in making predictions about the possible GSH conjugates produced from oxides, both carbonium ion stability and steric factors must be taken into account.

## 1,2,3,4-Tetrahydronaphthalene-1,2-oxide

Boyland and Sims have shown that when rabbits were treated with either 1,2-dihydronaphthalene or 1,2,3,4-tetrahydronaphthalene-1,2-oxide, N-acetyl-S-(2-hydroxy-1,2,3,4-tetrahydro-1-naphthyl)-L-cysteine was present in the urine [19]. Similar experiments using a rat-liver microsomal system produced the above compound in addition to the corresponding GSH conjugate [20]. Experiments with naphthalene resulted in the isolation of 1-naphthylmercapturic acid, and it was suggested that this arose from N-acetyl-S-(1,2-dihydro-2-hydroxy-1-naphthyl)-L-cysteine [22]. More recent experiments with the reaction of 1,2-dihydronaphthalene-1,2-oxide with model nucleophiles suggest that initial attack occurs at the 2-position [21] and not at the 1-position as suggested by the animal experiments [22]. In view of this apparent discrepancy, the GSH conjugation with 1,2,3,4-tetrahydronaphthalene-1,2-oxide has been investigated as a rigid model for the styrene oxides examined.

The $^{13}C$ NMR spectrum of the GSH conjugates produced by chemical synthesis is given in Figure 8. From initial inspection of this spectrum and from the SFORD spectrum, it is clear that only one of the two possible positional isomers is produced as a mixture of diastereoisomers. From $^{13}C$ NMR experiments on model compounds [31], the spectrum in Figure 8 is only consistent with *trans*-S-(1,2,3,4-tetrahydro-2-hydroxy-1-naphthyl)-L-glutathione (Figure 9). Chemical shift assignments are given in Figure 9. It has not been possible to assign absolute stereochemistry to the individual diastereoisomers. However, the mercapturic acid conjugates have been separated [19], and their $^{13}C$ NMR spectra have been obtained. The chemical shift assignments of the peaks in the individual GSH diastereoisomers is based on the corresponding assignments of the mercapturic acid conjugates.

The $^{13}C$ NMR spectrum of the enzymatically (rat-liver cytosol) produced GSH conjugates of 1,2,3,4-tetrahydronaphthalene-1,2-oxide is identical to

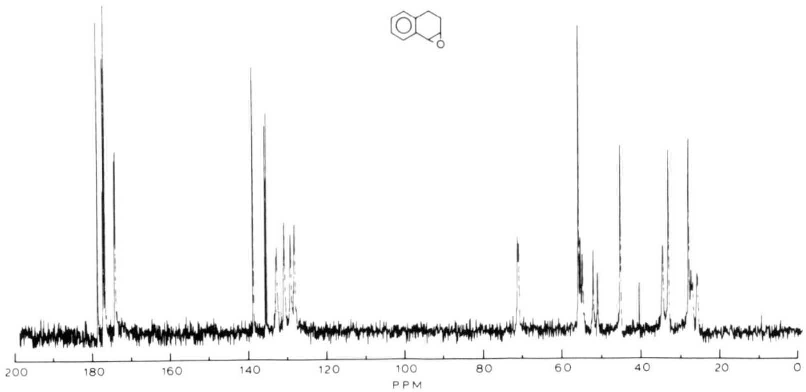


**Figure 8.** $^{13}C$ NMR spectrum of the glutathione conjugates derived chemically from 1,2,3,4-tetrahydronaphthylene-1,2-oxide.

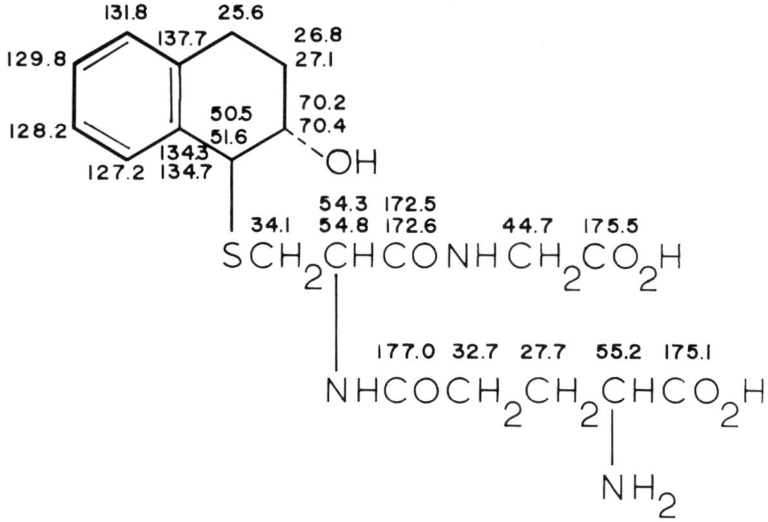


**Figure 9.** Structure and $^{13}C$ chemical shift assignments for the glutathione conjugates of 1,2,3,4-tetrahydronaphthalene-1,2-oxide. Two chemical shifts for a particular carbon are for the two diastereoisomers.

that given in Figure 8. For this oxide, both chemical and enzymatic conjugation produces only the benzylic thioether conjugate as a mixture of *trans*-diastereoisomers. These results are consistent with those reported earlier for animal feeding experiments [19]. The results are also consistent with those found for *trans*-$\beta$-methylstyrene oxide.

## Phenanthrene-9,10-oxide

Boyland and Sims have reported that phenanthrene [32] and phenanthrene-9,10-oxide [33] are converted by rats (urine) into *trans*-9,10-dihydro-9,10-dihydroxyphenanthrene and into one of the diastereoisomers of N-acetyl-S-(9,10-dihydro-9-hydroxy-10-phenanthryl)-L-cyteine (mercapturic acid). Correspondingly, a rat liver homogenate converts the oxide into the corresponding glutathione conjugate. The *n*-butyl ester (the butyl ester was used to aid in the isolation and solubility of the conjugates) of the mercapturic acid conjugates of phenanthrene-9,10-oxide has been examined as a model for the larger polycyclic hydrocarbon arene oxides. Because this is a symmetrical oxide, it was felt that the chemical shift differences observed between this oxide and its conjugates would serve as a useful model for the chemical shifts of the more complicated benzo[a]pyrene conjugates. The $^{13}$C NMR spectrum of the mercapturic acid *n*-butyl ester conjugates of phenanthrene-9,10-oxide prepared by chemical synthesis is given in Figure 10. The doubling of certain peaks in the spectrum (e.g., the hydroxyl-(71 ppm) and thiol-(50 ppm) bearing carbons) shows that the conjugate is produced as a mixture of diastereoisomers as expected. Chemical shift assignments, based on shifts of model compounds [31] and the SFORD

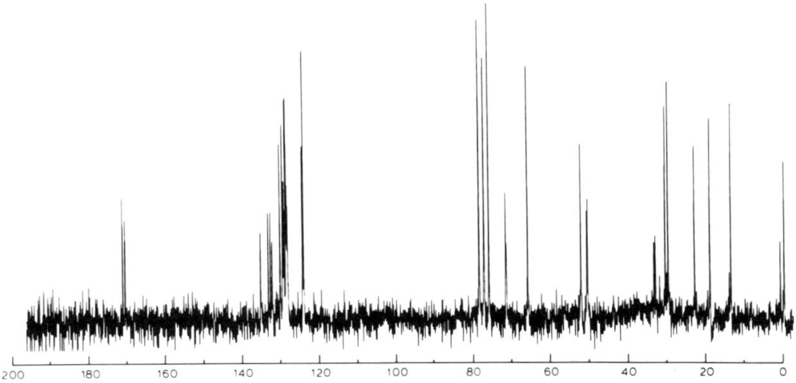


**Figure 10.** $^{13}$C NMR spectrum of the mercapturic acid-butyl ester conjugates derived chemically from phenanthrene-9,10-oxide.

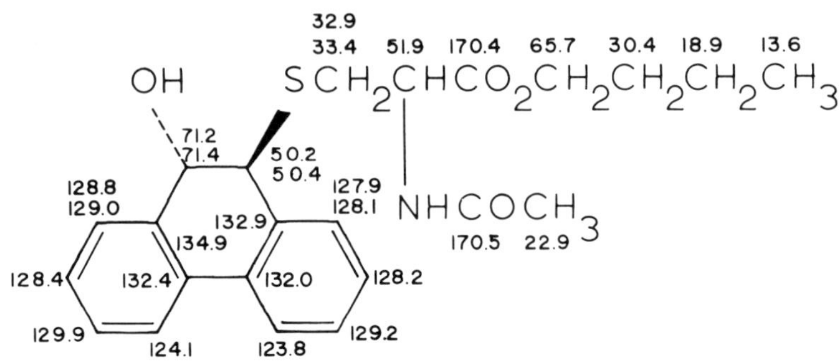


**Figure 11.** Structure and $^{13}$C NMR chemical shift assignments for the mercapturic acid-butyl ester conjugates derived chemically from phenanthrene-9,10-oxide. Two chemical shifts for a particular carbon indicate that separate peaks were resolved for the two diasteroisomers.

spectrum, are given in Figure 11. Interestingly, the *ortho* carbons (C-1 and C-8) also show individual peaks caused by the diastereoisomers. This was not observed for the phenyl carbons of the styrene oxide conjugates or the protonated carbons of the tetrahydronaphthalene oxide conjugates and may reflect the differences between a freely rotating aromatic moiety and a conformationally rigid system. This could be of diagnostic value in assigning the spectra of benzo[a]pyrene thioether conjugates.

In the reported animal experiments with this oxide, only one of the mercapturic acid diastereoisomers was isolated in the urine [32,33]. This is in contrast to the results with styrene oxide where both diastereoisomers were isolated [17]. Whether the differences observed for these two oxides represents a difference between alkene and arene oxides or a difference in the excretion and/or metabolism of the phenanthrene conjugates awaits further experimentation.

## Pyrene-4,5-oxide

When either rats or rabbits were treated with pyrene, the sulfuric acid and glucuronic acid conjugates of 1-hydroxypyrene, 1,6- and 1,8-dihydroxypyrene and *trans*-4,5-dihydro-4,5-dihydroxypyrene, together with the mercapturic acid conjugate resulting from the 4,5-oxide, were found in the urine [34]. The mercapturic acid *n*-butyl ester conjugates derived chemically from pyrene-4,5-oxide were examined. The doubling of peaks (Figure 12) for the hydroxyl-bearing carbon (71 ppm) and the thiol-bearing carbon (50 ppm) indicate that a mixture of diastereoisomers is formed in this reaction. Partial

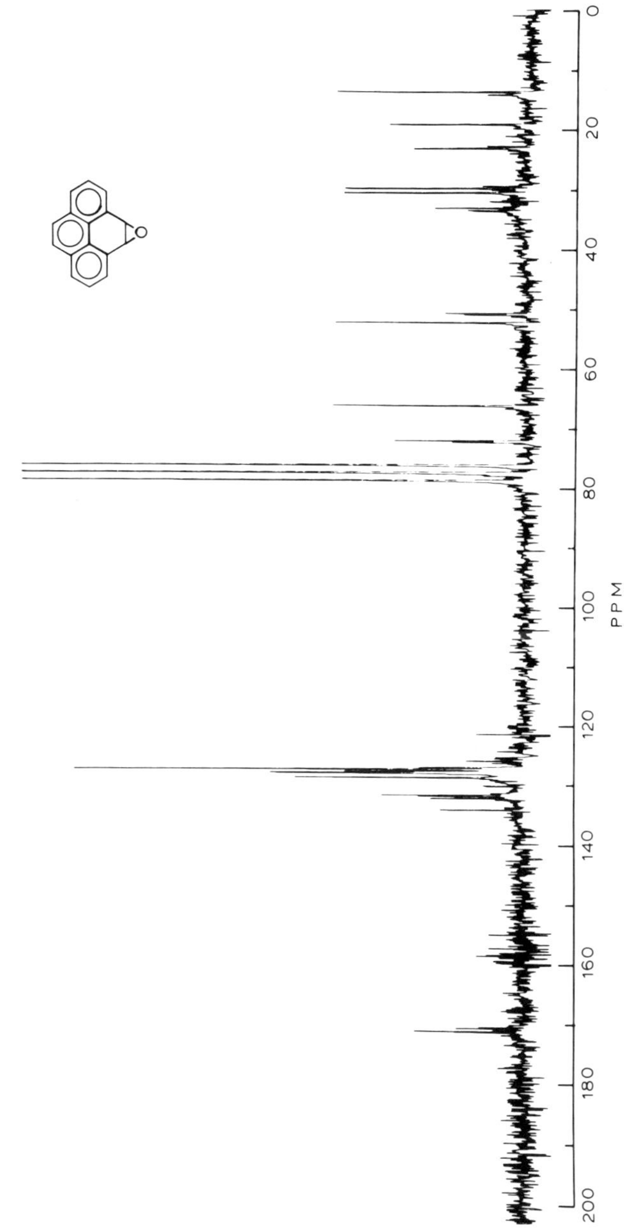


**Figure 12.** $^{13}$C NMR spectrum of the mercapturic acid-butyl ester conjugates derived chemically from pyrene-4,5-oxide.

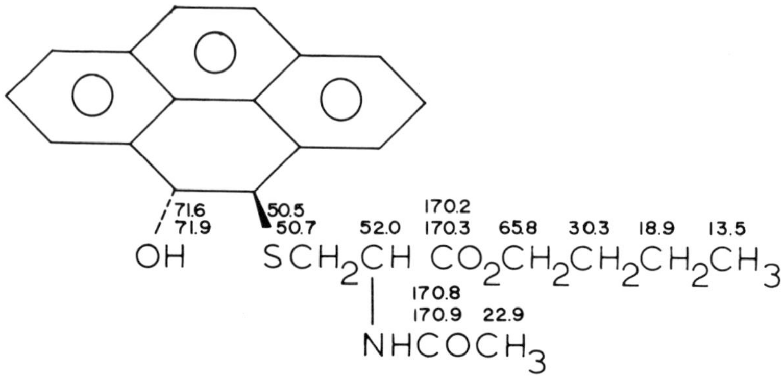


**Figure 13.** Structure and partial assignment of the $^{13}C$ NMR chemical shifts of the mercapturic acid-butyl ester conjugates derived chemically from pyrene-4,5-oxide.

assignment of the peaks is given in Figure 13. Because of the complexity of the resonances contributed by the aromatic carbons, it has not been possible at this point to assign completely all the peaks for these carbons.

### Benzo[a]pyrene-4,5-oxide

Previous studies with benzo[a]pyrene-4,5-oxide using rat and human hepatic glutathione s-transferases [35] and isolated perfused rat liver [36] have shown that GSH conjugates are formed. Preliminary studies of the $^{13}C$ NMR spectrum of the GSH conjugates of benzo[a]pyrene-4,5-oxide derived from chemical synthesis suggest that both positional isomers (4 and 5 thioether) are formed as a mixture of diastereoisomers. Furthermore, HPLC studies indicate that it may be possible to separate the positional isomers. Similar studies of the enzymatically (rat liver cytosol) produced GSH conjugates also suggest that both positional isomers are formed as a mixture of diastereoisomers. Further work with this oxide is in progress and will be reported at a later date.

## SUMMARY

The results presented here suggest a close parallel between the structure of the GSH conjugates derived chemically and enzymatically. In only one case (styrene oxide) did the product ratio vary significantly between the enzymatic and nonenzymatic conjugation reactions. In terms of predicting the structure of the products, it is clear that both carbonium ion stability and steric factors must be considered (*trans*-$\beta$-methylstyrene oxide vs $\alpha$-methylstyrene oxide). Whether this is a result of substrate binding to the transferases or other factors awaits further study. One final word of caution should be mentioned. The results presented here show that, substrate permitting, the GSH conjugates are formed as a mixture of diastereoisomers. In each case examined so far there appeared to be a 50-50 mixture of the diastereoisomers. However, this may not always be the case [32, 33] for the mercapturic acid conjugates isolated from urine. Different rates of metabolism of the GSH conjugates and/or different rates of excretion, and fractionation during the workup procedure may lead to the selective isolation of only one of the two possible diastereoisomers. This possibility should be kept in mind when drawing mechanistic conclusions from such urinary metabolite studies.

## ACKNOWLEDGMENTS

We wish to acknowledge the support of the U.S. Environmental Protection Agency under an interagency agreement relating to the Federal Interagency Energy/Environmental Research and Development Program.

## REFERENCES

1. Miller, E. C., and J. A. Miller. "Biochemical Mechanisms of Chemical Carcinogenesis," in *Molecular Biology of Cancer*, H. Busch, Ed. (New York: Academic Press, Inc., 1974), pp. 377-402.
2. Heidelberger, C. "Chemical Carcinogenesis," *Ann. Rev. Biochem.* 44:79-121 (1975).
3. Daly, J. W., D. M. Jerina and B. Witkop. "Arene Oxides and the NIH Shift: The Metabolism, Toxicity and Carcinogenicity of Aromatic Compounds," *Experientia* 28:1129-1149 (1972).
4. Miller, J. A. "Carcinogenesis by Chemicals: An Overview," *Cancer Res.* 30:559-576 (1970).
5. Gelboin, H. V., N. Kinoshita and F. J. Wiebel. "Microsomal Hydroxylases: Induction and Role in Polycyclic Hydrocarbons Carcinogenesis and Toxicity," *Fed. Proc.* 31: 1298-1309 (1972).
6. Sims, P., and P. L. Grover. "Epoxides in Polycyclic Aromatic Hydrocarbon Metabolism and Carcinogenesis," *Adv. Cancer Res.* 20:165-274 (1974).
7. Jerina, D. M., and J. W. Daly. "Arene Oxides: A New Aspect of Drug Metabolism," *Science* 185:573-582 (1974).
8. Jerina, D. M., and J. R. Bend. "Glutathione S-transferases," in *Biological Reactive Intermediates,* D. J. Jallow, J. J. Kocsis, R. Snyder and H.

Vainio, Eds. (New York: Plenum Publishing Corporation, 1977), pp. 207-236.

9. Weinstein, I. B., A. M. Jeffrey, K. W. Jennette, S. H. Blobstein, R. G. Harvey, C. Harris, H. Autrup, H. Kasai and K. Nakanishi. "Benzy[a]-pyrene Diol Epoxides as Intermediates in Nucleic Acid Binding *in vitro* and *in vivo*," *Science* 193:592-594 (1976).
10. Jeffrey, A. M., K. W. Jennette, S. H. Blobstein, I. B. Weinstein, F. A. Beland, R. G. Harvey, H. Kasai, I. Miura and K. Nakauishi. "Benzo[a]-pyrene-Nucleic Acid Derivative Found *in Vivo*: Structure of a Benzo[a]-pyrenetetrahydrodiol Epoxide-Guanosine Adduct," *J. Am. Chem. Soc.* 98:5714-5715 (1976).
11. Koreeda, M., P. D. Moore, H. Yagi, H. J. C. Yeh and D. M. Jerina. "Alkylation of Polyguanylic Acid at the 2-Amino Group and Phosphate by the Potent Mutagen (±) 7β,8α-Dihydroxy-9β, 10β-epoxy-7,8,9,10-tetrahydrobenzo[a]pyrene," *J. Am. Chem. Soc.* 98:6720-6722 (1976).
12. Wislocki, P. G., A. W. Wood, R. L. Chang, W. Levine, H. Yagi, O. Hernandez, D. M. Jerina and A. H. Conney. "High Mutagenicity and Toxicity of a Diol Epoxide Derived From Benzo[a]pyrene," *Biochem. Biophys. Res. Comm.* 68:1006-1012 (1976).
13. Regan, J. D., A. A. Francis, W. C. Dunn, O. Hernandez, H. Yagi, and D. M. Jerina. "Repair of DNA Damaged by Mutagenic Metabolites of Benzo-[a]pyrene in Human Cells," *Chem.-Biol. Interact.* 20:279-287 (1978).
14. Bruice, P. Y., T. C. Bruice, H. Yagi and D. M. Jerina. "Nucleophilic Displacement on the Arene Oxides of Phenanthrene," *J. Am. Chem. Soc.* 98:2973-2981 (1976).
15. Jeffrey, A. M., H. J. Yeh, D. M. Jerina, R. M. DeMarinis, C. H. Foster, D. E. Piccolo and G. A. Berchtall. "Stereochemical Course in Reactions Between Nucleophiles and Arene Oxides," *J. Am. Chem. Soc.* 96:6929-6937 (1974).
16. Beland, F. A., and R. G. Harvey. "Reactions of the K-Region Oxides of Carcinogenic and Related Polycyclic Hydrocarbons with Nucleophiles: Stereochemistry and Regioselectivity," *J. Am. Chem. Soc.* 98:4963-4970 (1976).
17. Seutter-Berlage, F., L. P. C. Delbressine, F. L. M. Smeets and H. C. J. Ketelaars. "Identification of Three Sulphur-Containing Urinary Metabolites of Styrene in the Rat," *Xenobiotica* 8:413-418 (1978).
18. Ryan, A. J., and J. R. Bend. "The Metabolism of Styrene Oxide in the Isolated Perfused Rat Liver, Identification and Quantitation of Major Metabolites," *Drug Metab. Disp.* 5:363-367 (1977).
19. Boyland, E., and P. Sims. "Metabolism of Polycyclic Compounds 16. The Metabolism of 1,2-Dihydronaphthalene and 1,2-Epoxy-1,2,3,4-tetrahydronaphthalene," *Biochem. J.* 77:175-181 (1960).
20. Booth, J., E. Boyland, T. Sato and P. Sims. "Metabolism of Polycyclic Compounds 17. The Reaction of 1,2-Dihydronaphthalene and 1,2-Epoxy-1,2,3,4-tetrahydronaphthalene with Glutathione Catalyzed by Tissue Preparations," *Biochem. J.* 77:182-186 (1960)
21. Jeffery, A. M., and D. M. Jerina. "Novel Rearrangements During Dehydration of Nucleophilic Adducts of Arene Oxides. A Reappraisal of Premercapturic Acid Structures," *J. Am. Chem. Soc.* 97:4427-4428 (1975).

22. Boyland, E., and P. Sims. "Metabolism of Polycyclic Compounds 12. An Acid-Labile Precursor of 1-Naphthylmercapturic Acid and Naphthol: An N-Acetyl-S-(1,2-dihydrohydroxynaphthyl)-L-cysteine," *Biochem. J.* 68:440-447 (1958).
23. Hernandez, O., B. Yagen, R. H. Cox, B. Smith, G. Foureman, J. R. Bend and J. D. McKinney. "Stereospecificity and Regioselectivity in the Reaction of Epoxides with Glutathione," Chapter 21, this volume.
24. "Styrene," *Chem. Eng. News.* (July 24, 1978) p. 11.
25. Leibman, K. C., and E. Ortiz. "Epoxide Intermediates in Microsomal Oxidation of Olefins to Glycols." *J. Pharmacol. Exp. Ther.* 173:242-246 (1970).
26. Dowty, B. J., D. R. Carlisle and J. L. Laseter. "New Orleans Drinking Water Sources Tested by Gas Chromatography-Mass Spectrometry, Occurrence and Origin of Aromatics and Halogenated Aliphatic Hydrocarbons." *Environ. Sci. Technol.* 9:762-765 (1975).
27. Loprieno, N., A. Abbondandolo, R. Barole, S. Baroncelli, S. Bonatti, G. Bronzetti, A. Cammellini, C. Corsi, G. Corti, D. Frezza, C. Leparini, A. Mazzaccaro, R. Nieri, D. Rosellini and A. M. Rossi. "Mutagenicity of Industrial Compounds: Styrene and Its Metabolite Styrene Oxide," *Mutat. Res.* 40:317-324 (1976).
28. Hayakawa, T., R. A. Lemahieu and S. Udenfriend. "Studies on Glutathione-S-arene Oxide Transferase: A Sensitive Assay and Partial Purification of the Enzyme from Sheep Liver," *Arch. Biochem. Biophys.* 162: 223-230 (1974).
29. Hayakawa, T., S. Udenfriend, H. Yagi and D. M. Jerina. "Substrates and Inhibitors of Hepatic Glutathione-S-epoxide Transferase," *Arch. Biochem. Biophys.* 170:438-451 (1975).
30. Milvy, P., and A. J. Garro. "Mutagenic Activity of Styrene Oxide (1,2-Epoxyethylbenzene), a Presumed Styrene Metabolite," *Mutat. Res.* 40:15-18 (1976).
31. Cox R. H. Unpublished results.
32. Boyland, E., and P. Sims. "Metabolism of Polycyclic Compounds 20. The Metabolism of Phenanthreme in Rabbits and Rats: Mercapturic Acids and Related Compounds," *Biochem. J.* 84:564-570 (1962).
33. Boyland, E., and P. Sims. "Metabolism of Polycyclic Compounds: The Metabolism of 9,10-Epoxy-9,10-dihydrophenanthrene in Rats," *Biochem. J.* 95:788-792 (1965).
34. Boyland, E., and P. Sims. "Metabolism of Polycyclic Compounds 23. The Metabolism of Pyrene in Rats and Rabbits," *Biochem. J.* 90:391-398 (1964).
35. Nemoto, N., H. V. Gelboin, W. H. Habig, J. N. Ketley and W. B. Jakoby. "K Region Benzo[a]pyrene-4,5-oxide is Conjugated by Homogeneous Glutathione S-Transferase," *Nature* 255:512 (1975).
36. Smith, B. R., and J. R. Bend. "Metabolism and Excretion of Benzo[a]-pyrene 4,5-Oxide by the Isolated Perfused Rat Liver," *Cancer Res.* 39: 2051-2056 (1979).

# CHAPTER 21

# STEREOSPECIFICITY AND REGIOSELECTIVITY IN THE REACTION OF EPOXIDES WITH GLUTATHIONE

**O. Hernandez, B. Yagen, R. H. Cox, B. R. Smith, G. L. Foureman, J. R. Bend and J. D. McKinney**

Laboratory of Environmental Chemistry and Laboratory of Pharmacology
National Institute of Environmental Health Sciences
Research Triangle Park, North Carolina

## INTRODUCTION

The oxidative metabolism of alkenes and arenes is known to proceed by formation of epoxides in a reaction mediated by the cytochrome P-450-dependent monooxygenase system [1]. This process, which has been referred to as Phase I metabolism, precedes another important aspect of drug metabolism, the conjugation and subsequent excretion (Phase II) of the primary metabolites [2] (Figure 1). Conjugation with glutathione is a major detoxication process for many electrophilic metabolites [3].

The conjugation of epoxides with glutathione ($\gamma$-glutamylcysteinylglycine [GSH]) is well documented [4]. The pioneering work of Boyland, Sims and co-workers has contributed much of the information available on the chemistry of these thioether conjugates [5]. In parallel experiments they demonstrated the in vivo formation of thioether metabolites from several hydrocarbons [6], which were thought to arise via arene oxide intermediates.

The reaction of GSH with epoxides and other electrophiles is catalyzed by a group of cytosolic, and to a lesser extent microsomal, enzymes known

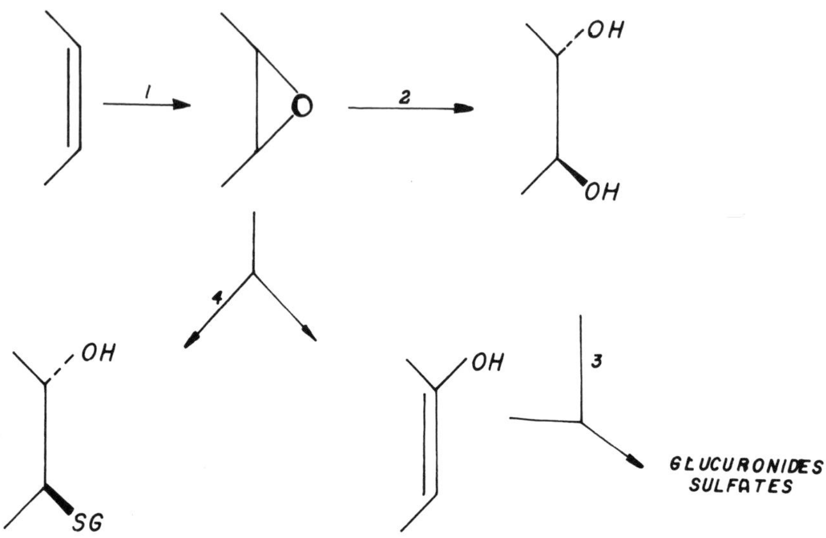


**Figure 1.** Representative biotransformation of an unsaturated compound. Phase I metabolism: (1) cytochrome P-450-dependent monooxygenase system; (2) epoxide hydrase; Phase II metabolism: (3) glucuronyl transferases; (4) glutathione S-transferases or sulfatransferases.

as the glutathione-S-transferases. Several of these proteins have been isolated and purified from different sources [7-9]. The pure enzymes isolated from rat liver have broad and overlapping substrate specificities [10]. The rates of catalysis of these enzymes in the conjugation of GSH with electrophiles are generally low, compared to other enzymatic reactions. This low level of activity, coupled with the high chemical reactivity and the natural abundance of GSH in tissues, has led to the suggestion that some of the GSH conjugates formed in vivo are produced in nonenzymatic reactions. The relative contribution of enzymatic and nonenzymatic conjugation with glutathione obviously depends on epoxide electrophilic reactivity and glutathione transferase specificity. The formation of GSH conjugates represents the first step in the in vivo excretion of many xenobiotics [3]. The intact conjugate is often eliminated in the bile, and undergoes further metabolism involving hydrolysis of the glutamic acid and glycine residues followed by N-acetylation of the S-substituted cysteine residue. These latter compounds (N-acetylcysteines) are commonly known as mercapturic acids and are excreted primarily in the urine (Figure 2) [11].

The participation of GSH in the detoxication and elimination of reactive intermediary metabolites stimulated interest in the chemistry of xenobiotic reaction products with this tripeptide. Since the chemical characterization of these types of thioether compounds has been rather fragmentary, the

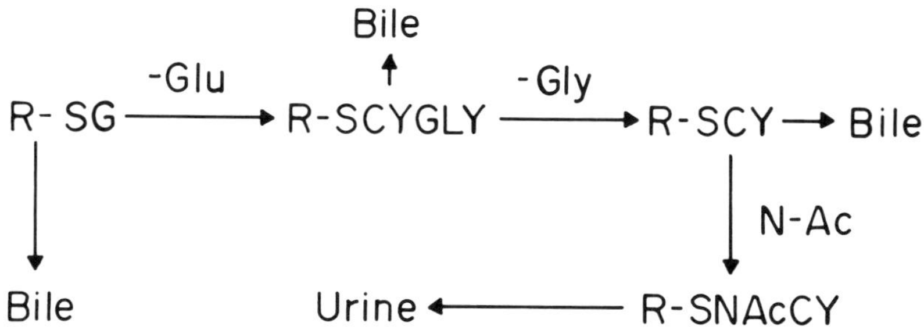


**Figure 2.** Biosynthesis of mercapturic acids (R-SNAcCy) from glutathione conjugates (R-SG) and predominant excretion routes for thioether metabolites.

initial approach was to prepare synthetic and biosynthetic samples of GSH conjugates and related thioether metabolites in sufficient quantities and purity to allow structural characterization.

As discussed in the preceding chapter, styrene oxide was chosen for good reasons as an important substrate for detailed investigation [12-16]. However, a complicating feature associated with styrene oxide is the inherent asymmetry of its oxirane ring. On reaction with GSH, two positional isomers are possible (Figure 3). Because of the chiral nature of the peptide moiety, each isomer will consist of a pair of diastereoisomers. In fact, a recent report describes the isolation of diastereomeric mixtures of mercapturic acids as urinary metabolites of styrene oxide in the rat [16]. For the above reasons, it was necessary to develop techniques to separate mixtures of isomeric glutathione conjugates, as well as to develop procedures for their synthesis. Once an efficient separation procedure was developed, the unsymmetrical nature of styrene oxide could be exploited, and the stereochemical preferences of some glutathione S-transferase enzymes could be studied.

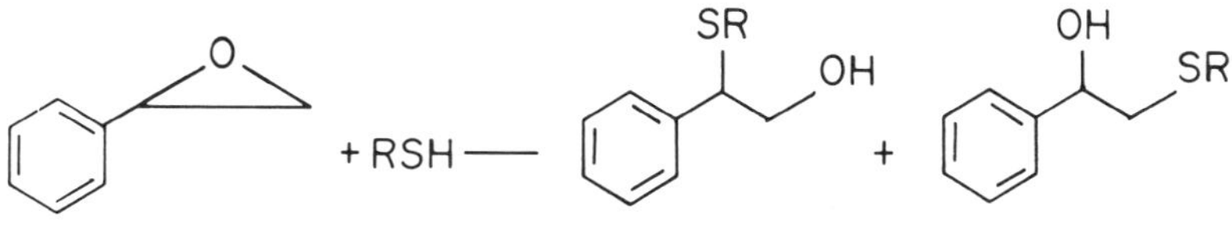


1 2

**Figure 3.** Reaction of styrene oxide with a thiol nucleophile to yield positional isomers, showing benzylic thioether (1) and benzylic alcohol (2) isomers.

## EXPERIMENTAL

### Spectral Determinations

A detailed description of the $^{13}C$ nuclear magnetic resonance (NMR) chemical shift assignments is given elsewhere in this volume [17]. Mass spectra were determined using direct probe insert samples in the chemical ionization mode with isobutane as reagent gas. All samples examined showed fragmentation patterns consistent with their structure.

### Synthesis

#### *Water-Soluble Epoxides*

An aqueous solution of GSH (1.2 equivalents) adjusted to pH 7-7.5 with NaOH was allowed to react with the epoxide under argon for 24 hr at room temperature. After acidification (pH 3.5) and extraction with ethyl acetate, the aqueous solution was adsorbed in a column packed with XAD-2 resin or C-18 bulk packing (37-75 $\mu$m Applied Science Laboratories, Inc.). Elution with water removed unchanged thiol amino acid and further elution with methanol provided the pure thioether conjugate.

#### *Phase-Transfer Preparation of Mercapturic Acids*

A solution of N-acetylcysteine (3 equivalents) and tetrabutylammonium bisulfate (4 equivalents) adjusted to pH 9-10 with NaOH was mixed with a chloroform solution of the epoxide substrate and the mixture was refluxed for 5-8 hr under argon. 1-Bromobutane (15-20 equivalents) was added and reflux continued for 4 hr. Aqueous workup gave a chloroform solution of the mercapturic acid butyl ester. Purification was accomplished by silica gel chromatography.

### Chromatography

Reverse-phase separations were carried out using a Waters Associates liquid chromatograph equipped with M6000A pumps, M660 programmer, U6K injector and a 440 ultraviolet (UV) detector. The column used was a $\mu$-Bondapak C-18 (0.39 $\times$ 30 cm), and peaks were monitored at 254 nm. Silica gel purifications were carried out in a Waters Associates Prep-500 liquid chromatograph equipped with refractive index and fixed wavelength ultraviolet (UV) (254 nm) detectors. The solvent system for the purification of esterified mercapturic acids was dichloromethane:ether (3:2 v/v).

### Enzymatic Incubations

The enzymatic conjugation of GSH with the epoxide substrates was performed with rat liver cytosol or purified skate liver transferase preparations according to established procedures [18,19]. The incubation conditions were adjusted to maximize formation of the glutathione conjugates and did not always give linear product formation.

## RESULTS AND DISCUSSION

### Synthesis and Purification

The preparation of glutathione conjugates from low-molecular-weight epoxides proceeds smoothly in aqueous solution. A small volume (1-2%) of organic solvent may be added in some cases to aid solubility of the epoxide. The preferred pH range for the reaction is 7-7.5. Reaction times are considerably shorter at higher pH (>9) but the quality of the products isolated suffers as compared to reactions at pH 7.5. The only water-soluble contaminant present at the end of the reaction is unchanged thiol and some oxidized glutathione. Purification of the glutathione derivative is readily achieved by adsorption on a column packed with XAD-2 resin or C-18 bonded phase (37-75 $\mu$m). Elution with water removes the amino acid and the desired conjugate is subsequently eluted with methanol. The conjugates eluting from the column are pure enough for spectral determinations and biological studies. This general procedure has also been applied to the preparation of cysteine, cysteinylglycine and N-acetylcysteine conjugates.

The synthesis of conjugates from higher-molecular-weight epoxides, particularly polycyclic arene oxides, by the above procedure is not entirely satisfactory. The solubility of these oxiranes in water is minimal requiring much larger concentrations of organic solvent ($\sim$50%) to achieve acceptable substrate concentrations in solution. This in turn is incompatible with dissociation of the thiol component, which itself is sparingly soluble in organic solvents. Despite these limitations, successful preparations of thioether adducts of arene oxides in mixed aqueous solution have been reported for GSH [20,21], N-acetylcysteine [20,21], cysteine [20-22] and model thiol nucleophiles [23-26]. However, structural parameters were not reported in detail with the exception of the model compounds, whose structures are fully documented [23-26].

An alternative approach which overcomes the contrasting solubility properties of thiol and substrate is the use of a phase-transfer procedure [27]. In this technique, anions generated in aqueous solution are transported to an organic phase by using a phase-transfer agent. The alkylation of these anions takes place in the organic phase or at the interface of the two-phase solvent system. In the work reported here, the use of tetrabutylammonium salts in combination with N-acetylcysteine has proved an efficient method for the preparation of mercapturic acid derivatives. The concept is illustrated in Figure 4. Purification of the mercapturic acid products is facilitated by esterification of the reaction mixture with 1-bromobutane. The resulting butyl esters are easily separated by silica gel chromotography from the side products S-butyl-N-acetylcysteine butylester and *bis*-N-acetylcysteine dibutylester. Yields obtained for the reaction are good (40–55%) considering that two steps are involved (Figure 5).

## Product Analysis

The reaction of GSH with styrene oxide produced, as anticipated, a mixture of positional isomers resulting from addition of the thiol group to either C-1 (carbon-bearing phenyl substituent) or C-2 (see Figure 3). The $^{13}C$ NMR analysis which allowed identification of these compounds is discussed elsewhere in this volume [17]. Integration of the $^{13}C$ NMR signals provided a 6:4 ratio for the benzylic thioether (attack of thio at C-1)

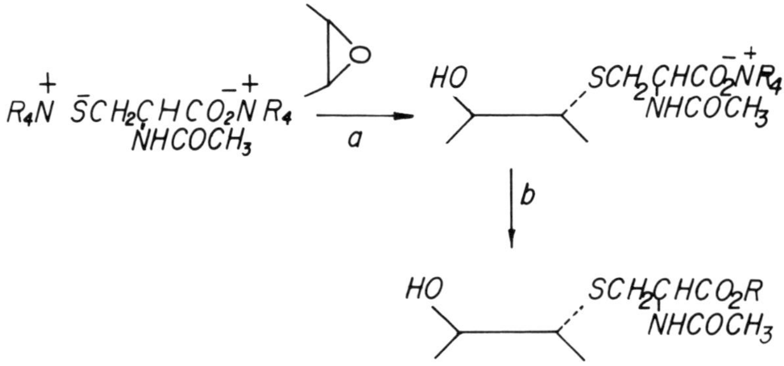


**Figure 4.** Phase-transfer synthesis of mercapturic acid *n*-butyl esters from alkene and arene oxides; (a) water-chloroform, pH 10, 56°C; (b) 1-bromobutane, 56°C, R = *n*-butyl, $R_4N$ = tetra-*n*-butylammonium ion.

and benzylic alcohol (attack at C-2) isomers. Additionally, the doubling of certain signals in the $^{13}C$ NMR spectrum clearly showed the presence of diastereomers for each positional isomer. A mixture of these isomers was not separated on silica gel thin-layer plates. The use of reverse-phase high-pressure liquid chromatography (HPLC) has been reported for the separation of underivatized peptides [28] and it seemed ideally suited for this analytical problem.

The use of an ion suppression system consisting of acetic acid (pH 3.4) or phosphoric acid (pH 2.2) solutions with various amounts of methanol was initially explored. The GSH conjugates of styrene oxide were adequately retained in a C-18 reverse phase column by using the above solvents. The acetic acid eluent gave two partly resolved peaks while at the lower pH baseline separation was obtained (Figure 6). Unfortunately, at pH $<3$, the conjugates proved unstable and partially decomposed during HPLC analysis.

By buffering the phosphoric acid solution with triethylamine the operating pH was increased to 3-3.5 without loss in resolution [29]. The efficiency of this alkylammonium buffer may be partly caused by ion pairing with the amine and carboxyl functions (Figure 6).

Integration of the chromatographic signals gave a relative ratio of 4:6 for the first and second eluting peaks, in apparent agreement with the values obtained from the $^{13}C$ NMR spectrum. However, after preparative separation of the styrene oxide conjugates, it was established that the first eluting peak consisted of a single compound, a diastereomer of benzylic thioether 1 (Figure 3). The second peak consisted of the second diastereomer of 1 and the two diastereomeric benzylic alcohols 2. Separation of diastereomeric peptides by HPLC is not without precedent [29,30]; the failure to separate the positional isomers 1 and 2 emerging in the second eluting peak is more surprising.

Examination of samples of chemically synthesized cysteinylglycine and cysteine conjugates as described above showed a similar pattern of stereoisomer distribution, a major difference being that the first eluting peaks contained the benzyl alcohol diastereomers (2) and one diastereomeric thioether 1, while the late eluting peaks contained a single diastereomeric benzyl thioether 1 (Figure 3).

Attempts to separate the corresponding N-acetylcysteine conjugates of styrene oxide in the reverse phase system were not entirely successful. However, on esterification with diazomethane the mixture of methyl esters was resolved into three components by silica gel chromatography (Figure 7A). The first peak was identified as the two benzyl alcohol stereoisomers 2 and the other two fractions each contained a single diastereomer of the benzyl thioether isomer 1. Previous workers had succeeded in separating only the positional isomers contained in this particular mixture [16]. The

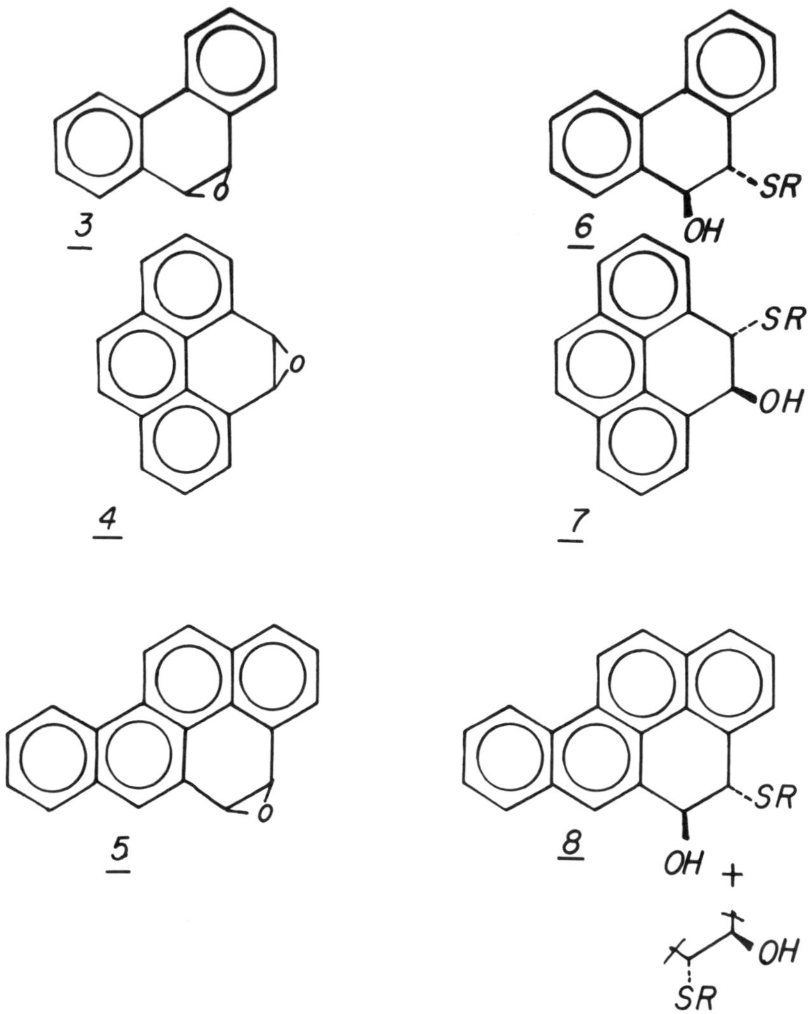


**Figure 5.** Chemical structures of some arene oxides and their corresponding mercapturic acids prepared by the phase-transfer procedure; R = -N-acetylcysteine butyl ester.

*n*-butyl esters of the mercapturic acid derivatives of styrene oxide prepared by the phase transfer method behaved equally well on silica gel chromatography. The styrene oxide mixture again separated into three well-resolved components as described above (Figure 7B). Interestingly, with the exception of benzo[a]pyrene 4,5-oxide (Figure 7C), all other arene oxide mercapturic acids chromatographed on silica gel as a single peak. This suggests that although diastereomers are not separated under these conditions, separation

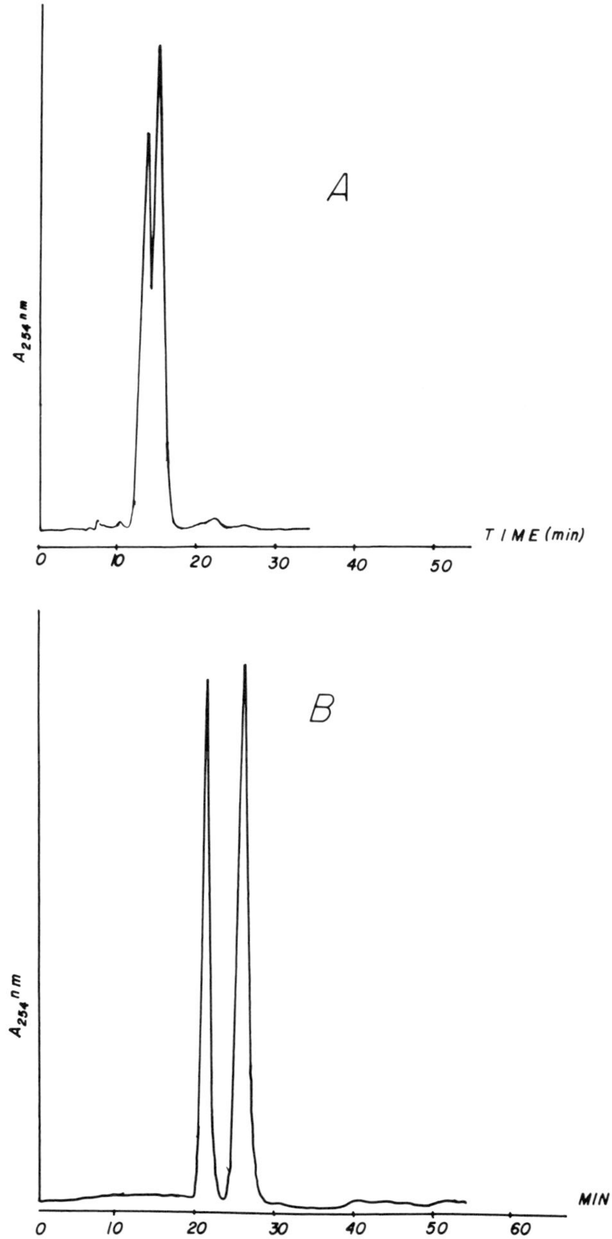


**Figure 6.** HPLC analysis of GSH conjugates of styrene oxide. The column used was a $\mu$-Bondapak $C_{18}$, 0.39 x 30 cm. The isocratic conditions were: trace A, 0.1% acetic acid in water/30% methanol, 1 ml/min; trace B, 0.05 *N* $H_3PO_4$ buffered with triethylamine to pH 3–3.5/15% methanol, 1 ml/min.

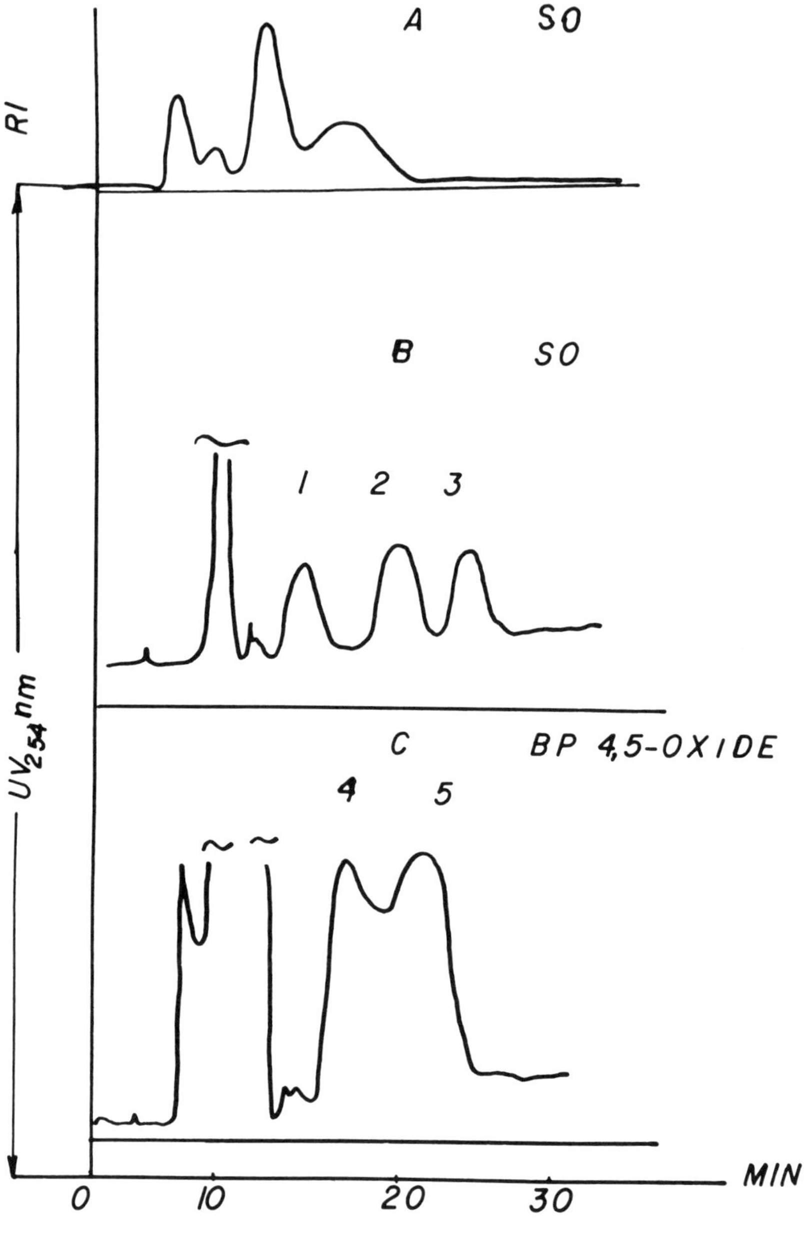


Figure 7. Preparative normal phase HPLC separation of mercapturic acid esters. See "Experimental" for separation conditions. Trace A, styrene oxide mercapturic acid methyl esters; trace B, styrene oxide mercapturic acid butyl esters, peak 1 was diastereomeric *2* (Fig. 3 R = -N-acetylcysteine), peaks 2 and 3 were diastereomerically pure *1* (Fig. 3); trace C, mercapturic acids (peaks 4 and 5) from benzo[a]-pyrene 4,5-oxide (5).

of positional isomers is more likely to occur. The chemical ionization mass spectra of the esterified mercapturic acids using isobutane as reagent gas were consistent with the postulated structures.

The information described above regarding stereoisomer distribution in the individual peaks allowed us to further refine the reverse phase HPLC system. Substitution of *tris*-(hydroxymethyl)aminomethane for triethylamine had a pronounced effect on the separation of the mercapturic acid isomers while maintaining resolution of the other thioether derivatives. By utilizing a gradient system, separation of all the potential major thioether metabolites of styrene oxide was readily accomplished (Figure 8), with the isomeric composition of each peak being the same as previously described. A recent application of this HPLC assay procedure allowed the identification of the cysteine conjugates of styrene oxide as major urinary metabolites in the winter flounder (*Pseudopleuronectes americanus*), a marine teleost [31].

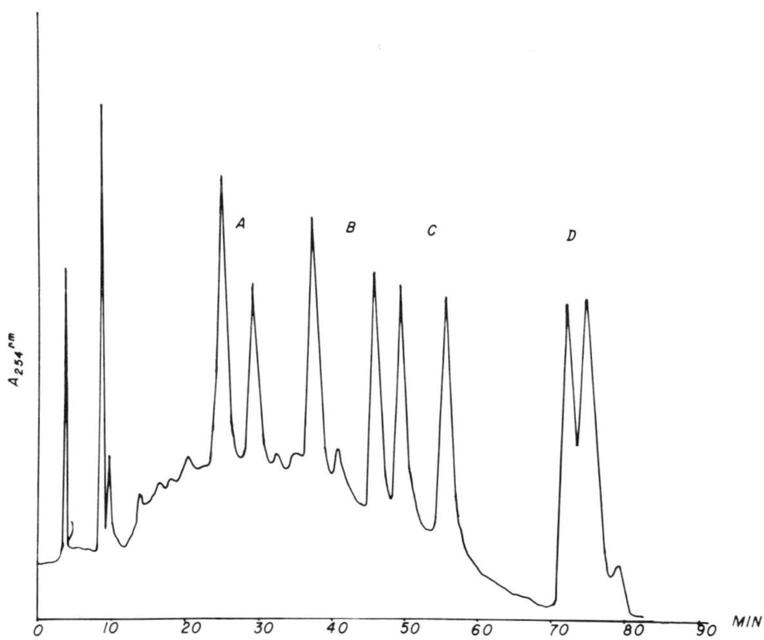


**Figure 8.** Reverse phase HPLC analysis of the thioether conjugates from styrene oxide. $\mu$-Bondapak $C_{18}$ column (0.39 x 30 cm). Solvent A, 0.05 $N$ $H_3PO_4$ buffered to pH 3.1 with Tris base; solvent B, 10% methanol in buffer A. Gradient conditions were linear from 0 to 100% B in 50 min after a 5 min delay. Flowrate was 1 ml/min. Peak identification, A:cysteine-, B:cysteinylglycine-, C:glutathione-, and D:N-acetylcysteine conjugates of styrene oxide.

## Stereochemistry and Mechanism

The information provided by the combined use of HPLC and $^{13}C$ NMR suggested a simple way for determining the stereochemistry of the GSH conjugates chemically produced from styrene oxide. A wide body of literature indicates that nucleophilic ring opening reactions of epoxides under neutral or basic conditions proceed with inversion of configuration [32]. Thus, enantiomerically pure styrene oxides should produce conjugates on reaction with L-GSH that are distinguishable by HPLC. Because mixtures of diastereomers are no longer possible with the pure enantiomers, the positional isomers 1 and 2 will appear on the chromatogram as either one or two peaks, depending on the styrene oxide enantiomer used. Accordingly, the optically pure styrene oxides were synthesized [33] and the HPLC traces of their GSH conjugates are shown in Figure 9. Two facts emerge from these chromatograms. First, the individual enantiomers on reaction with GSH gave rise to conjugate products which were either separated [(-)-oxide] or not separated [(+)-oxide] by HPLC. This is consistent with a stereospecific ring opening reaction, which validates our basic mechanistic assumption. Second, the positional glutathione isomers of the R-(-)-oxide are well resolved by this HPLC system, and it follows that this epoxide can be used to determine regioselectivity in the enzymatic formation of GSH conjugates because the ratio of positional isomers can be determined directly from the chromatogram. Conversely, the S-(+)-oxide may be used to determine stereospecificity (or lack of) in enzymatic reactions, when used in concert with the R-(-)-oxide.

Concerning the quantitation of the various isomeric glutathione conjugates of styrene oxide, an apparent discrepancy was found between the isomeric ratios for the (-)-styrene oxide conjugates determined by $^{13}C$ NMR and HPLC (absorbance at 254 nm). The latter method indicated a substantially higher concentration of benzyl thioether isomer 1. This inconsistency was eliminated by measuring the extinction coefficients for the individual positional isomers, isolated as the mercapturic methyl esters, at 254 nm. It was determined that absorption (254-nm) by the benzylic sulfur isomers was 2.5 times more intense than that of the corresponding benzylic oxygen isomers. When this correction factor was used, the isomer ratios obtained by both procedures were in good agreement.

The identity of the diastereomers formed in the reaction of racemic styrene oxide with glutathione was established as follows: the first eluting peak represented the benzylic thioether derived from the R-(-)-oxide; the second eluting peak was a composite of the two positional isomers of the S-(+)-oxide plus the benzylic alcohol from the levo rotating styrene oxide.

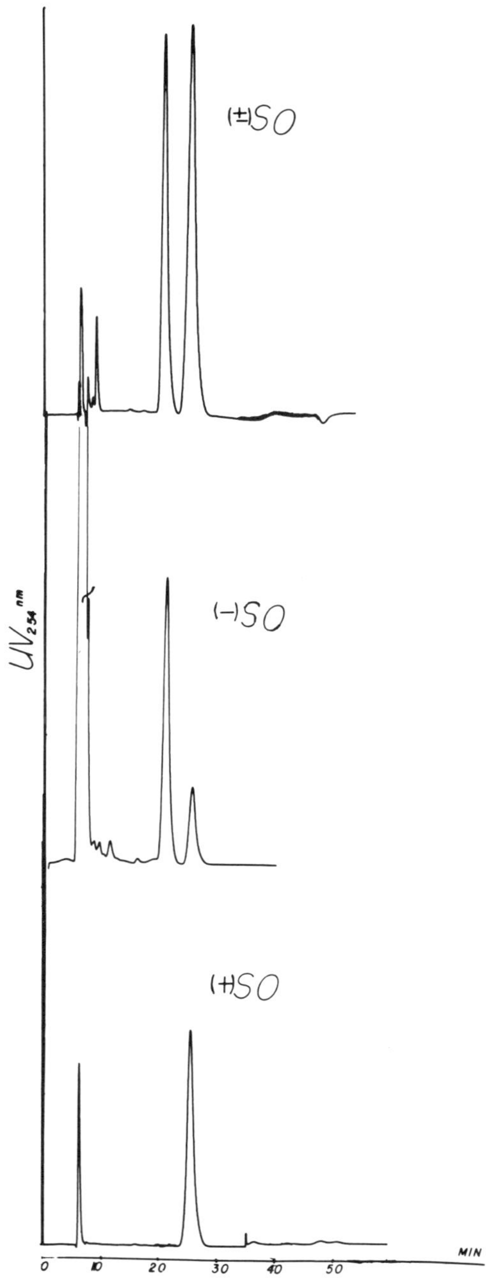


**Figure 9.** Reverse phase HPLC analysis of the glutathione conjugates from optically pure styrene oxides. Conditions were identical to those described in legend to Figure 6B.

The regioselectivity of the enzyme catalyzed conjugation of GSH with styrene oxide was examined with the optically pure epoxides as substrates (Table I). In the presence of a rat liver supernatant preparation [18] reaction of the (+)-oxide is regioselective affording 85% of benzylic sulfur conjugate as compared to 70% in the absence of enzyme. The enzymatic isomer ratios reported here have not been corrected for nonenzymatic contribution. A similar experiment conducted with the (-)-oxide showed that the regioselectivity for this enantiomer is identical (66-67%) for both enzymatic and non-enzymatic reactions. In addition, a small amount (8% total product mixture) of a diastereomer (benzylic sulfur) corresponding to the (+)-oxide was detected, indicating that racemization had occurred at some stage. By contrast, conjugation of (-)-oxide using a purified little skate liver glutathione-S-transferase [19] was highly regioselective (90% benzylic attack). Heat-denatured enzyme afforded benzylic thioether (69%) in the same proportion (67%) as the chemical reaction.

**Table I. Product Distribution in the Conjugation of Optically Pure Styrene Oxides with GSH**

| Oxirane | Conditions | % Substitution at C-1 | |
|---|---|---|---|
| | | Sulfur | Oxygen |
| S-(+)-Styrene Oxide | Chemical Reaction | 70 | 30[a] |
| | Rat Liver Cytosol | 85 | 15[a] |
| R-(–)-Styrene Oxide | Chemical Reaction | 67 | 32[a,b] |
| | Rat Liver Cytosol | 66 | 34[a,b,c] |
| | Purified Skate Liver Glutathione S-Transferase | 90 | 10[b] |
| | Boiled Skate Liver Transferase | 69 | 31[b] |

[a] $^{13}C$ NMR integration on mixture.
[b] Area integration of peaks from HPLC analysis.
[c] $^{13}C$ NMR showed 8% of benzylic thioether conjugate corresponding to S-(+)-styrene oxide.

The regioselectivity demonstrated in these enzymatic reactions is worthy of note. The role of the glutathione-S-transferases has been postulated to be binding of the substrate and GSH in close proximity such that the high reactivity of the thiol group suffices to complete the alkylation step without further enzymatic asssistance [10]. If only binding is responsible for the catalytic reaction observed, there must be a specific site(s) for these epoxides to bind to explain the higher regioselectivity found as compared to the nonenzymatic reactions. Denatured enzyme affords the same isomer distribution as the chemical reaction (Table I) and this finding eliminates non-specific protein binding as a factor affecting regioselectivity.

To extend these observations to other epoxides, the conjugations of 1,2,3,4-tetrahydronaphthalene 1,2-oxide (9), *trans*-β-methylstyrene oxide (11), and α-methylstyrene oxide (13) with glutathione were examined (Figure 10).

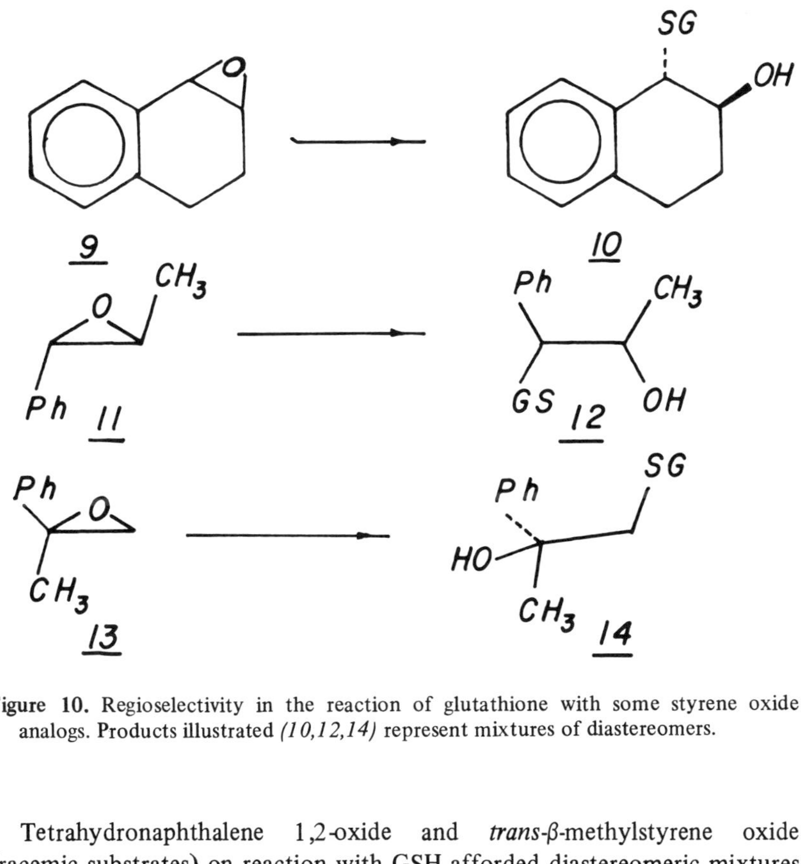


**Figure 10.** Regioselectivity in the reaction of glutathione with some styrene oxide analogs. Products illustrated *(10,12,14)* represent mixtures of diastereomers.

Tetrahydronaphthalene 1,2-oxide and *trans*-β-methylstyrene oxide (racemic substrates) on reaction with GSH afforded diastereomeric mixtures corresponding exclusively to benzylic attack by the thiol nucleophile. α-Methylstyrene oxide, on the other hand, afforded exclusively the product from nucleophilic attack at the unsubstituted carbon (Figure 10). In all three cases the product distribution is the same for both enzymatic and nonenzymatic reactions, as determined by $^{13}C$ NMR and HPLC analysis.

Two mechanisms emerge which are consistent with the stereospecificity and regioselectivity observed in the chemical reactions of the epoxides studied with glutathione. The first mechanism is a limiting $S_N2$ or direct displacement mechanism; the second involves nucleophilic trapping of an intimate ion pair. Both mechanisms are stereochemically equivalent, proceeding with net inversion of configuration. The reaction of phenanthrene 9,10-oxide with thiolate anions is kinetically consistent with either of the above mechanisms [26]. Assuming a Hammond-like reaction coordinate, the kinetic data suggested an early transition state for this reaction. The reaction of styrene oxide with glutathione offers a good test for both mechanisms. In an early transition state, polarization of the benzylic C-O bond would be anticipated to accelerate ion pair formation at this site, and the formation of a larger proportion of benzylic thioether would be expected. Simultaneously crowding in the transition by the phenyl substituent would discourage attack at the benzylic carbon, consistent with the significant alkylation observed at the primary carbon of styrene oxide (30-32%, Table I). When this steric factor is minimized, as in 1,2,3,4-tetrahydronaphthalene 1,2-oxide, where both oxirane carbons are sterically equivalent [32], the ion pair mechanism predominates as reflected by the product analysis (100% benzylic isomer). The methylated styrene oxides also fall within this scheme. In the case of *trans*-β-methylstyrene oxide, direct displacement at both carbons is sterically hindered, and the only product isolated results from the more favorable benzylic ring opening. Conversely, with a α-methylstyrene oxide, the ion pair trapping mechanism is inhibited by the presence of the methyl substituent (an early transition state is tetrahedral) and direct $S_N2$ displacement predominates with exclusive formation of the primary thioether adduct. These mechanistic speculations are based only on product analysis; kinetic confirmation is not available at this time.

The enzymatic reactions present a more complicated picture as the parameters increase in number and complexity. However, a qualitative picture emerges, again based on product analysis, which may explain the increased regioselectivity in enzymatic conjugations. The possible mechanisms by which the glutathione-S-transferases may catalyze the conjugations may be summarized as follows: (1) specific binding sites for both reactants [10,34]; (2) activation of the thiol nucleophile [10]; (3) activation of the oxirane oxygen [34]. The first possibility has been verified kinetically for transferase A isolated from rat liver [34]. The second possibility would involve base removal of the thiol proton, and the rate increase would follow from an increased concentration of thiolate anion. Finally, the third possibility calls for activation of the epoxide ring, perhaps by protonation. The binding mechanism is established [10,34], but it is not exclusive of reactant activation. Consequently, speculation will be limited to the latter two proposals. Relative substrate activities [34,36] and product distribution for styrene oxide and the two methylated oxides (11 and 13) are shown in Table II. The enzymatic rates were corrected by subtracting the nonenzymatic com-

**Table II. Product Distribution and Enzymatic Activity for Some Styrene Oxides**

| Oxirane | % Benzylic Thioether[a] | % Activity[b] |
|---|---|---|
| Styrene Oxide | 85-95 | 100 |
| *t*-β-Methylstyrene Oxide | 100 | 114 |
| α-Methylstyrene Oxide | 0 | 4 |

[a] Rat liver cytocol preparation was used, the incubation mixture was 2 m*M* in epoxide and 5 m*M* in GSH. Epoxide substrates were racemic.
[b] Data from Hayakawa et al. [35,36].

ponents. Among these compounds, the best substrate for the glutathione transferases is *trans*-β-methylstyrene oxide (11), and the worst is α-methylstyrene oxide (13). This opposing trend in activities is apparently reflected in the product distribution. Each epoxide forms a single positional isomer with glutathione (12 and 14) derived from attack at C-1 (β-methyl) or at C-2 (α-methyl). Thiol activation could account for increased activity in 11 but it cannot explain decreased activity in 13. Binding inhibition in the latter epoxide by the α-methyl group could be invoked to explain the decrease in substrate activity.

Oxygen activation by the enzyme could account for the increased activity in conjugation of the β-methyl epoxide (11) with glutathione, by lowering the activation energy in an ion pair mechanism. Similar activation of 13 (α-methyl) would not be expected to be significant because steric crowding by the methyl substituent would nullify the catalytic effect. Similar rationale may be used to explain the increased regioselectivity observed in the enzymatic conjugation of styrene oxide.

## SUMMARY

The main purpose of this work was not so much to establish or suggest a mechanism of action for the glutathione-S-transferase enzymes, but rather to stress the stereochemical complications implicit in the reaction of GSH with epoxides. Except for the simplest case, ethylene oxide, oxiranes are dissymmetric molecules, and on reaction with a chiral nucleophile (GSH) will give rise to diastereomeric mixtures of conjugates. The rates of excretion and metabolism of these conjugates may be influenced profoundly by stereochemical factors. As a consequence of this, conclusions drawn for a particular set of diastereomers may not entirely apply to seemingly related compounds. These stereochemical factors will be present regardless of the origin of these conjugates, enzymatic or nonenzymatic. The important thing to remember is that these compounds are formed in vivo; they have to be excreted and metabolized, and the better we understand the stereochemcial nature of the processes involved the better we will be able to evaluate detoxication mechanisms and hence toxic potential for specific compounds.

## REFERENCES

1. Daly, J. W. "Enzymatic Oxidation at Carbon," in *Handbook of Experimental Pharmacology, Vol. XXVIII, Part 2: Concepts in Biochemical Pharmacology,* B. B. Brodie and J. R. Gillette, Eds. (New York: Springer-Verlag, 1971), pp. 285-311.
2. Caldwell, J. "The Conjugation Reactions: the Poor Relations of Drug Metabolism," in A. Aitio, Ed. (Amsterdam: Elsevier/North-Holland Biomedical Press, 1978), pp. 477-485.
3. Boyland, E., and L. F. Chasseaud. "The Role of Glutathione and Glutathione S-Transferases in Mercapturic Acid Biosynthesis," *Adv. Enzymol.* 32:173-219 (1969).
4. Jerina, D. M., and J. R. Bend. "Glutathione S-Transferases," in *Biological Reactive Intermediates,* D. J. Jollow, J. J. Kocsis, R. Snyder and H. Vainio, Eds. (New York: Plenum Publishing Corporation, 1977), pp. 207-236.
5. Boyland, E., and P. Sims. "The Metabolism of 1,2-Dihydronaphthalene and 1,2-Epoxy-1,2,3,4-tetrahydronaphthalene," *Biochem. J.* 77: 175-181 (1960).
6. Boyland, E., and P. Sims. "The Metabolism of Phenanthrene in Rabbits and Rats: Mercapturic Acids and Related Compounds," *Biochem. J.* 84:564-570 (1972).
7. Asaoka, K., H. Ito, and K. Takahashi. "Monkey Glutathione S-Aryltransferases. I. Tissue Distribution and Purification from the Liver," *J. Biochem.* 82:973-981 (1977).
8. Kamisaka, K., W. H. Habig, J. N. Ketley, I. M. Arias, and W. B. Jakoby. "Multiple Forms of Human Glutathione S-Transferases and Their Affinity for Bilirubin," *Eur. J. Biochem.* 60:153-161 (1975).
9. Motoyama, N., and W. C. Dauterman. "Purification and Properties of Housefly Glutathione S-Transferase," *Insect Biochem.* 7:361-369 (1977).
10. Jakoby, W. B., W. H. Habig, J. H. Keen, J. N. Netley and M. J. Pabst. "Glutathione S-Transferases: Catalytic Aspects," in *Glutathione, Metabolism and Function,* I. M. Arias and W. B. Jakoby, Eds. (New York: Raven Press, 1976), pp. 189-211.
11. Boyland, E. "Mercapturic Acid Conjugation," in *Handbook of Experimental Pharmacology, Vol. XXVIII, Part 2: Concepts in Biochemical Pharmacology,* B. B. Brodie and J. R. Gillette, Eds. (New York: Springer-Verlag, 1971), pp. 584-608.
12. Bend, J. R., Z. Ben-Zvi, J. Van Anda, P. Dansette and D. M. Jerina. "Hepatic and Extrahepatic Glutathione S-Transferase Activity Toward

Several Arene Oxides and Epoxides in the Rat," in *Polynuclear Aromatic Hydrocarbons,* F. Fruedenthal and P. W. Jones, Eds. (New York: Raven Press, 1976), pp. 63-79.
13. Marniemi, J., and M. G. Parkki. "Radiochemical Assay of Glutathione S-Epoxide Transferase and its Enhancement by Phenobarbital in Rat Liver *in Vivo*," *Biochem. Pharmacol.* 74:1569-1572 (1975).
14. Leibman, K. C., and E. Ortiz. "Epoxide Intermediates in Microsomal Oxidation of Olefins to Glycols," *J. Pharmacol. Exp. Ther.* 173: 242-246 (1970).
15. Ryan, A J., and J. R. Bend. "The Metabolism of Styrene Oxide in the Isolated Perfused Rat Liver. Identification and Quantitation of Major Metabolites," *Drug. Metab. Disp.* 5:363-367 (1977).
16. Seuter-Berlage, F., L. P. C. Delbressine, F. L. M. Smeets and H. C. J. Ketelaars. "Identification of Three Sulphur-Containing Urinary Metabolites of Styrene in the Rat," *Xenobiotica,* 8:413-418 (1978).
17. Cox, R. H., O. Hernandez, B. Yagen, B. Smith, J. D. McKinney and J. R. Bend. "$^{13}$C Nuclear Magnetic Resonance Studies of the Structure and Stereochemistry of Products Derived from the Conjugation of Glutathione with Alkene and Arene Oxides," Chapter 20, this volume.
18. James, M. O., J. R. Fouts and J. R. Bend. "Hepatic and Extrahepatic Metabolism *in Vitro* of an Epoxide (8-$^{14}$C-Styrene Oxide) in the Rabbit," *Biochem. Pharmacol.* 25:187-193 (1976).
19. Aitio, A., and J. R. Bend. "Inhibition of Rat Liver Glutathione S-Transferase Activity by Aprotic Solvents," *FEBS Lett.* 101:187-190 (1979).
20. Boyland, E., and P. Sims. "The Metabolism of Pyrene in Rats and Rabbits," *Biochem. J.* 90:391-398 (1964).
21. Boyland, E., and P. Sims. "The Metabolism of 9,10-Epoxy-9,10-dihydrophenanthrene in Rats," *Biochem J.* 95:788-792 (1965).
22. Bucovax, E. T., J. C. Morrison, H. L. James, C. F. Dais and J. L. Wood. "Reaction of Polycyclic Hydrocarbon-Cysteine Conjugates with the Aminoacyl–RNA Synthetase System," *Cancer Res.* 30:155-161 (1970).
23. Beland, F. A. and R. G Harvey. "Reactions of the K-Region Oxides of Carcinogenic and Related Polycyclic Hydrocarbons with Nucleophiles: Stereochemistry and Regioselectivity," *J. Am. Chem. Soc.* 98:4963-4970 (1976).
24. Jeffrey, A. M., H. J. C. Yeh, D. M. Jerina, R. M. DeMarinis, D. H. Foster, D. E. Piccolo and G. A. Berchtold. "Stereochemical Course in Reactions Between Nucleophiles and Arene Oxides," *J. Am. Chem. Soc.* 96:6929-6937 (1974).
25. Jeffrey, A. M., and D. M. Jerina. "Novel Rearrangements During Dehydration of Arene Oxide Adducts," *J. Am. Chem. Soc.* 97:4427-4428 (1975).
26. Bruice, P. Y., T. C. Bruice, J. Yagi and D. M. Jerina. "Nucleophilic Displacements on the Arene Oxides of Phenanthrene," *J. Am. Chem. Soc.* 98:2965-2973 (1976).
27. Starks, C. M., and C. Liotta. *Phase Transfer Catalysis: Principles and Techniques* (New York: Academic Press, Inc., 1978).
28. Hancock, W. S., C. A. Bishop, R. L. Prestidge, D. R. K. Harding and M. T. W. Hearn. "High-Pressure Liquid Chromatography of Peptides and Proteins," *J. Chromatog.* 153:391-398 (1978).

29. Rivier, J. E. "Use of Trialkyl Ammonium Phosphate (TAAP) Buffers in Reverse Phase HPLC for High Resolution and High Recovery of Peptides and Proteins," *J. Liquid Chromatog.* 1:343-366 (1978).
30. Kroeff, E. P., and D. J. Pietrzyk. "High Performance Liquid Chromatographic Study of the Retention and Separation of Short Chain Peptide Diastereomers on a $C_8$ Bonded Phase," *Anal. Chem.* 50: 1353-1358 (1978).
31. Yagen, B., Z. Ben-Zvi, O. Hernandez, A. J. Ryan, G. L. Foureman, R. H. Cox and J. R. Bend. "The Metabolism of $^{14}$C-Styrene Oxide:Glutathione Conjugates in Winter Flounder (*Pseudopleuronectes Americanus*). Identification of S-Cysteine Conjugates as the Major Urinary Metabolites," (submitted).
32. Buchanan, J. G., and H. Z. Sable. "Stereoselective Epoxide Cleavages," in *Selective Organic Transformations, Vol. 2,* B. S. Thyagarajan, Ed. (New York: Wiley-Interscience, 1972), pp. 1-96.
33. Dupin, C., and J. -F. Dupin. "Etude Stereochimique de la Reactivite: Cours Sterique des Hydrolyses Baso et Acidocatalysees du Phenyl-1 epoxy-1,2 ethane S (+)," *Bull. Soc. Chim. France* (1970) pp. 249-251.
34. Mannervik, B., C. Guthenberg, I. Jakobson and M. Warholm. "Glutathione Conjugation: Reaction Mechanism of Glutathione S-Transferase A," in *Conjugation Reactions in Drug Biotransformation,* A. Aitio, Ed. (Amsterdam: Elsevier/North-Holland Biomedical Press, 1978), pp. 101-110.
35. Hayakawa, T., R. A. Lemahieu and S. Udenfriend. "Studies on Glutathione-S-Arene Oxidase Transferase–A Sensitive Assay and Partial Purification of the Enzyme from Sheep Liver," *Arch. Biochem. Biophys.* 162:223-230 (1974).
36. Hayakawa, T., S. Udenfriend, H. Yagi and D. M. Jerina. "Substrates and Inhibitors of Hepatic Glutathione-S-Epoxide Transferase," *Arch. Biochem. Biophys.* 170:438-451 (1975).

## CHAPTER 22

# MECHANISMS AND DETECTION OF PATHOLOGY CAUSED BY FREE RADICALS. TOBACCO SMOKE, NITROGEN DIOXIDE AND OZONE

**William A. Pryor**

Department of Chemistry
Louisiana State University
Baton Rouge, Louisiana

## INTRODUCTION

An important fraction of the harm caused to plants and animals in the modern urban environment results from pathological changes that are mediated by free radicals [1-15]. In this chapter I will review briefly the chemistry of several toxins that cause radical-mediated pathology, with special emphasis on the methods of proving that radicals are implicated in the cellular alterations that are observed [15] and the molecular-level mechanisms that are involved.

Historically, ionizing radiation was the first environmental threat to be recognized as affecting organisms because of the free radical reactions that it initiates [16-18]. Lethal amounts of radiation cause dramatic changes in the chromosomes of small mammals and humans; most of this damage results from free radical processes. Radiation is known to induce the autoxidation of lipids, and lipid peroxides are detected at toxic levels after high doses of radiation.

In recent years, it has become clear that a number of important environmental toxins also act via radical-mediated reactions. For example, both nitric oxide and nitrogen dioxide are themselves free radicals and react with bio-organic molecules to produce free radicals in the cell [19-21]. In addition, soot and smoke from cigarettes, automobile exhaust and similar combustion sources contain high concentrations of free radicals [22-24].

In addition to these toxins, a number of important pollutants, although not themselves free radicals, cause radicals to be formed in living systems. For example, ozone [25-30] and a number of carcinogens and toxins are believed to act by radical-mediated processes [31,32].

## METHODS OF DETECTING RADICALS AND RADICAL-MEDIATED PATHOLOGY

The most direct way of proving that radicals are involved in a biochemical transformation is through the use of electron spin resonance (ESR). Unfortunately, this technique cannot always be used at ambient temperatures because the concentrations of radicals involved in biological systems are usually below the detection limit (about $10^{-8}$ *M*) of the ESR method. In some cases, ESR spectra can be obtained by cooling the sample to low temperatures where radical lifetimes are greater. Another approach involves the use of spin traps; applications of this method will be described below [15,33-35].

One of the most frequently observed results of radical pathology is the autoxidation of lipids, which is often followed by membrane disruption, cellular leakage and, ultimately, cell death [10-15]. Thus, the detection of lipid autoxidation suggests that radicals were involved in the cellular changes that are observed [14,15]. The products of lipid autoxidation, conjugated diene hydroperoxides, can be detected by various titration methods or by the absorption at about 233 nm due to the diene function [14,15]. Less direct methods include the thiobarbituric acid (TBA) test and the detection of ethane and/or pentane in the expired breath of the exposed animal [11]. Fluorescent pigments also accumulate in cells that are exposed to toxins that initiate radical reactions [28].

## USE OF ESR TO STUDY RADICALS IN CIGARETTE TAR

In 1960, Lyons and Spence used ESR to show that free radicals are present in the total particulate matter (i.e., the "tar" or "soot") that can be condensed from the smoke from a variety of environmental sources [22,23]. They examined the smoke from cigarettes, gasoline- and diesel-powered automobiles, chimney soot, and smoke collected in urban air. In the years following their observations, a number of other workers have used ESR to probe the concentration of radicals in smoke. My research group [24,36], for example, has studied the particulate matter that is isolated from cigarette smoke using Cambridge filters (a glass fiber filter with an acrylic binder that retains more than 99.9% of the particles greater than 0.1 micron in diameter). We also have isolated tar by simply blowing the smoke over glass wool packed loosely into an ESR tube. The tar trapped on glass fiber filters by either of these two methods contains about $10^{17}$ free radicals per gram of tar, or more than $10^{15}$ free radicals per cigarette puff. Interestingly, approximately the same concentration of radicals is found in the tar filtered from mainstream and sidestream cigarette smoke. (Mainstream smoke is the smoke sucked through the cigarette and inhaled by the smoker; sidestream smoke is the smoke that rises from the cigarette into the air to be breathed by both smokers and nonsmokers in the vicinity.)

The radicals in tar are very long-lived [24,36]. Several authors have suggested that these long-lived radicals are "radical holes"; that is, free electrons localized in a conductance band of polynuclear aromatic hydrocarbons (PAH) that are known to be present in cigarette tar [23]. However, for the first time, we have been able to extract the free radicals in tar into organic solvents, and this has allowed us to fractionate the tar to determine what type of molecules are associated with the free radical signal [36]. (In addition, since the radical signal can be extracted into homogeneous solution, it is clear that discrete free radicals exist in tar, and the ESR signal observed does not result from some effect of the tarry matrix on a radical that would otherwise not be observable by ESR.) Fractionation of the solution containing the tar radicals shows that the radical signal is associated with the pigment fraction of the tar; this fraction derives from the tobacco leaf pigment that is produced from enzymatic oxidation of polymeric phenols in the tobacco leaf [36]. Because these tobacco leaf pigments bear a resemblance to melanin pigments, and because the ESR signal of the tar radical is very similar to the signal obtained from animal melanin pigments [37], we have suggested that the tar radical may in fact be a polymeric phenolic or semiquinone radical much like that found in melanin pigments. If this proves to be the case, it will suggest a potential involvement of radical chemistry in tar-induced carcinogenesis, because the tobacco leaf pigments are known to have cocarcinogenic properties.

## USE OF THE SPIN TRAP METHOD TO STUDY RADICALS IN GAS-PHASE CIGARETTE SMOKE

The spin trap method is a useful adjunct to the direct ESR method, and it has found increasing use in biology. In the spin trap technique, a diamagnetic molecule (the spin trap) is allowed to react with the paramagnetic radicals in the sample to form paramagnetic spin adducts. These spin adducts are more stable and more easily detected than are the original free radicals, and the spin adducts often have ESR properties that allow the structure of the original radical to be determined [33-35]. Equation 1 shows the reaction of a typical organic radical with nitroso-*t*-butane (NtB), a typical nitroso-type spin trap, and Equation 2 shows the reaction with phenyl *t*-butyl nitrone (PBN), a typical nitrone spin trap.

$$R\cdot + \text{t-Bu-N=O} \rightarrow \text{t-Bu-}\overset{O\cdot}{\overset{|}{N}}\text{-R} \qquad (1)$$

$$R\cdot + \text{PhCN=}\overset{O}{\overset{|}{N}}\text{-Bu-t} \rightarrow \text{Ph-}\underset{R}{\underset{|}{\text{CH}}}\text{-}\overset{O\cdot}{\overset{|}{N}}\text{-Bu-t} \qquad (2)$$

These two spin traps and two others in frequent use are shown below, with the commonly used abbreviation for each.

$t\text{-}C_4H_9\text{-N=O}$

NtB

$\text{PhCH=}\overset{O}{\overset{|}{N}}\text{-}C_4H_9\text{-t}$

PBN

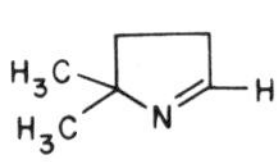


DMPO

$\text{HO-}C_6H_4\text{-CH=}\overset{O}{\overset{|}{N}}\text{-}C_4H_9\text{-t}$

OHPBN

We have used the spin trap method to determine the concentrations, lifetime and nature of the free radicals in the gas phase of cigarette smoke [24,36]. We find that mainstream smoke contains about $10^{17}$ free radicals per gram, and sidestream smoke contains about the same concentration of radicals. Thus, similar concentrations of radicals are found in both gas-phase smoke and in tar; however, the properties of the radicals in the gas phase and in tar are quite different. The gas-phase radicals are much shorter-lived and more reactive than are the tar radicals; for example, the tar radicals do not even react with highly reactive spin traps. The radicals in gas-phase smoke exist for about 10 min in the gas phase and have a half-life of approximately 10 sec in organic solvents. These radicals are stable enough to be able to diffuse great distances (over 200 cm) from the cigarette without appreciable reduction in concentration.

It is clear that a variety of types of radicals are present both in gas phase smoke and in tar, and the initial ESR spectra of the spin adducts from gas phase smoke and any of the spin traps we have studied are very complex because of overlapping signals from different types of radicals. However, we find that the spectra are greatly simplified if the smoke is allowed to age before it is bubbled into the spin trap solution, indicating that some of the radicals are shorter-lived than others. The spectra also are simplified if the spin adducts are aged, demonstrating that some of the spin adducts are less stable than others. We also have used computer simulation to dissect the initial complex spectrum into its component spin adducts.

Using these methods, we have shown that the radicals in gas phase smoke are primarily oxygen-centered, although a lower concentration of carbon-centered radicals also appears to be present. Among the oxygen radicals that are present are alkoxy (RO ·) and arylcarboxy ($ArCO_2$ ·) radicals. Evidence was also found for the superoxide (HOO ·) spin adduct at long times, indicating that this radical may be formed by one-electron reduction of oxygen by reducing agents in smoke [36].

The long lifetime of the radicals in smoke clearly presents a hazard not only to smokers, but also to nonsmokers in the vicinity of smokers. This long lifetime was a surprise to us, and we suggest that it can be rationalized in three ways. It is possible that some of the alkoxy radicals are tertiary (i.e., $R_3CO$ ·), since tertiary alkoxy radicals are longer-lived than primary or secondary. It also is possible that some are phenolic radicals, because these also can be long-lived.

The third possibility, and one that is currently being tested, is that the oxy radicals detected are the result of the reactions of nitrogen dioxide in smoke with other smoke constituents. Cigarette smoke contains a very high level (up to 800 ppm) of nitrogen oxides; most of this is in the form of nitric oxide, but nitrogen dioxide is also present. Both of these gases are, of course, highly toxic, although nitrogen dioxide is some 4–5 times more toxic than is nitric oxide. There also is a high concentration of olefins in cigarette smoke, and nitrogen dioxide is known to react with olefins to form carbon-centered radicals that can subsequently become oxygenated [38]. (As will be shown below, this reaction can occur by addition or by hydrogen abstraction.) Because nitrogen dioxide is a relatively stable free radical, the long lifetime observed could be a result of nitrogen dioxide diffusing downstream and continuously reacting with olefins in smoke to produce a flux of carbon- and oxygen-centered free radicals, as is shown in the following equations:

$$NO_2 + \;>C=C<\; \xrightarrow[\text{H-abstraction}]{\text{Addition or}} R\cdot$$

$$R\cdot + O_2 \longrightarrow ROO\cdot \xrightarrow[\text{mechanisms}]{\text{several}} RO\cdot$$

$$RO\cdot \xrightarrow[\text{Trap}]{\text{Spin}} \text{O} - \text{centered radical spin adduct}$$

$$R\cdot \longrightarrow \text{C} - \text{centered radical spin adduct}$$

## SUMMARY OF THE CHARACTERISTICS OF THE FREE RADICALS IN CIGARETTE SMOKE

In summary, the characteristics of the radicals in cigarette *tar* are as follows [24,36]:

1. They are long-lived.
2. They exhibit broad ESR absorbance without resolvable fine structure.
3. More than $10^{15}$ radicals per puff occur in the tar from either mainstream or sidestream smoke.
4. They can be extracted into organic solvents, where they also have a long life.
5. Fractionation shows that the radicals are associated with the pigment fraction that results from tobacco leaf pigment. Because this pigment is like a melanin pigment, and because the ESR characteristics of melanin pigments and the tar radical are similar, the tar radical may be a melanin-like polymeric phenoxy radical.

The characteristics of the radicals in the *gas phase smoke* can be summarized as follows:

1. They exist at least 10 min in the gas phase but have a 10-sec half-life in solution.
2. They diffuse far from the cigarette without appreciable decrease in concentration.
3. Radical concentrations in the gas phase smoke are very high, greater than $10^{15}$ radicals per puff, with approximately the same numbers of radicals in both mainstream and sidestream smoke,
4. They are mainly oxygen-centered radicals, but smaller concentrations of carbon-centered radicals also are detected. At long times, the superoxide radical is detected.

## REACTION OF GAS PHASE RADICALS WITH CIGARETTE TAR

Our preliminary evidence suggests that both gas-phase cigarette smoke radicals and the spin adducts produced from them react with cigarette tar. These reactions appear to be both chemically interesting and to have biological consequences. For example, we have suggested [9,24] that the peroxy radicals in tar may be converted to alkoxy radicals by reaction with the PAH molecules in tar, as shown below using benzene as a simplified model.

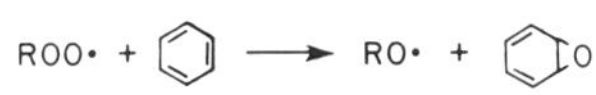

(3)

Because this gives an arene oxide, such a reaction would have obvious environmental significance. Although there is no precedent for this reaction, peroxy radicals are known to react with olefins to form alkoxy radicals and epoxides, as shown below [39]:

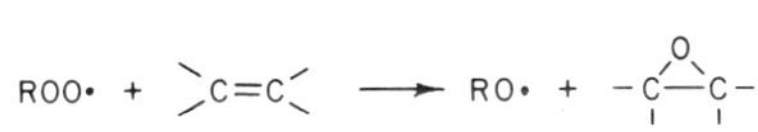

(4)

One indication that this reaction may occur is the recent finding by Marnett et al. that autoxidizing lipids convert aromatic compounds to carcinogenic arene oxides [40].

## NITROGEN DIOXIDE

Nitrogen oxides are produced as environmental contaminants when organic compounds undergo combustion; important environmental sources of these toxins include automobile exhaust, incinerators, fossil-fuel power plants and tobacco smoke. Both nitric oxide and nitrogen dioxide are themselves free radicals; therefore it would be expected that these two toxic gases would produce biological damage primarily by free radical mechanisms. In fact, there is considerable evidence that the principal, if not the exclusive, mechanism by which these toxins initiate damage involves free radicals.

The mechanisms of reactions of nitrogen dioxide have been studied more than nitric oxide, probably because nitrogen dioxide is more toxic.

Studies of in vitro models show that nitrogen dioxide initiates the autoxidation of polyunsaturated fatty acids (PUFA) [38]. The initiation of PUFA autoxidation by nitrogen dioxide has been demonstrated to occur in vivo by several methods. For example, Thomas et al. [19] have shown that 233-nm absorption is detected in pulmonary lipids from rats that have been exposed to nitrogen dioxide, indicating the presence of lipid hydroperoxides.

Classical studies by organic chemists over the past 60 years have shown that nitrogen dioxide adds very rapidly to olefins to produce an intermediate carbon-centered free radical [41-43]. This free radical can react with more nitrogen dioxide if the nitrogen dioxide concentration is high enough, or can be trapped by oxygen if air is present. One of these processes gives 1,2-dinitro and nitro-nitrite compounds and the other gives 2-nitro-1-hydroperoxides, as shown in the scheme below [38]:

$$NO_2 + \rangle C{=}C\langle \longrightarrow NO_2\text{-}\overset{|}{\underset{|}{C}}\text{-}\overset{|}{\underset{|}{C}}\cdot$$

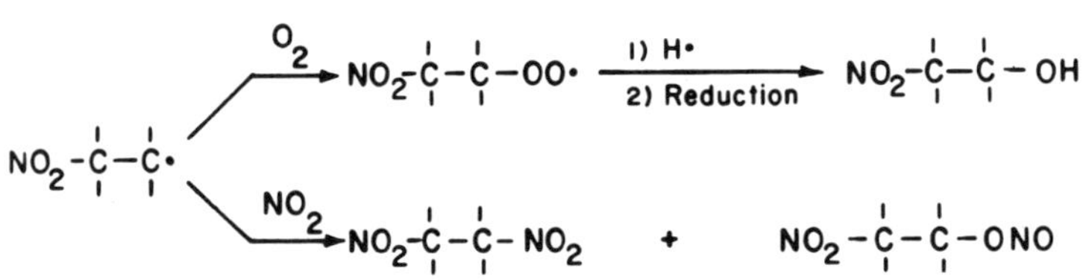

(5)

(6)

It is known that nitrogen dioxide also abstracts hydrogen from alkanes, such as cyclohexane, in the liquid phase but there was no evidence that nitrogen dioxide could abstract allylic hydrogens from an olefin in competition with addition to its double bond [44]. However, J. W. Lightsey in my laboratory [38] has shown that hydrogen abstraction even from simple olefins occurs in competition with addition. This hydrogen abstraction, shown in Equation 7, produces nitrous acid; in anhydrous media the nitrous acid disproportionates to form water, nitric oxide and nitrogen dioxide as shown in Equation 8:

$$NO_2 + -CH_2-CH{=}CH- \longrightarrow HONO + -\overline{C}H-\dot{\overline{C}}H-\overline{C}H- \quad (7)$$

$$2\ HONO \longrightarrow H_2O + NO + NO_2 \quad (8)$$

Hydrogen abstraction by nitrogen dioxide may have significant biological implications, since nitrous acid can nitrosate amines to form nitrosamines, which are extremely potent carcinogens.

$$HONO + R_2NH \longrightarrow R_2N-N=O + H_2O \tag{9}$$

Using the water produced in Equation 8 to estimate the fraction of the nitrogen dioxide that reacts via hydrogen abstraction, the data shown in Table I are obtained. Notice that very reactive dienes appear to react almost exclusively by hydrogen abstraction. Even simple olefins such as cyclohexene appear to react predominately by hydrogen abstraction in this simplified model system.

**Table I. Reaction of Nitrogen Dioxide by Hydrogen Abstraction and Addition for a Series of Olefins, Dienes and Polyenes in a Static System in the Absence of Oxygen [38]**

| | % H-abstraction[a] |
|---|---|
| 1,4-Cyclohexadiene | 115 |
| 1,3-Cyclohexadiene | 80[b] |
| Methyl Linolenate | 71 |
| Methyl Linoleate | 67 |
| Cyclohexene | 56 |
| 1,5,9-Cyclododecatriene | 52 |
| 1-Hexadecene | 38 |
| Methyl Oleate | 36 |

[a] Inferred from yield of $H_2O$.
[b] Benzene is observed as a product.

The percentages of hydrogen abstraction shown in Table I cannot be applied directly to biological systems for two reasons. First, the system used is initially anhydrous (some water is formed in Equation 8), and the concentrations of nitrogen dioxide used are very high (5-10%) to allow convenient analysis. Second, the isolation of water is not a satisfactory method to quantify the amount of Equation 7 that occurs. Nevertheless, the data in Table I clearly indicate that *both* addition and hydrogen abstraction must be expected when nitrogen dioxide reacts with even simple olefins in lipophilic media.

With the aim of proving that hydrogen abstraction competes with addition, we have identified the major products from the reactions of nitrogen dioxide with cyclohexene in the presence of either nitrogen or oxygen as the carrier gas [38]. Table II lists the major products that are formed in the order of decreasing volatility. As shown in the table, the hydrogen abstraction products are all of higher volatility than the products from addition. Hydrogen abstraction gives allylic alcohol (and the allyl ketone

Table II. Reaction of Cyclohexene in Pentane at 30°C With 20% Nitrogen Dioxide in Nitrogen or Oxygen as the Carrier Gas in a Gas Bubble Tower [38]

| Products from Hydrogen Abstraction | Percent | | Products from Addition | Percent | |
|---|---|---|---|---|---|
| | in $N_2$ | in $O_2$ | | in $N_2$ | in $O_2$ |
| | | | 1-Nitrocyclohexene | 17 | 4 |
| 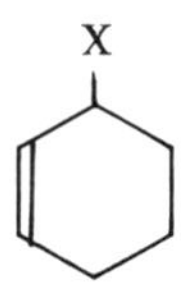 *X is* | | | 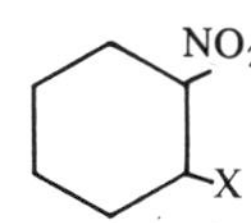 *X is* | | |
| $-OCH_3$ | 0 | 5 | -OH[a] | 38 | 56 |
| -OH[a] | 2 | 1 | -N=O[b] | 9 | 0 |
| $-O-NO_2$ | 2 | 3 | $-O-NO_2$ | 1 | 19 |
| $-NO_2$ | 8 | 1 | $-NO_2$ | 23 | 5 |
| Subtotals | 12 | 10 | | 88 | 84 |
| Totals | | | | 100 | 94 |

[a] Includes ketone.
[b] Measured as dimer
[c] Note the excellent material balance; from 94 to 100% of the cyclohexene that reacts is represented by the products that are isolated and identified.

that is its oxidation product) and the allyl nitro compound; these products result from capture of the allyl radical formed in Equation 7 by either oxygen or nitrogen dioxide.

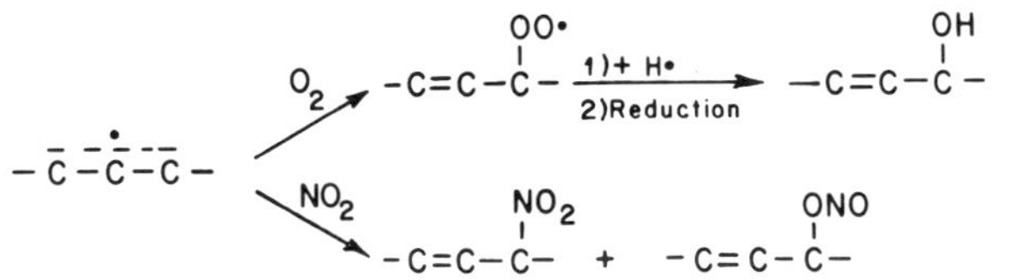

(10)

(11)

Allyl nitrite ester also is formed, as shown in Equation 11, but it is hydrolyzed to allyl alcohol by our workup procedure. Addition products consist predominantly of 1,2-dinitro compounds and 1-nitro-2-alcohols as well as other products [38].

There are significant changes in the product distribution caused by the presence of oxygen. For example, among the abstraction products, less allyl nitro compound is formed since oxygen competes with nitrogen dioxide to capture the allyl radical (see Equations 10,11). Among the addition products, oxygen leads to a lower yield of the 1,2-dinitro product and a lower yield of 1-nitrocyclohexene produced by elimination of HONO from the dinitro compound; however, the yield of the nitro-alcohol is greatly increased. These differences result from the competition shown in Equations 5 and 6. The nitro-nitrate ester is principally formed from the nitro adduct as shown below:

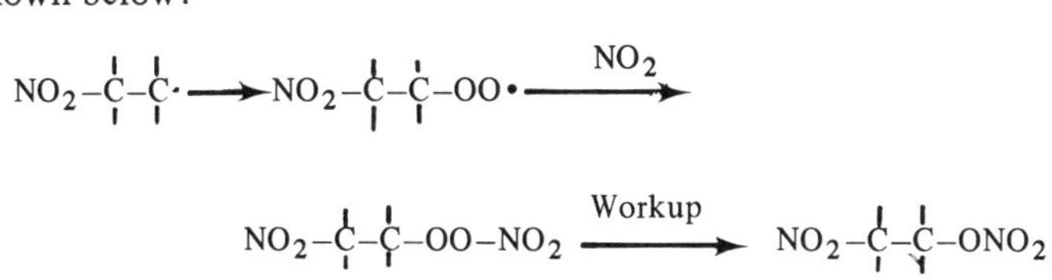

(12)

Alkyl Peroxynitrate

The data in Table I show that cyclohexene reacts 56% by hydrogen abstraction, whereas the data in Table II indicate just 12% abstraction. This difference arises from the fact that a very high level (about 20%) of nitrogen dioxide was used in the system reported in Table II, whereas that in Table I used about 5% nitrogen dioxide. In separate studies we have shown that more hydrogen abstraction is observed if the levels of nitrogen dioxide are low.

This undoubtedly results because addition is reversible whereas hydrogen abstraction is not [38].

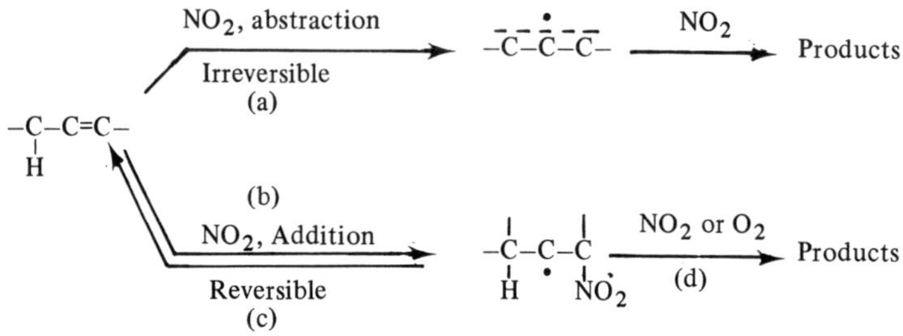


(13)

Thus, when concentrations of trapping species such as nitrogen dioxide are low, step 13d is slow, reversion occurs via step 13c, and less net addition is observed. (This explanation was originally applied to rationalize the fact that halogens give allylic substitution products at low concentrations and addition at higher concentrations (Pryor [39], p. 202).) Since $NO_2$ would be present at very low levels in biological exposures, a large amount of hydrogen abstraction might be expected; as remarked above, that implies that nitrous acid is formed with the potential for nitrosation of amines to produce carcinogenic nitrosamines.

We have studied the kinetics of the reaction of nitrogen dioxide with polyunsaturated fatty acids (PUFA) in a bubble tower reactor in which very efficient contact is made between the flowing gas stream containing ppm levels of nitrogen dioxide in air and the PUFA. With this design we have shown that each nitrogen dioxide initiates one kinetic chain in autoxidation. (It should be noted that either hydrogen abstraction or addition would initiate autoxidation; the products from the two initiation mechanisms are different but the kinetic consequences are the same.) First, using classical inhibitor methods [39] we have shown that each nitrogen dioxide initiates one kinetic chain. (The inhibitors used include α-tocopherol, α-naphthol, hydroquinone and 2,4,6-trimethylphenol.) Second, values of $k_p/(2k_t)^{0.5}$ for the autoxidation have been measured and the values obtained indicate that nitrogen dioxide behaves as a classical free radical initiator [38].

In summary, therefore, the data indicate that nitrogen dioxide reacts both with in vitro model systems and with intact animals virtually exclusively by free radical mechanisms. Studies of model systems indicate that nitrogen dioxide initiates the autoxidation of PUFA, with each nitrogen dioxide molecule starting one kinetic chain. Surprisingly, our studies have shown that nitrogen dioxide initiates autoxidation both by adding to the double bond of PUFA and by abstracting allylic hydrogen; either process initiates one kinetic chain. However, there is a significant difference between addition and abstraction: addition of nitrogen dioxide produces PUFA molecules containing a nitrogen dioxide group, whereas hydrogen abstraction yields a molecule of nitrous acid, a highly dangerous toxin because of its ability to nitrosate organic amines to form nitrosamines.

## OZONE: EVIDENCE FOR FREE RADICAL PRODUCTION IN BIOLOGICAL SYSTEMS

Ozone, unlike nitrogen dioxide, is not itself a free radical. Nevertheless, a very extensive literature indicates that the damage produced by ozone results at least in part from free radical processes [11,15,25-30]. For example, the exposure of intact animals to ozone leads to increased amounts of ethane and pentane in their expired breath, indicating the production of lipid hydroperoxides [45]. Antioxidants, including vitamin E, protect both in vitro systems and intact animals against the effects of ozone [25-30, 46-49].

In simplified lipophilic systems, we have shown that ozone shortens the induction period observed in the autoxidation of PUFA. Therefore, ozone produces radicals that initiate autoxidation and/or causes the formation of peroxidic materials (such as LOOH) by non free radical processes at a rate that is more rapid than would occur for air alone [50].

Antioxidants such as the tocopherols protect against the effects of ozone; this protection could arise either because ozone causes the formation of radicals that are scavenged by the antioxidants, or because ozone reacts directly with the antioxidants to destroy them. We have shown that ozone does destroy α-tocopherol, for example, but that the rate of this reaction cannot compete with the reaction of ozone with PUFA at the ratios of tocopherol to PUFA used in the study or that occur in cellular membranes [51]. It has also been shown that the induction period ends and the autoxidation phase begins after all the α-tocopherol has been used in sacrificial scavenging of initiating radicals [51].

As we have pointed out [11,15], it is not at all obvious how a nonradical like ozone can accelerate the production of radicals by interacting with another nonradical molecule such as PUFA, and several suggestions have been made. Ozone can abstract hydrogen atoms from certain types of molecules; reactions of this type are called molecule-assisted homolyses (MAH) reactions, and a large number of such reactions are known [52]. For example, ozone reacts with hydroperoxides in an MAH process, as shown in Equation 14 below [53,54]:

$$ROOH + O_3 \rightarrow ROO\bullet + O_2 + HO\bullet \qquad (14)$$

It is likely that the fastest reaction of ozone with olefins is addition to the double bond. This process produces an initial 1,2,3-trioxolane, which rearranges to form the Criegee ozonide [55]:

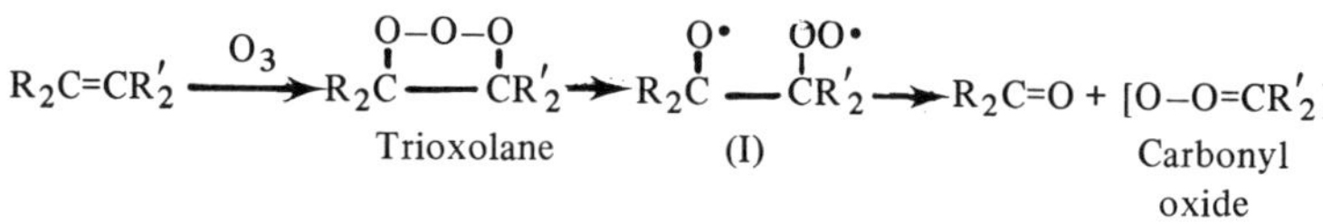

(15)

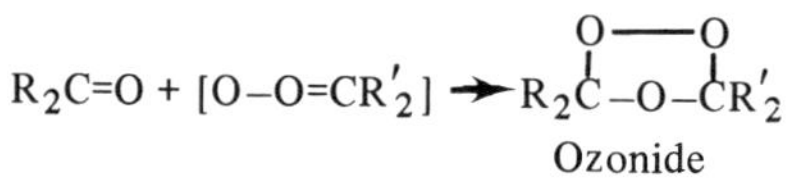

(16)

The carbonyl oxide has some diradical character, as represented by the resonance structures shown below [56]:

$$[R_2C{=}O{-}O \longleftrightarrow R_2\dot{C}{-}O{-}\dot{O} \longleftrightarrow R_2\overset{+}{C}{-}O{-}\overset{-}{O}\,] \qquad (17)$$

However, it is unlikely that the carbonyl oxide reacts as a radical to initiate autoxidation.

Diradical (I) rapidly decomposes by $\beta$-scission to form a carbonyl compound and the carbonyl oxide (Equation 15), and it is unlikely that it has sufficient lifetime to attack PUFA to initiate autoxidation. However, this diradical could undergo an intramolecular hydrogen atom abstraction (a "backbite" reaction) that would convert it to a more stable, longer-lived diradical that might have sufficient lifetime to initiate autoxidation. This backbite reaction, originally suggested by O'Neal and Blumstein [57] to rationalize the products formed from ozonation of simple olefins in the gas phase, also may occur for PUFA molecules in solution; in this case the abstracted hydrogen atom is allylic, as shown in the equation [11]:

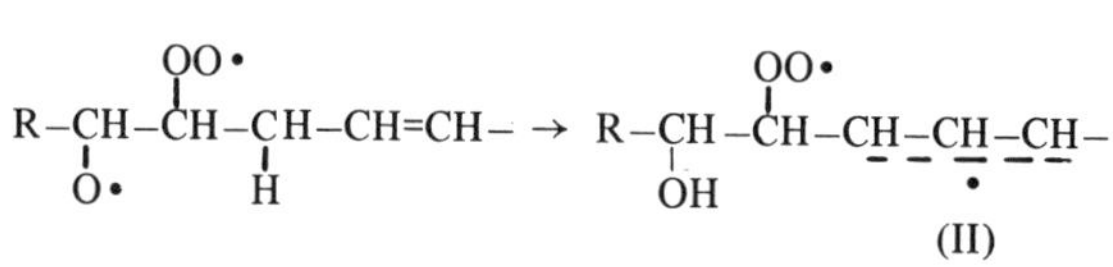

(18)

It seems possible that diradical (II), in contrast to diradical (I), may be sufficiently long-lived to initiate PUFA autoxidation.

## THE SQUARE-ROOT LAW FOR OZONE

Free radical processes generally follow the "square-root law"; that is, they show a kinetic order of one-half in the initiator species. In particular, autoxidations depend on the square-root power of the concentration of added organic free radical initiators (the derivation of this is given on p. 293 of [39]). We have recently found that the rate of development of absorption at 233 nm by methyl linolenate is proportional to the square root of the rate of absorption of ozone. This is shown in Figure 1. These data imply that the production of lipid hydroperoxides depends on the square root of the concentration of ozone, implying that ozone is acting as a free radical initiator. One important caveat, however, must be mentioned: Absorption at 233 nm may not be reliable as a measure of the concentration of PUFA hydroperoxides in the presence of ozonolysis products [15]; therefore, conclusions based on Figure 1 should be considered tentative.

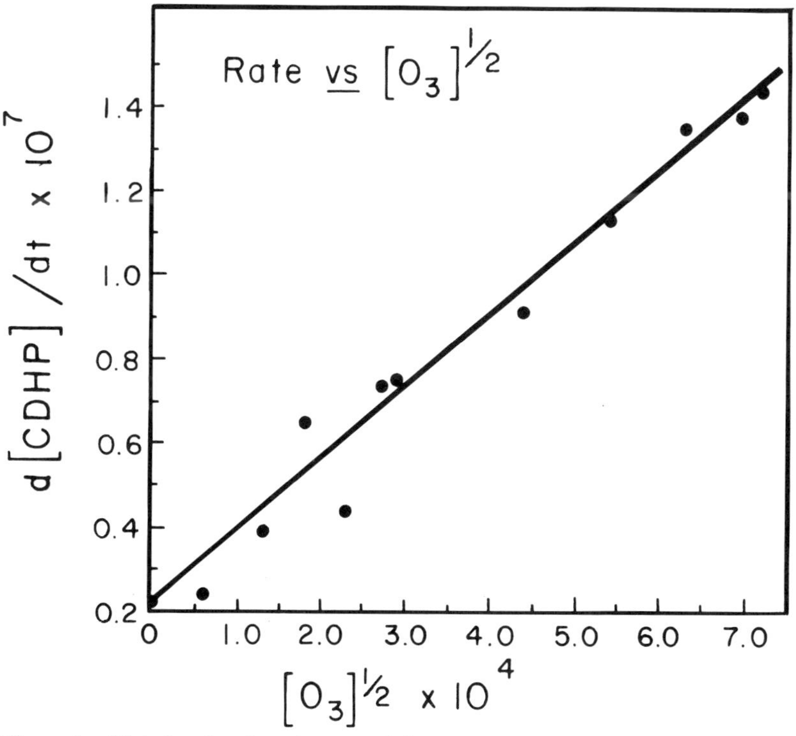


**Figure 1.** Plot showing that the rate of formation of conjugated diene hydroperoxide (CDHP) from methyl linolenate is proportional to the square root of the amount of ozone in the gas stream (using microimpingers [50]) during the induction period [51].

## ELECTRON SPIN RESONANCE (ESR) EVIDENCE FOR THE PRODUCTION OF RADICALS BY OZONE

The most direct technique to probe the mechanism of radical production by ozone is by ESR, a technique that detects radicals directly [58,59]. In 1968, Goldstein et al. [60] reported that ESR signals are observed when ozone is allowed to bubble through neat linoleic acid. This publication is often cited as proof that ozone does, in fact, cause the formation of radicals in PUFA; however, we have had reservations about this pioneering and extremely important publication for some time for the following reasons:

1. ESR signals were observed *only* while 40-ppm ozone in air was being bubbled through linoleic acid at 20 ml/min. However, $O_2$ is known to broaden organic ESR signals ("spin broadening"), and bubbles reduce ESR sensitivity.
2. The linoleic acid was only 95–97% pure and may have contained transition metal ion impurities, significant concentrations of lipid hydroperoxides, and a variety of other organic impurities. Three absorptions were observed at g-values of 2.014, 2.004 and 1.998 (each about 10 gauss in width), and absorptions at these g-values are not expected in pure organic materials. (The g = 2.014 signal could be due to peroxy radicals from hydroperoxide impurities.)
3. The signals appeared only after about 3 hr of bubbling ozone-air through the linoleic acid and disappeared within 3 min of the time the ozone was turned off. If one of the signals were due to transition metal ions (as seems reasonable and as suggested by Goldstein et al.), it is surprising that it disappears when the ozone is turned off.
4. The sample was observed to solidify after 3 hr of bubbling; in our experience, linoleic acid, methyl linoleate and similar PUFA do not solidify from this treatment.
5. The signal was extremely weak; Goldstein et al. state it was "near the limit" of detection.

For these reasons, we [36] repeated these experiments; a number of experiments modified from the original design were also performed. Both linoleic acid (greater than 99.9% pure) and methyl linoleate (purified and greater than 99% pure) were examined. Our method involves bubbling 40-ppm ozone in an oxygen stream at 20–40 ml/min through the substrate for 3.5 hr in an ESR tube held in the ESR cavity. We also bubbled ozone through the sample outside the cavity, quickly froze it in a dry ice bath, and then cooled it to liquid nitrogen temperatures; the sample was then allowed to thaw slowly in the cavity of the ESR instrument. For neither linoleic acid nor methyl linoleate was any ESR absorption observed. We conclude, therefore, that the previous result appears to be an artifact.

To eliminate the possibility that radicals were not observed although they were present, the linoleic acid radical L• was generated by the technique of

Krusic and Kochi [61]. *t*-Butyl peroxide was photolyzed using a 200-W Hg-Xe arc in deoxygenated linoleic acid while the sample was held in an ESR tube at -50°C. A complex spectrum was observed that computer simulation shows is consistent with the L• radical.

$$t\text{-Butyl peroxide} \xrightarrow{\text{Light}} 2t\text{-BuO}\bullet$$

$$\text{Linoleic acid} \xrightarrow{t\text{-BuO}\bullet} \text{R–CH}_2\text{–CH–CH–CH–CH–CH–CH}_2\text{–R}'$$

(L•)

## STUDIES OF RADICAL PRODUCTION FROM OZONE USING A SPIN TRAP TECHNIQUE

The method of spin trapping can very often be used to demonstrate the production of radicals when direct ESR methods fail, and the reaction of ozone with PUFA was therefore explored using a spin trap. It was necessary to develop a methodology that would allow the use of spin traps, which of course are extremely reactive, in the presence of ozone, a very strong oxidant. Our technique involves the following steps [36a]:

1. Ozone at 40–300 ppm in oxygen is allowed to bubble through the organic substrate in Freon-11 (or similar suitable solvent) held in an ESR tube at -78°C.
2. The sample is then thoroughly flushed with argon to remove all ozone. At this point no ESR signal can be observed. (Control experiments show that ozone reacts with spin traps to produce ESR signals; however, the argon flush removes all ozone.)
3. A solution of the spin trap in Freon-11 is then added so as to produce a final concentration of the spin trap of 0.1 *M*. At this point, no ESR signal due to any spin adduct is observed when linoleate is the substrate.
4. The sample is allowed to warm slowly in the cavity of the ESR instrument.

When methyl linoleate is studied in this way, the ESR signal of a spin adduct is observed beginning at approximately -50 to -40°C [36a]. The linoleate/ozone reaction has been studied using three different spin traps. PBN gives a signal which can best be interpreted as that of an alkoxy or peroxy spin adduct; DMPO gives a signal interpreted as that of an alkyl radical spin adduct superimposed over a weak background that could be caused by the less stable alkoxy radical spin adduct of DMPO; NtB gives a signal best interpreted as an alkyl spin adduct, with the alkyl radical having the structure consistent with that of the allylic L· radical. (See Table III.)

**Table III. Spin Adducts from Ozone and Methyl Linoleate [36a]**

| Spin Trap | $a_N$ | $a_H$ | Identification of radical(s) trapped |
|---|---|---|---|
| PBN | 13.7 | 1.8 | RO• and /or ROO• |
| DMPO | 13.9 | 20.4 | R• and a weaker background signal that could be due to the less stable RO• adduct |
| NtB | 15.2 | 1.8 | An alkyl radical with one α-hydrogen, suggestive of the allylic L• radical |

A few experiments have also been performed with small olefins using the same technique. All were found to produce both carbon- and oxygen-centered radical spin adducts. The oxygen-centered radicals were only spin-trapped if the solution was oxygenated after addition of the spin trap. 2-Methyl-2-pentene, a tri-substituted olefin, gives the largest yield of radicals of any olefin we have studied to date.

Thus low-temperature studies of the reactions of ozone with methyl linoleate indicate that intermediates are formed at -78°C that are stable at that temperature both to homolysis and to reaction with spin traps. On warming to temperatures near -50°C, the intermediate(s) decompose to form both carbon- and oxygen-centered radicals that react with spin traps to form spin adducts. Although the nature of the intermediate(s) that are formed cannot be identified, it seems reasonable to speculate that they are peroxygenated compounds. It is known, for example, that ozone reacts with *tert*-butyl hydroperoxide to produce di-*tert*-butyl trioxide, ROOOR and di-*tert*-butyl tetroxide, ROOOOR (where R is a *tert*-butyl group) [62, 63]. Ozone also is known to react with several types of organic compounds to form hydrotrioxides, ROOOH [54]. Table IV shows the bond dissociation energies and temperatures of decomposition of a series of peroxy compounds. Dialkyl peroxides, ROOR and hydroperoxides, ROOH, are much too stable to be the intermediate that we observed. Tetroxide species of both the $RO_4R$ and $RO_4H$ types are far too unstable to be responsible for these observations. Thus, at present it appears that ozone reacts with methyl linoleate to form either dialkyl trioxides, ROOOR, or alkyl hydrotrioxides, ROOOH, or similar trioxide species, and that these materials decompose at about -50°C to produce the spin adducts that we observe.

These observations appear to prove conclusively that ozone reacts with PUFA to form radicals, despite the failure to observe ESR signals directly from ozone-PUFA reaction mixtures at room temperature. The detailed mechanism for the reactions of ozone with PUFA, the nature of the inter-

Table IV. Bond Dissociation Energies (BDE) and Temperatures of Decomposition of Various Peroxygenated Species [62-64]

| Compound (R is tert-butyl) | BDE (kcal/mol) | Approximate Temperature Where Decomposition Becomes Fast (°C) |
|---|---|---|
| $RO_2R$ | 38 | 120 |
| $RO_3R$ | 23 | -30 |
| $RO_4R$ | 8 | -80 |
| $RO_2H$ | 42 | |
| $RO_3H$ | 23 | |
| $RO_4H$ | 8 | |

mediates that are formed, the pathways of their decomposition, and the nature of the radicals that are formed are the subject of our current investigation.

## REFERENCES


1. Pryor, W. A., Ed. *Free Radicals in Biology, Vol. I* (New York: Academic Press, Inc., 1976).
2. Pryor, W. A., Ed. *Free Radicals in Biology, Vol. II* (New York: Academic Press, Inc., 1976).
3. Pryor, W. A., Ed. *Free Radicals in Biology, Vol. III* (New York: Academic Press, Inc., 1977).
4. Pryor, W. A. Ed. *Free Radicals In Biology, Vol IV* (New York: Academic Press, Inc., 1980).
5. Slater, T. F. *Free Radical Mechanisms in Tissue Injury* (London, England: Pion Ltd., 1972).
6. Pryor, W. A. "Free Radicals in Biological Systems," *Sci. Am.* 223(8): 70-83 (1970).
7. Pryor, W. A. "Free Radical Pathology," *Chem. Eng. News* 49:34-51 (June 7, 1971).
8. Pryor, W. A. "Free Radical Reactions and Their Importance in Biochemical Processes," *Fed. Proc.* 32:1862-1869 (1973).
9. Pryor, W. A. "The Involvement of Free Radical Reactions in Aging and Carcinogenesis," in *Medicinal Chemistry, Vol. V*, J. Mathieu, Ed. (Amsterdam: Elsevier, 1977), pp. 331-359.
10. Pryor, W. A. "The Role of Free Radical Reactions in Biological Systems," in *Free Radicals in Biology, Vol. I*, W. A. Pryor, Ed. (New York: Academic Press, Inc., 1976), p. 1.
11. Pryor, W. A. "The Formation of Free Radicals and the Consequences of the Reactions *in Vivo*," *Photochem. Photobiol.* 28:787-801 (1978).

12. Mead, J. F. "Free Radical Mechanisms of Lipid Damage and Consequences for Cellular Membranes," in *Free Radicals in Biology, Vol. I,* W. A. Pryor, Ed. (New York: Academic Press, Inc., 1976), p. 51.
13. Tappel, A. L. "Lipid Peroxidation," in *Pathological Aspects of Cell Membranes, Vol. I,* B. F. Trump and A. Arstila, Ed. (New York: Academic Press, Inc., 1972).
14. Gray, J. I. "Measurement of Lipid Oxidation: A Review," *J. Am. Oil Chem. Soc.* 55:539-546 (1978).
15. Pryor, W. A. "Methods of Detecting Free Radicals and Free Radical-Mediated Pathology in Environmental Toxicology," in *Molecular Basis of Environmental Toxicity,* R. S. Bhatnager, Ed., (Ann Arbor, MI: Ann Arbor Science Publishers, Inc., 1980), pp. 3-36.
16. Altman, K. I., G. B. Gerber and S. Okada. *Radiation Biochemistry, Vol. I and II* (New York: Academic Press, Inc., 1970).
17. Phillips, G. O., Ed. *Energetics and Mechanisms in Radiation Biology* (New York: Academic Press, Inc., 1968).
18. Smith K. C., Ed. *Aging, Carcinogenesis and Radiation Biology* (New York: Plenum Publishing Corporation, 1975).
19. Thomas, K. V., P. K. Meuller and R. L. Lyman. "Lipoperoxidation of Lung Lipids in Rats Exposed to Nitrogen Dioxide," *Science* 159: 532-534 (1968).
20. Estefan, R. M., E. M. Guase and J. R. Rowlands. "Electron Spin Resonance and Optical Studies of the Interaction Between $NO_2$ and Unsaturated Lipid Components," *Environ. Res.* 3:62-78 (1970).
21. Fletcher, B. L., and A. L. Tappel. "Protective Effects of Dietary Tocopherol in Rats Exposed to Toxic Levels of Ozone and Nitrogen Dioxide," *Environ. Res.* 6:165-175 (1973).
22. Lyons M., and J. Spence, "Environmental Free Radicals," *Brit. J. Cancer* 14:703-708 (1960).
23. Ingram, D. J. E. *Free Radicals as Studied by Electron Spin Resonance* (New York: Academic Press, Inc., 1958).
24. Pryor, W. A., K. Terauchi and W. H. Davis. "An Electron Spin Resonance Study of Cigarette Smoke Using Spin Trapping Techniques," *Environ. Health Persp.* 16:161-176 (1976).
25. Menzel, D. B. "Toxicity of Ozone, Oxygen, and Radiation," *Ann. Rev. Pharmacol.* 10:379-394 (1970).
26. Roehm, J. N., J. C. Hadley and D. B. Menzel. "Oxidation of Unsaturated Fatty Acids by Ozone and Nitrogen Dioxide: A Common Mechanism of Action," *Arch. Environ. Health.* 23 (142) (1971).
27. Menzel, D. B. "The Role of Free Radicals in the Toxicity of Air Pollutants (Nitrogen Oxides and Ozone)," in *Free Radicals in Biology, Vol. II,* W. A. Pryor, Ed. (New York: Academic Press, Inc., 1976), p. 181.
28. Tappel, A. L. "Lipid Peroxidation," in *Pathological Aspects of Cell Membranes, Vol. I,* B. F. Trump and A. Arstila, Eds. (New York: Academic Press, Inc., 1972).
29. Goldstein, B. D. "Hydrogen Peroxide in Erythrocytes. Detection in Rats and Mice Inhaling Ozone," *Arch. Environ. Health* 26:279-280 (1973).
30. Chow, C. K., and A. L. Tappel. "An Enzymatic Protective Mechanism

Against Lipid Peroxidation Damage to Lungs of Ozone Exposed Rats," *Lipids* 7:518-524 (1972).
31. Ts'o, P. O. P., W. J. Caspary and R. J. Lorentzer. "Free Radicals Associated with Carcinogens and Carcinogenesis," in *Free Radicals in Biology, Vol. III,* W. A. Pryor, Ed. (New York: Academic Press, Inc., 1977).
32. Recnagel, R. O., E. A. Glende, Jr. and A. M. Hruszkewycz. "Chemical Mechanisms in Carbon Tetrachloride Toxicity," in *Free Radicals in Biology, Vol. III,* W. A. Pryor, Ed. (New York: Academic Press, Inc., 1977).
33. Janzen, E. G. "Spin Trapping," *Acct. Chem. Res.* 4:31-40 (1971).
34. Janzen. E. G. "A Critical Look at Spin Trapping in Biological Systems," in *Free Radicals in Biology, Vol. IV,* W. A. Pryor, Ed. (New York: Academic Press, Inc., 1980).
35. McCay, P. B. et al. "Production of Radicals from Enzyme Systems and the use of Spin Traps," in *Free Radicals in Biology, Vol. IV,* W. A. Pryor, Ed. (New York: Academic Press, Inc., 1980).
36. Pryor, W. A., and D. G. Prier. In preparation.
36a. Pryor, W. A., D. G. Prier and D. F. Church. *Environ. Res.* (in press).
37. Swartz, H. et al. "Structure and Reactivity of Melanins: Influence of Free Radicals and Metal Ions," in *Free Radicals in Biology, Vol. IV,* W. A. Pryor, Ed. (New York: Academic Press, Inc., 1980).
38. Pryor, W. A., and J. W. Lightsey. In preparation.
39. Pryor, W. A. *Free Radicals* (New York: McGraw-Hill Book Co., 1966).
40. Marnett, L. J., and G. A. Reed. "Peroxidatic Oxidation of Benzo(a)-pyrene and Prostaglandin," *Biochemistry* 18:2923-2929 (1979).
41. Schechter, H. "The Chemistry and Mechanisms of Reactions of Oxides of Nitrogen and Olefins," *Rec. Chem. Prog.* 25:55-76 (1964).
42. Titov, A. I. "The Free Radical Mechanism of Nitration," *Tetrahedron* 19:557-580 (1963).
43. Topchiev, A. V. *Nitration of Hydrocarbons* (New York: Pergamon Press, 1959).
44. Dechaux, J. C. "Nitration of Alkanes in the Gas Phase," *Oxidation Combust. Rev.* 6:47-74 (1973).
45. Tappel, A. L. "Measurement of *In Vivo* Lipid Peroxidation," in *Free Radicals in Biology, Vol. IV,* W. A. Pryor, Ed. (New York: Academic Press, Inc., 1980).
46. Roehm, J. N., J. C. Hadley and D. B. Menzel. "Antioxidants vs Lung Disease," *Arch. Intern. Med.* 128:88-93 (1971).
47. Goldstein, B. D., R. D. Buckley, R. Cardenas and O. J. Balchum. "Ozone and Vitamin E," *Science* 169:605-606 (1970).
48. Roehm, J. N., J. C. Hadley and D. B. Menzel. " The Influence of Vitamin E on the Lung Fatty Acids of Rats Exposed to Ozone," *Arch. Environ. Health* 24:237-242 (1972).
49. Goldstein, B. D., M. R. Levine, R. Cuzzi-Spada, R. Cardenas, R. D. Buckley and O. J. Balchum, "p-Aminobenzoic Acid as a Protective Agent in Ozone Toxicity," *Arch. Environ. Health* 24:243-247 (1972).
50. Pryor, W. A., J. P. Stanley, E. Blair and G. B. Cullen. "Autoxidation of PUFA. I. Effect of Ozone on the Autoxidation of Neat Methyl Linoleate and Linolenate," *Arch. Environ. Health* 31:201-210 (1976).

51. Pryor, W. A., and D. F. Church. Unpublished.
52. Pryor, W. A. "Radical Production from the Interaction of Closed-Shell Molecules," in *Organic Free Radicals,* W. A. Pryor, Ed. (Washington, DC: American Chemical Society, 1978).
53. Pryor, W. A., and M. E. Kurz. "Radical Production from the Interaction of Closed-Shell Molecules. VIII. The Mechanism of the Reaction of Ozone with *tert*-Butyl Hydroperoxide; 1,3-Dipolar Insertion, Electron Transfer or Molecule-Assisted Homolysis," *Tetrahedron Lett.* (1978) pp. 697-700.
54. Pryor, W. A., and M. E. Kurz. "Radical Production from the Interaction of Closed-Shell Molecules. IX. Reaction of Ozone with *tert*-Butyl Hydroperoxide," *J. Am. Chem. Soc.* 100:7953-7959 (1978).
55. Bailey, P. S. *Ozononation in Organic Chemistry, Vol. I, Olefinic Compounds* (New York: Academic Press, Inc., 1978).
56. Wadt, W. R., and W. A. Goddard. "The Electronic Structure of the Criegee Intermediate.Ramifications for the Mechanisms of Ozonolysis," *J. Am. Chem. Soc.* 97:3004-3021 (1975).
57. O'Neal, G. E., and C. Blumstein. "A New Mechanism for Gas Phase Ozone-Olefin Reactions," *Int. J. Chem. Kinetics* 5:397-413 (1973).
58. Swartz, H. M., J. R. Bolton and D. C. Borg, Eds. *Biological Applications of Electron Spin Resonance* (New York: John Wiley and Sons, 1972).
59. Borg, D. C. "Applications of ESR in Biology," in *Free Radicals in Biology, Vol. I,* W. A. Pryor, Ed. (New York: Academic Press, Inc., 1976).
60. Goldstein, B. D., O. J. Balchum, H. B. Demopoulos and P. S. Duke, "Electron Paramagnetic Resonance Spectroscopy: Free Radical Signals Associated with Ozonization of Linoleic Acid," *Arch. Environ. Health* 17:46-49 (1968).
61. Krusic, P. J., and J. K. Kochi. "Electron Spin Resonance of Aliphatic Hydrocarbon Radicals in Solution," *J. Am. Chem. Soc.* 90:7155-7157 (1968).
62. Bartlett, J. D., and M. Lehav. "Crystalline Di-*tert*-Butyl Trioxide and Dicumyl Trioxide," *Israel J. Chem.* 10:101-109 (1972).
63. Bartlett, J. D., and G. Guaraldi. "Di-t-Butyl Trioxide and Di-t-Butyl Tetroxide," *J. Am. Chem. Soc.* 89:4799-4801 (1967).
64. Benson, S. W. *Thermochemical Kinetics,* 2nd ed. (New York: John Wiley and Sons, 1976).

## CHAPTER 23

# TOXICITY AND METABOLISM OF METAL COMPOUNDS: SOME STRUCTURE-ACTIVITY RELATIONSHIPS

**Robert P. Hanzlik**

Department of Medicinal Chemistry
University of Kansas
Lawrence, Kansas

## INTRODUCTION

It has become quite apparent that metal compounds in the workplace and the environment can pose a significant hazard to human health. Numerous reviews, monographs and symposia dealing with various toxicological problems associated with specific metals have been published. This discussion of metal toxicity and metabolism will not deal with such case histories. It will attempt to construct a framework of chemical considerations for use in interpreting the biological properties of a wide variety of metal containing compounds. It is hoped that this attempt at unification and generalization will be useful in suggesting further experimentation in systems already under study, and perhaps eventually as a guide for predicting or anticipating the biological properties of metallic compounds. Much of our present knowledge of the mechanisms by which foreign chemicals affect biological systems is derived from studies with organic compounds. From this has come a number of fundamental principles, described briefly below, which help one to understand, and sometimes to predict, the biological effects of a given organic chemical. While this is probably not the only way one can integrate chemical and toxicological information, it has proven to be a very useful approach. This discussion will therefore parallel it whenever possible in attempting to arrive at some generalizations about metal toxicity.

## PROCESSES BY WHICH FOREIGN CHEMICALS AFFECT LIVING SYSTEMS

When foreign chemicals and living systems encounter one another, they usually interact, i.e., they affect each other in some way. For organic chemicals, some features of this interaction process can now be predicted fairly well. Thus, one can often anticipate the course of absorption, distribution and elimination of a xenobiotic organic compound by a mammalian system based simply on knowledge of the physicochemical properties of the compound, such as its solubility, partitioning behavior and pKa. The latter are usually determined simply by the functional groups present in the molecule. Compared to the enzymes of intermediary metabolism, most enzymes which biotransform xenobiotic compounds are more specific for functional groups than overall molecular structure, and the ability to predict the major metabolites of a compound from its chemical structure is steadily improving.

On the other hand, predicting the effects of a foreign compound on a living system is more complicated. Most living systems are dynamically balanced in a steady-state and tend to resist changes from outside influences. Drug metabolism and excretion are only two mechanisms for this; these processes prevent foreign compounds from reaching sites where they might act. But, assuming these barriers are overcome, what about predicting the biological action or effect that will be induced?

Many of the toxic as well as beneficial effects of organic compounds can be traced to their action at specific pharmacological receptors or at the catalytic or regulatory sites of enzymes. The toxicities of such diverse compounds as carbon monoxide, fluoroacetate, strychnine and poison ivy constituents can be understood in these terms. Within the limits of the specificities of such receptors, structurally related compounds may be predicted to have similar biological effects. Clearly the factor which limits our predictive ability in this area is incomplete knowledge of all possible receptor or effector sites.

Nonspecific interactions may also play an important role in determining the biological properties of foreign organic compounds. Membranous structures which form much of the cellular and subcellular organization of living systems may be altered by compounds which are detergent-like. A wide variety of lipid-soluble compounds which can complex protons, metal cations or anions can function as ionophores within biological membranes and wastefully discharge essential electrochemical gradients produced by expenditure of metabolic energy. Many compounds in this class are toxic to plant and animal cells.

A model for the production of toxic responses to chemicals which has received much attention [1] in the last decade is the covalent binding hypothesis. According to this model, chemically reactive substances react nonenzymatically with cellular macromolecules such as proteins and nucleic acids; presumably this results in the "denaturation" or disabling of the macromolecule. The biological consequences of this depend on the types of macromolecules damaged, the critical nature of the functions lost, the time course over which damage is produced and the ability of the cell to cope either through biochemical repair processes or by resorting to alternative processes not involving the damaged macromolecules. Generally, chemically reactive toxins are electrophiles or free radicals. Reactive hard nucleophiles are protonated under biological conditions, but soft nucleophiles such as cyanide or phosphine can disable critical metalloenzymes, particularly in the respiratory chain.

Thus in the broadest sense, predicting the biological activities of a given organic molecule or its metabolites usually involves one of two basic approaches:

1. Recognition of structural similarities to compounds known to have a role in intermediary metabolism (i.e., the concepts of lethal synthesis and antimetabolites) or action at discrete pharmacological receptors (i.e., the concept of pharmacophores). If such similarities are apparent, prediction of at least part of the biological outcome may be relatively straightforward.
2. Anticipating nonspecific effects based on the physicochemical properties and reactivity of the moelcule. In this case a number of precedents are available, but it is still difficult to make predictions of target organs, interspecies variability and the actual manifestation of the toxic effect. The latter may range from selective loss of specialized cell functions without cell death to cytotoxicity (i.e., defects in essential cell functions) to gene-related defects such as carcinogenesis, mutagenesis or teratogenesis.

In attempting to extend the above considerations to metal compounds two things immediately become apparent. The first is that much less is known about the normal physiological functioning of metals, as compared to organic compounds, in biological systems. It is encouraging to note that this area has been getting considerable attention during the past decade or so, and that descriptions and models for normal metal function and metabolism are emerging [2-4]. The second immediate realization is that the range of chemical properties and reactivities offered by metal compounds of various types is considerably greater than that of simple organic compounds. Fortunately, one can draw a number of parallels between the biochemical toxicology of organic and inorganic chemicals based on key chemical properties or processes which may be common to both groups. It is these parallels which will be the major focus of the discussion.

## BONDING AND BINDING: METALS AS ALKYLATING AGENTS

The covalent binding model for the toxicity of reactive organic compounds is a convenient point of departure for analyzing the toxic effects of metal compounds. Certainly one of the most important criteria which differentiate metal ions from each other and from electrophilic organic species is the chemistry of their bonding to biological ligands (for a general review see Hanzlik [5]). Metal-ligand bonds can be as strong in a thermodynamic sense as bonds formed when a reactive epoxide alkylates a nitrogen base in DNA or a sulfhydryl group in an enzyme. In this light the legendary toxicity of the "heavy metals" is readily understandable at least in general terms. However, the apparent strength of a metal ligand bond may result from either thermodynamic or kinetic considerations, or both. Thus, it is worthwhile to review briefly some of the features of metal-ligand bonding and ligand exchange at metal centers. In doing so some interesting patterns with predictive utility can be seen to emerge.

In 1953 Irving and Williams observed [6] that for a variety of ligands, the stabilities of their complexes with a series of divalent first-row transition metal ions usually fell into the sequence Mn<Fe<Co<Ni<Cu>Zn. This behavior was soon recognized to derive principally from the energetics of two processes, the ionization of the metal atoms and the ligation of the resulting ions. Soon afterwards the biological implications of this rather fundamental chemistry were pointed out by Shaw [7], who demonstrated that the toxic effects of transition metal ions on living organisms as well as isolated enzymes followed the Irving-Williams sequence (Figure 1).

Before going further into the biological side it may useful to restate some other factors which govern bonding and substitution at metal centers [5]. From a thermodynamic or equilibrium viewpoint the ability of some ligands to form more than one bond to a given metal, i.e., chelation by multidentate $\sigma$-donor ligands, can greatly increase the strength of the interaction. A second type of multiple bonding not to be confused with chelation in $p\pi$-$d\pi$ bonding or back-bonding involving overlap of filled d-orbitals on the metal with empty n or $\pi^*$ orbitals on unsaturated or heavy-atom donor ligands such as $R_3P$, $R_2S$, CO, $CN^-$, imidazole, porphyrins and similar systems. Ligands already

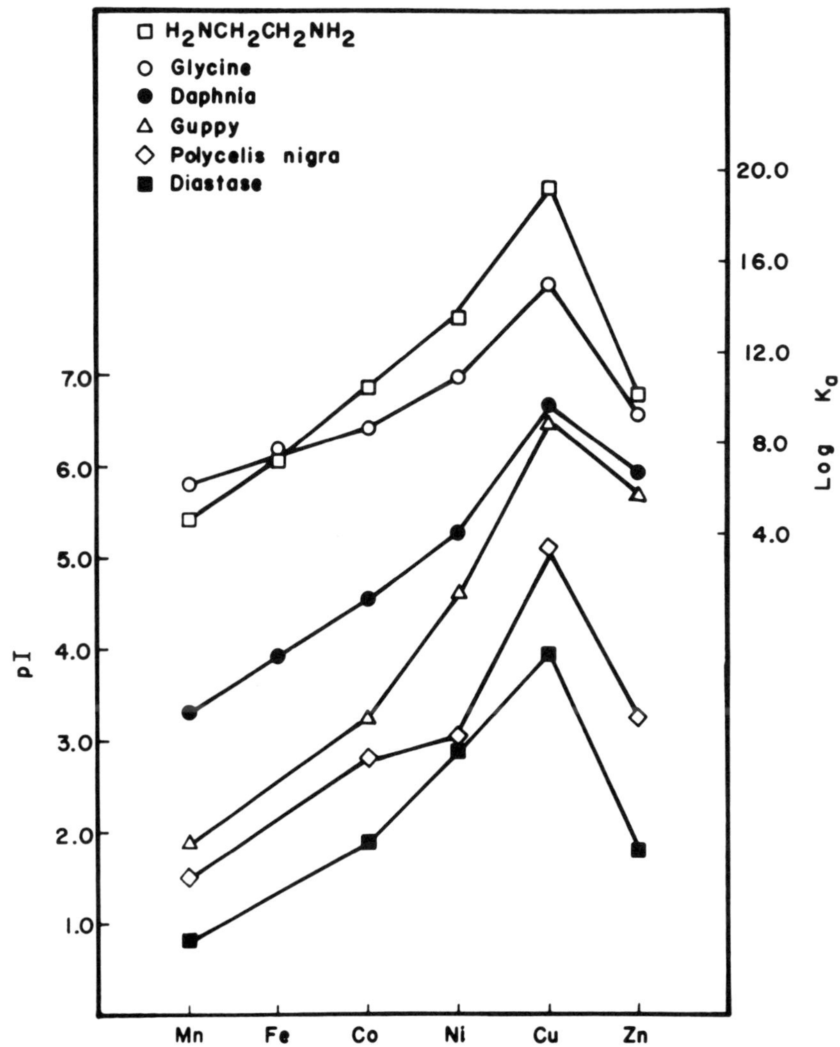


**Figure 1.** Correlation of transition metal complex stability and toxicity. Data from Shaw [7].

bound to a metal can influence the subsequent binding of another ligand in several ways. Metal ions are Lewis acids, and one very important determinant of their affinity for ligands is their charge/radius ratio. Increasing the oxidation state of the metal increases its Lewis acidity and its affinity for a given ligand (provided that the ligand is not oxidized by the metal in its higher oxidation state). Conversely, strongly coordinating Lewis base ligands ($\sigma$-

donors) will reduce the apparent Lewis acidity of the metal and hence its affinity for other ligands, although unsaturated $\pi$-bonding ligands which drain electron density away from the metal may actually increase its affinity for $\sigma$-donor ligands.

The number and geometric relationship among coordination sites in a metal complex can also have a considerable influence on its biological activity. For example, while both *cis*- and *trans*-$Pt(NH_3)_2Cl_2$ interact irreversibly with one or more nonessential sulfhydryl groups on the enzyme thymidylate synthetase [8], only the *trans* isomer interacts with the one SH group essential for catalysis. In contrast, the monovalent agent *p*-hydroxymercuribenzoate titrates all four of the free SH groups on each molecule of enzyme (Table I). Diethyltin ($Et_2Sn^{2+}$), phenylarsenious acid ($PhAs(OH)_2$) and arsenite ($AsO_2^-$) have very high avidity for chelating dithiol ligands.

**Table I. Effects of Stereochemistry and Chelation on the Biological Effects of Metal Compounds**

| Inactivation of Thymidylate Synthetase by | Target Groups | Respiratory Poison | Blocking Agent |
|---|---|---|---|
| *cis*-$Pt(NH_3)_2Cl_2$ | ~1 nonessential SH | $Et_2SnCl_2$, $PhAs(OH)_2$ | Dithiols |
| *trans*-$Pt(NH_3)_2Cl_2$ | ~2 SH groups, one essential | $Ph_2AsCl$ | Monothiols |
| *p*-Hydroxymercuribenzoate | All 4 SH groups | $Et_3SnCl$ | None |

They have similar toxicities in vivo and are powerful inhibitors of $\alpha$-ketoacid oxidation by lipoate-dependent enzymes; the inhibition is reversed by small chelating dithiol ligands like BAL (2,3-dimercaptopropanol) but not by the monothiol glutathione [9,10]. The monovalent compounds triethyltin chloride and chlorodiphenylarsine are also very toxic but in a very different manner. The latter is a powerful inhibitor of sulfhydryl enzymes such as isocitric dehydrogenase, and its inhibition is prevented by glutathione. In contrast, triethyl tin has little affinity for sulfhydryl groups and its toxicity is not affected by BAL or glutathione. The mechanism of its action as a respiratory poison is discussed below.

At the kinetic level, many features of metal-ligand exchange reactions are reminiscent of substitution reactions of organic compounds [5]. A small but important group of metal complexes react by an associative pathway analogous to Sn2 displacements or acyl transfer reactions involving intermediates with increased coordination number. Most members of this group are four-coordinate square planar complexes (Table I), whose low coordination number and coordinative unsaturation (i.e., presence of 16 or fewer valence shell electrons rather than the 18 required for an inert gas-like configuration) invite nucleophilic attack on the metal by Lewis base ligands. Apart from this group, most other metal complexes undergo ligand exchange by processes involving a dissociative rate-limiting step analogous to the Sn1 solvolysis of alkyl halides. Although the rates of the dissociative processes vary over more than a dozen orders of magnitude within this group, several unifying themes can be identified. For a given metal, the rates are quite sensitive to the nature of the departing ligand and essentially independent of the entering group. The major factor in determining the reaction rates is the strength of the bond being broken, which in turn depends on charge/radius effects, oxidation state of the metal, and the effects of coligands. Flexible multidentate ligands (like EDTA) dissociate in a stepwise process, but net dissociation may be slow unless protons are present to trap the free ligand because the reverse reaction, chelation, is entropically favored. However, dissociation of a rigid multidentate ligand, such as a porphyrin or perhaps a protein or apoenzyme, may be extremely slow because several metal-ligand bonds must be broken simultaneously to effect dissociation.

In the case of transition metal ions with partially filled $\alpha$-orbitals, crystal field stabilization energies can have profound (inhibitory) effects on the rates of ligand exchange via dissociative processes. These effects are quite important, and their basis is reasonably straightforward, but their discussion is beyond the current scope [5]. We will simply accept them and consider their consequences. However, it should first be noted that there are several special mechanisms for ligand dissociation from so-called "inert" or substitutionally nonlabile complexes which may be important in a biological context. One of these is acid catalysis, i.e., a protonated carboxylate ligand is a better leaving group than the carboxylate anion. Of course, carboxylate, phosphate and sulfate complexes can be cleaved by pathways involving either substitution (M-O bond cleavage) or hydrolysis (C-O, P-O or S-O bond cleavage), and examples of both processes are known. Lastly, base catalysis can greatly facilitate leaving group departure if the complex contains amine or hydroxylic ligands with dissociable protons, particularly if the latter are *trans* to the leaving group. In this so-called Snlcb mechanism the deprotonated conjugate base forms ($H_2N^-$, $HO^-$) are much more powerful Lewis bases and decrease the "effective" Lewis acidity of the metal and thus the strength of the metal-leaving group bond.

In light of the foregoing discussion, and the analogy drawn earlier between metals and organic alkylating agents as modifiers of macromolecule structure and function, it should be clear that a metal-macromolecule interaction may persist long enough to have biological consequences if either the equilibrium constant or the rate constant for dissociation of the complex is very small. Metals for which the latter condition obtains are listed in Table II. Most

**Table II. Substitutionally Nonlabile Metals**

| Octahedral | | | | | Square planar | | |
|---|---|---|---|---|---|---|---|
| V(II)[a] | Cr(III) | | Co(III) | Ni(II) | | Ni(II) | |
| | | Ru(II,III) | Rh(III) | Pd(IV)[b,c] | Rh(I) | Pd(II) | |
| | | | Ir(III) | Pt(IV)[b,c] | | Pt(II) | Au(III)[c] |

[a]Easily oxidized under biological conditions.
[b]Requires two-electron reduction for reactivity toward ligand exchange.
[c]Strong oxidant under biological conditions.

conspicuous among these perhaps is Pt (II), some complexes of which still appear to have promise as antitumor agents [11]. The testing of Pt (II) complexes for antitumor activity was prompted by the observation that Pt (II) complexes, formed in situ by electrolysis of solid platinum electrodes, caused growth of a filamentous form of the bacterium *Escherichia coli*, an action also caused by alkylating agents and certain antibiotics and thought to result from impairment of cell division at the level of DNA synthesis [12]. Numerous studies of the biological effects and chemical properties of Pt (II) compounds have been carried out with the general result that their biological effects correlate reasonably well with two chemical parameters, complex geometry and ligand exchange rate [11,12]. Compounds which were extremely inert to ligand exchange did not cause filamentous growth of *E. coli* and lacked antitumor and cytotoxic activity, while complexes with highly labile ligands were highly cytotoxic. Pt (II) compounds having *cis* geometry and ligands of intermediate lability toward exchange (e.g., cis-$(NH_3)_2PtCl_2$) had a more favorable ratio of antitumor to cytotoxic activity. Complexes of other transition metals were soon screened for similar activities, and the results reinforced in a general way the correlations between complex geometry, ligand substitution rates and interference with cellular processes involving DNA which had developed from the platinum work (compare Tables II and III). Thus, complexes of metals which undergo ligand exchange at slow but not insignificant rates commonly elicit such biological effects as inhibition of cell division leading to filamentous growth in bacteria, suppression of immune responses in vivo, inhibition of lymphocyte blastogenic responses in vitro, antitumor, and carcinogenic, mutagenic and teratogenic effects (Table III). All of these actions are, of course, well known for a variety of organic alkylating agents. The dependence of biological activity on ligand exchange rates is simply an expression of the fact that the complex must be sufficiently inert to survive long enough in vivo to reach critical reactive target molecules and yet be sufficiently labile to react once having reached those sites. The dependence of biological activity on geometry

**Table III. DNA-Related Biological Effects of Substitutionally Nonlabile Transition Metal Complexes[a]**

| Biological Response | Transition Metal Complex | | | | | |
|---|---|---|---|---|---|---|
| | Cr | Ru | Co | Rh | Ni | Pt |
| Filamentous growth of *E. coli* | 18 | 16 | 18 | | | 11,12 |
| Immunosuppression; inhibition of blastogenic response in vitro | | 16 | | 16,17 | | 12,16 |
| Mutagenesis in bacteria | 19-21 | 13 | | | | 13 |
| Carcinogenesis; in vitro transformation | 21-23 | | 23 | | 22,23 26,27 | 14 |
| Antitumor activity | | | | 28 | | 11-13 |
| Teratogenesis | | | | | 24,25 | 15 |
| Infidelity or inhibition of DNA synthesis | 23 | | 23 | 17 | 23 | |

[a]References are given where a positive response has been reported.

indicates geometric specificity on the part of the target, as is well known for the different actions of mono- and difunctional organic alkylating agents with varying chain lengths.

Although Ni(II) is included in the above discussion for the sake of generality, it should be noted that it is by far the most labile of the metals in Table II, and that mechanisms for its carcinogenic effects involving modification of proteins (particularly RNA polymerase) as opposed to DNA have also been suggested [29]. Ni (II)-protein interactions are probably of considerable biological importance in the virtually unique property of Ni (II) as an allergen [30]. Ni (II) ions, which may be released by corrosion of jewelry, might act as hapten-like modifiers of protein structure and thus provoke the immune system. In fact, in contrast to Pt (II) and functionally similar complexes, Ni (II) actually stimulates rather than inhibits the lymphocyte blastogenic response in vitro [24]. It should be noted that Pd (II) complexes, whose ligand exchange rates are intermediate between those of Ni (II) and Pt (II), also lack the antitumor effects of the latter [31].

## ISOMORPHOUS INTERCHANGE

Both bacterial and mammalian cells require folic acid as a coenzyme for a number of enzymatic reactions involving "one-carbon metabolism." Mammals cannot synthesize folic acid and thus require it in their diet, whereas bacteria cannot absorb folic acid and must therefore synthesize it. The discovery that sulfanilamide was selectively toxic to bacteria because it blocked the biosynthetic incorporation of *p*-aminobenzoic acid into folic acid formed the basis of the antimetabolite concept, a principle which still guides important research in intermediary metabolism, enzymology, biochemical toxicology and drug design [32]. Essentially, an antimetabolite is a compound having structural features which allow it to be recognized and bound by an enzyme as if it were the natural metabolite, but will not function as the normal metabolite would. The key words here are "structure" and "function." In more general terms "antimetabolites" can be primarily inorganic as well as organic compounds, although the latter are perhaps better known. Similarly the "structural recognition site" need not be the catalytic site of an enzyme but may be any site at which a reversibly bound moiety affects some biochemical or biological function, for example the carrier site of an active transport system or the allosteric site of an enzyme or gene regulator.

Mineralogists and crystallographers have long known that when ions are substituted for one another in a crystal lattice, their relative sizes are more important than their net charges, or in other words, that the best substitutions are isomorphous rather than isoelectronic. Important applications of this principle in biochemical studies have involved isomorphous replacement of physiologically important but "silent" ions such as $K^+$ and $Zn^{2+}$ with metal ions whose spectral properties are "reporters" of the chemical environment of the ion [3,5,33,34]. Replacement of the former by "probe ions" may or may not affect biological or biochemical function in the system being studied. With metalloenzymes for example, most substitutions of unnatural metals (e.g., $Cd^{2+}$ for $Zn^{2+}$) lead to substantial decreases in catalytic activity, and such substitutions have been suggested to underlie, at least in part, the toxicities of various metals not generally found in biological systems. However, this is only one example of the many ways in which isomorphous interchange may figure into the overall picture of toxicity from metal compounds.

Structural similarities between toxic metal species and important physiological substrates may allow the former to gain access to biological systems intended for the latter. Thus methyl-mercury derivatives of cysteine and homocysteine may be transported into cells by an amino acid transport system, [35], after which very rapid ligand exchange will lead to redistribution of the $CH_3Hg^+$ moiety inside the cell. Chromate ion may enter cells via an active transport system intended for sulfate ion, after which it is enzymatically reduced to the carcinogenic Cr(III) oxidation state, salts of which are absorbed very poorly if at all [21,36].

Sodium, potassium, magnesium and calcium are particularly important to biological systems, which have an almost uncanny ability to differentiate these ions from each other as well as many other potentially competing alkali, alkaline earth, lanthanide and transition metal ions. However even these systems may be fooled. Thus the toxic thallous ion ($Tl^+$) competes effectively with potassium ion for active transport in some systems, while it is preferentially selected over potassium in others [37,38]. Similarly, lithium ion interferes with active reuptake of sodium in kidney tubules, leading to electrolyte imbalances which can progress to fatal consequences [39]. Several important reviews give many other examples of biochemical applications and biological consequences of this type of isomorphous exchange of metal ions [34,40-42]. In general, most chemical as well as biological systems conform to one of a rather small number of selectivity sequences for mono- and divalent cations as well as anions, and the chemical principles which govern these are reasonably well understood. This knowledge often gives a good basis for retrospective rationalization of specific toxic effects caused by a certain metal ion in a certain organism. Unfortunately, it is not in itself sufficient for predicting toxicity; one must first know the complementary chemistry of the particular biological system, and this is where the real difficulty arises.

Isomorphous interchange of metal and nonmetal species can also have interesting biological consequences, and an elegant example of this with potentially far-reaching consequences has been unfolding for the past several years [43-48]. Phosphorylation and phosphoryl group transfer reactions play extremely important roles in the overall scheme of cellular metabolism [43]. Interference in various of these reactions by other anions such as arsenate, molybdate, tungstate and, especially, vanadate, has long been known. One key functional difference is that in these species the metal-oxygen bonds are kinetically more labile and thermodynamically weaker than corresponding P-O bonds [43,44]. Thus, in the case of arsenate, its participation in reactions which normally form phosphate esters leads to arsenate esters which are labile to spontaneous hydrolysis via As-O bond cleavage. The arsenate ion thus released can recycle in competition with phosphate, with the result that metabolic pathways and the flow of high energy phosphate intermediates (e.g., glucose-l-phosphate, 1,3-diphosphoglycerate and ATP) is disrupted, with detrimental consequences for the cell. Similar considerations apply to molybdate [44].

The essential mechanistic feature of nucleophilic phosphoryl transfer reactions is a trigonal bipyramidal transition state with entering and leaving groups in axial positions with the equatorial plane containing a metaphosphate moiety ($HOPO_2^-$) (Figure 2). The inhibitory action of transition metal oxoanions on phosphoryl transfer and phosphatase enzymes is rationalized [44-47] in terms of their ability (in contrast to phosphorus) to form relatively stable complexes with trigonal bipyramidal geometry. Thus, they apparently

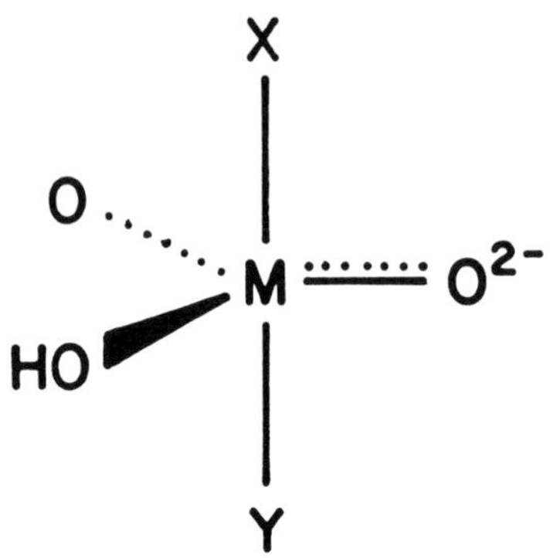


| Metal | M-O (Å) |
|---|---|
| P | 1.52 |
| As | 1.65 |
| V | 1.66-1.68 |
| Mo | 1.74 |

**Figure 2.** Transition state model for phosphoryl group-transfer reactions and ground state bond lengths for phosphate and related transition metal oxoanions. Data from VanEtten et al. [47].

act as transition state analog inhibitors of enzymes such as ribonuclease, alkaline phosphatase, and (Na,K)-ATPase. Subtle differences in these inhibitory interactions result from variations in M-O bond lengths and exchange rates with the different metals, and the closeness in match between various metal species and the particular enzyme active-site structure (Figure 2). As discussed earlier, metal oxidation state can be a major factor in determining bond lengths and ligand exchange rates. It is thus not surprising that vanadium in its $5^+$ oxidation state (vanadate, $VO_4^{3-}$) is more inhibitory than vanadyl complexes ($VO^{2+}$). The potential significance of this comes from recent studies [47] indicating that vanadate may be physiologically important in regulating (Na,K)-ATPase activity. The observation [48] of the reduction of vanadate to vanadyl complexes in vivo suggests the possible existence of a mechanism for coupling biological oxidation-reduction pathways to ion transport and the control of membrane potential, a possibility with intriguing implications.

## METAL COMPOUNDS AS INITIATORS OR CATALYSTS IN VIVO

### Metals and Gene Expression

It is not difficult to envision that inhibition of enzyme molecules by stoichiometric quantities of tightly bound metal ions could reduce the flow of vital metabolites through a pathway and thus lead to toxicity. This is especially plausible if the particular enzyme is rate-limiting in the pathway, and if the normal concentration of substrate can exceed its $K_m$; in this situation increments of toxic metal lead directly to decreases in the activity of the pathway. However, another important factor in the modulation of enzymatic pathways is regulation of the concentration of enzyme by altered rates of synthesis and degradation. For enzymes which are normally abundant and active, repression of their synthesis by metals would produce effects on the pathway of a magnitude comparable to those from direct metal-inhibition of a certain fraction of the existing enzyme. In contrast, metal-induced synthesis of enzymes which have low abundance in normal cells can lead to vary large changes in the activity of certain pathways and consequently, perhaps, to toxicity.

One physiological prototype for this type of metal-induced effect is provided by the iron-ferritin system [49]. Ferritin is a very large complex of 24 protein subunits wrapped around a ferric oxyhydroxide core containing 3000-4500 iron atoms. It is a major storage site for nonheme iron in mammals and other organisms, and administration of iron salts or complexes such as iron-dextran initiates the rapid synthesis of ferritin protein. Ferritin is also an enzyme of sorts, in that it accepts ferrous iron and oxidizes it to the ferric state, which is much less soluble as an oxide-hydroxide polymer within the protein shell.

Thionein is another cytoplasmic metal-binding protein present in many mammalian and other tissues [50]. It contains a very high proportion of cysteine, and apparently has no internal disulfide bonds. Thus, it is very well endowed as a macroligand for soft mono- and divalent cations such as zinc, cadmium, mercury, silver and copper; the metal-laden protein is called metallothionein [51]. As discussed below, metallothionein complexes and stores toxic metal ions and probably prevents them from exerting their toxic effects, even though thionein itself is a rapidly turning-over protein (as is ferritin). Its synthesis is induced [50,52] by excesses of copper and zinc and by subtoxic doses of cadmium and mercury. Evidence is beginning to accumulate that this induction can protect animals from subsequent toxic doses or accumulation of toxic levels of metal ions.

Another very important cytoplasmic sulfhydryl compound is the tripeptide glutathione (γ-glu-cys-gly [GSH]) [53]. Acute treatment of animals with a variety of toxic metal salts leads to rapid falls in intracellular GSH detectable as soluble sulfhydryl equivalents by a chromogenic disulfide exchange reaction [54,55]. However, this is soon followed by a rebound increase in free GSH to values well above the original or control concentration; similar effects are also seen after depletion of GSH by chemically reactive metabolites of organic compounds [56]. This probably indicates that GSH controls its own synthesis, and serves to emphasize the parallelism between metal ions and electrophilic organic compounds alluded to earlier.

A wide variety of metal ions have been found to affect heme biosynthesis and degradation [55]. The rate-limiting enzymes in these pathways are δ-aminolevulinic acid synthetase (ALA-S) and heme oxygenase, respectively, and the synthesis of these enzymes is regulated by heme. Increases in free intracellular heme, such as might follow an episode of hemolysis, leads to repression of ALA-S synthesis, induction of heme oxygenase synthesis, and a consequent fall in heme concentration. Metal ions including $Fe^{2+}$, $Co^{2+}$, $Ni^{2+}$, $Cu^{2+}$, $Zn^{2+}$, $Cd^{2+}$, $Sn^{2+}$, $Pt^{2+}$, $Pt^{4+}$ (reduced to $Pt^{2+}$ in vivo?), $Hg^{2+}$ and $Pb^{2+}$ have been shown to induce heme oxygenase in a variety of tissues for up to 96 hr after a single dose of the metal compounds [55]. The relative ability of these metal ions to induce heme oxygenase varies substantially from tissue to tissue, but there is no readily apparent explanation for this aspect of their action. One practical significance of this action, however, is a general depletion of cellular heme proteins, including respiratory cytochromes and cytochrome P-450 mixed function oxidases. Thus, for example, children with chronic lead intoxication may display reduced capability for oxidative biotransformation of drugs [57]. $CoCl_2$-treatment is commonly used to deplete hepatic cytochrome P-450 levels in animals in connection with drug metabolism studies, and recent unfortunate incidents of cardiotoxicity involving cobalt [58] as an additive to preserve the foamy head on beer might have involved depletion of respiratory cytochromes in myocardial mitochondria. It is quite clear the $Co^{2+}$ induces heme oxidase, and that this is probably responsible for at least the majority of the decrease in heme enzymes; $Co^{2+}$ may also inhibit directly or repress the synthesis of ALA-S, but this matter is not completely resolved [59].

One final example of a metal ion which can influence both the action and the synthesis of enzymes is beryllium. Salts of beryllium are very toxic, yet beryllium is a metal with a wide variety of industrial and military applications. Beryllium is the lightest alkaline earth metal, and one with almost unique chemical and biological properties. It is a hard divalent ion that hydrolyzes and polymerizes readily in base and interacts strongly with oxyanions such as phosphate. It also undergoes ligand exchange reactions rather slowly, in accord with its relatively large charge/radius ratio.

The biological effects of beryllium depend on the species and route of administration. In the beryllium industry, workers' health problems include contact dermatitis (compare earlier discussion of nickel allergy), pneumonitis and lung granulomatosis [60-62]. In rabbits, intravenous $BeSO_4$ leads to rapid splenic atrophy and development of osteosarcoma, whereas in rats it produces massive and fatal midzonal hepatic necrosis. Inhaled beryllium leads to lung carcinoma in rats, but guinea pigs develop contact hypersensitivity and no neoplasia. It has been suggested that the immunologic status of the animal may determine or limit the carcinogenicity of beryllium [60].

At the molecular level, beryllium shows relatively little affinity for nucleic acids or proteins in general, although there are some important and striking exceptions to this. It is not a general enzyme inhibitor, but it is a very potent inhibitor of alkaline phosphatase [61]. (Is it only coincidental that $Be^{2+}$ deposits in bone, that alkaline phosphatase is important in bone metabolism and that $Be^{2+}$ causes osteosarcoma in rabbits?) At micromolar concentrations it inhibits phosphoglucomutase irreversibly. The onset of inhibition follows first-order kinetics and is halted but not reversed by addition of $Mg^{2+}$ or substrate. The original reports [63,64] characterizing the beryllium inhibition of these two enzymes make fascinating reading, and this problem clearly invites further investigation with modern instrumentation, particularly high-resolution nuclear magnetic resonance (NMR) spectroscopy. In vitro, beryllium also inhibits DNA synthesis and causes an increase in the frequency of base substitution errors (compare Table III). Although $Be^{2+}$ does not directly inhibit thymidine kinase or thymidylate kinase, it blocks and rises in levels of these enzymes in liver which are normally induced by partial hepatectomy [65]. It does not inhibit protein synthesis in general, and did not prevent rises in other liver enzymes after partial hepatectomy. Thus it was concluded that $Be^{2+}$ selectively blocks the synthesis of thymidine kinase and thymidylate kinase. It is regrettable that despite the industrial importance of beryllium and its unique and specific effects on living systems, the study of its biochemistry and toxicology is currently at a low ebb.

## Chemical Catalysis by Metal Ions in Vivo

In addition to stimulating or inhibiting the synthesis of enzymes, as well as the enzymes themselves, many simple metal ions and compounds have catalytic activity in their own right. In some cases, expression of this activity in a living cell can have deleterious consequences. As one example of this we may consider the important electrochemical gradients across biological membranes associated with such processes as oxidative phosphorylation, muscle contraction, nerve impulse propagation, photosynthesis, kidney function and others. Several cases were mentioned earlier in which isomorphous substitution of a foreign metal ion for an endogenous substrate could lead to an "antimetabolite" effect and toxicity. Transport of ions across biological membranes generally requires some sort of "ionophore," and the search for the endogenous ionophores of cellular or organellar membranes, and the processes which regulate them, is a very active area of biological chemistry today [66]. Encouraging this search is a growing family of fermentation-derived natural ionophores, the so-called ionophoric antibiotics [67], and a growing group of synthetic ion-binding agents, the crown-ether and cryptate ligands [68].

The ionophorous antibiotics are generally toxic to mammalian cells and mitochondria because they dissolve in plasma membranes and act as a passive transport system for monovalent cations, thereby discharging critical electrochemical gradients. As yet they have no use in human medicine, but they are used in animal feeds becuase they are poorly absorbed from the digestive tract. The crown-ethers also appear to have some mammalian toxicity, but this group of compounds has received relatively little study to date [69,70]. Interestingly, some cryptate ligands have been found to increase urinary lead excretion in lead-poisoned rats. [71].

Organotin compounds, particularly the trialkyl derivatives such as triethltin chloride have a long history of use in agriculture and industry [72, 73]. Early studies of the mammalian toxicity of these compounds revealed major effects on the central nervous system, first on its function and ultimately at the histopathological level [74-76]. Shortly thereafter it was found that triethyltin was a potent inhibitor of respiration in tissue slices and, in accordance with its selective toxicity, brain was much more sensitive to its effects than liver, kidney or muscle tissue [77]. More recently the trialkyltins have been shown to derange mitochondrial function in various ways [78-81]. It might have been expected that "binding to a critical sulfhydryl group" would have been a major mechanism for the effects on mitochondria (compare Table I), but this does not really follow from the chemistry of organotin compounds. The latter by and large do not have very high affinity for O- N-, or S-donor ligands of halide ions, and tend to dissociate fairly easily, especially at lower pH. This property, which is closely shared by related trialkyllead compounds [82,83], might have foretold the biological properties of this class: trialkyltins act in mitochondrial membranes as lipid soluble inonophores for anions such as hydroxide and especially chloride. Because of the cyclincal nature of the ion-exchange process (Figure 3), major biological changes can potentially be wrought by only catalytic amounts of the tin derivative.

Methylmercury, $CH_3Hg^+$, also shares some of the chemical properties of trialkyltin and trialkllead compounds, especially reversible binding to halide ions and O-, N-, or S-donor ligands. It is also toxic to the nervous system [84-86], but unlike the trialkyltin and trialkyllead compounds, its effects develop over a period of weeks to months. Thus, it is unlikely that the same biochemical mechanisms are involved. However, an interesting proposal has been offered to relate the chemical properties of $CH_3Hg^+$, a soft Lewis acid, to the biological lesion, which involves extensive lysis of cell membranes. Segal and Wood [87] have observed in vitro that methylmercuric ion dissolves in a class of membrane phospholipids known as plasmalogens, and catalyzes the hydrolysis of an enolether linkage in these molecules (Figure 4). The likelihood of this occurring in vivo remains to be established, but the in

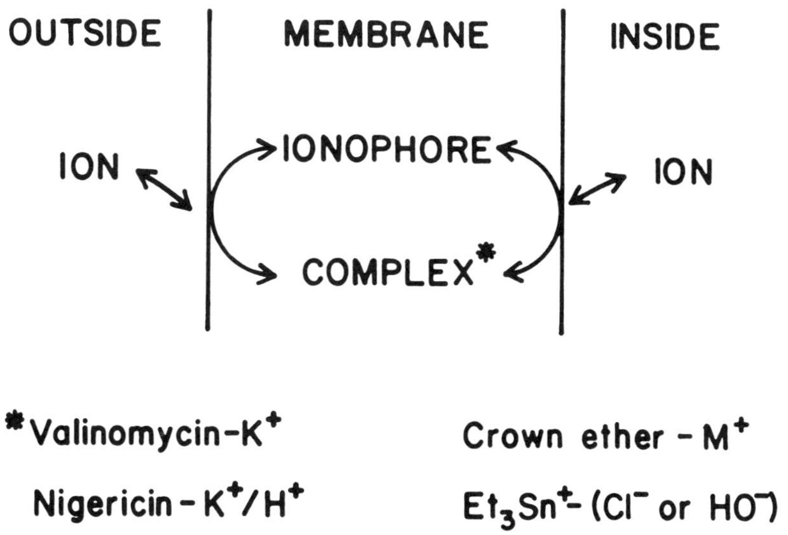


**Figure 3.** Model for ion translocation across biological membranes by ionophores.

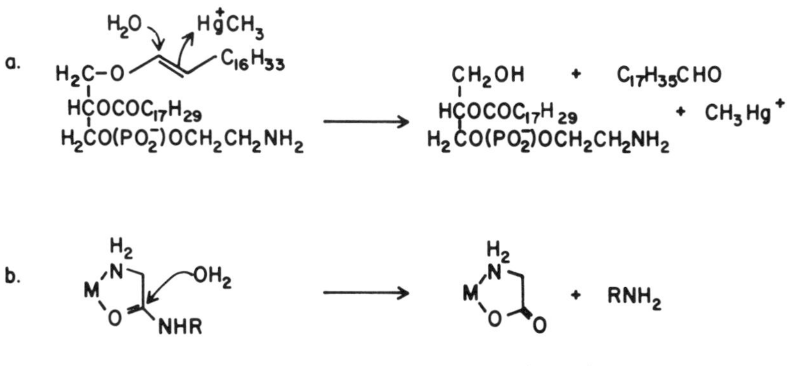


**Figure 4.** Mechanisms of hydrolytic reactions catalyzed by transition metal complexes.

vitro study was a very clever conception. Methylmercuric ion has also been shown to catalyze the cleavage of disulfide bonds in chemical systems [88].

Two remaining examples of chemical reactions which might be catalyzed by metal ions in vivo may be cited. The first involves the action of certain *cis*-$[L_4Co(OH)(OH_2)]^{2+}$ complexes as "aminopeptidases" or "ATP-ases" [5,89]. The aquo and hydroxo ligands in these complexes are labile at around physiological pH, and can be replaced by a pyrophosphate moiety of ATP or the amino and carbonyl groups of the N-terminal amino acid in a peptide. The phosphoric anhydride or peptide bonds involved are then susceptible to hydrolysis under very mild conditions. The second example involves the clearly demonstrated ability of a variety of metal-nitrosyls or metal nitrites to diazotize and/or nitrosate organic amines and to nitrosate active aromatic rings (e.g., tyrosine and tryptophan) under physiologically relevant conditions [90]. Secondary nitrosamines, which are toxic and carcinogenic, can be formed readily this way. The question which remains to be answered is how important is this process in vivo. For example, could hemoglobin or cytochrome P-450 activate nitrite ion or gaseous oxides of nitrogen, leading to diazotization of primary amines and nitrosation of secondary amines?

## COMPLEXATION AND REDOX PROCESSES IN ABSORPTION, STORAGE, METABOLISM AND EXCRETION OF METAL COMPOUNDS.

Iron is an essential element for life, and the mechanisms which have evolved for its uptake and storage exemplify the roles which redox processes and complexation chemistry can play in modulating the biological effects of metals [91]. In an oxidizing environment, iron exists in its ferric form, largely as insoluble oxides and hydroxides. Certain microorganisms have circumvented this difficulty by secreting a variety of iron-complexing ligands, known as siderophores, which bind ferric iron tightly enough to solubilize it. Iron solubilized in this way is diffusible and can be recovered by the cell through one of several mechanisms, depending on the particular siderophore and microorganism. In the simplest case the ferric-siderophore complex, which is much more lipid-soluble than simple iron salts, is absorbed by the cell and reduced enzymatically to the ferrous form. The latter is much less stable and dissociates, releasing the iron for use in cellular metabolism and the siderophore for resecretion.

The intracellular release of metal ions through biotransformation of lipid-soluble precursor complexes represents an important mechanism of entry for toxic as well as physiologic metals. Mercury vapor probably represnets the simplest example of this [84-86]. Elemental mercury is monatomic in the gas phase, and partitions readily between lipid and aqueous phases in solution. From the vapor phase it readily crosses alveolar membranes and enters plasma, from which it rapidly distributes to tissues, including the erythrocyte, brain and placenta. Injected mercury vapor also crosses alveolar membranes and is readily exhaled. However, a large fraction of mercury vapor reaching the plasma is retained in the body rather than being exhaled. The observation that ethanol increases the exhalation of administered mercury vapor led to the discovery that the major system responsible for its oxidation in vivo is catalase-$H_2O_2$, which is particularly active in erythrocytes. Thus the uptake of mercury by brain, placenta and fetus is much greater after mercury vapor than after an equivalent dose of mercuric chloride.

Similar factors may be involved in the toxicity and metabolism of $Ni(CO)_4$, an intermediate in the Mond process for nickel ore refining. Nickel carbonyl is a volatile liquid with extrordinary toxicity, particularly to the lungs [24]. The mechanism of this toxicity is not known, but the lungs play a major role in both absorption of $Ni(CO)_4$ vapors and excretion of parenterally administered $Ni(CO)_4$ [92,93]. Thus, 60 min after intravenous administration of $^{14}C$- or $^{63}Ni$- labeled $Ni(CO)_4$, 25% was exhaled unchanged, 11% was exhaled as $^{14}CO$ (with only traces of $^{14}CO_2$ detected), 10% was present as $^{14}C$-carbon-monoxyhemoglobin and 6.5% was present as unchanged $Ni(CO)_4$ in whole blood. Translocation of $^{63}Ni$ from erthrocytes to plasma correlated with the disappearance of $Ni(CO)_4$ from whole blood. Since metal-CO bonds are greatly weakened by oxidation of the central metal, it is conceivable that $Ni(CO)_4$, like $Hg^\circ$, might be biotransformed in vivo by the catalase-$H_2O_2$ system, as outlined below:

$$Ni(CO)_4 \xrightarrow[\text{(enzyme)}]{-2e^-} [Ni(CO)_4{}^{2+}] \xrightarrow[\text{fast}]{} 4CO + Ni^{2+}$$

The widely used gasoline additive tetraethyllead is a volatile liquid which easily crosses biological membranes. Its toxicity resembles that of the trialkyltin and trialkyllead compounds discussed in the previous section, and indeed it is converted in vivo to its $Et_3Pb^+$ derivative, which very likely is the true toxic species [94]. A similar situation obtains for $Et_4Sn$, and in fact the biotransformation pathways and associated nonenzymatic decomposition reactions which have been elucidated for the alkyltin group can probably be generalized to most alkyl and aryl derivatives of mercury (except possibly $CH_3Hg^+$) and lead as well as tin. Casida and co-workers [95,96] have thoroughly investigated the biotransformation of tetrabutyltin and related tri- and dialkyl derivatives. They found that the essential reactions involved cytochrome P-450 mediated hydroxylations of the alkyl chain, followed in

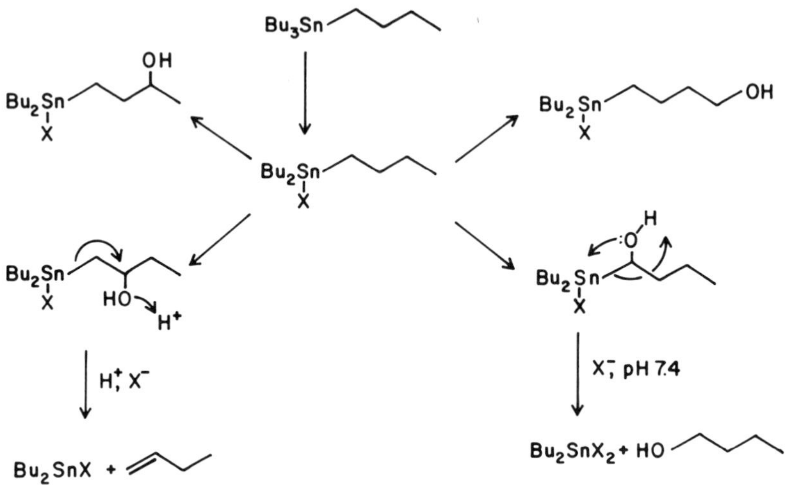

**Figure 5.** Biotransformation of organotin compounds by cytochrome P-450 enzymes.

certain cases by spontaneous or acid-catalyzed decompositions involving C-Sn bond cleavage (Figure 5).

Protodemetallation reactions are well precedented in organometallic chemistry, and are apparently involved in governing the biological fate of other alkyl and aryl derivatives of mercury and lead. Thus, the main toxicities of aryl and β-alkoxyethyl derivatives of mercury (including the mercurial diuretics) apparently stem from the rapid release of $Hg^{2+}$ in vivo by reversal of the familiar "oxymercuration" reactions used to synthesize such derivatives [97,98]. In contrast alkyl mercuric compounds (RHgX) are much more toxic because they do not decompose in the stomach, and they distribute differently in vivo, undergoing metabolic dealkylation rather slowly; $CH_3Hg^+$ is particularly troublesome in this respect. With aryllead compounds, similar chemistry is involved. Thus triphenyllead acetate has an LD50 of 6 mg/kg for intraperitoneal administration to rats, whereas for oral administration it is 200 mg/kg. In the latter case, most of the lead is not absorbed, and a considerable amount of benzene is either exhaled or converted to phenolic metabolites and excreted [99].

Cytochrome P-450 also plays a role in the biotransformation of transition metal cyclopentadienyl compounds such as ferrocene and the related manganese compound MMT (Figure 6). Early studies with ferrocene [100,101] indicated that it was well absorbed when given orally to a variety of mammals, relatively nontoxic and very efficiently reversed iron-deficiency anemia in animals and man. Recently it was found that ferrocene undergoes "aromatic

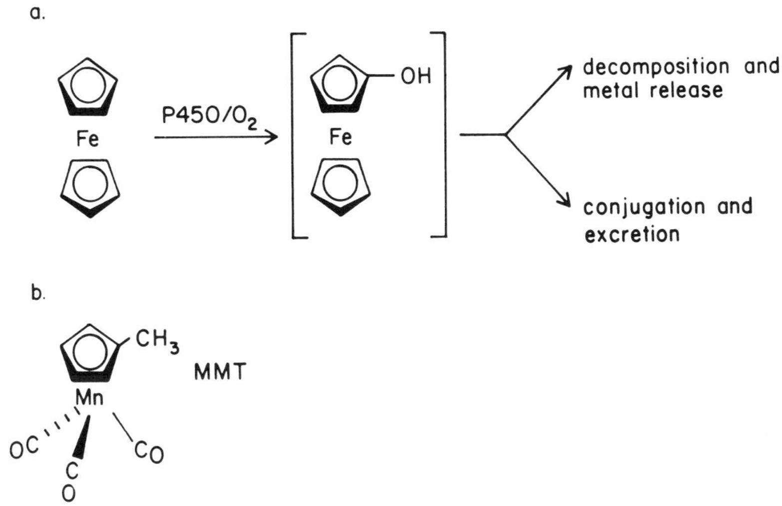


**Figure 6.** Structures and biotransformations of organometallic $\pi$-complexes.

hydroxylation" in vivo, followed by conjugation of the resultant "phenol" with sulfate or glucuronic acid. However, a portion of the rather unstable hydroxyferrocene decomposes with release of iron before it can be stabilized by conjugation [102].

Methylcyclopentadienyl manganese tricarbonyl (MMT) is currently being used as an antiknock additive in unleaded gasolines [103]. Rats metabolize tritiated MMT extensively and excrete at least five urinary metabolites containing tritium; two major urinary metabolites also contain manganese in approximately the same $^{3}$H:Mn ratio as the MMT administered, while the others are apparently devoid of manganese [104]. In contrast to ferrocene, MMT is a very toxic compound, producing a severe hemorrhagic lung edema [105-106]. It is unclear whether the toxicity is due to MMT itself or its biotransformation products. However, the lesion it produces is not caused by inorganic manganese compounds nor by doses of methylcyclopentadiene as high as 1 g/kg. Thus it appears that MMT toxicity must be due either to the complex itself, or to a biotransformation product which has not completely dissociated to separate metal- and ligand-derived fragments [105].

Regardless of the mechanism by which a metal ion enters a biological system, complexation will undoubtedly play an extremely important role in both its distribution within and elimination from the organism. Fortunately, a great deal is already known about the chemistry of metal ion complexation. For small, hard cations such as lithium, complexation involves mainly hydration. At the other extreme large soft cations, the so-called heavy metals, prefer soft donor ligands such as sulfur. Soft cations which have sufficient Lewis acid character may also undergo a unique vitamin $B_{12}$-dependent methylation; included in this category are mercury, platinum, arsenic, gold and thallium, but not lead and probably not tin or cadmium salts [35,107].

Biological systems have at their disposal a number of agents for complexing or sequestering both physiological and aphysiological metal ions. Glutathione, ferritin and thionein have already been discussed, but it is also worth mentioning transferrin and ceruloplasmin in this context. Albumin, the major protein in plasma, also serves as an important ligand for metals such as copper and nickel [24,108]. Human, rabbit, rat and bovine serum albumins bind copper or nickel ion at a single high-affinity site, although additional ions may be weakly bound at secondary sites. The primary site is furnished by the terminal amino group, the nitrogens of the two terminal peptide bonds, and an imidazole of histidine in the third position from the end (i.e., $H_2N$-asp-thr-his-). Canine and procine albumin have an altered N-terminal sequence ($H_2N$-asp-thr-tyr-), and have a much lower affinity for copper and nickel.

In addition to albumin and other proteins, plasma contains a large number of small peptide fragments and even free amino acids which can complex metal ions [24,109]. Although there is relatively little specific information about the identity of these complexes, it is clear that they provide one important mechanism for elimination of metal ions, namely filtration through the glomerular membrane and excretion in the urine.

Biliary secretion is another route of elimination for metals such as copper, arsenic lead and manganese [110]. In fact, for manganese, biliary excretion is the only significant route of elimination [111]. Methylmercury in bile is found as a glutathione adduct [112], but, in general, little is known of the chemical forms of other metals in bile, and whether the metal ions or their complexes are the actively secreted forms. Although the metal may be more concentrated in bile than in plasma, this route of elimination is not always efficient because of reabsorption of the metal from the intestinal tract. Attempts to prevent this reabsorption by oral administration of chelating- or ion-exchange resins have met with mixed results [84]; the same can be said for chelation therapy as a general approach to metal poisoning and disorders of metal metabolism such as Wilson's disease [71,109,113,114]. However, this is an area which holds much promise, and the recent activity with iron chelators may help to define better the problems which must be solved.

In many cases apparently nonessential metals which are absorbed into an organism are not eliminated at all, but are simply concentrated in granular deposits as insoluble complexes with or without accompanying proteinaceous material. Deposits of this kind are especially common with many kinds of algae and lower animals, and may contain manganese, barium, strontium, iron, zinc, aluminum, boron, copper, tin or arsenic [115]. Metallic concretions may also be found in mammalian cells. One example is the "nuclear inclusion bodies" observed in kidney cells and long regarded as pathognomonic for chronic lead poisoning. These structures have recently been shown to contain large amounts of both lead and proteins [116]. The occurrence of such deposits is often interpreted as an adaptive response to a metal-polluted environment, although metal exclusion as an adaptive response is also known [117]. It has been noted [115] that intracellular deposits of metals are often associated with the endoplasmic reticulum and/or Golgi apparatus in cells of tissues which are connected in some direct way to the exterior of the organism, suggesting that these packages of metals may ultimately be destined for elimination from the organism. It is also interesting to speculate that bones, teeth, shells and other hard structures of higher organisms may have evolved from such a primitive beginning. Many metals other than calcium may deposit in bone and reside there indefinitely, but because bone is a metabolically active tissue, metal ions trapped in bone should not be regarded as permanently detoxified.

## CONCLUSION

Present knowledge of the mechanisms by which xenobiotic chemicals affect living organisms is derived largely from studies with organic compounds. A good deal of this knowledge has been organized around a small number of basic generalizations pertaining to the chemical interactions between foreign and endogenous substances, and to the consequences these interactions may have for a cell and its processes. The above discussion has attempted to extend these considerations to metal compounds by relating similarities between organic and metallic compounds existing at the level of structure and reaction mechanism to similarities in the ways in which these two broad classes of compounds interact with, and thus affect, biological systems. In closing it is perhaps worth emphasizing that toxicity is not an intrinsic property of a given metal, but a consequence of the way in which the metal compound and the cell interact. It is this interaction which is governed by intrinsic chemical properties, both those of the metal complex and those of the cell.

## ACKNOWLEDGMENT

The preparation of this manuscript, as well as the author's research mentioned here, was carried out with financial support provided by the National Institutes of Health through research grant ES-01375.

## REFERENCES


1. Jollow, D. J., J. J. Kocsis, P. Snyder, and H. Vainio, Eds. *Biological Reactive Intermediates: Formation Toxicity and Inactivation* (New York: Plenum Publishing Corporation, 1978).
2. Eichhorn, G., Ed. *Inorganic Biochemistry* (Amsterdam: Elsvier, 1973).
3. Sigel, H., Ed. *Metal Ions in Biological Systems Volumes 1-7*, (New York: Marcel Dekker, Inc., 1972-1978).
4. Ochiai, E. *Bioinorganic, Chemistry: An Introduction* Boston: Allyn and Bacon, Inc., 1977).
5. Hanzlik, R. P. *Inorganic Aspects of Biological and Organic Chemistry* (New York: Academic Press, Inc., 1976).
6. Irving, H., and R. J. P. Williams. "The Stability of Transition-Metal Complexes," *J. Chem. Soc.* (London, 1953) pp. 3192-3210.
7. Shaw, W. H. R. "Cation Toxicity and the Stability of Transition-Metal Complexes," *Nature* 192:754-755 (1961).
8. Aull, J. L., A. C. Rice and L. A. Tibbetts. "Interactions of Platinum Complexes With Essential and Nonessential Sulfhydryl Groups of Thymidylate Synthetase," *Biochemistry* 16(4):672-677 (1977).
9. Aldridge, W. N., and J. E. Cremer. "The Biochemistry of Organo-Tin Compounds," *Biochem. J.* 61:406-418 (1955).
10. Armstrong, J., and M. Webb. "The Reversal of Phenylarsenoxide Inhibition of Keto Acid Oxidation in Mitochondrial and Bacterial Suspensions by Lipoic Acid and other Disculfides," *Biochem. J.* 103:913-922 (1967).
11. Leh, R. K. V., and W. Wolf. "Platinum Complexes: A New Class of Antineoplastic Agent," *J. Pharmacol. Sci.* 65(3):315-328 (1976).
12. Gale, G. R. "Platinum Compounds," *Handbuch Exp. Pharmakol.* 38(2): 829-840 (1975).
13. Monti-Bragadin, C., M. Tamaro and E. Banfi. "Mutagenic Activity of Platinum and Ruthenium Complexes," *Chem.-Biol. Interact.* 11:469-472 (1975).
14. Leopold, W. R., E. C. Miller, and J. A. Miller. "Carcinogenicity of Antitumor *cis*-Platinum (II) Coordination Complexes in the Mouse and Rat," *Cancer Res.* 39:913-918 (1979).
15. Lazar, R., P. C. Conran and I. Domjanov. "Embryotoxicity and Teratogenicity of *cis*-Diamminedichloroplatinum," *Experientia* 35(5):647-648 (1979).
16. Klugmann, R. B., B. Pani, and G. Castellani. "Effects of Transition Metal Complexes on Human Lymphocyte Blastogenesis in Vitro," *Pharmacol. Res. Comm.* 9(2):149-154 (1977).
17. Giraldi, T., G. Zassinovich and G. Mestroni. "Antitumor Action of Planar, Organometallic Rhodium (I) Complexes," *Chem.-Biol. Interact.* 9:389-394 (1974).
18. Theodotou, A., R. J. Stretton, A. H. Norbury and A. G. Massey. "Morphologicol Effects of Chromium and Cobalt Complexes on Bacteria," *Bioinorg. Chem.* 5:235-239 (1976).
19. Petrilli, F. L., and S. DeFlora. "Oxidation of Inactive Chromium to the Mutagenic Hexavalent Form," *Mutat. Res.* 58:167-173 (1978).

20. Petrilli, F. L., and S. DeFlora. "Metabolic Deactivation of Hexavalent Chromium Mutagenicity," *Mutat. Res.* 54:139-147 (1978).
21. Jennette, K. W. "Chromate Metabolism in Liver Microsomes," in *Biological Trace Element Research* (in press).
22. "OSHA Issues Tentative Carcinogen List" *Chem. Eng. News* (July 31, 1978), pp 20-22.
23. Sirover, M. A., and L. A. Loeb. "Infidelity of DNA Synthesis in vitro: Screening for Potential Metal Mutagens or Carcinogens," *Science* 194: 1434-1436 (1976).
24. Sunderman, F. W. "The Metabolism and Toxicology of Nickel," in *Clinical Chemistry and Chemical Toxicology of Metals,* S. S. Brown, Ed. (New York: Elsevier/North-Holland, 1977), pp 231-259.
25. Sunderman, F. W., P. R. Allpass, J. M. Mitchell, R. C. Baselt and D. M. Albert. "Eye Malformations in Rats: Induction by Prenatal Exposure to Nickel Carbonyl," *Science* 203:550-553 (1979).
26. Sunderman, F. W. "The Current Status of Nickel Carcinogenesis," *Ann. Clin. Lab. Sci.* 3(3):156-180 (1973).
27. Sunderman, F. W., and R. M. Maenza. "Comparisons of Carcinogenicities of Nickel Compounds in Rats," *Res. Comm. Chem. Pathol. Pharmcol.* 14(2):319-330 (1976).
28. Erck, A., L. Rainen, J. Whileyman, I.-M. Chang, A. P. Kimball and J. Bear. "Studies of Rhodium (II) Carboxylates as Potential Antitumor Agents," *Proc. Soc. Exp. Biol. Med.* 145:1278-1283 (1974).
29. Sunderman, F. W., K. S. Kasprzak, T. J. Lau, P. P. Minghetti, R. M. Maenza, N. Becker, C. Onkelinx and P. J. Goldblatt. "Effects of Manganese on Carcinogenicity and Metabolism of Nickel Subsulfide," *Cancer Res.* 36:1790-1800 (1976).
30. Wahlberg, J. E. "Sensitization and Testing of Guinea Pigs with Nickel Sulfate," *Dermatologica* 152:321-330 (1976).
31. Cleare, M. J., and J. D. Hoeschele. "Studies on the Antitumor Activity of Group VIII Transition Metal Complexes. Part I. Platinum (II) Complexes," *Bioinorg. Chem.* 187-210 (1973).
32. Rogers, E. F. "The Antimetabolite Concept in Drug Design," *Ann. Rep. Med. Chem.* 11:233-241 (1976).
33. Horrocks, W. DeW., and D. R. Sudnick. "Lanthanide Ion Probes of Structure in Biology. Laser-Induced Luminescence Decay Constants Provide a Direct Measure of the Number of Metal-Coordinated Water Molecules," *J. Am. Chem. Soc.* 101(2):334-340 (1979).
34. Williams, R. J. P. "The Biochemistry of Sodium, Potassium, Magnesium, and Calcium," *Quart. Rev. Chem. Soc.* 24:331-365 (1970).
35. Wood, J. M. "Biological Cycles for Elements in the Environment," *Naturwissenschaft.* 62:357-364 (1974).
36. Gruber, J. E., and K. E. Jennette. "Metabolism of the Carcinogen Chromate by Rat Liver Microsomes," *Biochem. Biophys. Res. Comm.* 82(2):700-706 (1978).
37. Melnick, R. L., L. G. Monti and S. Motzkin. "Uncoupling of Mitrochondrial Oxidative Phosphorylation by Thallium," *Biochem. Biophys. Res. Comm.* 69(1):68-73 (1976).
38. Gehring, P. J., and P. B. Hammond. "The Interrelationship Between

Thallium and Potassium in Animals," *J. Pharmacol. Exp. Ther.* 155(1): 187-201 (1967).
39. Thomsen, K. "Renal Elimination of Lithium in Rats with Lithium Intoxication." *J. Pharmacol. Exp. Ther.* 199(3):483-489 (1976).
40. Frausto da Silva, J. J. R., and R. J. P. Williams. "The Uptake of Elements by Biological Systems," *Structure Bonding* 29:67-121 (1976).
41. Wright, E. M. and J. M. Diamond. "Anion Selectivity in Biological Systems," *Physiol. Rev.* 57(1):109-156 (1977).
42. Diamond, J. M., and E. M. Wright. "Biological Membranes: The Physical Basis of Ion and Nonelectrolyte Selectivity," *Ann. Rev. Physiol.* 31:581-646 (1969).
43. Byers, L. D., H. S. She and A. Alayoff. "Interaction of Phosphate Analogs with Glyceraldehyde-3-phosphate Dehydrogenase," *Biochemistry* 18(12):2471-2480 (1979).
44. Lindquist, R. N., J. L. Lynn and G. E. Lienhard. "Possible Transition State Analogs for Ribonuclease. The Complexes of Uridine with Oxovanadium (IV) Ion and Vanadium (V) Ion," *J. Am. Chem. Soc.* 95(26): 8762-8768 (1973).
45. VanEtten, R. L., P. P. Waymack and D. M. Rehkop. "Transition Metal Ion Inhibition of Enzyme-Catalyzed Phosphate Ester Displacement Reactions," *J. Am. Chem. Soc.* 96(21):6782-6785 (1974).
46. Lopez, V., T. Stevens and R. N. Lindquist. "Vanadium Ion Inhibition of Alkaline Phosphatase-Catalyzed Phosphate Ester Hydrolysis," *Arch. Biochem. Biophys.* 175:31-38 (1976).
47. Cantley, L. C., L. G. Cantley and L. Josephson. "A Characterization of Vanadate Interactions with the (Na,K)-ATPase," *J. Biol. Chem.* 253: 7361-7368 (1978).
48. Cantley, L. C., and P. Aisen. "The Fate of Cytoplasmic Vanadium," *J. Biol. Chem.* 254:1781-1784 (1979).
49. Munro, H. N., and M. C. Linder. "Ferritin: Structure, Biosynthesis, and Role in Iron Metabolism," *Physiol. Rev.* 58:317-396 (1978).
50. Cherian, M. G., and R. A. Goyer. "Metallothioneins and their Role in the Metabolism and Toxicity of Metals," *Life Sci.* 23:1-10 (1978).
51. Chen, R. W., H. E. Ganther and W. G. Koekstra. "Studies on the Binding of Methylmercury by Thionein," *Biochem. Biophys. Res. Comm.* 51(2): 383-390 (1973).
52. Rudd, C. J., and H. R. Herschman. "Metallothionein in a Human Cell Line: The Response of HeLa Cells to Cadmium and Zinc," *Toxicol. Appl. Pharmacol.* 47:273-278 (1979).
53. Chasseand, L. F. "The Nature and Distribution of Enzymes Catalyzing the Conjugation of Glutathione with Foreign Compounds," *Drug Metab. Rev.* 2:185-220 (1974).
54. Maines, M. D., and A. Kappas. "Regulation of Heme Pathway Enzymes and Cellular Glutathione Content by Metals That Do Not Chelate with Tetrapyrroles: Blockade of Metal Effects by Thiols," *Proc. Nat. Acad. Sci.*, U.S.A. 74(5):1875-1878 (1977).
55. Maines, M. D., and A. Kappas. "Metals as Regulators of Heme Metabolism," *Science* 198:1215-1221 (1977).
56. Thor, H., P. Moldeus, A. Kristofferson, J. Hogberg, D. J. Reed and S. Orrenius. "Metabolic Activation and Hepatotoxicity," *Arch. Biochem. Biophys.* 188:114-121 (1978).

57. Anderson, K. E., A. Fischbein, D. Kestenbaum, A. Sassa, A. P. Alvares and A. Kappas. "Plumbism from Airborne Lead in a Firing Range," *Am. J. Med.* 63:306-312 (1977).
58. Alexander, C. S. "Cobalt and the Heart," *Ann. Intern. Med.* 70:411-413 (1969).
59. DeMatteis, F., and A. H. Gibbs. "Inhibition of Heme Synthesis Caused by Cobalt in Rat Liver," *Biochem. J.* 162:213-216 (1977).
60. Reeves, A. L. "Beryllium Carcinogenesis," *Adv. Exp. Med. Biol.* 91: 13-27 (1978).
61. Thomas, M., and W. N. Aldridge. "The Inhibition of Enzymes by Beryllium," *Biochem. J.* 98:94-99 (1966).
62. Vacher, J., and H. B. Stoner. "The Transport of Beryllium in Rat Blood," *Biochem. Pharmacol.* 17:93-107 (1968).
63. Aldridge, W. N., and M. Thomas. "The Inhibition of Phosphoglucomutase by Beryllium," *Biochem. J.* 98:100-104 (1966).
64. Hashimoto, R., J. G. Joshi, C. Del Rio and P. Handler. "Phosphoglucomutase. IV. Inactivation by Beryllium Ions," *J. Biol. Chem.* 242: 1671-1679 (1967).
65. Witschi, H. P. "Effects of Beryllium on Deoxyribonucleic Acid-Synthesizing Enzymes in Regenerating Rat Liver," *Biochem. J.* 120:623-634 (1970).
66. Shamoo, A. E., and D. A. Goldstein. "Isolation of Ionophores from Ion Transport Systems and Their Role in Energy Transduction," *Biochim. Biophys. Acta* 472:13-53 (1977).
67. Westley, J. W. "The Polyether Antibiotics: Monocarboxylic Acid Ionophores," *Ann. Rep. Med. Chem.* 10:246-256 (1975).
68. Lehn, J. M. "Cryptates: The Chemistry of Macrobicyclic Inclusion Complexes," *Accts. Chem. Res.* 11(2):49-57 (1978).
69. Leong, B. K., T. O. T. Ts'O and M. B. Chenoweth. "Testicular Atrophy from Inhalation of Ethylene Oxide Cyclic Tetramer," *Toxicol. Appl. Pharmacol.* 27:342-354 (1974).
70. Talsayama, K., S. Hasegawa, S. Sasagowa, N. Nambu and T. Nagai. "Apparent Oral Toxicity of 18-Crown-6 in Dogs," *Chem. Pharmacol. Bull.* (Tokyo) 25(11):3125 (1977).
71. Baudot, Ph., M. Jacque and M. Robin. "Effect of a Diaza-Polyoxa-Macrobicyclic Complexing Agent on the Urinary Elimination of Lead in Lead-Poisoned Rats," *Toxicol. Appl. Pharmacol.* 41:113-118 (1977).
72. Smith, P. and L. Smith. "Organotin Compounds and Applications," *Chem. Brit.* 11(5):208-212 (1975).
73. Zuckerman, J. J., Ed. *Organotin Compounds: New Chemistry and Applications, Adv. Chem. Ser. Vol. 157,* (Washington DC: American Chemical Society, 1976).
74. Stoner, H. B., J. M. Barnes and J. I. Duff. "Studies on the Toxicity of Alkyl Tin Compounds," *Brit. J. Pharmacol.* 10:16-25 (1955).
75. Stoner, H. B., and C. J. Threlfall. "The Biochemistry of Organotin Compounds," *Biochem. J.* 69:376-385 (1958).
76. Magee, P. N., H. B. Stoner and J. M. Barness. "Experimental Production of Edema in the Central Nervous System of the Rat by Triethyltin Compounds," *J. Pathol. Bacteriol.* 73:107-117 (1957).
77. Cremer, J. E. "The Metabolism in vitro of Tissue Slices from Rats given Triethyltin Compounds," *Biochem. J.* 67:87-96 (1957).

78. Aldridge, W. N. "The Influence of Organotin Compounds on Mitochondrial Function," in *Organotin Compounds: New Chemistry and Applications, Adv. Chem. Ser., Vol. 157*, J. J. Zuckerman, Ed. (Washington DC: American Chemical Society, 1976), pp. 186-196.
79. Selwyn, M. J. "Triorganotin Compounds as Inonophores and Inhibitors of Ion Translocating ATPases," in *Organotin Compounds: New Chemistry and Applications, Adv. Chem. Ser., Vol. 157,* J. J. Zuckerman, Ed. (Washington, DC: American Chemical Society, 1976), pp. 204-226.
80. Bygrave, F. L., C. Ramachandran, and R. N. Robertson. "The Interaction of Tributyltin with the Mitochondrial Calcium Transport System of Rat Liver," *Arch. Biochem. Biophys.* 188(2):301-307 (1978).
81. Aldridge, W. N., J. E. Casida, R. H. Fish, E. C. Kimmel and B. W. Street. "Action on Mitochondria and Toxicity of Metabolites of Tri-n-Butyltin Derivatives," *Biochem. Pharmacol.* 26:1997-2000 (1977).
82. Shapiro, H. and F. W. Frey. "The Organic Compounds of Lead," (New York: Wiley Interscience, 1968).
83. Greninger, D., V. Kollonitsch and C. H. Cline. "Lead Compounds," International Lead-Zinc Research Organization (1978).
84. Clarkson, T. W. "Factors Involved in Heavy Metal Poisoning," *Fed. Proc.* 36(5):1634-1639 (1977).
85. Gerstner, H. B. and J. E. Huff. "Clinical Toxicology of Mercury," *J. Toxicol. Environ. Health* 2:491-526 (1977).
86. MacGregor, J. T., and T. W. Clarkson. "Distribution, Tissue Binding, and Toxicity of Mercurials," *Adv. Exp. Med. Biol.* 48:463-503 (1974).
87. Segal, H. J., and J. M. Wood. "Reaction of Methylmercury with Plasmalogens Suggests a Mechanism for Neurotoxicity of Metal-Alkyls," *Nature* 248(5447):456-458 (1974).
88. Bach, R. D., and S. J. Rajan. "Kinetics of Disulfide Cleavage by Methylmercury. Evidence for a Concomitant Electrophilic and Nucleophilic Mechanism," *J. Am. Chem. Soc.* 101(11):3112-3113 (1979).
89. Suzuki, S., S. Kimura, T. Higashiyama and A. Nakahara. "Hydrolysis of Adenosine 5′-Triphosphate in the Presence of Some Cobalt (III) Chelates," *Bioinorg. Chem.* 3:183-186 (1974).
90. McCleverty, J. A. "Reactions of Nitric Oxide Coordinated to Transition Metals," *Chem. Rev.* 79(1):53-76 (1979).
91. Raymond, K. N., and C. J. Carrano. "Coordination Chemistry and Microbial Iron Transport," *Accts. Chem. Res.* 12:183-190 (1979).
92. Sunderman, F. W., and C. E. Selin. "The Metabolism of Nickel-63 Carbonyl," *Toxicol. Appl. Pharmacol.* 12:207-218 (1968).
93. Kasprzak, K. S., and F. W. Sunderman. "The Metabolism of Nickel Carbonyl-$^{14}$C," *Toxicol. Appl. Pharmacol.* 15:295-303 (1969).
94. Cremer, J. E. "The Biochemistry of Organotin Compounds," *Biochem. J.* 68:685-692 (1958).
95. Fish, R. H., E. C. Kimmel and J. E. Casida. "Bioorganotin Chemistry: Biological Oxidation of Organotin Compounds," in *Organotin Compounds: New Chemistry and Applications, Adv. Chem. Ser., Vol. 157,* J. J. Zuckerman, Ed. (Washington, DC: American Chemical Society, 1976), pp. 197-203.
96. Fish, R. H., J. E. Casida and E. C. Kimmel. "Bioorganotin Chemistry: Situs and Stereoselectivity in the Reaction of Cyclohexyltriphenyltin

with a Cytochrome P-450 Dependent Monoxygenase Enzyme System" *Tetrahedron Lett.* (40):3515-3518 (1977).

97. Daniel, J. W., J. C. Gage and P. A. Lefevre. "The Metabolism of Methoxyethylmercury Salts," *Biochem. J.* 121:411-415 (1971).
98. Daniel, J. W., J. C. Gage and P. A. Lefevre. "The Metabolism of Phenylmercury by the Rat," *Biochem. J.* 129:961-967 (1972).
99. Williams, B., L. G. Dring and R. T. Williams. "The Fate of Triphenyllead Acetate in the Rat," *Toxicol. Appl. Pharmacol.* 46:567-578 (1978).
100. Yeary, R. A. "Chronic Toxicity of Dicyclopentadienyliron in the Dog," *Toxicol. Appl. Pharmacol.* 15:666-676 (1969).
101. Golberg, L., and L. E. Martin. "The Absorption, Distribution, and Utilization of Iron in Fat-Soluble Form," *Life Sci.* 3:1465-1471 (1964).
102. Hanzlik, R. P., and W. H. Soine. "Enzymatic Hydroxylation of Ferrocene," *J. Am. Chem. Soc.* 100:1290-1291 (1978).
103. *Chem. Eng. News,* (May 21, 1979) p.8; (April 16, 1979) p. 4.
104. Hanzlik, R. P., P. Bhatia, R. Stitt and G. J. Traiger. "Biotransformation and Excretion of Methylcyclopentadienyl Manganese Tricarbonyl (MMT) in the Rat," *Drug. Metab. Disp.* (in press).
105. Hanzlik, R. P., R. Stitt and G. J. Traiger. "Toxic Effects of Methylcyclopentadienyl Manganese Tricarbonyl (MMT) in Rats. Role of Metabolism," *Toxicol. Appl. Pharmacol.* (in press).
106. Hysell, D. K., W. Moore, J. F. Stara, R. Miller and K. I. Campbell. "Oral Toxicity of Methylcyclopentadienyl Manganese Tricarbonyl (MMT) in Rats," *Environ. Res.* 7:158-168 (1974).
107. Wood, J. W. "Biological Cycles for Toxic Elements in the Environment," *Science* 183:1049-1052 (1974).
108. Osterberg, R. "Metal Ion-Protein Interactions in Solution," in *Metal Ions in Biological Systems, Vol. 3,* H. Sigel, Ed. (New York: Marcel Dekker, Inc., 1974), pp. 45-88.
109. Perrin, D. D., and R. P. Agarwal. "Multimetal-Multiligand Equilibria: A Model for Biological Systems," in *Metal Ions in Biological Systems, Vol. 2,* H. Sigel, Ed. (New York: Marcel Dekker, Inc., 1973), pp. 167-206.
110. Klaassen, C. D. "Biliary Excretion of Xenobiotics," *CRC Crit. Rev. Toxicol.* 2:1-29 (1975).
111. Cotzias, G. C., and J. J. Greenough. "The High Specificity of the Manganese Pathway through the Body," *J. Clin. Invest.* 37:1298-1305 (1958).
112. Omata, S., K. Sakimura, T. Ishii and H. Sugano. "Chemical Nature of a Methylmercury Complex with a Low Molecular Weight in the Liver Cytosol of Rats Exposed to Methylmercury Chloride," *Biochem. Pharmacol.* 27:1700-1702 (1978).
113. Yoshida, A., B. E. Kaplan and M. Kimura. "Metal-Binding and Detoxification Effect of Synthetic Oligopeptides Containing Three Cysteinyl Residues," *Proc. Nat. Acad. Sci., US* 76(1):486-490 (1979).

114. Grady, R. W., and A. Cerami. "The Current Status of Iron Chelation Therapy," *Ann. Rep. Med. Chem.* 13:219-226 (1978).
115. Sinkiss, K. "Metal Ions in Cells," *Endeavour New Ser.* 3:2-6 (1979).
116. Choie, D. D., and G. W. Richter. "Lead Poisoning: Rapid Formation of Intranuclear Inclusions," *Science* 177:1194-1195 (1972).
117. Foster, P. L. "Copper Exclusion as a Mechanism of Heavy Metal Tolerance in a Green Alga," *Nature* 269:322-323 (1977).

# CHAPTER 24

# SOME SPECIATION AND MECHANISTIC ASPECTS OF TRACE METALS IN BIOLOGICAL SYSTEMS

**Duane R. Boline**

Department of Chemistry
Emporia State University
Emporia, Kansas

## INTRODUCTION

Trace metals have an important role in the proper functioning of biological systems. This fact is well documented. The mechanisms by which these substances influence the chemical reactions occurring in living organisms are not completely understood. This is partially caused by a dependence on the chemical species of the metal present. Trace metals can exist in three basic forms: (1) the free hydrated ion; (2) bound to a ligand in a manner that allows the metal to remain labile and subject to dissociation by changes in concentration of free metal, pH, presence of other chelating groups or changes in ionic strength of the medium; and (3) tightly bound metal chelates in which the metal is not exchanged or dissociated readily. These categories do not imply the existance of a rigid method for classifying metals or organmetallic complexes, but merely emphasize the need for analytical methods which are capable of distinguishing between different chemical species of a metal in a biological system. Unfortunately, such methods are not readily available.

The analytical techniques that have been developed for the determination of metals at the subnanogram levels often encountered in environmental and biological samples do not distinguish between different species of the element. Knowledge of the total amount of a metal present in a sample has increased awareness of the importance of these elements in our environment. The number of essential trace metals has been expanded as studies of the growth rate and abnormal skeletal and tissue development of animals fed diets that are deficient in a particular metal have been performed. Knowledge of the toxicity of metals to biological systems has been enhanced as the ability to measure accurately trace quantities of these substances in blood, urine and tissue has improved. However, the mechanisms by which these elements enhance or inhibit body functions are not well defined. Enough information has been obtained to make some general comments about the role of trace metals. The rate of absorption into the body, mode of transport, ultimate storage site or excretion, and biological half-life of the element are quite dependent on the chemical species of the metal. The minimum amount of an essential metal required for proper functioning of metabolic processes and the concentration at which symptoms of toxicity begin to appear are often within a narrow range. The actual amounts of a substance which will invoke a toxic response in an organism is difficult to determine because of the ability to store some metals in a relatively inert form in skeletal tissue (e.g., lead) or bind it to a low-molecular-weight protein (e.g., Cd-metallothione). The toxicity of a metal is normally related to the concentration of the free ion or an alkylated molecule such as methylmercury or tetraethyllead. These species are more readily transported through the biological system than are the chelated forms of the metal.

The reason for the present lack of knowledge in trace element speciation and reaction mechanisms is actually twofold. Analytical instrumentation currently available for the determination of trace metals at the concentration levels encountered in biological samples is usually not capable of distinguishing between different chemical species of a metal. Only the total metal content is determined, and any interactions with the organic compounds in the sample is referred to as matrix interference. The analytical techniques commonly used for trace analysis (atomic absorption and atomic emission spectroscopy, neutron activation, and X-ray fluorescence) provide data related to the total amount of a metal present in the sample. Any information related to the chemical species must be obtained by separation procedures or isolation methods used to prepare the sample for analysis. Gas chromatographic techniques have been used to separate the different species of volatile organic compounds of lead and mercury, but most metal-organic molecules are not suitable for this type of speciation. Advances in the use of liquid chromatographic techniques and the capability of combining high-performance liquid chromatograph (HPLC) with an electrically heated atomic absorption (HVAA) device, such as the graphite tube atomizer, holds a great deal of promise for advancing the knowledge of trace metal species found in biological systems.

Electrochemical methods have some distinct advantages over spectroscopic methods for differentiating between chemical species of a metal. Specific ion electrodes are capable of measuring only the free ion concentration of a system containing both free and bound metal ions, but the sensitivity and precision normally obtained in practice does not approach that predicted in theory.

Polarographic methods, incuding square wave, pulsed polarography and electrode plating techniques, are also capable of determining trace quantities of metals. Speciation is possible through the difference in half-wave and redox potentials of free and bound metal ions.

The second and possibly more difficult task related to chemical speciation is the procurement of a sample in a form suitable for analysis without disrupting the chemical environment in a manner that will alter the form or relative amounts of each chemical species of a metal present in the original system. Changes in the ionic strength, pH and temperature can influence the stability of an organometallic complex or the oxidation state of a metal. The development of procedures for obtaining a sample with minimal disruption of the chemical species will need to be the first advancement in the quest to advance our knowledge of the mechanisms by which trace metals influence biological processes.

The purpose of this review is to summarize the present knowledge of the role of trace metals in biological systems. An attempt has been made to emphasize the need for further study to determine the mechanisms by which these elements function as the active sites of metalloenzymes or as enzyme activators.

This is not a comprehensive review of all known functions of each metal, but an attempt has been made to present an accurate account of what is currently known about each of the metals discussed in regard to their chemical activity in mammals. Emphasis has been placed on proposed reaction mechanisms and chemical speciation of the metal ions.

More emphasis has been placed on the chemistry of the enzymes containing metals of the first period of transition elements (Mn, Fe, Co, Cu and Zn) than on the metals that are more commonly considered important because of their toxicity (Pb, Hg, Cd and As). This is consistent with the theory that one must first understand what is normal before abnormal effects can be explained. Unfortunately, the normal mechanisms by which cellular metabolism, self-maintenance and replication occur are still not completely defined, despite recent advances in these areas. The ability to identify the biochemically active species of trace metals should significantly advance our knowledge of these processes.

If one is to attempt to explain the apparently complex interactions of enzymes, coenzymes, cofactors and substrates encountered in biological systems, consideration of the chemistry of coordination compounds is imperative. Crystal field stabilization energies, redox potentials of complexes, geometric orientation of bonding orbitals, polarizability and ionic radii of metallic ions all have a part in determining the function and stability of a metalloenzyme.

Thermodynamic stability of a complex is often considered when one attempts to explain the selectivity of a metal ion for a particular ligand base. However, in biological systems one must also consider the kinetics of a reaction before proposing a mechanism for a particular function.

This review is not intended to provide the answers to the question of how trace metals are involved in biological reactions. It is an attempt to focus attention on and accelerate expansion of this area of health-related research. It further emphasizes the need for identification of the metal species that control the normal functions of living organisms in developing a knowledge base for understanding what is abnormal for these species.

## TRANSITION METAL COMPLEXES

The predominance of coordination compounds formed from transition metal ions and ligand groups of porphyrins, amino acids and proteins found in all biological species makes a basic understanding of coordination chemistry quite desirable. The ability of a metal ion to bind to a chelate depends not only on its physical size, but also on the geometric arrangement of the bonding orbitals of the metal. There is some reason to debate whether a particular metalloenzyme has a specificity for a metal ion because of the positions of the ligating groups, or if the position of the ligating groups is established by the presence of the metal during synthesis (template effect). Regardless of which is more important, the ability of a metal to replace another that occurs naturally in an enzyme and to restore enzymatic activity appears to depend to a great extent on the geometric orientation of the bonding orbitals of the metals.

The splitting of d orbital energies by the electrostatic fields of neutral or anionic ligands influences the electron distribution in the orbitals, and thus the binding energy and electrochemical potential are affected.

The crystal field theory provides a model by which these changes can be described. If one considers an octahedral arrangement of six negative ligands about a transition metal ion containing only one electron in the d orbitals, the degree of repulsion experienced by the electron will be determined by the proximity of the orbital lobes to one of the regions of negative charge. Both the $d_{z^2}$ and $d_{x^2-y^2}$ orbitals will have lobes that are very near the negative charge as shown in Figure 1. The lobes of the $d_{xy}$, $d_{xz}$ and $d_{yz}$ orbitals will be between the ligand sites. Thus, the electron would experience a greater

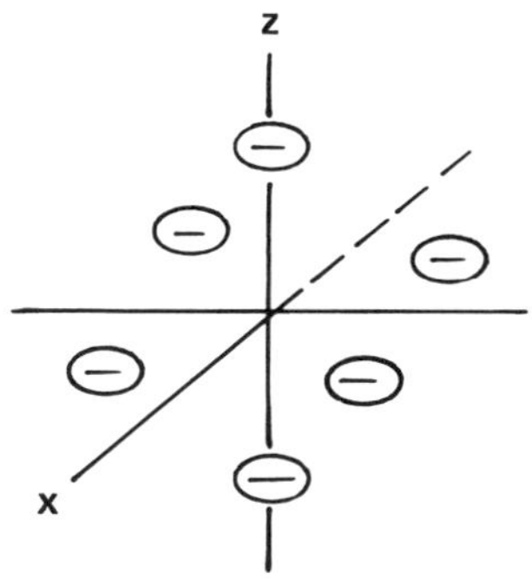


**Figure 1.** Octahedral arrangement of six negative ligands about a transition metal ion containing one electron in the d orbital.

force of repulsion if it were in the $d_{z^2}$ or $d_{x^2-y^2}$ orbitals than if it were in $d_{xy}$, $d_{xz}$ or $d_{yz}$. The degeneracy of the five orbitals is thus split into two degenerate sets (Figure 2) if all the ligands are identical. The magnitude of the energy difference between the degenerate sets will depend on the strength of the ligand field.

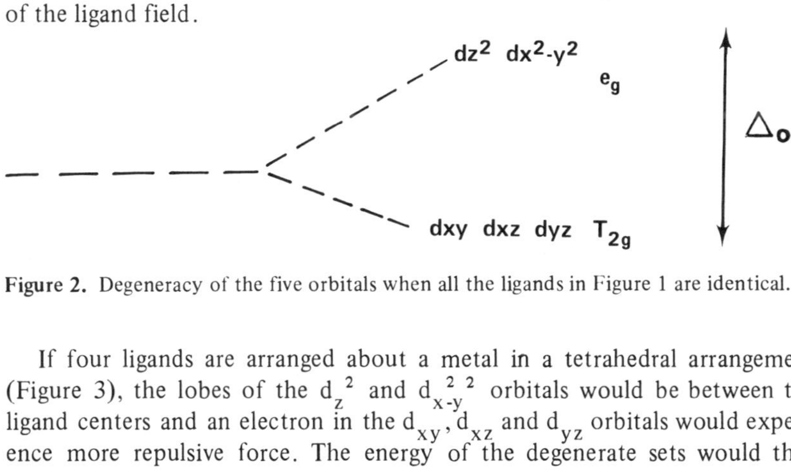


**Figure 2.** Degeneracy of the five orbitals when all the ligands in Figure 1 are identical.

If four ligands are arranged about a metal in a tetrahedral arrangement (Figure 3), the lobes of the $d_{z^2}$ and $d_{x^2-y^2}$ orbitals would be between the ligand centers and an electron in the $d_{xy}$, $d_{xz}$ and $d_{yz}$ orbitals would experience more repulsive force. The energy of the degenerate sets would thus be inverted. The value of $\Delta_t$ (tetrahedral energy differences) is about half that of $\Delta_o$ (octahedral energy difference):

$$\Delta_t = \frac{4}{9}\Delta_o$$

The other geometric arrangement normally encountered in biological systems is a square planar arrangement of the ligands about the central metal atom. In this case, the d orbital splitting is more complex, and the relative energies of each orbital, particularly the $d_{xy}$ and $d_{z^2}$ orbitals, depend on the properties of the metal ion and ligand involved.

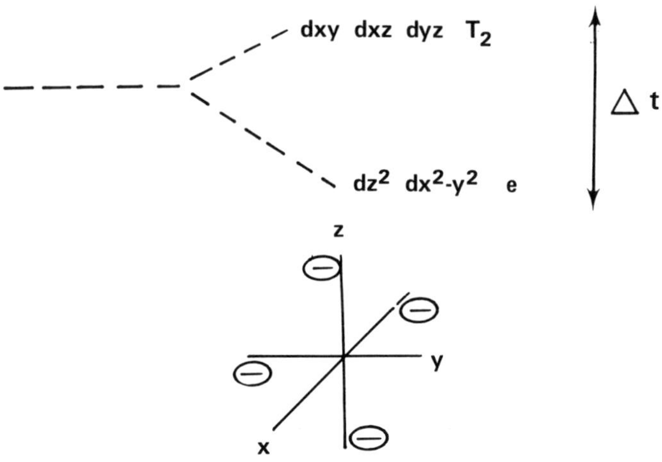


**Figure 3.** Degeneracy of orbitals in tetrahedral arrangement of four ligands about a metal.

A generalized diagram based on the square complexes of Co II, Ni II and Cu II is shown in Figure 4.

An interesting correlation is observed if one considers the elongation of the ligand bonds along the z axis of an octahedral complex. Tetragonal distortion is observed, and the d orbital energies shift (Figure 5) until at the extreme case of complete removal of the axial ligands a square planar arrangement is obtained. The distribution of electrons in the d orbitals of a transition metal will follow Hund's rule. If the orbitals are all degenerate, the electrons will half fill each orbital, before spin pairing in any one orbital. If crystal field splitting occurs, the picture becomes more complex. The magnitude of the energy difference between the lower and next higher energy orbitals ($\Delta$E) relative to the repulsion energy encountered when two electrons are placed in the same orbital must be considered.

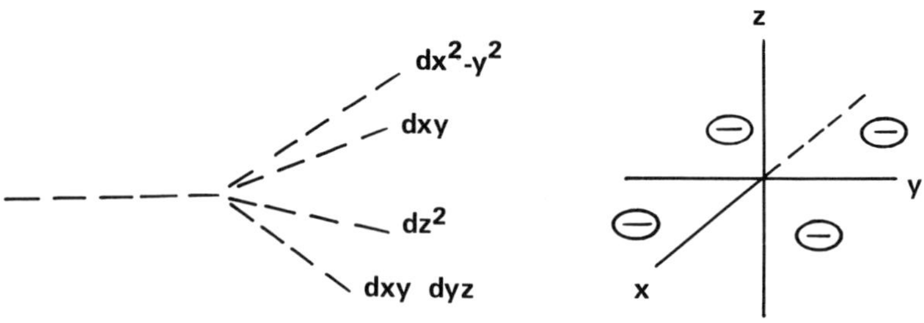


**Figure 4.** Degeneracy of orbitals in square planar arrangement of ligands about a metal.

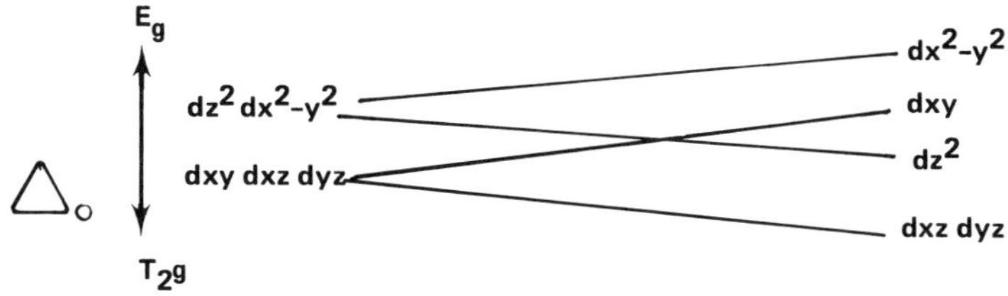


**Figure 5.** Increasing "Z" axis displacement of ligands in an octahedral complex.

Octahedral complexes with one, two or three electrons in the d orbitals will have the three $T_{2g}$ orbitals occupied forming high-spin complexes. Ions with eight, nine or ten electrons also have only one way in which the orbitals can be occupied. Ions with $d^4$, $d^5$, $d^6$ and $d^7$ orbital occupancy can have two possible configurations, and the ground state orientation depends on the difference in energy of $\Delta_o$ and the electron-electron repulsion energy. Compounds with a minimum number of paired electrons are high-spin, and those with maximum spin pairing (i.e., greater $\Delta_o$) are low-spin. Properties of both the metal and the ligand will determine the configuration of the ground state.

Tetrahedral complexes with electron populations of $d^1$, $d^2$, $d^7$, $d^8$ and $d^9$ in the transition metal ion form only high-spin compounds. Those with $d^3$, $d^4$, $d^5$ or $d^6$ populations will be low-spin. This can be rationalized by realizing that low-spin complexes will form only if $\Delta_t$ is greater than the electron-electron repulsion forces. Because $\Delta_t$ is about 0.5 $\Delta_o$, this is not likely to occur.

Square planar orientation of the ligands about a transition metal will remove the degeneracy of all but the $d_{xz}$ and $d_{yz}$ orbitals. The relative energies of these lowest energy orbitals and $d_{z^2}$, $d_{xy}$, and the highest energy orbital $d_{x^2-y^2}$ will determine the spin state of the complex.

It is of some interest to note the changes that occur when an octahedral complex undergoes tetragonal distortion with the related change in energy of the $d_z{}^2$ and $d_{xy}$ orbitals. A high spin complex can shift to the low spin state. Any correlation of this phenomenon and the observed activity of the "entatic" state of metalloenzymes is worthy of speculation.

The changes that occur in the oxidation potential of a transition metal as a consequence of the type of ligand bound to it is of particular importance in charge transfer reactions of a biological system. Likewise, the stereochemical changes accompanying an oxidation state change seem to be of some consequence in determining the activity of an enzyme center. In the same manner, geometric conformation of the ligands about a bound metal or loosely bound metal ion cofactor, may influence the selectivity of the enzyme for one metal over another, and makes it possible to predict which other metals would be most likely to compete for the coordinating site.

Metabolism in plants and animals can be simplified by relating it to the oxygen cycle. The overall processes involve the oxidation of water to molecular oxygen in plants (an endergonic process) and the reduction of $O_2$ in animal metabolism (an exergonic process). Both processes involve a series of redox reactions which are catalyzed by enzymes. In fact, a major function of metalloenzymes is charge transfer.

The release of energy as $O_2$ is reduced to the divalent state is analogous to combustion. The biological organism provides a pathway of intermediate steps to facilitate the slow release and rapid dissipation or transfer of this energy.

The stepwise reduction of oxygen involves the formation of some very reactive intermediates such as superoxide ($O_2^{\dot{-}}$), peroxides ($H_2O_2$, ROOH and ROOR) and singlet oxygen. Accumulation of these species would result in damage or destruction of the cells in which they are contained. Fortunately, a number of enzymes (catalase, and superoxide disumatases for example) are available for transfer of the energy stored in these molecules to other less toxic substances.

The reduction of 0.5 mol oxygen will be accompanied by the formation of 3 mol adenosine triphosphate (ATP). Assuming an average value of 8 kcal/mol ATP, about 24 kcal of energy is stored of a theoretically available 52 kcal released. This is an efficiency of 46%. The remaining energy is lost to the surroundings.

Inorganic charge transfer reactions normally involve an electron exchange between ions or between ions and atoms. The process is quite rapid. One might expect a similar type of rapid exchange in reactions involving metalloenzymes, but this is not always the case. Because the oxidation of a metal is associated with the removal of an electron, one might also expect a correlation between the redox potential and the ionization energy. As a general rule, this tendency is observed for nontransition-series metals, but the energy of hydration of the metal ion must also be considered. Lithium would be expected to be the poorest reducing agent of the alkali metals because of its higher ionization potential. In aqueous solution it is the best reducing agent in this family from the large hydration energy of the $Li^+$ ion. The total free energy change between the oxidized and reduced forms and their environment must be considered for prediction of redox potentials.

The kinetics of a reaction must also be taken into account when attempting to predict the feasibility of a reaction as part of a charge transfer process. Copper I is an unstable ion in aqueous solution. It disproportionates rapidly to copper II and metallic copper, accompanied by a free energy change of -8.53 kcal/mol. Hydrogen peroxide also disproportionates to form $O_2$ and $H_2O$. The free energy change is -56.5 kcal/mol. The rate of disproportionation of hydrogen peroxide is very slow if the solution is pure. This would appear to be a contradiction, if the comparatively high activation energy of the $H_2O_2$ decomposition were not considered. The presence of a catalyst will cause the disproportion reaction of $H_2O_2$ to occur rapidly, as can be observed in inorganic as well as biological systems.

The free energy change accompanying a redox reaction will depend on the activity of the species in solution. This is a function of the total ionic strength of the medium and the concentration of the reacting species. Thus, a comparison of the redox potentials of a system at unit activity ($E^\circ$) and the actual potential observed in a biological system can be quite different.

The Nernst equation ($E = E^\circ - RT/nF\ ln\ K$) must be used to calculate the actual emf of a reaction and corresponding free energy change:

$$\Delta G = -nF\Delta E$$

Oxidation-reduction reactions involving transition metal complexes present another complication. The electrons occupying unfilled d orbitals are normally involved in the redox reaction. The ligand affects the energy of the orbital, and thus the stability of the electron occupying it, by the manner in which the ligand splits the energies of the d orbitals, and the effect of crystal field stabilization energy on the energy of hydration. In general, the lower the energy of an orbital the more difficult it is to remove an electron, thus changing the value of $E_o$.

Iron III will form complexes with water, $Fe(H_2O)_6{}^{+3}$ and with *ortho*-phenanthroline, $Fe(O\text{-phen})_3{}^{+3}$. The hexaaquo complex is high-spin (one electron in each 3d orbital) and the O-phenanthroline complex is low-spin (two filled and a half-filled 3d orbitals). The reduction of these complexes requires the introduction of an electron into a $T_{2g}$ orbital; however, the orbital is of lower energy in the low-spin complex than the high spin-one. Thus, the reduction potential of the $FE(O\text{-phen})_3{}^{+3}$ complex is greater than that of $Fe(H_2O)_6{}^{+3}$. The charge on a complex can also have an effect on the reduction potential. A low-spin $Fe(CN)_6{}^{-3}$ ion has a much lower reduction potential than the $Fe(O\text{-phen})_3{}^{+3}$ complex because of "resistance" of the negative charge on the ion to the introduction of an electron.

$$Fe(CN)_6{}^{-3} \rightarrow Fe(CN)_6{}^{-4}$$

$$E^\circ = 0.36\ V$$

The redox potential of a complex in which rearrangement of the geometric shape (i.e., orbital hybridization) can occur easily will not be the same as is observed if the metal is complexed with ligands whose positions are difficult to change (as in a protein molecule). Copper I tends to form complexes that are most stable in a tetrahedral orientation. A square planar configuration is favored for copper II complexes.

Oxidation of bound copper I to copper II will result in distortion of the tetrahedron to a square planar arrangement, or a "squashed" tetrahedral form if relocation of the ligands is restricted. The energy required for reorientation of the ligands will effect the apparent redox potential. To further complicate matters, some metalloenzymes contain copper for which the oxidation state can not be determined readily because of delocalization of the charge on the ligands.

The bond length, if not bond angle, can be expected to change as the oxidation state of a metal changes. Bond lengths normally decrease as the oxidation state increases. If redox reactions are considered an electronic change, they should be governed by the Franck-Condon principle just as are the electronic changes observed in absorption spectroscopy. Because electrons pass between orbitals at a much faster rate than stretching or bending vibrations occur, the electron transfer occurs without a change in the relative position of the nucleii. The reduced form of a metal would thus be formed before bond elongation could occur. A reduced ion in an excited state would thus be formed, and rearrangement to the ground state would occur with a subsequent electronic change to a lower-energy orbital.

Another possibility that is perhaps more feasible would require rearrangement of the ligand centers before reduction of the metal. If only a low-activation barrier were encountered, the reduction could occur readily. However, if the activation energy is high, the reduction of the metal would be hindered. The reverse arguments can be made for oxidation of a bound metal, and it could be stabilized in the reduced state.

All of these factors must be considered when one attempts to predict the mechanism by which a metalloenzyme catalyses a charge transfer reaction in a biological system.

The ability of similar metals to occupy the same site in a metalloenzyme is related to the angular distribution of molecular orbitals. The orientation of binding orbitals about the nucleus is determined by the electronic configuration of the ion, and is independent of the element. Thus, one might suspect an antagonistic effect between the absorption and metabolism of isoelectronic ions.

Using this reasoning, one would expect Cu I, Zn II, Cd II and Hg II to compete for binding sites on metalloproteins. Each of these metal ions has a completely filled set of "d" orbitals. Copper II would not be expected to be antagonistic to any of these metals, but should be similar to silver I which also has a $d^9$ configuration.

This type of interaction has been studied, and the hypothesis appears to be valid [1]. The difference in ionic radii is found to decrease the antagonistic effect of Hg II on Cu I metabolism, as might be anticipated.

Similar comparisons can be made between anionic radicals. Phosphate and arsenate have identical electronic distributions and selenate is quite similar (having two $\pi$d bonds rather than one). The involvement of these ions in the metabolic process is influenced by their relative concentrations in the biological system. Other factors, such as ionic radius, electronegativity and redox potentials, can also influence the tendency of similar ions to compete for binding sites, but the orientation of binding molecular orbitals appears to be a major factor.

The Pauling electronegativity values of some biologically important elements must be considered. It should be noted that selenium is more like sulfur in terms of electronegativity than like the heavy metals (Hg, Pb and Cd). The first-row transition metals show little variation in electronegativity.

The radius of a hydrated metal ion is difficult to determine accurately. Therefore, the crystal ionic radius can be used for comparisons. Several similarities can be observed. Zinc II ions have a radius of 0.74 Å. Cobalt II, which has been shown to restore the activity of the apoenzyme carboxypeptidase after removal of zinc, has an ionic radius of 0.72 Å. Copper II, which does not restore the activity of the apoenzyme, also has a radius of 0.72 Å. The zinc II ion forms tetrahedral complexes, as will cobalt II, but copper II complexes are normally square planes.

The polarizability of an ion is related to its charge-to-size ratio. The similarity between the dipositive ions of Co, Cu, Fe and Zn is of interest.

Several metals have been selected for further discussion to illustrate their importance in biological systems. The list is not comprehensive, as it has been suggested that all the elements of the periodic chart may have some essential role in a particular organism. However, emphasis has been placed on some metals that are known to be essential to mammals, and others that are more commonly thought of in the context of their toxicity.

A general treatment has been used, with some specific examples incorporated to illustrate the degree of knowledge that has been obtained in some cases, and lack of it in others.

This review presents a summary of the available literature, and a bibliography is included to direct the reader to the original papers for a more complete discussion. One of the major problems in preparing a review of this type is the selection of papers to be included. An attempt has been made to limit the discussion to the research that has contributed to a proposed mechanism for the function of a metal or structural elucidation of a metalloenzyme.

## ZINC

The importance of zinc for the normal functioning of most organisms can be anticipated because of its high concentration, as compared to other trace metals, in the cell. The only transition element that is present in the cell in higher concentrations is iron. Zinc deficiency has been associated with retardation of normal growth of animals, impaired bone development, impaired protein and carbohydrate metabolism, hindrance of the development and functioning of reproductive organs and processes, retardation of learning capacity, formation of dermal lesions in rats, and parakeratosis in swine. This metal has been used to promote the healing of skin wounds, and is suspected of having therapeutic value in the treatment of atherosclerosis.

A deficiency of zinc in the diet is normally rapidly apparent. The concentration of zinc in serum drops rapidly apparently from the inability of the body to mobilize zinc reserves. Zinc deficiency in the human diet has been associated with hypophosphatasia. Alkaline phosphatase is low in concentration or absent and high levels of phosphoethanolamine (a substrate for the enzyme) are found in blood. Zinc is also suspected of having a role in DNA replication and protein synthesis [23,] and being involved with the action of nucleotidyl transferase enzymes. The metal has been shown to be present in DNA polymerase I and RNA polymerase from *Escherichia coli* [4,5].

Purified zinc metalloproteins show that the apoenzyme has a preference for binding zinc relative to Co II, Ni II and Cu II ions. The binding ligands are usually nitrogen or oxygen. These Lewis bases would normally be expected to have a greater coordinating affinity for these other metals. One would expect that zinc binding sites would contain sulfur ligands, but this does not seem to be the normal complex present in most zinc metalloproteins.

There are three well-established zinc-binding ligands in metalloproteins. These are: the imidazole nitrogen, the gamma carboxyl of glutamic acid and the sulfhydryl group of cysteine. Carboxypeptidase A and thermolysin both bind zinc in a somewhat distorted tetrahedral structure. The imidazole nitrogen of two separate histidyl residues and the $\gamma$ carbonyl of a glutamyl residue occupy three of the available coordination sites. A water molecule or hydroxide ion (depending on pH) occupies the fourth site. Zinc is bound to sulfhydryl groups in metallothionein.

The apoenzyme of alkaline phosphatase has been synthesized in the absence of zinc. Enzymatic activity is obtained when zinc is added, indicating that the zinc binding site is present even in the absence of the metal, but catalytic activity does depend on its presence.

The function of zinc in a metalloenzyme would be expected to involve Lewis acid reactions. This has been shown to be the case in carboxypeptidase, (a reaction which will be discussed in detail). In aspartate transcarbamylase, however, the zinc ion is not located at the active site. It seems to be involved with maintaining the structure of the regulatory subunit. A similar situation exists in superoxide dismutase. The active catalytic site contains a copper ion, but a zinc ion is located in close proximity.

Classification of metalloenzymes, in which the metal is tightly bound to the protein, and metal activated enzymes, in which a correlation between the metal concentration and a specific activity is apparent, is a somewhat nebulous task. The normal distinction is based on the ability to separate and purify the enzyme without dissociation of the ligand-metal complex. Zinc metalloproteins have been bound to have dissociation constants of about $10^{-10}$ *M* or less. However, the dissociation of the enzyme into an equilibrium between the metal ion, apoenzyme and metal-enzyme complexes depends on the procedures used in obtaining the purified substance. A method of obtaining a purified enzyme without loss of a loosely bound metal ion is needed. A method involving the maintenance of an isotropic ion concentration during separation has recently been reported and needs to be investigated further [6].

Enzymes that are activated by zinc are thought to contain zinc. However, if the metal is loosely bound, the activation may depend only on the presence of a divalent cation, and could be related to the available amounts of Mg II, Ca II, Fe II, Co II, Ni II, Cu II or Zn II. Further study in this area is needed before a specific mechanism for the activity of metal activated enzymes is proposed.

There are 37 functionally distinguished proteins that have been reported to contain zinc II as a component after isolation. Some of these have been shown to be zinc II metalloproteins [7-24]. Others have been reported to contain zinc, but there is less evidence available in regard to its function [4,5,25-51].

The essential nature of zinc in metalloenzymes has been investigated by several methods. The enzymes have been dialyzed to remove the metal ion and the activity of the apoenzyme measured. Chelating agents, 1,10-phenanthroline, ethylene diamine tetracetic acid (EDTA) and 8-hydroxyquinoline, have been used to complex the metal. These bi- and polydentates have been found to remove the metal from carboxypeptidase A, themolysin, alkaline phosphatase and carbonic anhydrase. Mixed complexes of the enzyme and chelating agent have not been found, indicating that a dissociation of the enzyme-metal complex occurs as the free metal ion concentration is decreased by formation of a metal-chelate complex. An exception has been noticed in the formation of a ligand-Zn-enzyme complex when 1,10-phenanthroline reacts with alcohol dehydrogenase.

In addition to the use of organic chelating agents to remove zinc from an enzyme, other metal ions have been substituted for the zinc. The stabilities of the metallocarboxypeptidase complexes of Cu II and Cd II are about the same as zinc, and that of Hg II is greater.

In addition to the stability of these metalloenzyme complexes, it is of interest to compare the relative activities of the enzymes to determine what functional changes occur if another divalent metal ion is substituted for zinc. Some general comments that can be made in regard to the activity of the enzyme after substitution are: (1) some enzymes that normally contain zinc show activity when other divalent metals are present; (2) cobalt seems to be more closely associated with zinc than any of the other metals investigated; (3) cobalt activity is consistently higher than that of zinc except in those cases where activity is limited to the presence of these two metals only.

Carboxypeptidase A is a hydrolytic enzyme whose structure has been determined by X-ray diffraction and chemical sequence analysis [52]. The enzyme has a molecular weight of 34,472 and contains 307 amino acids. A zinc II ion is bonded to a glutamic acid-72 and two histidine-69-196 amino acid residues. The fourth bonding site is occupied by a water molecule as hydroxyl group (depending on pH). Three amino acid residues that are involved with binding and catalysis of the substrate are: arginine-71, the binding site of the carboxyl end of the substrate; glutamic acid, the promoter of general base hydrolysis or the nucleophile; and tyrosine-248, whose primary function appears to be protonation of the N-H group in the peptide.

The function of each component is shown by the reaction sequence shown in Figure 6.

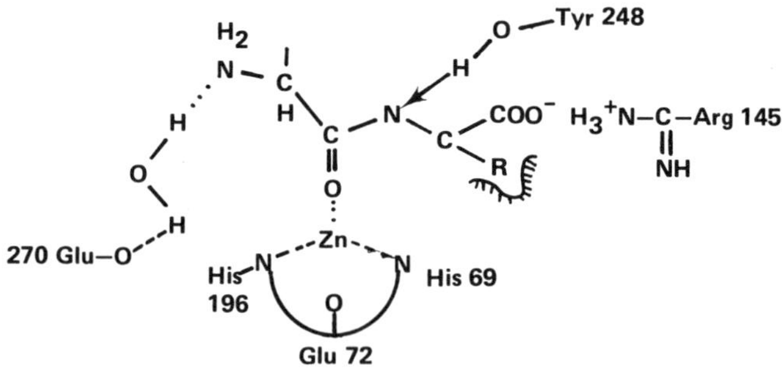


**Figure 6.** Proposed reaction mechanism for carboxypeptidase A.

The carboxyl terminal of the substrate is bonded to Arg-145. The carbonyl oxygen of the peptide undergoing hydrolysis replaces the water molecule in the fourth coordination site of zinc, and the α amino group of this same amino acid is H-bonded through a water molecule to glutamic acid-270. The four ligands around zinc form a somewhat distorted tetrahedron. It should be noted that the substrate lies in a "groove" in the enzyme containing the zinc ion. A "pocket" adjacent to this groove that does not appear to contain any specific binding sites is large enough to accommodate a tryptophan side chain.

The replacement of the water molecule coordinated to zinc by the carbonyl oxygen of the substrate lowers the dielectric constant of the medium surrounding the zinc ion. The net charge of +1 on zinc induces a dipole in the substrate, the magnitude of which is enhanced by the H-bonding of the α amino group to Glu-270. The uncompensated charges in the substrate can induce proton transfer reactions. Tyrosine-248 donates a proton to the peptide nitrogen, and hydrolysis of the peptide occurs.

Substitution of Cd II or Hg II for zinc will destroy the peptidase activity of carboxypeptidase A, but the estrase activity is enhanced [53,54]. The hydrolysis of a peptide requires protonation of the nitrogen, but this is not as essential for the hydrolysis of an ester. It would appear that the tyrosine-248 position is changed relative to the bonded substrate when these metals are substituted for zinc II. The replacement of zinc by copper II ions inhibits the hydrolytic function of this enzyme. Zinc II will tend to form a tetrahedral complex because of its filled "d" orbitals, but copper II tends to form a square planar complex ($d_{sp^2}$). The distortion of the three coordinating groups to approach a square planar configuration obviously alters the activity of the enzyme.

Cobalt II seems to be more similar to zinc in its ability to restore carboxypeptidase activity than are Mn II, Fe II, Ni II, Cu II, Cd II and Hg II. A comparison of the ionic radius and electronegativity of Co II, Cu II and Zn II shows some similarities between these ions.

| Metal Ion | Electronegativity | Ionic Radius Å | Complex Shape |
|---|---|---|---|
| Zn II | 1.6 | 0.74 | Tetrahedral |
| Cu II | 1.8 | 0.72 | Square Planar |
| Co II | 1.8 | 0.72 | Tetrahedral |

The geometric shapes of the metal-ligand complex would appear to be the dominant feature governing the ability of the enzyme to retain its hydrolytic function when another ion is substituted for zinc II.

Zinc has been shown to be involved in the maintenance of the structure of superoxide dismutase [55,56]. This enzyme has an important role in the dismutation of the $O_2^{\bar{\cdot}}$ radical to $O_2$ and $H_2O_2$. The active center for the catalysis of the redox reaction is a copper II ion bound to four amino acid residues (histidine-44, histidine-46, histidien-61 and histidine-118). The histidines are bound in a square planar configuration, leaving one side of the copper ion exposed to easy access by the solvent medium. The zinc II ion is bound to histidine-61, histidine-69, histidine-78 and aspartic acid-81. The coordination of histidine-69 to both copper II and zinc II indicates the importance of the zinc ion in maintaining the orientation of the functional group. The two metal ions are separated by only 6 Å. Replacement of zinc with cobalt II does not inhibit the activity of the enzyme; however, replacement of zinc with a copper II ion decreases the activity by 50-75% [57,58]. This is consistent with the activity changes observed when these two metal ions were substituted for the zinc in carboxypeptidase A. It would seem reasonable to assume that the change from a tetrahedral to a square planar configuration could restrict the availability of the copper II ion at the active site to the solvent in which the $O_2^{\bar{\cdot}}$ is contained. The imidazole ring of histidine-61 would have both the pyridinium and pyrole protons displaced because of coordination with the two metal ions. Further discussion of this enzyme will be reserved for the section pertaining to copper. It should be noted, however, that although zinc has not been shown to be actively involved in the catalytic function of this enzyme, it is reasonable to expect some contribution from polarization effects.

Zinc has been shown to be present in DNA polymerase. Manganese has a major role in the action of this enzyme, but it does not bind directly to the DNA molecule. It has been proposed that a zinc II ion bound to the enzyme bonds to the 3′-hydroxyl terminus of DNA [59]. The binding of a deoxynucleoside triphosphate occurs by coordination of the α-phosphonyl group by the 3′-hydroxyl group at the end of the primer strand with a concerted displacement of pyrophosphate. Zinc is believed to facilitate this process by promoting the loss of a proton from the hydroxyl group. Manganese II coordinates with the α-phosphonyl group, thereby enhancing its susceptibility to nucleophilic attack by electron withdrawal and charge neutralization [60]. The nucleotide transfer is thus completed, and relocation of the primer is required. Slater et al. [59] proposed the replacement of the two phosphodiester oxygens, bound to the manganese II, by water molecules. The 3′-hydroxyl group of the newly added nucleotide substitutes for that of the 3′-oxygen atom of the previous nucleotide. Thus, the enzyme has been relocated for addition of the next nucleoside.

This mechanism is an oversimplification of the process, but is sufficient to indicate the essential role of both zinc and manganese. Magnesium can be substituted for manganese in the enzyme, but no data are currently available for the effects observed by substitution of cobalt or copper for zinc. If a similarity of behavior exists between the results observed in the two previously discussed enzymes, one would expect copper II to inhibit the polymerization and cobalt II to behave in a manner similar to zinc.

The role of zinc in these three selected metalloenzymes indicates the types of mechanisms and specificity encountered in cellular reactions. Similarities in ionic radius, electronegativity, polarizability and Lewis acid activity are to be considered when attempting to replace a metal ion of an enzyme with an ion of a similar metal.

The orientation of the ligands about the metal is obviously a major factor influencing the inhibitory nature of a metal that is otherwise similar to the metal normally present in the enzyme. The stability of complexes formed between oxygen and nitrogen ligands and zinc are normally less stable than those formed by these Lewis bases and divalent ions of other first row transition metals. The zinc-metalloenzymes seem to preferentially bind this metal in contradiction to the expected order of stability. The reason for this preference has not been explained, but it may be caused by the particular orientation of the ligands about the metal. One must remember that the complex does not necessarily exist in a regular tetrahedral shape, but seems to be in an entatic state. A low symmetry is often observed with considerable distortion of the proposed regular geometric form [61,62].

## COPPER

A soluble copper protein was isolated by Mann and Keilin in 1938 [63]. This blue copper protein, hemocuprein, contained 0.34% copper and had a molecular weight of 34,000. It was isolated from bovine erythrocytes. A similar copper protein was isolated from human erythrocytes and named erythrocuprein [64,65]. These metalloproteins did not have any known enzymatic function until Fridovich attempted to determine the nature of a competitive inhibitor for the reduction of cytochrome C (another copper-containing enzyme) by xanthine oxidase [66,67]. It was found that neither the cytochrome C nor the suspected protein inhibitors were bound to xanthine oxidase, but the reduction of cytochrome C was controlled by the superoxide radical [68]. The superoxide was apparently being destroyed by a trace impurity in the solution. This substance was purified and has been identified as erythrocuprein (hemocuprein), also known as superoxide dismutase [69]. The crystal structure of this copper enzyme has been reported by Richardson et al. [56]. The classification of cytochrome C as a copper enzyme has been the subject of considerable controversy [70-80]. However, evidence presented by Griffiths and Warton seems to support strongly the role of this metal in the action of the enzyme [81]. Copper is found in both plants and animals. It has been shown to be present in ascorbic acid oxidase. cytochrome oxidase, tyrosinases and hemocyanin. Ascorbic acid oxidase catalyzes the oxidation of ascorbic acid to dehydroascorbic acid with $O_2$ as the electron-acceptor. Cytochrome oxidase contains heme and copper in a 1:1 ratio. It is the terminal electron acceptor of the mitochondrial pathway. Tyrosinases, which catalyze the formation of melanin pigments, were the first enzymes for which the essential nature of copper was shown. Hemocyanin (which does not contain heme) is a high-molecular-weight protein. There is evidence that it is involved in $O_2$ transport with one molecule of $O_2$ being bound per two copper atoms.

Before discussing the structure of these copper compounds, a brief review of the properties of this element should be helpful in understanding its enzymatic activity.

The copper I, copper II and Fe II, Fe III systems are the most common metallic redox groups found in biological systems. The copper II ion forms stronger complexes with most ligands than are formed with other divalent metals.

The functional groups found in amino acids can be classified according to their specificity for copper in each of its normal oxidation states:

1. copper II specific ligands–$COO^-$, $ArO^-$ (Tyr), $RO^-$ (Ser,Thr), $HNC(NH)NHCH_2$ (Arg), CONH (peptide), $NH_2$ (Lys) (most Cu II complexes are five or six-membered rings);
2. copper I specific ligands–$R_2S$ (Met), RSSR (cystine), and
3. nonspecific copper ligands–immidazole (Hist), R-S (cysteine).

From this list, it would seem reasonable to predict the most probable ligands binding copper in a redox system would be the nonoxidation state-specific groups of histidine and cysteine. One should also notice that ligands containing oxygen as the only functional group do not bind Cu I. The only exception is $O^{-2}$.

Cuprous compounds are diamagnetic and colorless; unless charge transfer bonds are present the color is caused by the anion.

The relative stability of the copper I and copper II oxidation states is indicated by their electrochemical potentials.

$$Cu^{\circ} \rightarrow Cu^{+} + e^{-} \qquad E^{\circ} = -0.52 \text{ V}$$
$$Cu^{+} \rightarrow Cu^{2+} + e^{-} \qquad E^{\circ} = -1.153 \text{ V}$$
$$Cu^{\circ} + Cu^{2+} \rightarrow 2Cu^{+} \qquad E^{\circ} = -0.37 \text{ V}$$

$$Keq = \frac{[Cu^{+2}]}{[Cu^{+1}]^2} \cong 10^6$$

In aqueous solution, only low concentrations of copper I can exist ($<10^{-2}$ *M*). The copper I halides and cyanide are the most stable compounds, but have low water solubility.

The equilibrium of the disproportionation reaction—$2Cu^+ \rightleftarrows Cu^{2+} + Cu^\circ$—can be shifted in either direction by the anion present in solution. The formation of copper I from copper II is favored in the presence of $CN^-$, $I^-$, and $Me_2S$. With anions that do not form covalent bonds or bridging groups (i.e., $C1O_4^-$ or $SO_4^{2-}$) or complexing agents that are specific for copper II, the higher oxidation state is favored.

Copper I, with a $d^{10}$ electron configuration, can exhibit coordination numbers of 2 (linear), 3 (planar) and 4 (tetrahedral). The last is favored when coordination to simple ligands (i.e., halide ions and amines) are bound. The $Cu(CN)_2^-$ ion does not exist as a linear molecule, but has a spiral polymeric structure in which each copper I ion is bound to two carbon atoms and one nitrogen atom in a coplanar array.

The copper II ion ($d^9$) is the most stable ionic form of this metal. Its chemistry has been studied extensively, and it forms a large number of compounds and complexes. It has been shown to exhibit coordination numbers of 5 (trigonal bipyramidal and square pyramidal); 4 (distorted tetrahedral and square); and 6 (distorted octahedral). The normal distortion of the octahedral complex is an elongation of the bonds along the fourfold rotation axis.

The distorted tetrahedral complex can be obtained in halide solutions containing large cations. A "squashed" tetrahedron of $CuX_4^{-2}$ complex ions (Figure 7) is formed. The distorted tetrahedral shape has also been observed in *bis*-salicylaldiminato complexes (Figure 8) in which the R group attached to the nitrogen is large.

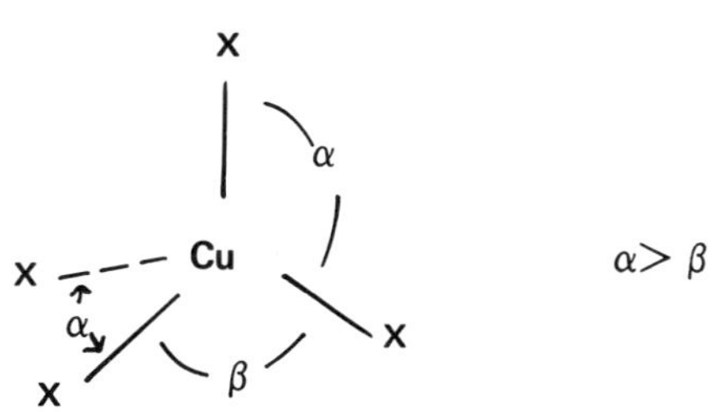


**Figure 7.** Distorted tetrahedral complex containing large metal cation.

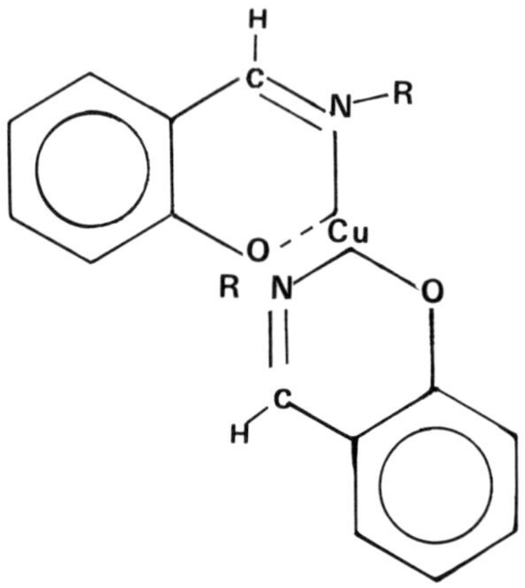


**Figure 8.** Distorted tetrahedral shape of Cu II in *bis*-salicylaldiminato complexes.

This distorted tetrahedral shape should be considered when the inability of copper II ions to restore the catalytic activity of the apoenzymes which normally contain a tetrahedrally bonded zinc II ion is attempted. The normal structure of a neutral four-ligand copper II complex is planar. In this regard, it is more like nickel II than like zinc II.

The copper II ion forms a hexaaquo complex in water solutions, $Cu(H_2O)_6{}^{2+}$. The water molecules can be replaced by other ligands up to four. Replacement of the remaining two water molecules is more difficult. They occupy the axial position of a distorted octahedron. The water molecules in the planar position of the molecule are not more loosely bound, but the competing ligands can normally occupy these sites preferentially to the axial sites. The axial water molecules are loosely bound, but interact with copper more readily than do most other Lewis bases.

Copper forms dinuclear compounds in which there are short Cu-Cu distances, but Cu-Cu bonds have not been observed. The $Cu_2(CH_3COO^-)_4{\circ}(H_2O)_2$ complex has one oxygen of each carboxyl group bound to each copper ion. A similar compound is formed with 1,3-triazinato compounds.

Nitrogenous monodentate ligands form complexes with copper I which have two favored orientations depending on the nature of the ligand. Ammonia forms a pyramidal complex, but a trigonal configuration is obtained with pyridine. The trigonal complex is more stable due to a greater degree of S orbital character of the ligand bonding orbital. This favors copper I affinity.

The most biologically important nitrogen ligand is imidazole (ImH). Only two ImH ligands associate with a copper I ion in dilute solutions. In basic solution a proton is lost from one of the imidazole ligands and a neutral, insoluble polymer is formed.

$$\underset{}{Cu^+} + \underset{(excess)}{ImH_2^+} \overset{pH\ 4}{\rightleftharpoons} Cu(ImH)_2^+ + 2H^+ \overset{pH\ 8}{\rightleftharpoons} \frac{1}{n}(CuIm)_n + 3H^+ + ImH$$

The second step does not occur if mon-alkalyted imidazole is used. The amino group of histamine or histidine apparently does not compete for a coordination site on copper to form a six-membered ring, but the acid dissociation constant of the $NH_3^+$ group is increased by the presence of the metal ion. If the ImH group is attached to a charged residue such as histamine or histidine, the polymer (Figure 9) is soluble.

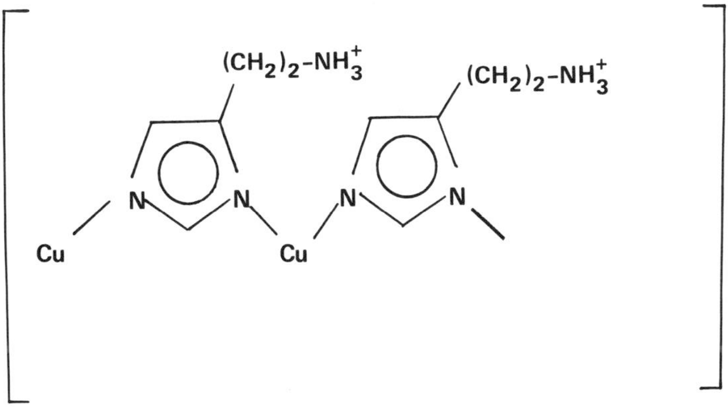


**Figure 9.** Charged histamine-Cu I polymer.

Chelating ligands do not form more than monodentate complexes with copper I unless considerable delocalization of d electrons toward low-lying empty antibonding d or $\pi$ orbitals of the ligand is allowed. Examples of this type of chelate are oxinate, bipyridine and O-phenanthroline. Ligands that exhibit redox behavior themselves are particularly good chelators for copper 1. Riboflavin is a good example of this type of compound. 1,2-Dioximes and disulfides that have a second ligand group, such as cystine and cystamine, also form copper I chelates.

1,4-Bidentate ligands will cause rapid disproportionation (Figure 10) of copper I to copper II and free copper atoms. 1,5-Bidentate ligands exhibit monodentate coordination with copper I. Hydrolysis occurs at high pH, but no disproportionation takes place, probably due to the relative instability of copper II five-membered rings.

Reactions of copper I with sulfur-containing ligands show a complicated behavior. If the sulfur group is part of a ligand that does not have $\pi$ bonds, a linear complex is favored over the formation of a chelate. Complexation with

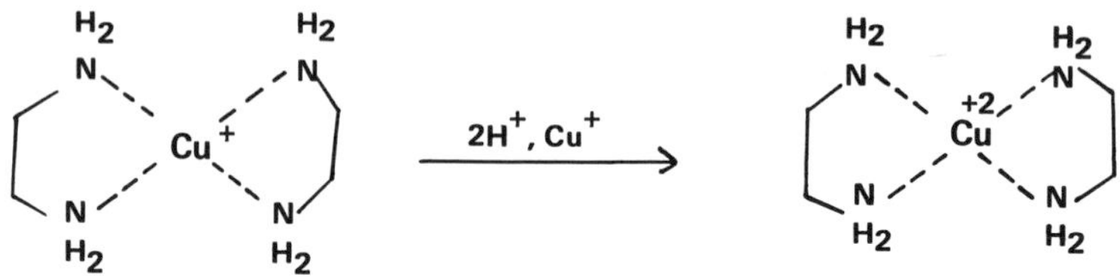


**Figure 10.** Disproportionation of Cu I to Cu II and Cu° in 1,4-bidentate complexes.

excess mercaptide ion $RS^-$ will result in the formation of a linear polymer-type structure which is quite insoluble if there are no ionic groups present in the "R" group.

$$Cu^+ + \underset{(excess)}{RSH} \rightleftarrows [\overset{R}{\overset{|}{S}}\text{-}Cu\cdot\cdot\cdot\overset{R}{\overset{|}{S}}\text{-}Cu\text{-}\overset{R}{\overset{|}{S}}]^{-1} + 1.5H^+ \text{ per Cu}$$

If excess $Cu^+$ is present the reaction will normally proceed as:

$$\frac{1}{n}(\overset{R}{\overset{|}{S}}Cu)_n + \underset{(excess)}{Cu^+} \rightleftarrows Cu\text{-}\overset{R}{\overset{|}{S}}\text{-}Cu^+$$

If there are no $\pi$ bonds between sulfur and the ligand residue, a coordination number of 3 occurs for the Cu-coordinated sulfur. Should the ligand contain a $Cu^{2+}$-specific group (i.e., $COO^-$), disproportionation will occur:

$$Cu^+\overset{R}{\overset{|}{S}}\text{-}Cu^{2+}$$

If a second coordinating group is not present, partial hydrolysis will occur in aqueous solution.

The presence of $\pi$ bonds in the ligand will give rise to two types of complexes, depending on the presence of an acidic proton. If a full negative charge can be generated on the sulfur, the system will behave like $RS^-$. Such is the case with a thiosemicarbazone [82]:

$$R\text{-}CH{=}N\text{-}NH\text{-}\overset{NH_2}{\overset{|}{C}}{=}S + Cu^+ \rightarrow \frac{1}{n}R\text{-}CH{=}N\text{-}N{=}\overset{NH_2}{\overset{|}{C}}\text{-}(SCu)_n + H^+$$

Thiourea, which does not have a readily dissociable proton, will form a complex in which up to four ligands will bind to the copper I ion [83].

Thioethers are quite specific for copper I ions over copper II. Thus, methionine and S-alkylcysteine will form rather stable $R\text{-}S\text{---}Cu^+\text{---}S\text{-}R$ complexes. If an amino group is present in the ligand, hydrolysis and disproportionation is suppressed up to very high pH values if the ligand-to-metal ratio is at least 2:1. This indicates the presence of a chelate structure (Figure 11), rather than a monodentate one.

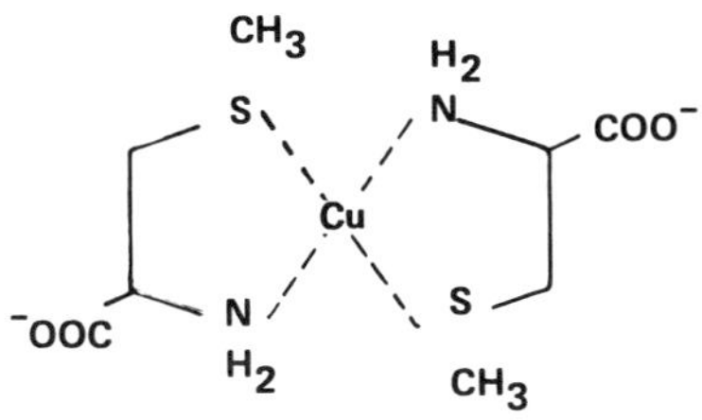


**Figure 11.** Thioether chelate structure with Cu I.

Compounds containing the disulfide group present a very interesting phenomenon when complexed with copper. In a complex of the general formula ($R_2S_2Cu$) the copper I and copper II chelates are practically indistinguishable. Valence mesomerism plays a large role in biologically important redox systems (heme-Fe-$O_2$, nonheme Fe-$S_2R_2$, RS-Mo-flavin and copper complexes).

If copper I is to form a stable complex with a disulfide ligand, a second chelating group must be present as it is in thioether type complexes.

The equilibria reactions of copper-disulfide complexes can be summarized by the reaction sequence shown in Figure 12.

If a polydentate disulfide is considered, state I does not contribute greatly to the equilibrium. If cystine is titrated with $Cu^+$ (stabilized in $CH_3CN$), one $H^+$ ion is liberated reversibly per copper I ion if cystine is in excess, giving rise to state II. If the pH is less than 7, disproportionation does not occur. The reaction state I → state V liberates only 0.5 $H^+$ per $Cu^+$, and on addition of additional $Cu^{2+}$, the cystine system acquires a violet color due to state IV if a cystamine system is used, and two Cu per RSSR are present. However, state V is highly favored over state IV if the Cu II cystine system is observed. This is due to the Cu II specificity of α-amino acid bidentate residues.

States III, IV and V imply a Cu-Cu interaction, whereas states I and II do not. State II is, therefore, of general importance in enzymes containing one copper atom, and state III would be considered only in two copper enzymes.

The preceding discussion of ligand specificity for different oxidation states of copper can perhaps be somewhat better understood if one considers the theory of hard and soft acids and bases proposed by Pearson [84]. This theory has not received general acceptance, perhaps because of its somewhat

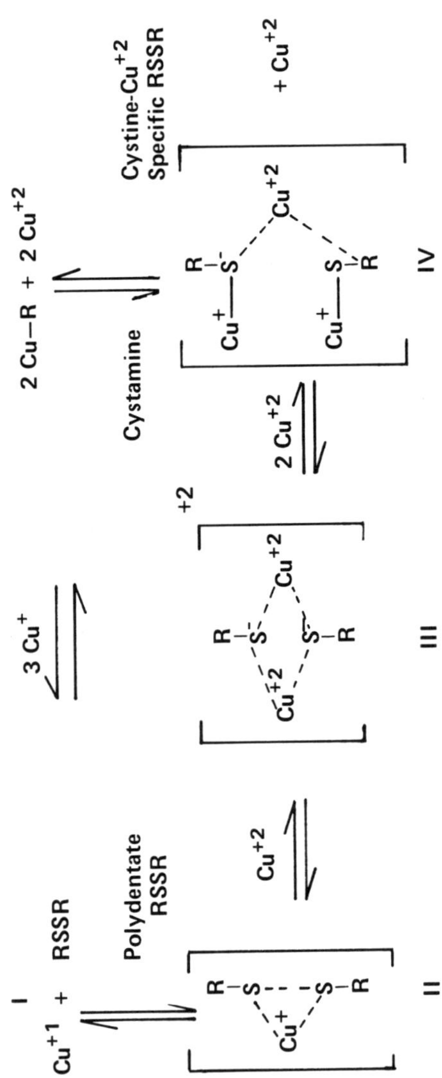


**Figure 12.** Equilibria reactions of copper-disulfide complexes.

ambiguous nature; but it is interesting to consider in relation to the interaction of copper with various bases.

A "hard" ligand or base is one for which the interaction with metal ions can be described by electrostatic interaction or a sigma covalent interaction that does not disrupt the normal electron configuration of the metal. Complexes formed by "soft" ligands involve extensive delocalization of electrons. Additional bonding may occur by the formation of $\pi$ bonds; $(d,P)_\pi$ or $(d,d)_\pi$. The metal always contributes d orbitals and the ligand p orbitals or, in the case of sulfur, d orbitals are vacant. Complicated molecular ligands can contain empty $\pi$ orbitals into which electrons from the metal can be delocalized. The terms hard and soft are not to be confused with strong and weak ligands. Strong and weak refer to the basicity of the ligand, hard and soft notation concerns electron delocalization or orbital polarizability. The terms polarizable and nonpolarizable are more analogous to hard and soft, but the meaning is not exactly the same.

Water will form a stable complex with copper II, but not with copper I. Water is a hard ligand but becomes softer after loss of a proton. Copper I is a soft acid, but copper II is considered borderline between hard and soft. In general, hard acids form more stable complexes with hard bases, and soft acids tend to complex with soft bases.

The classification of a metal depends on its oxidation state. Normally the hardness increases as the oxidation state of the metal ion increases. A partial listing of metal ions of interest in biological systems according to Pearson [84] would include:

| Hard Acids | Borderline | Soft Acids |
|---|---|---|
| $H^+$, $Li^+$, $Na^+$, $K^+$<br>$Mg^{2+}$, $Ca^{2+}$, $Al^{3+}$, $Cr^{3+}$<br>$Co^{3+}$, $Fe^{3+}$ | $Fe^{2+}$, $Co^{2+}$, $Ni^{2+}$<br>$Cu^{2+}$, $Zn^{2+}$, $Pb^{2+}$ | $Cu^+$, $Cd^{2+}$, $CH_3Hg^+$ |

If one considers the base groups essential to proteins, $NH_2$, $COO^-$ and carbonamide are all hard bases. Soft ligands would include the thioether groups found in methionine or ethionine. These groups exhibit a preference for the soft acid copper I over copper II, which is harder. Mercaptide is the softest ligand found in proteins. Disulfide is also very soft and is sometimes called "noninnocent" because it can accommodate donated electrons. It can be stable with one or two electrons added, because it can assume a mecaptide configuration.

The increase in hardness as copper I is oxidized to copper II in enzymes should influence the relative stability of the complex, unless a corresponding change occurs in the ligand molecule which alters its hardness. The same phenomena should be observed for the iron II, iron III systems.

If one were to compare the copper I specific ligands with those that favor formation of copper II complexes, the soft acid-soft base theory holds true. The imidazole group of histidine is moderately soft. It should also be noted that this base is deprotoned at a pH only slightly below the physiological range. Thus, it is present in rather high concentration relative to amino nitrogens, and is softer than amino nitrogen. This group was classified as nonspecific for copper I and copper II, and is often found bound to the metal in metalloenzymes involved in redox reactions.

The nonspecific nature of cysteine can be related to valence mesomerism in addition to the relative softness of the group.

## Copper Metalloenzymes

Superoxide dismutase has been shown to catalyze the conversion of superoxide ions to oxygen and hydrogen peroxide [69]:

$$2O_2^{\overline{\cdot}} + 2H^+ \rightarrow O_2 + H_2O_2$$

This enzyme is also known as hemocuprein (isolated from bovine erythrocytes) and erythrocuprein (obtained from human erythrocytes). The amino acid sequence of this metalloenzyme has been determined. Two apparently identical subunits of 151 amino acid residues have been described. An electron density map at 3-Å resolution has also been obtained for this enzyme [56], and the alpha carbon coordinates have been determined [55].

Each subunit contains one copper II and one zinc II ion. The copper ions are about 34 Å apart. The ligands bonded to the copper are histidine residues 44, 46, 61 and 118 arranged in a distorted square planar configuration. One side of the copper ion is readily available to solvent access perpendicular to the coordination plane. A zinc II ion lies about 6 Å from the copper and is bonded to histidine residues 61, 69 and 78. The fourth coordinating position of zinc is occupied by aspartic acid 81. The four ligands are in the nearly tetrahedral configuration normally associated with zinc II ion. The bonding of histidine 61 to both the copper and zinc ion is somewhat unusual. Replacement of zinc by cobalt II does not significantly decrease the activity of the enzyme, but the presence of copper is essential.

Almost all of the residues bonded to the metal ions have potential hydrogen-bonding groups located nearby. Thus, a second shell of interactions extending from the metal centers is possible.

The oxidation of copper I to copper II involves a one electron change. These are the only oxidation states normally considered for copper ions. There is an increasing amount of evidence for the existence of stable Cu III complexes in biological systems [85].

The possibility of a two-electron transfer reaction between copper I and copper III in a biological system could avoid the need to postulate the existence of high-energy free radical intermediates. Further study of the phenomena is needed, but as investigators accept the possibility of the existence of a tripositive copper ion, the probability of finding such a species is increased.

## IRON

Iron is the most abundant metal found in biological systems. The metal is quite well suited for the formation of complexes, exhibiting coordination numbers of 4, 5 and 6; and can exist in either the 2+ or 3+ oxidation states. An attempt to include the chemistry of all iron containing compounds in living organisms would be beyond the scope of this review. Thus, only a few representative systems will be discussed.

Iron containing proteins can be categorized in the following manner:

1. Ferrodoxins–simple iron-containg proteins that are not well understood. This structure is thought to contain a series of Fe-S linkages bound to a simple protein (Figure 13). Ferrodoxins occur in all photosynthesizing cells and have a molecular weight range of 6000–30,000. They have a significant role in photosynthesis and are also involved in nitrogen fixation.
2. Ferritin–this soluble iron-storage protein is found in all cells.
3. Hemosiderin–granules of this iron-protein can contain amorphous deposits of iron and geometrically oriented ferritin molecules.
4. Iron-sulfur proteins–some examples of this type of protein are aconitase, xanthine oxidase, succinate dehydrogenase and NADH dehydrogenase.
5. Transferrin and lactoferrin–proteins which are involved with iron transport.
6. Hemoproteins–these iron proteins can be classified according to their function: (1) oxygen carriers (hemoglobin and myoglobin); and (2) charge transfer (cytochromes).

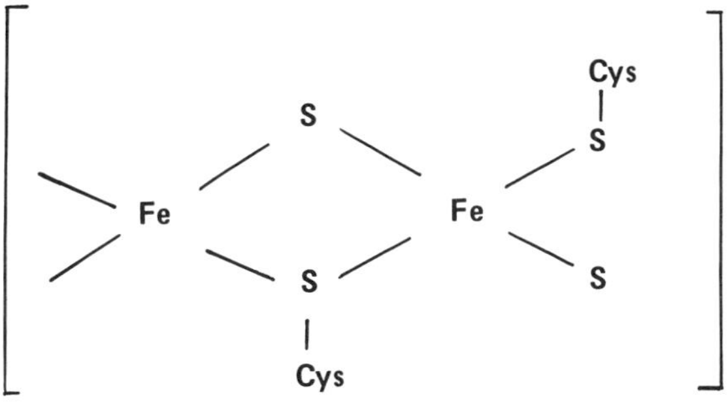


**Figure 13.** Repeating unit in the structure of ferrodioxins.

The hemoproteins have rather well known structures. The basic heme structure is a porphyrin with four nitrogen groups lying in a plane. An iron II ion is coordinated to nitrogen ligands and lies slightly above the plane. Oxidation of the iron II to iron III results in the formation of hemin. The iron in all hemoproteins is five or six coordinate. The protein donates at least one ligand, usually an imidazole nitrogen from a histidine residue.

Hemoglobin and myoglobin have the sixth coordination site available for bonding to oxygen. Cytochrome a is also five-coordinate but rather than reversibly binding oxygen the iron II-cytochrome is oxidized to the iron III state. The iron in b and c cytochromes is six-coordinate, with another base group of the protein occupying the final coordination site. In general, the b cytochrome has a lower oxidation potential than the c type, which is in turn lower than the a cytochrome. The flow of electrons in respiration will normally follow the pattern $b \rightarrow c \rightarrow a \rightarrow O_2$. Thus, a series of small energy changes is available for stepwise transfer of electrons.

Iron can influence biological reactions in a variety of ways. In the cytochrome it is tightly bound to the enzyme at the active center. Xanthanine oxidase, a flavoprotein, contains flavin, iron and molybdenum at the active site. All these substances seem to function in the electron transport process [86].

Aconitase requires loosely bound iron, apparently to bind the substrate in a position to facilitate the addition or removal of a water molecule. In succinate dehydrogenase, iron is bound in the enzyme and is also required as a hydrated ion.

Iron will normally be present in the tripositive oxidation state unless it is stabilized in the divalent state by chelation. It is transported in the higher oxidation state, bound to transferrin, to the site of erythrocyte formation [87-90].

The trivalent iron is transferred to protoporphyrin, forming heme, after reduction to the divalent state by cytochrome oxidase. The addition of iron II to protoporphyrin is catalyzed by ferrochelatase [91,92]. The chelated iron II remains in the divalent state and is capable of binding reversibly to oxygen.

The cytochromes (a, b and c) contain iron in the 3+ state, coordinated to the four planar nitrogen ligands of a porphyrin. They differ in terms of the type of constituent groups attached to the prophyrin and the manner of attachment to the protein portion of the molecule.

Protoheme IX, designated as Heme B, is the porphyrin found in hemoglobin, myglobin, catalase and the b-type cytochromes. It is bound to the protein by ionic and hydrophobic interactions. A similar structure is found in c-type cytochromes, except the alkene structures in the side groups have been reduced and a thioether bridge to the protein is present. The major distinguishing feature of the a-type cytochromes is the long unsaturated side chain.

The a-type cytochromes have two heme units, two copper atoms per molecule and a molecular weight of range of $1\text{-}2 \times 10^5$. The b-type have a molecular weight range of $1.3\text{-}4 \times 10^4$, with one protoheme unit; and c-type cytochromes have a range in molecular weights of $1.2\text{-}3.7 \times 10^4$, and contain only one heme C unit.

Most of the iron in humans is found in hemoglobin (60-70%) [93]. Only a relatively small amount (0.2-0.4%) is found in the cytochromes, catalase, peroxidase and nonheme compounds. The metal is stored in ferritin and hemosiderin (7-15%), and about 0.1% is bound to transferrin.

Absorption of iron in man usually occurs with the ion in the divalent state [94,95]. This ion is readily oxidized to iron III by dissolved oxygen at a rate that is pH-dependent. At neutral or physiological pH, iron III forms a hydroxide of very low solubility ($10^{-17}$ *M*). Chelation of iron III by citrate or fructose can prevent precipitation of the hydroxyl compound [96,97]. These iron III chelates can be absorbed, but incorporation of iron II into hemoglobin occurs more readily than iron III [98]. Transferrin-bound iron III is readily absorbed. Reduction of the iron by a copper-protein results in dissociation of the transferrin-iron complex and incorporation of the iron II into a hemoglobin molecule. Histidine and lysine have also been shown to bind iron in a form suitable for absorption [99,100].

Iron is of such an essential nature for all living organisms that means of solubilizing the metal are present in some bacteria and plants. Complexing agents, specific to trivalent metal ions, are secreted from the organism.

The complexing agent binds to iron (due to relative abundance) or other trivalent metal ions (Al, Cr), and diffuses back into the organism. Some plants secrete organic acids (malonic and citric) from their roots which bind iron and form a soluble complex. Specific enzymes are available within the cells of the organism to hydrolyze the complex and convert iron to a usable form [101-104].

Divalent metals (Mn, Co, Zn and Cu) have been found to interfere with the absorption of iron, possibly by competition for the binding site of the ligands [105]. Zinc has also been shown to interfere with the storage of iron in ferritin [106,107].

The transport of $O_2$ by hemoglobin and transfer to myglobin is basic to the existence of an animal cell. Hemoglobin consists of four subunits, each containing a heme group. Myglobin is similar to one of the subgroups of hemoglobin.

The mechanism of oxygen transport has been described by Peurtz [108]. Deoxyhemoglobin contains iron II in a high spin state. With electrons occupying each of the $e_g$ orbitals, the radius of the iron II ion is too large to fit between the nitrogen ligands of the porphyrin. It lies about 0.75 Å out of the nitrogen plane and is bonded to each of the four porphyrin nitrogens (Fe-N distance ~2.2 Å) and an imidazole nitrogen of histidine. When an $O_2$ molecule binds to the sixth coordination site of the iron II, both electrons in the $e_g$ orbital go into the $T_{2g}$ orbitals, forming a low-spin complex. The radius of the metal ion decreases with the electron orbital change, and fits into the middle of the porphyrin ring.

This change in position causes a corresponding shift in the location of several amino acid residues in the subunit, and the charge is transmitted to other subunits through interfacial rearrangements. The binding of oxygen to other heme units is facilitated by this structural change.

Hemoglobin binds oxygen as well as myglobin at high oxygen partial pressures, but the binding to myglobin is favored at the low oxygen pressures occurring in the cells. The relative binding tendency is thus proportional to the "need" for $O_2$ in a particular tissue. The formation of $CO_2$ in the cell causes a reduction of pH, which also favors release of $O_2$ from hemoglobin. Both the decreased pH and partial pressure of $O_2$ are important phases of $O_2$ transport. The $CO_2$ binds to amino acids in the protein portion of hemoglobin and is transported to the lungs.

### Nonheme Iron Proteins

Ferredoxins are small proteins containing iron, cysteine-sulfur and "inorganic sulfur." They occur in all green plants and photosynthetic bacteria. Their major function is electron transfer at the low-potential end of the photosynthesis process, but the exact specificity of this action is not known [109,110].

Rubredoxin has about the same molecular weight as the ferredoxins. It contains one iron atom, four cysteine units and no "inorganic" sulfur and it seems to function in a manner similar to the ferrodoxins [111,112].

## COBALT

Cobalt is an essential trace element for mammals, but except for its role in vitamin $B_{12}$, its function is not well known. The element normally exhibits either a divalent or trivalent positive oxidation state. The trivalent ion is a good oxidizing agent, and the divalent form is the most stable. Both cobalt II and cobalt III form stable complexes with nitrogen- or oxygen-containing ligands, but the only ones known to be biologically active are porphyrin-like corrinoid structures of cobalamin, vitamin $B_{12}$ and the $B_{12}$

derivatives. These contain cobalt II, which has coordination numbers of four or six. Five-coordinate compounds have also been reported [113], and the five-coordinate structure has been proposed as an intermediate in $B_{12}$-catalyzed reactions [114,115].

There are only about ten reactions that are known to be catalyzed by $B_{12}$. Of these, only the conversion of methylmolonyl-coenzyme A to succinyl-coenzyme A is known to occur in mammals. All of the reactions involve the rearrangement of groups on the carbon skeletal chain of the substrate molecule:

$$\begin{array}{c} -C_1-C_2- \\ \begin{array}{cc} | & | \\ X & H \end{array} \end{array} \rightarrow \begin{array}{c} -C_1-C_2- \\ \begin{array}{cc} | & | \\ H & X \end{array} \end{array}$$

Some group "X" migrates to an adjacent carbon atom and a hydrogen moves in the opposite direction. It has been shown that proton exchange with the solvent does not occur except in the reaction where $B_{12}$ is a coenzyme with ribonucleotide reductase [116]. The mechanisms of $B_{12}$ coenzyme catalyzed reactions are not thoroughly established, but several possible pathways have been proposed [115,117,118].

Only one enzyme, other than those for which $B_{12}$ is a coenzyme, that requires cobalt specifically has been isolated from animals [119]. This is glycylglycine dipeptidase. There is no known requirement for the free divalent ion; however, it would seem probable that it could activate enzymes that have a nonspecific divalent cation cofactor requirement.

Cobalt has been used to replace other metals (i.e., zinc in carbonic anhydrase) in metalloenzymes to aid in elucidating the location and function of the metal in the natural enzyme. The $d^8$ configuration of electrons in cobalt II makes it a very useful ion for spectroscopic measurements.

Cobalt is absorbed from the intestine readily if small doses (30-50 $\mu$g/kg) are ingested and less efficiently for large amounts. It appears to be transported across the intestinal mucosa in a manner similar to that of iron II [120].

Small doses of cobalt salts injected into tissue are dissipated from the site rather slowly, but if injected intravenously, the metal binds to $\alpha$ globulins and is distributed rapidly to tissues. Cobalt salts are accumulated primarily in the bone marrow, pancreas, liver, spleen, kidneys and heart. It is eliminated from mammals in the form of a histamine complex [121].

Cobalt toxicity appears to be related to improper erythrocyte formation by its presence in bone marrow and inhibition of precursors required for hemoglobin formation [122]. The metal has also been implicated in heart disorders [123-125]. The ability of cobalt salts to produce cancer in animals has been demonstrated [126,127], but no evidence of such action in man is available.

## MANGANESE

Manganese exhibits oxidation states of +3 to +7. The trivalent ion is the biologically active form often found in mammals. It chelates more readily than the divalent ion, because it is fairly stable as a complex at physiological pH. Manganese binds readily to oxygen-containing ligands. The divalent ion forms complexes that are less stable than other transition metals. Its ligand-field stabilization energy is weak because of the $d^5$ configuration.

Despite its many oxidation states, there is no evidence of direct involvement of manganese in electron transfer reactions in mammals. However, a superoxide dismutase enzyme isolated from *E. coli* contains tightly bound manganese [128,129]. This enzyme is similar in function to the copper- and zinc-containing enzyme found in mammals, but quite different in amino acid content, molecular weight and bound metal. The actual oxidation state of manganese is not known, but the Mn III ion is thought to be present, because of the purple color of the enzyme [130]. The redox function of superoxide dismutase makes it likely that a reversible oxidation state reaction occurs as a result of enzymatic activity.

Manganese is found as a tightly bound part of only a few enzymes, but there are a large number of enzymes that can be activated by the metal ion, such as transferases, decarboxylases, hydralases and kinases [131]. The variety of functions catalyzed by these enzymes and the ability of other divalent ions to stimulate their activity makes it probable that the manganese is required only as a divalent cation rather than possessing any unique catalytic feature.

The essential nature of manganese was shown in 1931. It is needed for proper growth and reproduction of rats and mice [132,133]. One symptom of manganese deficiency was skeletal defects. This led to several fruitless investigations to find a role of manganese in bone formation. Leach [134] discovered a correlation between manganese deficiency and a reduction in tissue mucopolysaccharide content, which is in turn related to the appearance of skeletal defects. Chondroitin sulfate is the mucopolysaccharide most severely affected by manganese deficiency. Two enzymatic systems are affected by the deficiency of this metal: (1) the polymerase system responsible for polysaccharide chain building; and (2) the galactosyltransferase system which incorporates galactose into the trisaccharide (gal-gal-xyl) that connects the polysaccharide to the protein portion of the molecule.

Many glycosyltransferases require divalent manganese for the transfer of a sugar molecule from a diphosphonucleotide to substrate forming a polysaccharide, glycoprotein or glycolipid. The catalytic action of this cation has been described in detail for two reactions involving galactosyltransferase [135,136].

Manganese is bound to isocitrate dehydrogenase, and is thought to form a coordination bond to the C-2 carbonyl of oxalosuccinate, thus forming a stable enolate intermediate of $\alpha$-ketoglutarate during the decarboxylation of isocitrate [137-139].

One of the more thoroughly studied manganese-metalloenzymes is pyruvate carboxylase [140,141]. A manganese ion is coordinated to three ligands of the protein and three water molecules in its other positions. The mechanism of the reaction and interference by oxalate after interaction of the biotin residues with avidin has been studied by the use of nuclear magnetic resonance (NMR) proton relaxation techniques. The manganese is very tightly bound to the enzyme, and functions as the active site. The enzyme contains four moles of biotin and four moles of manganese per molecule of enzyme.

The addition of a carboxyl group to pyruvic acid to form oxaloacetate takes place in two steps. The first reaction requires magnesium, acetyl CoA and the conversion of one mole of ATP to ADP. It has been proposed [142-144] that a biotin, attached to the enzyme by a long flexible hydrocarbon chain, binds a $CO_2^-$ group from bicarbonate. Pyruvate binds to manganese (at a separate site on the enzyme) through its $\alpha$ carbonyl ligand. The biotin-$CO_2$ complex "pivots" into a position in which an oxygen of the $CO_2^-$ group bonds to a second orbital of manganese. The manganese is not readily complexed by large chelating molecules (EDTA), but oxalate ion interferes with the second reaction. Thus, the metal ion is protected by steric hindrance of the enzyme. The coordinated activity of two separated enzymatic active sites is of considerable interest, and may provide a clue to the mechanisms of other metalloenzyme catalyzed reactions.

Manganese has been shown to occupy an active site in succinyl-CoA synthetase [145], and aminoacyl-tRNA synthetase [146]. It is a cofactor in the activation of RNA polymerase [147,148] and phosphoglycerate kinase [149]. The metal is normally found in the divalent state unless it is tightly bound by an enzyme. Then the trivalent state is stabilized. When manganese is coordinated to a metalloenzyme, it has an octahedral geometry with three sites occupied by the enzyme; the remaining orbitals are occupied by electrons from loosely bound water molecules. Thus, much of the information which has been accumulated about the mechanisms and rates of reactions catalyzed by manganese-metalloenzymes has been obtained from proton magnetic resonance studies [145,146,148,149].

A protein-containing manganese in the high-spin Mn III state has been isolated by Scrutton [150]. It has been given the name "avimanganin," but no enzymatic function has been determined for it.

A study of metal-polynucleotide interactions has shown that manganese II and cadmium II can cause mispairing of bases. Magnesium and zinc, similar to Mn and Cd, respectively, do not show mispairing effects [151]. The possibility of a direct metal-nucleic acid interaction in metal-induced carcinogenesis is proposed, but conclusive evidence is not available.

Manganese is closely associated with enzymes of the citric acid cycle. Considering the number of oxidation states that this metal can exhibit, it is surprising not to find it involved in charge transfer reactions in mammals. The ligand field stabilization energy may contribute to the fact, however, that the ligands to which the metal is bound have not been identified. Further study of the mechanisms of catalysis and structures of manganese-metalloenzymes is needed.

## CADMIUM

Cadmium has an electronic configuration similar to that of zinc. It forms tetrahedral complexes, but is also capable of forming complex anions in solutions containing a high concentration of halide ions (e.g., chloride). The hydroxide is amphoteric, and stable cadmate salts can be formed.

The metal has a greater affinity for thiol ligands than does zinc, but the latter forms more stable complexes with oxygen- or nitrogen-containing groups. It binds to sulfur-containing ligands more tightly than the first-row transition metals other than copper, but mercury and lead both form more stable sulfur complexes than does cadmium.

The cadmium II ion is similar to calcium II in size and charge density. It is not surprising therefore to find a relationship between decalcification of bone and the cadmium content of the diet fed to laboratory rats [152]. The mechanism by which cadmium interferes with the bone structure is not known, but it has been reported to interfere with the synthesis of 1,25-dihydroxycholecalciferol, which is the activated form of vitamin D [153].

Cadmium has been found bound to metallothionein [51] and other proteins isolated from kidney, liver and mammary glands [154,155].

The metal inhibits the action of ATPase [156] and increases the rate of formation of the AMP-synthesizing enzyme in rats [157]. It has been shown to decrease the zinc content of serum, and have an adverse effect on serum insulin levels and glucose tolerance, which can be prevented in rats by increased zinc intake [158].

The correlation of "itai-itai" disease in Japan with cadmium intake has led to numerous reviews of the symptoms related to the toxicity of the metal [159,160]. Unfortunately, little is known about the mechanisms by which these toxic effects occur.

Cadmium accumulates in the liver and kidneys. It has been shown to be related to the degree of renal retention of sodium ions, and thus can be associated with hypertension [161]. Primary carcinogenicity of cadmium has been shown to occur in animals, but conclusive evidence is not available for man. The metal has been shown to accumulate in cancerous tissue of humans suffering from cadmium intoxication [162]. Ingested cadmium has not been found to be carcinogenic [126] but malignant tumors have been found to form at the site of injection into laboratory animals [163,164].

The toxicity of cadmium in a marine environment is related to the concentration of the free ion. Increasing the salinity of the medium decreases the toxic effect on mollusks through the formation of anionic chloride complexes of the metal. Low-molecular-weight proteins bind cadmium up to a saturation point, then it appears to bond to sensitive sites on membranes and enzymes. The low-molecular-weight proteins found in mollusks have a high ratio of dicarboxylic amino acids relative to cysteine residues, indicating that chelation may occur through carbonyl groups rather than at sulfydryls as occurs in vertebrate metallothionein [165].

Cadmium from inorganic salts [160] or Cd-metallothionein [166] is absorbed from the gastrointestinal tract. The Cd-metallothionein undergoes degradation during renal deposition.

The appearance of cadmium in the intestine apparently triggers the formation of thionene. Because this protein can bind other metals (e.g., zinc) as well as cadmium, the disturbance of the metabolism of zinc, copper and iron may be related to the competitive binding of these cations [167,168].

Inhalation of cadmium is followed by absorption of all but the sulfide salt through the lungs. The sulfide salt is quite insoluble and remains as a solid antagonist in the lung cavity. Oral administration of the metal can lead to emphysema in rats, but this affect can be reversed by the addition of zinc to the diet [168].

The injection of selenium into rats apparently does not prevent absorption of cadmium, but diverts it from binding to low-molecular-weight proteins to those of higher molecular weight. Addition of selenium to the diet decreases the accumulation of cadmium in liver, but increases the amount in the testes [169].

The similarity of ionic radius and charge between cadmium ion and calcium ion suggests a possible relationship between the absorption and transport of the two metals. A low-cadmium diet will stimulate an increase in the production of calcium binding protein (CaBP) in the intestinal mucosal cells [170]. During periods of low calcium intake, cadmium will also bind to this protein [171,172]. As mentioned previously, the renal deposition of cadmium appears to interfere with the conversion of vitamin D to its activated form. This action, possibly through interaction with 25-hydroxycholecoliferol-1-hydrolase, will influence calcium metabolism [173,174].

Although the exact mechanism by which cadmium interacts with the metabolism of calcium, zinc and other essential metals is not known, a pathway of transport and interaction has been proposed [167]. Cadmium, in the form of metallothionein is absorbed by the intestinal mucosal cells. It is transported via plasma to the liver and stored as hepatic metallothionein. From here it is slowly degraded, and possibly interacts with other cell components. It is eventually transported to the kidney and deposited. The ability of the kidney to synthesize metallothionein makes it doubtful if the metal is transported from the liver to the kidney as the Cd-metallothionein complex, however, the exact mechanism is unknown.

## LEAD

More has been written about the toxicity of lead than any other heavy metal, but little is actually known about the mechanisms by which it influences body functions. The metal has been used by man since ancient times, and has even been implicated as a factor related to the decline of the Roman empire.

The lack of knowledge about the biological effects of lead could once have been the result of the lack of a sensitive analytical method for the determination of trace quantities of the metal, but this is no longer a valid excuse. Clinical methods using atomic absorption spectroscopy (AAS) [175, 176] and the Delves cup AAS technique [177] have been available to researchers for several years. The results obtained by flameless AAS methods often lacked precision and accuracy because of improper ashing temperatures and vaporization parameters, but these errors have been identified, and improvements have been made [178]. A microsampling cup has been used for the determination of lead in homogenized tissue. A sensitivity of $10^{-2}$ $\mu$g/g tissue has been achieved [179].

Lead is introduced into the body primarily through oral ingestion; however, tetraethyllead is readily absorbed through the skin. It is absorbed from the intestine presumably by binding to high-molecular-weight mucosal proteins. Iron and lead have been shown to compete for binding sites on these proteins, primarily to a fraction which has a molecular weight of about 370,000. This may be related to the increased rate of lead absorption when iron is deficient in the diet [180].

Rats fed a low-calcium diet and 200 ppm of lead in the drinking water show an increase in lead absorption, urinary excretion and lead content in blood, soft tissue and bone [181]. The authors postulate that of the three factors they investigated in relationship to lead absorption (vitamin D, phosphorus and calcium), it was calcium which exhibited the greatest influence. The rats that received lead in their drinking water also showed a decrease in serum calcium, regardless of the calcium level in the diet, and an increase in both calcium and lead in the kidneys. This implies a possible competition between these two metals for a common transport mechanism. The kidneys of rats receiving lead in their water develop intranuclear inclusion bodies in the renal cells. These consist of a lead-protein complex that also contains an unusually high amount of calcium. These intranuclear inclusion bodies have been observed in rats fed smaller amounts of lead than is required to show other physiological changes. The amount of lead in the renal cell nucleus has been observed to be 30 times greater than normal while the level in the mitochondria is increased by only 3–4 times [182]. The formation of Pb-protein inclusion bodies in the nucleus of renal cells may be a defensive mechanism of the body against heavy metal poisoning.

The development of symptoms of lead toxicity is closely related to the concentration of the metal in blood and soft tissue. The ability of the body to store the metal in a relatively immobile form in bone makes it difficult to determine a minimum toxic or lethal dose, or even to predict the maximum allowable body burden.

Lead toxicity influences a number of body functions, but one of the most dramatic appears to be the interference with heme synthesis. The first and slowest step in the formation of heme is the reaction of glycine and succinyl-coenzyme A. This reaction is catalyzed by δ-aminolevulinic acid (ALA) synthetase. The product of this reaction (ALA) reacts with the enzyme ALA dehydrase (ALA-D) to form porphobilinogen (PBG). Uroporphyrinogen, (URO III) is formed by enzymatically catalyzed reactions from PBG. It then enters the mitochondria, undergoes decarboxylation and oxidation to form protoporphyrin IX, which reacts with iron II ions, catalyzed by ferrochelatase, to form heme. Heme is transported to the endoplasmic reticulum where apocytochromes are synthesized. These combine with the heme molecule to form hemoproteins. The hemoproteins play a major role in the metabolic process in cells.

Lead has been shown to inhibit the activity of ALA-D [183-185]. In fact, the presence of increased ALA in urine has been used as an indirect test for lead ingestion. Zinc is an essential element for ALA-D activity and an increase of zinc concentration appears to modify some of the effects of lead on the enzyme [186]. There is a logarithmatic correlation between the lead concentration in blood and the amount of erythrocyte ALA-D, within the lead concentration range 0.05–0.95 ppm [184].

Allain et al. [187] examined the relationship between ALA-D and zinc concentration of human erythrocytes from healthy individuals and those suffering from cirrhosis. In the latter group, they found lower concentrations of zinc and albumin and a decrease in the activity of ALA-D. An increased concentration of lead in the blood was also observed. This was assumed to be related to the decreased amount of zinc, but a mechanism was not proposed.

The action of ferrochelatase is also inhibited by lead. The mechanism is not known, but the similarity between lead and iron as shown by their competition for binding sites on proteins may be a factor. It should be noted, however, that cobalt and manganese inhibit the action of ferrochelatase to a greater extent than does lead [188].

Lead poisoning in children is often associated with iron-deficiency anemia. Rats fed iron-deficient diets and 200 $\mu$g Pb/ml of drinking water developed typical lead poisoning symptoms. The lead content increased in the liver, kidney and bone. Urinary excretion of both lead and ALA increased [189].

In the liver, lead is almost exclusively bound to membrane proteins and is not found in phospholipids. Intranuclear lead is associated with histone fractions and other basic or weakly acid proteins [190]. It has been found in chromatographically purified DNA, but whether it is bound to the molecule is not known. It has been reported to induce DNA replication by stimulating the synthesis of RNA and protein [191].

Lead storage in bone can delay the appearance of poisoning symptoms for several years. The metal can be stored in a relatively inert form in bone matter, but it is released into the blood on metabolic disturbance resulting in osteolysis, in cases of chronic infection or if a fracture should occur.

It will accumulate in areas of active bone formation and become less mobile with elapsed time.

The storage of lead in bone and its subsequent release is affected by several factors, including calcium, phosphorus and vitamin D in the diet. Studies involving the amounts of these substances in the diet fed to rats that had previously received lead in their water showed the following relationships [192]:

1. A high-calcium, low-phosphorus diet produced a rapid loss of lead from bone and an increase in the blood-lead level.
2. A low-calcium, high-phosphorus diet produced slow loss of lead from bone and low blood-lead levels.
3. The addition of vitamin D to the diet enhances the absorption of lead, but also decreases the rate at which it is lost from bone.

Parathyroid hormone adminstered to humans increases the amount of both lead and calcium in the urine [181]. The mobilization of calcium from bone is apparently accompanied by a release of lead also. This would imply that the two metals are bound in a similar manner.

The toxicity of lead in biological systems has been studied extensively [192]. The metal binds quite readily to phosphate, sulfydryl and carboxylic groups of the erythrocyte membrane. It can alter membrane permeability, block potassium permeability of the cell and inhibit active transport of Na and K.

Lead is also toxic to the central nervous system. Neural tissue is quite sensitive to lead toxicity. The passage of a metal ion across the blood-brain barrier requires a lipid-soluble form of the metal to be present. Thus, tetraethyllead should be suspect in this area.

Stillbirths and sudden infant death cases have been investigated by Coumbis [193]. Large amounts of both lead and cadmium have been found in several organs of the infant's body. Lead concentrations in the brain above the lethal level have been found. Apparently, the metal passes through the placental barrier.

Despite all the incriminating evidence of lead toxicity, it has also been mentioned as a possible essential growth factor in rats [194].

## MERCURY

Mercury is unique in serveral ways. It is the only metal to exist as a liquid at normal temperature (25°C), and has a vapor pressure of about $4 \times 10^{-3}$ torr at this temperature. The metallic ion does not form cyclic chelates because of the large angle between bonding orbitals (180°), but does form tetrahedral complexes with monodentate ligands. It has the greatest affinity for sulfhydryl groups of all metals (pK ∿17) and bonds to other ligands in the order of $SH > CONH_2 > NH_2 > COOH > PO_4{}^{3-}$.

The high affinity of mercury II for sulfur-containing amino acid residues is responsible for the rather selective binding of the metal to protein structures. This results in agglutination of the protein and inhibition of the activity of enzymes containing thiol groups.

The ingestion of mercury can occur through oral consumption, inhalation of vapors containing mercury or mercuric components, or through the skin. The absorption of mercury salts from the intestine is slow to moderate, depending on the solubility of the salt. Inhaled mercury vapor is absorbed rapidly and is oxidized in the blood. It is loosely bound to erythrocytes and diffuses readily into soft tissues and even the brain.

Methylmercury ($CH_3Hg^+$) is one of the more toxic species of the element found in biological systems. It can permeate cell membranes readily, binds loosely to sulfhydryl groups in blood-proteins from which it can disassociate and dissolve in lipid membrane. The high and rather specific toxicity of methylmercury in the central nervous system is attributed to its binding to nerve cell membranes and reducing the RNA content of nerve cells in the dorsal root ganglia and cerebellum [195].

An experiment conducted on three male volunteers showed that methylmercury accumulates primarily in the liver (∿50%) and brain (∿10%). The uptake of orally ingested $^{203}Hg$ by erythrocytes was found to be quite rapid (within 15 min). The half-life in the body was found to be 70–74 days, with excretion primarily in the feces; but urinary excretion increased with time up to 30 days. Chang et al. [196] studied the effect of methylmercuric chloride and mercuric chloride on enzymes in the liver, kidney and cerebellum of rats. The activities of glucose-6-phosphatase, alkaline phosphatase, ATPase and succinic anhydrase decreased, and a slight increase in activity was observed for acid phosphatase in all tissues examine. Methylmercuric chloride had a greater effect on the enzymes of the liver and cerebellum, but mercuric chloride had a greater effect on the kidneys. This is consistent with the observation that about 80% of an inorganic mercuric salt will collect in theproximal renal tubules of rats [197]. Methylmercury has also been found to inhibit the action of ALA-D and cholinesterase [198,199].

Lactating mammals have been shown to contain methylmercury in their milk after intoxication with the compound. It tends to accumulate in the brain of the suckling [200,201]. Some of the results obtained from studies involving poisoning of laboratory animals with mercury salts or methylmercury seem somewhat contradictory. The species of mercury and the manner in which it is ingested both affect the distribution in the body. Inorganic salts of mercury do not easily pass the blood-brain barrier, but methylmercury passes into the central nervous system rather readily [202]. Mercury vapor also accumulates in the brain, but ingested mercury does not [203]. The release of mercury from the brain occurs at a slower rate than from other organs. The primate brain can concentrate the metal to levels that are four to five times that found in the blood [204].

The high affinity of methylmercury for sulfhydryl groups seems to imply the formation of a strong ligand-metal bond. Contrary to the thermodynamic stability of the complex, methylmercury is rather labile [205]. It exchanges with other sulfhydryl groups, and has been extracted by chemotherapeutic agents [206]. Glutathione displaces methylmercury from protein or peptide sulfhydryl ligands very rapidly. A mechanism involving second-order reaction kinetics has been proposed to account for the mobility of methylmercury in its protein complexes [205].

Biosynthesis of metal-alkyls is a microbiological response to heavy metal poisoning. Local concentrations of inorganic salts are diluted by the formation of the more rapidly diffusing metal-alkyl compounds. There are three major coenzymes known to catalyze the formation of these compounds. These are S-adenoxylmethionine, $N^5$-methyltetrahydrofolate derivatives and methylcorrinoid derivatives [80]. The mechanisms for the formation of methylmercury have been thoroughly studied [207-209], and the reaction has been shown to proceed rapidly [210].

Tuna and swordfish tend to accumulate mercury in excess of the maximum allowable level (0.5 ppm) established by the U. S. Food and Drug Administration. Ganther et al. [211] reported that tuna, mixed in the diet of Japanese quail, reduced the toxicity of methylmercury. They proposed that selenium could be responsible for the effect. Similar observations have been reported in rats [212], and seals [213].

The binding affinity of methylmercury to various ligating groups containing selenium and sulfur has been investigated with proton magnetic resonance spectroscopy [214]. The order of binding affinity was found to be SeH> SH>Se-Se>$NH_2$>S-S, $SeCH_3$, $SCH_3$.

The protective capability of selenium [215] has been the subject of several studies [214,216-219], but the actual mechanism involved remains unknown. Fang [217] suggested that induction of enzyme formation, such as glutathione peroxidase, C-Hg cleavage enzyme [216] and the diversion of mercury from binding to critical proteins by formation of selenoproteins with a high mercury affinity may all have a role in such protective action. The enhanced production of metallothionein is a possible, but rather poor protective mechanism against mercury poisoning.

Several theories have been formulated to explain the toxicity of mercury. These are summarized as follows:

1. The high affinity for the sulfhydryl groups of functional proteins causes deactivation of these enzymes.
2. The binding of mercury to phosphate ligands changes the cellular membrane permeability and conformational changes in macromolecules.
3. Mercury inhibits the uptake of iodide by the thyroid.
4. The metal acts as an antimetabolite to zinc.
5. Mercury decreases the liver micromosal detoxification systems and thus indirectly enhances the harmful effects of other toxic substances.

There is sufficient reason to believe that any or all of the above are important actions of mercury. However, further study is needed to gain an understanding of the complex mechanism by which this metal alters normal body functions.

## ARSENIC

Arsenic is the most misunderstood and maligned element in the periodic chart. The almost synonymous use of the name with poison has had a more historical than clinical development. In fact, the toxic effects of arsenic-containing compounds are rather slow to appear, making it much less desirable for homicidal purposes than many other more lethal substances.

One of the most deceiving practices concerning arsenic is the tendency to list it as a heavy metal along with mercury, lead and cadmium. The purpose of this review in including it with these elements is to dispel the myth. Arsenic is not a heavy metal; in fact, it can hardly be considered as a metal at all. Logically, it is considered a metalloid. Chemically, it is similar to phosphorous and selenium. It normally exhibits a +3 or +5 oxidation state in the oxides or sulfides it forms. The arsenite and arsenate radicals are the most important forms of the element found in biological systems. It does exhibit a -3 oxidation state in arsine ($AsH_3$), which is very toxic gas. Arsine is quite reactive, and exposure to the substance is unlikely, but should be avoided. Much of the confusion about the toxicity of arsenic is caused by a lack of understanding of its chemistry. The pentavalent arsenate ion is not readily absorbed by the body, and thus is not considered toxic. The trivalent arsenite form is more readily absorbed, and distributes into soft tissue [220]. The oxidative processes occurring in animal cells will convert arsenite to arsenate. The arsenate ion does inhibit the action of several enzymes including α-glycerophosphate dehydrogenase, DNA polymerase, cytochrome oxidase and alkaline phosphatase [221]. It should be noted that the similarity of structure between arsenate and phosphate can be related to the tendency of the two ions to have an antagonistic relationship. Phosphorus is present in the body in a ratio of about 10,000 to 1 (excluding bone) over arsenic; thus, competitive interference is not a normal event [222]. Arsenate is capable of inhibiting the synthesis of ATP in liver mitochondria through its ability to replace the phosphoryl group. The arsenic analog hydrolyzes quite readily.

Arsenite accumulates in leukocytes, and can bind readily to thiol-containing enzymes, thus decreasing their activity. In the tripositive oxidation state, arsenic relaxes and increases the permeability of capillaries and arterioles, causing circulatory changes which can result in inflammation and changes in function [223].

Inorganic arsenic salts are more toxic than its organic compounds. Tryparsamide and atoxyl have been used for their therapeutic effects. These compounds can pass the blood-brain barrier and have been used for the treatment of neurosyphilis [224]. A side effect often encountered with such treatment is a deterioration of the peripheral area of the ganglion cell layer of the eye. Arsenic has been a suspected carcinogen for well over a hundred years [225,226]. Many attempts to substantiate these claims have not met with success [227-231]. On the other hand, inhalation or exposure to arsenic compounds has been shown to result in chronic and acute toxic results, including cancer [222,232,233].

Stone [234] has proposed that arsenic V can act as a cocarcinogenic agent by suppressing the resistance factors of the host, thus increasing the probability of survival of a tumor. In light of the antagonistic relationship between arsenate and selenate ions, this possibility is worthy of further consideration.

At the present, the most accurate statement that can be made in regard to the carcinogenic properties of arsenic and its compounds is that the metal is highly suspect, but no convincing evidence has yet been obtained to establish it as a carcinogen or cocarcinogen.

## SELENIUM

Selenium has been shown to be essential for animals [235-237], but its essentiality for man has not been proven. The chick has been shown to have a requirement for selenium even if all other nutrients, including vitamin E, are present in the diet. The selenium requirement is somewhat lower in chicks receiving high amounts of vitamin E than in those fed vitamin E–deficient diets [236]. The major effects observed in chicks fed a selenium-deficient diet are stunted growth, poor feathering and degeneration of the pancreas. The blood level of vitamin E is lowered. This may be caused by the degeneration of the pancreas. Poor fat absorption is observed, which could be responsible for the decreased absorption of vitamin E. A similar effect should be observed for other vitamins and lipid-soluble nutrients. The turnover rate of vitamin E is quite rapid. The effect of the decreased absorption of other lipid-soluble nutrients may be balanced somewhat by the reserves in the tissue, but the effects of a decreased vitamin E level are readily apparent [237].

Selenium has been shown to have a role in the enzymatic action of glutathione (GSH) peroxidase [238]. There is evidence for the binding of selenium as an integral part of the enzyme, but conclusive proof has not yet been obtained.

Glutathione peroxidase catalyzes the reduction of hydroperoxides formed in the metabolism of fatty acids and other substances. The general equation for this reaction is:

$$\mathrm{ROOH + 2GSH \rightarrow ROH + H_2O + GSSG}$$

A similar protection against accumulation of peroxides is provided by vitamin E. Thus, although the mechanism is not necessarily the same for the peroxide reduction, vitamin E and GSH peroxidase deficiencies would tend to have similar effects.

If vitamin E prevents fatty acid hydroperoxide formation and GSH (including Se) is involved in destruction of these compounds, similar biochemical results would be observed for deficiencies of either substance. Likewise, an increase in the activity of either substance could partially compensate for a deficiency of the other.

The oxidation of glutathione by peroxidases, catalyzed by GSH peroxidase, is followed by reduction of the oxidized form by NADPH. The reduction reaction is catalyzed by glutathione reductase. The reduction of NADP occurs in mature erythrocytes, accompanied by the oxidation of glucose by the hexose monophosphate shunt. Thus, a deficiency of selenium in the system can be related to the inhibition of a number of other charge transfer reactions.

The ingestion of foreign particles or bacteria in the body is counteracted by the action of phagocytic cells. These cells rapidly increase the rate of peroxide production and lipid metabolism when a foreign particle is present. Oxygen consumption increases rapidly, and the hexose monophosphate shunt activity increases [12]. Very reactive forms of oxygen, singlet oxygen and superoxide radicals are generated. The cell can destroy itself in attempting to combat the foreign matter. It is protected to some extent by the presence of catalase, superoxide dismutase and glutathione peroxidase [239,241]. The latter enzyme has not been found in bacteria, and thus phagocytes may have an advantage. A deficiency of selenium, and thus a reduced activity of GSH peroxidase, would diminish the ability of the cell to decrease the high level of peroxidases formed in this process, and thus destruction of the phagocyte is possible.

Glutathione reduction of peroxides is an important reaction in lens cells of the eye [242,243]. The activity of the enzyme diminishes with a decrease in selenium content. One of the effects of this decreased activity is the appearance of cataracts. Swanson and Truesdale report a selenium content in cataractous lenses that is about 16% of that in normal lenses from similar age groups [244].

A possible correlation of the selenium content in the diet and a decrease in the toxicity of mercury compounds has been suggested [211]. Japanese quail fed a corn-soya diet, with varied amounts of tuna containing trace amounts of mercury and differing amounts of added mercury, showed a significant retardation of the toxic effects of mercury in the birds fed a higher ratio of tuna. The selenium content of the tuna was suspected of being a significant factor. Further evidence for the role of selenium in decreasing methylmercury toxicity was obtained by feeding rats a purified diet containing 20% casein or the same diet supplemented with 0.5 ppm selenium. Various amounts of methylmercury were added to the drinking water. Selenium was found to decrease the rate at which mercury toxicity became apparent.

Selenium and mercury are both associated with sulfur-containing proteins. In addition, selenium will form complexes with mercury, as does sulfur. The exact mechanism by which selenium reduces the toxicity of mercury, and if this can be observed for other heavy metals remains to be explained.

Koeman et al. [213] determined a stoichiometric 1:1 mole ratio of selenium to mercury in aquatic mammals, even those fed a fish diet containing 40 times as much selenium as mercury. The 1:1 mole ratio is apparently established in the mammal and not just related to the relative amounts of each metal found in the marine environment.

## REFERENCES


1. Hill, C. H., and G. Matrone. "Chemical Parameters in the Study of in Vivo and in Vitro Interactions of Transition Elements," *Fed. Proc.* 29:1474-1481 (1970).
2. Eichorn, G. L. *Inorganic Biochemistry, Vol. II*, (Amsterdam: Elsvier, 1973), pp. 1191-1209.
3. Wacker, W. E. C. "Nucleic Acids and Metals. III. Changes in Nucleic Acid, Protein, and Metal Content as a Consequence of Zinc Deficiency in Euglena gracilis," *Biochemistry* 1:859-865 (1962).
4. Scrutton, M. C., C. W. Wu and D. A. Goldthwait. "The Presence and Possible Role of Zinc in RNA Polymerase Obtained from *Escherichia coli*," *Proc. Nat. Acad. Sci.*, U.S. 68:2497-2501 (1971).
5. Springgate, C. F., A. S. Moldvan, R. Abramson, J. L. Engle and L. A. Loeb. "*Escherichia coli* Deoxyribonucleic Acid Polymerase I, a Zinc Metalloenzyme," *J. Biol. Chem.* 248:5987-5993 (1973).
6. Evans, G. W., P. E. Johnson, J. G. Brushmiller and R. W. Ames. "Detection of Labile Zn-Binding Ligands in Biological Fluids by Modified Gel Filtration Chromatography," *Anal. Chem.* 51:839-843 (1979).
7. Vallee, B. L., and H. Neurath. "Carboxypeptidase, A Zinc Metalloenzyme," *J. Biol. Chem.* 217:253–261 (1955).
8. Cox, D. J., E. Wintersberger and H. Neurth. "Bovine Pancreatic Procarboxypeptidase B. II. Mechanism of Activation," *Biochemistry* 1:1078-1082 (1962).
9. Latt, S. A., B. Holmquist and B. L. Vallee. *Biochem. Biophys. Res. Commun.* 37:333–339 (1969).
10. McConn, J. D., D. Tsuru and K. T. Yasunobu. "Bacillus Subtilis Neutral Proteinase I. A Zinc Enzyme of High Specific Activity," *J. Biol. Chem.* 239:3706-3715 (1964).
11. Wagner, F. W., and J. M. Prescott. "Purification and Some Characteristics of a Snake Venom Proteinase," *Fed. Proc.* 25:590 (1966).
12. Klebanoff, S. *Ann. Rev. Med.* 22:39–62 (1971).
13. Himmelhoch, S. R. *Arch. Biochem. Biophys.* 134:597-602 (1969).
14. Wacker, H., P. Lehkg, E. H. Fischer and E. A. Stein. *Helv. Chem. Acta.* 54:473-485 (1971).
15. Plocke, D. J., C. Levinthal and B. J. Vallee. "Alkaline Phosphatase of Escherichia coli: A Zinc Metalloenzyme," *Biochemistry* 1:373-378 (1962).
16. Rickli, E. E., S. A. S. Ghanzanfar, B. H. Gibbons and J. T. Edsatt. "Carbonic Anhydrases from Human Erythrocytes," *J. Biol. Chem.* 239:1065-1078 (1964).
17. Lindskag, S., and B. G. Malmström. "Metal Binding and Catalytic Activity in Bovine Carbonic Anhydrase," *J. Biol. Chem.* 237:1129-1137 (1962).

18. Drum, D. E., J. H. Harrison, T. K. Liu, J. L. Bethune and B. L. Vallee. *Nat. Acad. Sci.*, U.S. 57:1434-1440 (1967).
19. Keele, B. B., J. M. McCord and I. Fridovich. "Further Characterization of Bovine Superoxide Dismutase and its Isolation from Bovine Heart," *J. Biol. Chem.* 246:2875-2880 (1971).
20. Kobes, R. D., R. T. Simpson, B. L. Vallee and W. J. Rutter. "A Functional Role of Metal Ions in a Class II Aldolase," *Biochemistry* 8:585-588 (1969).
21, Schwartz, N. B., and D. S. Feingold. *Bioinorg. Chem.* 1:233 (1972).
22. Nelbach, M. E., V. P. Pigiet, J. C. Gerhardt and H. K. Schachman. "A Role for Zinc in the Quarternary Structure of Asparate Transcarbamylase from Escherichia coli," *Biochemistry* 11:315-327 (1972).
23. Northrop, D. B., and H. G. Wood. "Transcarbosylase V: The Presence of Bound Zinc and Cobalt," *J. Biol. Chem.* 244:5801-5807 (1969).
24. Slater, J. P., A. S. Mildvan and L. A. Leob. "Zinc in DNA Polymerase," *Biochim. Biophys. Res. Commun.* 44:37-43 (1971).
25. Corder, C. N., and O. H. Lowry. *Biochim. Biophys. Acta.* 191:579-587 (1969).
26. Haroz, R. K., J. S. Twu and R. K. Bretthaver. "Purification and Properties of a Yeast Nucleotide Pyrophosphatase," *J. Biol. Chem.* 247:1452-1457 (1972).
27. Dvorak, H. F., and L. A. Heppel. "Metalloenzymes Released from Escherichia coli by Osmotic Shock," *J. Biol. Chem.* 243:2647-2653 (1968).
28. Gracy, R. W., and E. A. Noltmann. "Studies on Phosphomannose Isomerase," *J. Biol. Chem.* 243:4109-4116 (1968).
29. Hirose, M., E. Sergiomoto and H. Chiba. *Biochim. Acta.* 289:137-146 (1972).
30. Snaith, S. M., G. A. Levvy and A. J. Hay. *J. Biochem.* 117:129-137 (1970).
31. Sabath, L. D., and M. Finland. *J. Bacteriol.* 95:1513-1519 (1968).
32. Yonetoni, T. *Biochem. Biophys. Res. Commun.*, 3:549-553 (1960).
33. Seifter, S., S. Takahaski and E. Harper. *Biochim. Biophys. Acta.* 214:559-561 (1970).
34. Feder, J., and L. R. Garrett. *Biochem. Biophys. Res. Commun.* 43:943-948 (1971).
35. Campbell, B. J., Y. C. Lin, R. V. Daivs and E. Ballew. *Biochim. Biophys. Acta.* 118:371-386 (1966).
36. Ottolenghi, A. C. *Biochim. Biophys. Acta.* 106:510-518 (1965).
37. Hayman, S., and E. K. Patterson. "Purification and Properties of a Mouse Ascites Tumor Dipeptidase: A Metalloenzyme," *J. Biol. Chem.* 246:660-669 (1970).
38. Vallee, B. L., E. A. Stein, W. N. Sumerwell and E. H. Fisher. "Metal Content of α-Amylases of Various Organs," *J. Biol. Chem.* 234:2901-2905 (1959).
39. Vallee, B. L., and W. E. C. Wacker. "Zinc, A Component of Rabbit Muscle Lactic Dehydrogenase," *J. Am. Chem. Soc.* 78:1771-1772 (1956).
40. Mattauch, J. *Phys. Rev.* 50:617 (1936).
41. Keleti, T. *Biochem. Biophys. Res. Commun.* 22:640-643 (1966).

42. Murphy, M. K., S. A. Clyburn and C. Veillon. "Comparison of Lock-in Amplification and Photon Counting with Low Background Flames and Graphite Atomizers in Atomic Fluoresence Spectrometry," *Anal. Chem.* 45:1468-1473 (1973).
43. Harrison, J. H. "Participation of $Zn^{++}$ in Mechanism of Action of Malic Dehydrogenase," *Fed. Proc.* 22:493 (1963).
44. Adelstein, S. J., and B. L. Vallee. "Zinc in Beef Liver Glutamic Dehydrogenase," *J. Biol. Chem.* 233:589-593 (1958).
45. Scrutton, M. C., M. R. Yound and M. F. Utter. "Pyruvate Carboxylase from Baker's Yeast," *J. Biol. Chem.*, 245:6220-6227 (1970).
46. Vachek, H., and J. L. Wood. *Biochim. Biophys. Acta.* 258:133-146 (1972).
47. Volini, M., F. Detoma and J. Westley. "Dimeric Structure and Zinc Content of Bovine Liver Rhodanese," *J. Biol. Chem.* 242:5220-5225 (1967).
48. Wilson, E. L., P. E. Burger and E. B. Dowdle. *Eur. J. Biochem.* 29:563-571 (1972).
49. Parisi, A. F., and B. L. Vallee. "Isolation of a Zinc $\alpha_2$-Macroglobulin from Human Serum," *Biochemistry* 9:2421-2426 (1970).
50. Kägi, J. H. R., and B. L. Vallee. "Metallothionein: A Cadmium and Zinc-Containing Protein from the Renal Cortex," *J. Biol. Chem.* 236: 2435-2442 (1961).
51. Pulido, P. A., J. H. R. Kagi and B. L. Vallee. "Isolation and Some Properties of Human Metallothionein," *Biochemistry* 5:1768-1777 (1966).
52. Lipscomb, W. N., J. A. Hartsuck, F. A. Quiocho and G. N. Reeke, Jr. "The Structure of Carboxy Peptidase A. IX. The X-Ray Diffraction Results in the Light of the Chemical Sequence," *Proc. Nat. Acad. Sci., U.S.* 64:28-35 (1969).
53. Coleman, J. E., and B. L. Vallee. "Metallocarboxypeptidases," *J. Biol. Chem.* 235:390-395 (1960).
54. Henkens, R. W., and J. S. Sturtevant. "The Kinetics of the Binding of Zinc II by Apocarbonic Anhydrase," *J. Am. Chem. Soc.* 90:2669-2676 (1968).
55. Richardson, J. S., K. A. Thomas and D. C. Richardson. "Alpha Carbon Coordinates for Bovine Cu, Zn Superoxide Dismutase," *Biochem. Biophys. Res. Commun.* 63:986-992 (1975).
56. Richardson, J. S., K. A. Thomas, B. H. Rubin and D. C. Richardson. "Crystal Structure of Bovine Cu, Zn Superoxide Dismutase at 3Å Resolution: Chain Tracing and Metal Ligands," *Proc. Nat. Acad. Sci., U.S.* 72:1349-1353 (1975).
57. Calabrese, L., G. Ratilio and B. Mondovi. "Properties of the Apoprotein and Role of Copper and Zinc in Protein Conformation and Enzyme Activity of Bovine Superoxide Dismutase," *Biochemistry* 11:2182-2187 (1972).
58. Calabrese, L., G. R. Ratilio and B. Mondovi. "Properties of the Apoprotein and Role of Copper and Zinc in Protein Conformation and Enzyme Activity of Bovine Superoxide Dismutase," *Biochemistry* 11:2182-2187 (1972).
59. Slater, J. P., I. Tamis, L. A. Loeb and A. S. Mildvan. "The Mechanism

of Escherichia coli Deoxyribonucleic Acid Polymerase I, *J. Biol. Chem.* 247:6784-6794 (1972).

60. Mildvan, A. S. In: *The Enzymes, Vol. II*, 3rd ed., P. D. Bayer, Ed. (New York: Academic Press, Inc., 1970), p. 445.
61. Vallee, B. L., and R. J. P. Williams. *Chem. Br.* 4:397-402 (1968).
62. Vallee, B. L., and R. J. P. Williams. *Proc. Nat. Acad. Sci., U.S.* 59:498-505 (1968).
63. Mann, T., and D. Keilin. *Proc. Roy. Soc. (London), Ser. B.* 126:303-315 (1939).
64. Porter, H., and J. Folch. *J. Neurochem.* 1:260-271 (1957).
65. Porter, H., and J. Folch. *J. Neurochem.* 5:91-98 (1959).
66. Fridovich, I. "Competitive Inhibition by Myoglobin of the Reduction of Cytochrome C by Xanthine Oxidase," *J. Biol. Chem.* 237:584-586 (1962).
67. Fridovich, I. "A Reversible Association of Bovine Carbonic Anhydrase with Milk Xanthine Oxidase," *J. Biol. Chem.* 242:1445-1449 (1967).
68. McCord, J. M., and I. Fridovich. "The Reduction of Cytochrome C by Milk Xanthine Oxidase," *J. Biol. Chem.* 243:5753-5760 (1968).
69. McCord, J. M., and I. Fridovich. "Superoxide Dismutase, An Enzymatic Function for Erythrocuprein (Hemocuprein)," *J. Biol. Chem.* 244: 6049-6055 (1969).
70. Castor, L. N., and B. Chance. "Photochemical Action Spectra of Carbon Monoxide-Inhibited Respiration," *J. Biol. Chem.* 217:453-465 (1955).
71. Chance, B. "The Carbon Monoxide Compounds of the Cytochrome Oxidases. I. Difference Spectra," *J. Biol. Chem.* 202:383-396 (1953).
72. Chance, B. "The Carbon Monoxide Compounds of the Cytochrome Oxidases. II. Photo Dissociation Spectra," *J. Biol. Chem.* 202:397-406 (1953).
73. Chance, B. "The Carbon Monoxide Compounds of the Cytochrome Oxidases. III. Molecular Extinction Coefficients," *J. Biol. Chem..* 202: 407-416 (1953).
74. Chance, B., L. Smith and L. N. Castor. *Biochim. Biophys. Acta.,* 12: 289-298 (1953).
75. Eichel, B., W. W. Wainio and S. J. Cooperstein. "A Partial Separation and Characterization of Cytochrome Oxidase and Cytochrome b," *J. Biol. Chem.* 183:89-103 (1950).
76. Keilen, D., and E. F. Hartree. *Nature* 141:870 (1938).
77. Keilen, D., and E. F. Hartree. *Proc. Roy. Soc. (London), Ser. B.* 127: 167-191 (1939). Cytochrome and Cytochrome Oxidase
78. Person, P., W. Waino and B. Eicheal. "The Prosthetic Groups of Cytochrome Oxidaseand Cytochrome b," *J. Biol. Chem.* 202:369-381 (1953).
79. Wainio, W. W., C. V. Wende and N. F. Shimp. "Copper in Cytochrome Oxidase," *J. Biol. Chem.* 234:2433-2436 (1959).
80. Wood, J. M., A. Cheh, L. J. Dizikes, W. P. Ridley, S. Rakow and J. R. LaKowilz. "Mechanisms for the Biomethylation of Metal and Metalloids," *Fed. Proc.* 37:16-21 (1978).
81. Griffiths, D. E., and David C. Warton. "Studies of the Electron Transport System: Properties of Copper in Cytochrome Oxidase," *J. Biol. Chem.* 236:1857-1862 (1961).

82. Gingras, B. A., and A. F. Sirianni. *Can. J. Chem.* 42:17-19 (1964).
83. Onstatt, E. I., and H. A. Laitinen. "Polarography of Copper Complexes. II. Dipyridyl, Orthophenanthroline, and Thiourea Complexes, A Double Complex System," *J. Am. Chem. Soc.* 72:4724-4728 (1950).
84. Pearson, R. G. "Hard and Soft Acids and Bases," *J. Am. Chem. Soc.* 85:3533-3539 (1963).
85. Drykacz, G. R., R. D. Libby and G. A. Hamilton. "Trivalent Copper as a Probable Intermediate in the Reaction Catalyzed by Galactose Oxidase," *J. Am. Chem. Soc.* 98:626-628 (1976).
86. Handler, P., K. V. Rajogopalan and V. Aleman. "Structure and Function of Iron-Flavoproteins," *Fed. Proc.* 23:30-38 (1964).
87. Morgan, E. H. *J. Physiol. (London)* 171:26-41 (1964).
88. Morgan, E. H. *Brit. J. Haematol.* 10:442-452 (1964).
89. Morgan, E. H., and E. Baker. *Biochim. Biophys. Acta.* 184:442-454 (1969).
90. Morgan, E. H., and C. B. Laurell. *Brit. J. Haematol.* 9:471-483 (1963).
91. Green, S., A. K. Saha, A. W. Carleton and A. Mazur. *Fed. Proc.* 17: 920 (1958).
92. Rimington, C. *Brit. Med. Bull.* 15:19-26 (1959).
93. Underwood, E. J. *Trace Elements in Human and Animal Nutrition*, 3rd ed. (New York: Academic Press, Inc., 1971), p. 17.
94. Niccum, W. L., R. L. Jackson and G. Stearns. *Am. J. Dis. Child.* 86: 558-567 (1953).
95. Stewart, W. B., C. L. Yuile, H. A. Clairborne, R. T. Snowman and G. H. Whipple. *J. Exp. Med.* 92:375-382 (1950).
96. Fritz, J. C., G. W. Pla, T. Roberts, J. W. Bachne and E. L. Have. *Agric. Food Chem.* 18:647-651 (1970).
97. Spiro, T. G., L. Pape and P. Saltman. "The Hydrolytic Polymerization of Ferric Citrate. I. Chemistry of the Polymer," *J. Am. Chem. Soc.* 89:5555-5559 (1967).
98. Underwood, E. J. *Trace Elements in Human and Animal Nutrition*, 4th ed. (New York: Academic Press, Inc., 1977).
99. Kroe, D. J., N. Kaufman, J. V. Klavins and T. D. Kinney. *Am. J. Physiol.* 211:414-418 (1966).
100. Van Campen, D., and E. Gross. *J. Nutr.* 99:68-74 (1969).
101. Brown, J. C., and L. D. Tiffen. *Plant Physiol.* 40:395-400 (1965).
102. Bryce, G. F., and N. Brot. *Arch. Biochem. Biophys.* 142:399-406 (1971).
103. Neilands, J. B. *Science* 156:1443-1447 (1967).
104. O'Brien, I. G., G. B. Cox and F. Gibson. *Biochim. Biophys. Acta.* 237: 537-549 (1971).
105. Pollack, S., J. N. George, R. C. Reba, R. Kaufman and W. H. Crosby. *J. Clin. Invest.* 44:1470-1473 (1965).
106. Settlemire, C. T., and G. Matrone. "In Vivo Interference of Zinc with Ferritin in the Rat," *J. Nutr.* 92:153-158 (1967).
107. Settlemire, C. T., and G. Matrone. "In Vivo Effect of Zinc on Iron Turnover in Rats and Lifespan of the Erythrocyte," *J. Nutr.* 92:159-164 (1967).
108. Perutz, M. F. "Stereochemistry of Cooperative Effects in Haemoglobin," *Nature* 228:726-734 (1970).

109. Hall, D. O., and M. C. W. Evans. "Iron-Sulphur Proteins," *Nature* 223: 1342-1348 (1969).
110. Malkin, R., and J. C. Rabinowitz. *Ann. Rev. Biochem.* 36:113-148 (1967).
111. Herriott, J. R., L. C. Sieker, L. H. Jensen and W. Lovenberg. *J. Mol. Biol.* 50:391-400 (1970).
112. Long, T. V., Jr., T. M. Loehr, J. Allkins and W. Lovenberg. "Determination of Iron Coordination in Nonheme Iron Proteins Using Laser-Raman Spectroscopy. II. Clostridium Pasteurianum Rubrodoxinin Aqueous Solution," *J. Am. Chem. Soc.* 93:1809-1811 (1971).
113. Earnwhaw, A., P. C. Hewlitt and L. F. Larkworthy. "Five-Coordinate Compounds of Cobalt," *Nature* 199:483-484 (1963).
114. Babior, B. M., and D. C. Gould. *Biochem. Biophys. Res. Commun.* 34: 441-447 (1969).
115. Retey, J., C. J. Suckling, D. Arigoni and B. M. Babior. "The Stereochemistry of the Reaction Catalyzed by Ethanolamine Ammonium Lyase, an Adenosylcobalamin Dependent Enzyme," *J. Biol. Chem.* 249:6359-6360 (1974).
116. Abeles, Robert H. In: *Biological Aspects of Inorganic Chemistry*, A. W. Addison, W. R. Cullen, D. Dolphin and B. R. James, Eds. (New York: John Wiley & Sons, Inc., 1977).
117. Silverman, R. B., and D. Dolphin. "A Model for the Mechanism of Action of Coenzyme $B_{12}$ Dependent Enzymes. Evidence for $\sigma \rightleftharpoons \pi$ Rearrangements in Cobaloximes," *J. Am. Chem. Soc.* 94:4028-4030 (1972).
118. Walling, C., and R. A. Johnson. "Fenton's Reagent VI Rearrangement During Glycol Oxidations," *J. Am. Chem. Soc.* 97:2405-2407 (1975).
119. Dixon, M., and E. C. Webb. *Enzymes*, 2nd ed. (New York: Academic Press, Inc., 1964).
120. Valbert, L. S. In: *Intestinal Absorption of Metal Ions, Trace Elements and Radionuclides,* S. C. Skoryna and D. Waldron-Edward, Eds. (Oxford: Pergamon Press, 1971), p. 257.
121. Hatem, S. *Compt. Rend.* 247:1681-1684 (1958).
122. Warren, C. O., Q. D. Schubmehl and I. R. Wood. *Am. J. Physiol.* 142: 173-178 (1944).
123. Grice, H. C., T. Goodman, I. C. Munn, G. S. Wiegerg and A. B. Morrison. *Ann. N.Y Acad. Sci.* 156:189-194 (1969).
124. Grice, H. C., I. C. Munro, G. S. Wieberg and H. A. Heggtreit. *Clin. Toxicol.* 2:273-287 (1969).
125. Wieberg, G. S., I. C. Munro, J. C. Meranger, A. B. Morrison, H. C. Grice and H. A. Heggtreit. *Clin. Toxicol.* 2:257-271 (1969).
126. Suderman, F. W. *Food Cosmet. Toxicol.* 9:105–120 (1972).
127. Weaver, J. C., V. M. Kaslainsek and P. D. N. Richards. *Calif. Med.* 85: 110-112 (1956).
128. Fee. J. A., E. R. Shapiro and T. H. Moss. "Direct Evidence for Manganese III Binding to the Manganosuperoxide Dismutase of Escherichia coli b," *J. Biol. Chem.* 251:6157-6159 (1976).
129. Keele, B. B., Jr., J. M. McCord and I. Fridovich. "Superoxide Dismutase from Escherichia coli b," *J. Biol. Chem.* 245:6176-6181 (1970).

130. Sastry, G. S., R. E. Hamm and K. H. Pool. "Spectrophotometric Determination of Dissolved Oxygen in Water," *Anal. Chem.* 41:857-858 (1969).
131. Vallee, B. L., and J. E. Coleman. In: *Comprehensive Biochemistry, Vol. 12*, M. Florkin and E. H. Stolz, Eds. (Amsterdam: Elsevier, 1964), p. 165.
132. Kemmer, A. R., C. A. Eluehjem and E. B. Hart. *J. Biol. Chem.* 92:623-630 (1931).
133. Orent, E. R., and E. V. McCollum. *J. Biol. Chem.* 92:651-678 (1931).
134. Leach, R. M., Jr., and A. M. Munester. *J. Nutr.* 78:51-56 (1962).
135. Morrison, J. F., and K. E. Ebner. "Studies on Galactosyltransferase: Kinetic Investigations with N-Acetylglucosamine as the Galactosyl Group Acceptor," *J. Biol. Chem.* 246:3977-3984 (1971).
136. Morrison, J. F., and K. E. Ebner. "Studies on Galactosyltransferase: Kinetic Investigations with Glucose as the Galactosyl Group Acceptor," *J. Biol. Chem.* 246:3985-3991 (1971).
137. Levy, R. S., and J. J. Villafranca. "Structure-Function Relationships in TPN-Dependent Isocitrate Dehydrogenase. I. EPR Studies of the Interaction Enzyme-Bound MnII and Substrates, Cofactors and Substrate Analogues," *Biochemistry* 16:3293-3301 (1977).
138. Villafranca, J. J., and R. F. Coleman. "Frequency and Temperature Dependence of the Proton Relaxation Rates of Solvent and Substrate Interaction with Isocitrate Dehydrogenase Bound MnII," *Biochemistry* 13:1152-1159 (1974).
139. Villafranca, J. J., R. S. Levy, J. Kernich and T. Vickroy. "TPN and Mn-Isocitrate Protect Isocitrate Dehydrogenase Against Inactivation but Increase the Number of Modified Sulfhydral Groups," *Biochem. Biophys. Res. Commun.* 77:457-463 (1977).
140. Scrutton, M. C., P. Griminger and J. C. Wallace. "Pyruvate Carboxylase: Bound Metal Content of the Verterbrate Liver Enzyme as a Function of Diet and Species," *J. Biol. Chem.* 247:3305-3310 (1972).
141. Scrutton, M. C., and A. S. Mildvan. "Pyruvate Carboxylase XI Nuclear Magnetic Resonance Studies of the Properties of the Bound Manganese After Interaction of the Biotin Residues with Avidin," *Biochemistry* 7:1490-1505 (1968).
142. Green, N. M. *Biochem. J.* 89:585-591 (1963).
143. Scrutton, M. C., and M. F. Utter. "Pyruvate Carboxylase. V. Interaction of the Enzyme and Adenosine Triphosphate," *J. Biol. Chem.* 240: 3714-3723 (1965).
144. Scrutton, M. C., M. F. Utter and A. S. Mildvan. "Pyruvate Carboxylase. VI. The Presence of Tightly Bound Manganese," *J. Biol. Chem.* 241: 3480-3487 (1966).
145. Lam, Y.-F., W. A. Bridger and G. Kotowycz. "Nuclear Magnetic Resonance Relaxation Time Studies on the Manganese II Ion Complex with Succinyl Coenzyme A. Synthetase from Escherichia coli," *Biochemistry* 15:4742-4748 (1976).
146. Backer, J. M., S. V. Vocel, L. M. Weiner, S. I. Oshevskii and O. T. Lavrik. "Coordination of $Mn^{++}$ Ions at Contact Sites Between +RNA and Aminoacyl+RNA Synthetase," *Biochem. Biophys. Res. Commun.* 63:1019-1026 (1975).

147. Burgess, R. R. *Ann. Rev. Biochem.* 40:711-740 (1971).
148. Koren, R. and A. S. Mildvan. "Magnetic Resonance and Kinetic Studies of the Role of the Divalent Cation Activator of RNA Polymerase from Escherichia coli," *Biochemistry* 16:241-249 (1977).
149. Chapman, B. E., W. J. O'Sullivan, R. K. Scapes and G. H. Reed. "Magnetic Resonance Studies on Manganese-Nucleotide Complexes of Phosphoglyceiate Kinase," *Biochemistry* 16:1005-1010 (1977).
150. Scrutton, M. C. "Purification and Some Properties of a Protein Containing Manganese (Avimanganin)," *Biochemistry* 10:3897-3905 (1971).
151. Mildvan, A. S., M. C. Scrutton and M. F. Utter. "Pyruvate Carboxylase. VII. A Possible Role for Tightly Bound Manganese," *J. Biol. Chem.* 241:3488-3498 (1966).
152. Kobayashi, J. In: *Trace Substances in Environmental Health, Vol. VIII,* D. D. Hemphill, Ed. (Columbia, MO: University of Missouri, 1974), pp. 295-304.
153. Feldman, S. L., and R. J. Cousins. "Inhibition of 1,25-Dihydroxycholecalciferol Synthesis by Cadmium in Vitro," *Fed. Proc.* 32:918 (1973).
154. Shaikh, Z. A., and O. J. Lusic. *Arch. Environ.. Health* 24:418-425 (1972).
155. Shaikh, Z. A., and O. J. Lucis. *Experentia* 27: 1024-1025 (1971).
156. Cross, C. E., I. B. Ibrahim, N. Ahmeb and M. G. Mustafa. *Environ. Res.* 3:512 (1970).
157. Merali, Z., S. Kacew and R. L. Singhla. *Can. J. Physicol. Pharmacol.* 53:174-184 (1975).
158. Book, R. L. M., T. Shirley and L. Srivastava. "Effects of Cadmium on Glucose Tolerance and Serum Insulin Zinc and Copper in Male Rats," *Fed. Proc.* 32:468 (1973).
159. Flick, D. F., H. F. Kraybill and J. M. Dimitruff. "Toxic Effects of Cadmium: A Review," *Environ. Res.* 4:71-85 (1971).
160. Friberg, L., M. Piscator and G. Nordberg. *Cadmium in the Environment* (Cleveland, OH: CRL Press, 1971).
161. Perry, H. M., Jr., E. F. Perry and J. E. Purifoy. *Proc. Soc. Exp. Biol. Med.* 136:1240-1244 (1971).
162. Butt, E. M., R. E. Nusbaum, T. C. Gilmour and S. L. Didio. *Am. J. Clin. Pathol.* 30:479-499 (1958).
163. Haddow, A., F. J. C. Roe, C. E. Duker and D. C. V. Mitchly. *Brit. J. Cancer* 18:667-673 (1964).
164. Roe, F. J. C. *Brit. J. Cancer* 18:674-681 (1964).
165. Engel, D. W., and B. A. Fowler. *Environ. Health Persp.* 28:81-88 (1979).
166. Cherian, M. G. "Metallothioneins and Their Role in the Metabolism and Toxicity of Metals," *Environ. Health Persp.* 28:127 (1979); *Life Sci.* 23(1):1-10 (1978).
167. Cousins, R. J. *Envion. Health Persp.* 28:131-136 (1979).
168. Pertering, H. G., H. Choudhury and K. L. Stemmer. *Environ. Health Persp.* 28:97-106 (1979).
169. Whanger, P. D. *Environ. Health Persp.* 28:115-121 (1979).
170. Bar, A., and R. H. Wasserman. *Biochem. Biophys. Res. Commun.* 54: 191-196 (1973).

171. Washki, P. W., and R. J. Cousins. *J. Nutr.* 107:920-928 (1977).
172. Washko, P. W., and R. J. Cousins. "Metabolism of $^{109}$Cd in Rats Fed Normal and Low-Calcium Diets," *J. Toxicol. Environ. Health* 1:1055-1066 (1976).
173. Feldman, S. L., and R. J. Cousins. *Nutr. Rep. Int.* 8:251-260 (1973).
174. Lorentzon, R. and S. E. Larsson. *Clin. Sci. Mol. Med.* 53:439-446 (1977).
175. Berman, E. *Atomic Abs. Newsl.* 3:111-114 (1964).
176. Einarsson, O., and G. Lindstedt. *Scand. J. Clin. Lab. Invest.* 23:367-371 (1969).
177. Delves, H. T. *Analyst* 95:431-438 (1970).
178. Nise, G. and O. Vesterberg. "Blood Lead Determination by Flameless Atomic Absorption Spectroscopy," *Clin. Chem. Acta.* 84:129-136 (1978).
179. Jackson, K. W., E. Marzak and D. G. Mitchell. "Rapid Determination of Lead in Biological Tissues by Microsampling-Cup Atomic Absorption Spectroscopy," *Anal. Chim. Acta.* 97:37-42 (1978).
180. Barton, J. C., M. E. Conrard, S. Nuby and L. Harrison. "Effects of Iron on the Absorption and Retention of Lead," *J. Lab. Clin. Med.* 92:536-547 (1978).
181. Six, K. and R. A. Goyer. "Experimental Enhancement of Lead Toxicity by Low Dietary Calcium," *J. Lab. Clin. Med.* 76:933-942 (1970).
182. Goyer, R. A., D. L. Leonard, J. F. Moore, B. Rhyne and M. R. Krigman. "Lead Dosage and the Role of the Intranuclear Inclusion Body," *Arch. Environ.. Health* 20:705-711 (1970).
183. Davies, J. R., R. H. Abrahams, W. I. Gishbein and E. A. Fevrega. *Arch. Environ. Health* 17:164-171 (1968).
184. Hernberg, S., J. Nikkanen, G. Mellin and H. Lilius. "δ-Aminolevulinic Acid Dehydrase as a Measure of Lead Exposure," *Arch. Environ. Health* 21:140-145 (1970).
185. Kao, R. L.C., and R.M. Forbes. "Effects of Lead on Heme-Synthesizing Enzymes and Urinary δ-Aminolevulinic Acid in the Rat," *Proc. Soc. Exp. Biol. Med.* 143:234-237 (1973).
186. Border, E. A., A. C. Contrell and T. A. Kilroe-Smith, *Brit. J. Intern. Med.* 33:85-87 (1976).
187. Allain, P., E. Foussard and J. Boyer. *J. Lab. Clin. Med.* 79:128 (1972).
188. Tephly, T. R., G. Wagner, R. Sedman and W. Piper. "Effects of Metals on Heme Biosynthesis and Metabolism," *Fed. Proc.* 37:35-39 (1978).
189. Six, K. M., and R. A. Goyer. "The Influence of Iron Deficiency on Tissue Content and Toxicity of Ingested Lead in the Rat," *J. Lab. Clin. Med.* 79:128-136 (1972).
190. Sabbioni, E., and E. Marafante. "Identification of Lead Binding Components in Rat Liver: In Vivo Study," *Chem.-Biol. Interact.* 15:1-20 (1976).
191. Choie, D. D., and G. W. Richter. "Cell Proliferation in Mouse Kidney Induced by Lead. II. Synthesis of Ribonucleic Acid and Protein," *Lab. Invest.* 30:652-656 (1972).
192. Sobel, A. E., and M. Burger. "Calcification: The Influence of Calcium, Phosphorus, and Vitamin D on the Removal of Lead from Blood and Bone," *J. Biol. Chem.* 212:105-110 (1955).

193. Coumbis, J. T. *Environmenta* 17:21 (1975).
194. Schwarz, K. In: *Trace Elements Metabolism in Animals,* W. G. Hoekstra, J. W. Suttie, H. E. Ganther and W. Mertz, Eds. (Baltimore, MD: University Park Press, 1974), pp. 355-380.
195. Venugopal, B., and T. D. Luckey. *Metal Toxicity in Mammals, Vol. 1,* (New York: Plenum Publishing Corporation, 1978), p. 86.
196. Burrows, K. C., M. P. Brindle and M. C. Hughes. "Modification of Pulse Polarograph for Rapid Scanning and its Use with Stationary Electrodes," *Anal. Chem.* 49:1459-1461 (1977).
197. Iverson, F., R. H. Downie, C. Paul and H. L. Trenholm. *Toxicol. Appl. Pharmacol.* 24:545-554 (1973).
198. Aberg, B., L. Ekman, R. Persson and J. O. Sniks. "Metabolism of Methyl Mercury Compounds in Man," *Arch. Environ. Health* 19:478-484 (1969).
199. Osamu, W., K. Toyokawa, T.-Y. Suzuki, Y. Yano and N. Nakao. *Arch. Environ. Health* 19:485-488 (1969).
200. Garrett, N. E., R. J. B. Garrett and J. W. Archdeacon. *Toxicol. Appl. Pharmacol.* 22:649-654 (1972).
201. Neathery, M. W., W. J. Miller, R. P. Gentry, O. M. Blackburn and P. E. Stake. *J. Dairy Sci.* 56:309 (1973).
202. Clarkson, T. W., L. Amin-Zaki and S. Al-Tikriti. "An Outbreak of Methyl Mercury Poisoning Due to Consumption of Contaminated Grain," *Fed. Proc.* 35:2395-2399 (1976).
203. Berlin, M. In: *Effects and Dose-Response Relationships of Toxic Metals*, G. F. Nordberg, Ed. (Amsterdam: Elsevier, 1976), pp. 235-245.
204. Weiss, B. "The Behavioral Toxicology of Metals," *Fed. Proc.* 37:22-27 (1978).
205. Robenstein, D. L., and C. Evans. "The Mobility of Methyl Mercury in Biological Systems," *Bioinorg. Chem.* 8:107-114 (1978).
206. Arseth, J. *Acta. Pharmacol Toxicol.* 39:289 (1976).
207. Bertilsson, L., and H. Neujohr. "Methylation of Mercury Compounds by Methyl Cobalamin," *Biochemistry* 10:2805-2808 (1971).
208. Imura, N., S. Sakegawa, E. Paq, K. Nagaro, J. Kin, T. Kwan and T. Ukita. *Science* 172:1248-1249 (1971).
209. Schmidt, U., and F. Huber. "Methylation of Organolead and Lead II Compounds to $(CH_3)_4Pb$ by Microorganisms," *Nature* 259:157-158 (1975).
210. DeSimone, R. E., M. J. Penley, L. Charbonneau, S. G. Smith, J. M. Wood, H. A. D. Hill, S. Ridsdale, J. M. Pratt and R. J. P. Williams. *Biochim. Biophys. Acta.* 304:851-863 (1973).
211. Ganther, H. E., C. Goudie, M. L. Sunde, M. J. Kopecky, P. Wagner, S.-H. Ho and W. G. Hoekstra. "Selenium: Relation to Decreased Toxicity of Methyl Mercury Added to Diets Containing Tuna," *Science* 175:1122-1124 (1972).
212. Potter, S. D., and G. Matrone. "Effect of Selenite on the Toxicity and Retention of Dietary Methyl Mercury and Mercuric Chloride," *Fed. Proc.* 32:929 (1973).
213. Koeman, J. H., W. H. M. Peters, C. H. M. Koudstool-Hol, P. S. Tjioe and J. J. M. DeGoeij. "Mercury-Selenium Correlations in Marine Mammals," *Nature* 245:385-386 (1973).
214. Sugiura, Y., Y. Tamai and H. Tanaka. "Selenium Protection Against

Mercury Toxicity: High Binding Affinity of Methyl Mercury by Selenium-Containing Ligands in Comparison with Sulfur-Containing Ligands," *Bioinorg. Chem.* 9:167-180 (1978).
215. Parizek, J., and I. Ostadalova. *Experientia* 23:142–143 (1967).
216. Fang, S. C. "Induction of C-Hg Cleavage Enzymes in Rat Liver by Dietary Selenite," *Res. Commun. Chem. Pathol. Pharmacol.* 9:579-582 (1974).
217. Fang, S. C. "Interaction of Mercury and Selenium in the Rat," *Chem.-Biol. Interact.* 17:25-40 (1977).
218. Fang, S. C., R. W. Chen and E. Fallin. "Influence of Dietary Selenite on the Binding Characteristics of Rat Serum Proteins to Mercurial Compounds," *Chem.-Biol. Interact.* 15:51-57 (1976).
219. Robenstein, D. L., and M. T. Fairhurst. "Nuclear Magnetic Resonance Studies of the Solution Chemistry of Metal Complexes. XI. The Binding of Methyl Mercury by Sulfhydryl-Containing Amino Acids by Glutathione," *J. Am. Chem. Soc.* 97:2086-2092 (1975).
220. Schrieber, M., and E. A. Brouwer. "Metabolism and Toxicity of Arsenicals," *Fed. Proc.* 23:199 (1964).
221. Gardner, J. H., and L. D. Byers. "Enzymic Reactions of Phosphate Analogs," *J Biol. Chem.* 252:5925-5927 (1977).
222. Vallee, B. L., D. D. Ulmer and W. E. C. Wacker. *Arch. Ind. Health* 21:132-151 (1960).
223. Venugopol, B., and T. D. Lucky. *Metal Toxicity in Mammals, Vol. 2,* (New York: Plenum Publishing Corporation, 1978), p. 207.
224. Henricksen, J. *Veneral Dis. Inform.* 20:293-324 (1939).
225. Hutchinson, J. *Brit. Med. J.* 2:1280 (1887).
226. Paris, J. A. *Pharmacologia,* 3rd ed. (London: W. Phillips, 1820), p. 132.
227. Baroni, C., G. J. Van Esch and V. Saffiotic. *Arch. Environ. Health* 7: 668-674 (1963).
228. Boutwell, R. K., *J. Agric. Food Chem.* 11:381-385 (1963).
229. Byron, W. R., G. W. Bierbower, J. B. Brower and W. H. Hansen. *Toxicol. Appl. Pharmacol.* 10:132-147 (1967).
230. Hueper, W. C., and W. W. Payne. *Arch. Environ. Health* 5:445-462 (1962).
231. Kennaway, E. L. *Lancet* 243:769-772 (1942).
232. Buchannan, M. D. *Toxicity of Arsenic Compounds* (Amsterdam: Elsevier, 1961).
233. Pinto, S. S., and B. M. Bennett. *Arch. Environ. Health* 7:583-591 (1963).
234. Stone, O. J. *Tex. St. J. Med.* 65:40-43 (1969).
235. McCoy, K. E. M., and P. H. Weswig. "Some Selenium Responses in the Rat Not Related to Vitamin E," *J. Nutr.* 98:393-389 (1969).
236. Thompson, J. N., and M. L. Scott. "Role of Selenium in Nutrition of the Chick," *J. Nutr.* 97:335-342 (1969).
237. Thompson, J. N., and M. L. Scott. "Impaired Lipid and Vitamin E. Absorption Related to Atrophy of the Pancreas in Selenium-Deficient Chicks," *J. Nutr.* 100:797-809 (1970).
238. Rotuck, J. T., A. L. Pope, H. E. Ganther, A. B. Swanson, D. G. Hafeman and W. G. Hoekstra. "Selenium: Biochemical Role as a Component of Glutathione Peroxidase," *Science* 179:588-590 (1973).
239. Baehner, R. L. *Pediat. Clin. North Am.* 19:935-956 (1972).

240. Flohe, L., B. Eisle and A. Wendel. *Hoppe-Zeyler's J. Physiol. Chem.* 352:151-158 (1971).
241. Fridovich, I. *New England J. Med.* 290:624-625 (1974).
242. Kinoshita, J. H. *A.M.A. Arch. Opthalmol.* 72:554-572 (1964).
243. Pirie, A. *Biochem. J.* 96:244-253 (1964).
244. Swanson, A. A., and A. W. Truesdale. *Biochem. Biophys. Res. Commun.* 45:1488-1496 (1971).

# Section 4

# Chemistry Aspects of Toxicological Testing

# CHAPTER 25

# OVERVIEW OF THE NATIONAL TOXICOLOGY PROGRAM

**J. A. Moore, J. E. Huff, L. Hart and D. B. Walters**
National Toxicology Program
Public Health Service
Department of Health and Human Services
Research Triangle Park, North Carolina

## INTRODUCTION

The National Toxicology Program (NTP), established in November 1978 [1], develops scientific information about potentially toxic and hazardous chemicals which can be used for protecting the health of the American people and for the primary prevention of chemically induced disease. NTP centralizes and strengthens the Department of Health and Human Services (DHHS, formerly DHEW) activities in toxicology research, testing and test development/validation efforts, and provides toxicological information needed by research and regulatory agencies [2]. Three specific goals have been identified:

1. to expand the toxicological profiles of the chemicals nominated, selected and being tested;
2. to increase the number and rate of chemicals under test; and
3. to develop, coordinate and validate a series of tests/protocols more appropriate for regulatory needs.

## NATIONAL TOXICOLOGY PROGRAM CHARTER AGENCIES

To accomplish these three major aims, the NTP was formed by bringing together the relevant toxicological programs, people and resources from Public Health Service. Presently, the four DHHS agencies that comprise the NTP are:

1. National Cancer Institute, National Institutes of Health;
2. National Institute of Environmental Health Sciences, National Institutes of Health;
3. National Center for Toxicological Research, Food and Drug Administration; and
4. National Institute for Occupational Safety and Health, Center for Disease Control.

The scientific capabilities and resources of the NTP member agencies encompass a broad range of toxicologic expertise and research/testing activities: each agency, for instance, conducts lifetime toxicological and carcinogenicity studies as well as some mutagenicity testing and test development; three agencies are involved in neurobehavioral testing; and two agencies study pulmonary toxicity [3-6]. Progress continues on the integration of these activities. The proportionate funding committed to NTP from the member agencies was $41 million in fiscal year (FY) 1979 and $69 million for FY 1980.

The technical information capabilities of the NTP have been augmented through an interagency agreement with the National Library of Medicine, National Institutes of Health.

Other agencies with a toxicology-oriented mission are invited to participate as active members of the NTP.

## NTP PROGRAMS AND PROJECT LEADERS

The program segments of the National Toxicology Program are grouped into two categories–toxicologic research and testing, and coordinative management activities (Table I). To allow a reasonable estimate of the levels of activity within particular NTP disciplinary components, the FY 1979 funding levels allocated to each of the NTP program areas are diagrammed in Figure 1 [5,7]. Individual NTP scientists have been appointed as leaders of major program segments. Each scientist serves as the center for a particular program activity and is responsible for developing (in collaboration with other NTP colleagues) the subprogram objectives and the implementation

**Table 1. NTP Program Areas**

| Toxicologic Research and Testing | Coordinative Management |
|---|---|
| Carcinogenesis | Bioassay Coordination |
| Short-Term Test Development | Chemical Nomination |
| Tumor Pathology | Chemical Repository |
| Chemical Disposition | Data Management and Analysis |
| General Toxicology | Carcinogenesis |
| Toxicopathology | Mutagenesis |
| Genetic Toxicology | Toxicology |
| Immunologic Toxicology | Toxicology Data Management System (TDMS) Development |
| Neurobehavioral Toxicology | Information Dissemination |
| Pulmonary Toxicology | Laboratory Animal Quality Control |
| Reproductive and Developmental Toxicology | Laboratory Health and Safety |
| | Technical Information |

plan, as well as the coordination and supervision of the program work. Further, the program leaders are responsible for the development and supervision of contracts that extend these activities or that perform in-depth toxicologic characterization of chemicals.

## NTP EXECUTIVE COMMITTEE

The NTP Executive Committee provides linkage between DHHS research and regulatory agencies to ensure that toxicology research, testing and test development carried out under the aegis of the NTP are responsive to the needs of those agencies and to the wants of the public [5,7]. This unique aspect of the NTP brings together the research and regulatory agencies doing fundamental biomedical research. The governmental offices and agencies that comprise the NTP Executive Committee are:

1. Chairman, Consumer Product Safety Commission;
2. Assistant Secretary for Health, Department of Health and Human Services;
3. Administrator, Environmental Protection Agency;
4. Commissioner, Food and Drug Administration;
5. Director, National Cancer Institute;
6. Director, National Institute for Occupational Safety and Health;
7. Director, National Institute of Environmental Health Sciences;
8. Director, National Institutes of Health; and
9. Assistant Secretary of Labor, Occupational Safety and Health Administration.

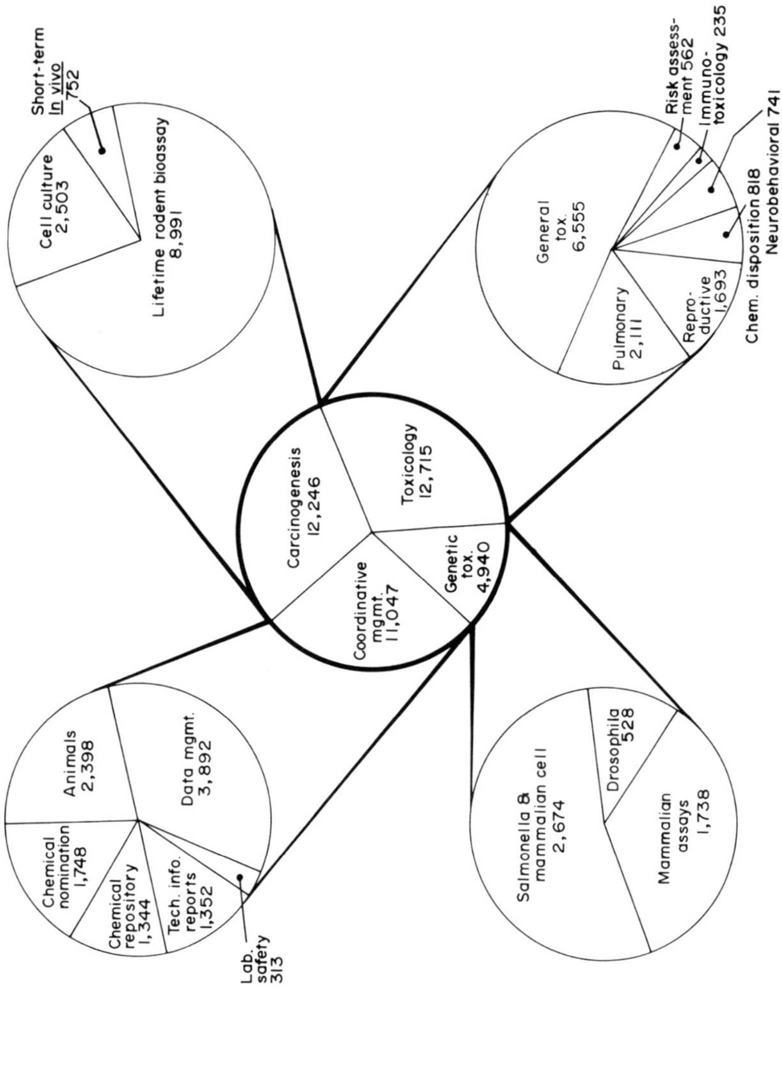


**Figure 1.** FY 1979 funding levels by NTP program activity (thousands of dollars).

## NTP BOARD OF SCIENTIFIC COUNSELORS

The NTP Board of Scientific Counselors provides scientific oversight of the NTP; advises the NTP Director and the NTP Executive Committee on scientific content, philosophy and policy; and evaluates the merit and overall quality of the science conducted in the NTP components. Eight scientists have been appointed by the Secretary of the Department of Health and Human Services (term ends during year shown in parentheses):

1. Joseph C. Dunbar, PhD, Associate Professor of Physiology, Wayne State University School of Medicine (1982);
2. Curtis Harper, PhD, Associate Professor of Pharmacology, University of North Carolina School of Medicine (1981);
3. Margaret Hitchcock, PhD, Assistant Professor of Pharmacology, Yale University Medical School (1983);
4. Marjorie G. Horning, PhD, Professor of Biochemistry, Baylor College of Medicine (1983);
5. Mortimer L. Mendelsohn, MD, PhD, Director, Biomedical Sciences Division, Lawrence Livermore Laboratory, University of California (1982);
6. Norton Nelson, PhD (Chairperson), Professor, Environmental Medicine, New York University School of Medicine (1983);
7. Thomas H. Shepard, MD, Professor of Pediatrics and Head of Central Laboratory for Human Embryology, University of Washington School of Medicine (1981); and
8. Alice S. Whittemore, PhD, Adjunct Professor of Family, Community, and Preventive Medicine, Stanford University (1983);

## NTP CHEMICAL SELECTION

More chemicals are nominated for NTP consideration than can be selected for study (Figure 2). Early recognition of this pending asymmetry led the NTP Executive Committee to formulate a set of program guidelines [5,7,9,10]. These resultant eight chemical selection criteria motivate an NTP matrix which operates throughout the NTP. All research, testing and test development/ validation efforts start here.

The NTP Executive Committee operates under the principle that industry will test chemicals for health and environmental effects as intended and mandated by Congress under legislative authorities. Therefore, the NTP, acting under its chemical selection principles, will test:

1. chemicals found in the environment that are not closely associated with commercial activities;
2. desirable substitutes for existing chemicals, particularly therapeutic agents, that might not be developed or tested without federal involvement;

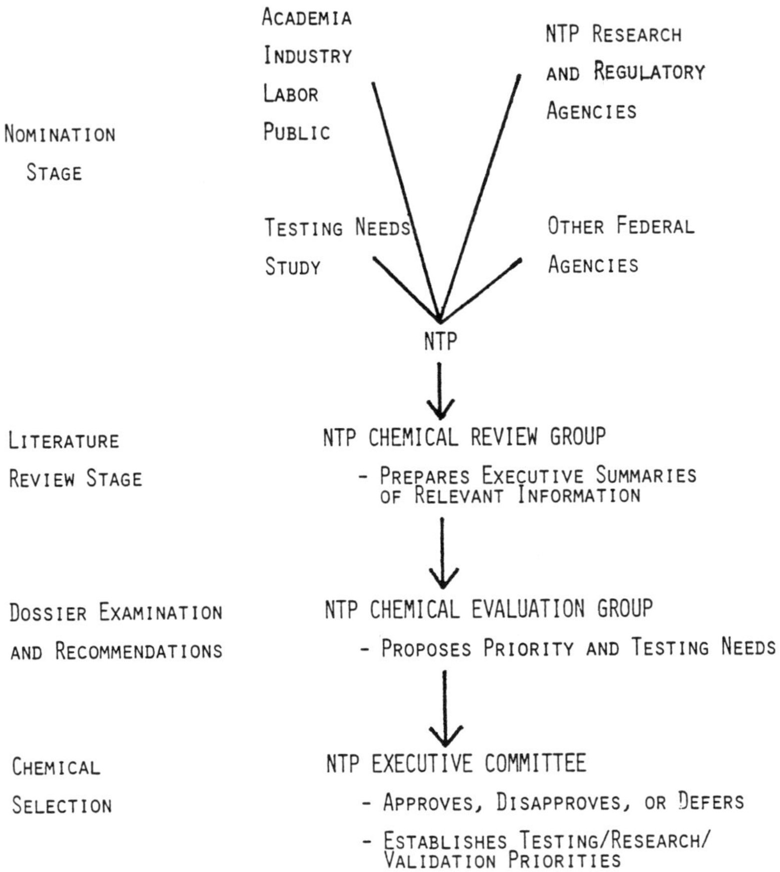


**Figure 2.** NTP chemical selection process.

3. chemicals that should be tested to improve scientific understanding of structure-activity relationships and thereby assist in defining groups of commercial chemicals that should be tested by industry;
4. certain chemicals tested by industry, or by others, the additional testing of which by the federal government is justified to verify the results;
5. previously tested chemicals for which other testing is desirable to cross-compare testing methods;
6. "old chemicals" with the potential for significant human exposure which are of social importance but which generate too little revenue to support an adequate testing program (some of these may be "grandfathered" under FDA laws);

7. two or more chemicals together, when combined human exposure occurs (such testing probably cannot be required of industry if the products of different companies are involved); and
8. in special situations, as determined by the Executive Committee, marketed chemicals which have potential for large-scale and/or intense human exposure, even if it may be possible to require industry to perform the testing.

Most chemicals are nominated and selected for testing because toxicologic information is lacking and because the potential exists for human exposure. Other important criteria include production levels, physical and chemical properties, agency interests and significance to society. The NTP toxicology testing strategy: identify with assurance the major toxic effects for each chemical studied. This includes (in addition to identifying chemical mutagens and carcinogens) damage to critical target organs such as the lungs, liver and nervous system. Thus, Phase I tests (Table II) result in a core of toxicology data essential to the proper design of more extensive studies. As an example, using the information from the Phase I rodent toxicologic screen, Phases II and III testing can be started with increased capabilities to confirm and better define toxicities identified in the screen.

Nomination and selection of test chemicals receives more attention in Chapter 26 of this volume [11].

**Table II. NTP Interactive Testing Phases**

| Program Area | Phase I Identify Toxic Potential | Phase II Corroborate Toxic Effect | Phase III Confirm and Define Toxicity | Phase IV Scientific and Public Health Assessment |
|---|---|---|---|---|
| Genetic Toxicology | *Salmonella* assay mammalian cell culture | *Drosophila* Spp | Mammalian assays (mouse heritable translocation)[b] | Total evaluation of all data, and publication and desemination of information from all program areas |
| General Toxicology | Rodent toxicology | Confirmation of organ system toxicities[a] | In-depth characterization; specific toxic effects[a] | |
| Carcinogenesis | Cell culture transformation[b] | Short-term in vivo (mouse lung adenoma)[b] | Lifetime rodent bioassays | |

[a]Some in validation phase.
[b]Test validation.

## TEST DEVELOPMENT AND VALIDATION

The strategy for test development and validation examines existing and emerging methodologies to identify those which may be adequately sensitive and reproducible. Those offering improvements over older methods will be selected for validation. When basic research findings suggest new areas of toxicology testing, NTP will undertake the appropriate methods development and validation. Existing methodologies that are being examined for modification include techniques used to detect impaired liver or kidney function and neurobehavioral toxicity; and new areas for methods development and validation include behavioral teratology, immunotoxicology and short-term tests for presumptive carcinogenic potential. Fertility, reproductive and cardiovascular toxicology continue to be addressed inadequately within NTP; new test systems need to be developed and are being pursued.

Test methods validation signals a two-stage process: (1) Does the procedure(s) yield test results that are reproducible within and between laboratories? (2) Does the test(s) predict for toxic potential in humans? The latter demands that NTP continue to keep abreast of and examine closely any results from human epidemiologic studies that correlate or contrast with experimental test data. The NTP approach to testing directs toward developing new and better test methods. This overture does not imply flaws in traditional toxicology and regulatory test requirements, but reflects rapid advancements in testing methodology and expanding boundaries of scientific knowledge. Thus, NTP plans to validate possible alternatives that may be performed more reliably, yield new toxicologic data, give results relevant to human disease and develop a testing approach that produces equivalent results in a faster, more economical manner. Often, testing results affect regulatory or public health issues, and the NTP will meld these innovative techniques with "standard" methods to ensure results that are germane and of utility to regulatory and public health needs. When standard methods are used, the NTP will attempt to incorporate those standards presently advocated by regulatory agencies, such as the life-time rodent bioassay.

## TOXICOLOGY RESEARCH AND TESTING

Toxicology research and testing within NTP divides into three major disciplines: genetic toxicology, general toxicology and carcinogenesis [12-14]. Other program areas have been arbitrarily assigned to one of these three, even though much interchange occurs; for example, interprogram utility of *Salmonella* mutation assays within the genetic toxicology and the carcinogenesis programs.

The screening program consists of four phases or tiers that progress in complexity from simple systems composed of microbial or mammalian cells in culture to *Drosophila* systems to specific whole-animal mammalian systems to data evaluation and technical report preparation.

Table II depicts the four ongoing and interacting testing/research phases. These are summarized in the following sections on genetic toxicology, general toxicology and carcinogenesis.

## Genetic Toxicology

Mutagenicity assays identify structural and functional DNA perturbations in germinal and somatic cells. Effects in germ cells are important for predicting potential undesirable effects on fertility, on the developing conceptus and on subsequent generations. Somatic mutation may predict physiological alterations in the exposed person and may forecast for potential induction of cancer.

In FY 1980 the NTP will increase the rate of in vitro microbial mutagenesis testing to 300 chemicals, commence parallel testing in cultured mammalian cells for 70 chemicals and begin Phase II testing utilizing *Drosophila* systems at a rate of 30 chemicals per year. All chemicals selected for general toxicology and for life-time carcinogenesis bioassays will be first tested using the *Salmonella* mutagenesis screen.

The Phase I *Salmonella* mutagenicity assay was established in FY 1979, and uses *Salmonella typhimurium* tester strains TA-98, -100, -1535 and -1537 (with and without metabolic activation).

Tests with cultured mammalian cells are the second component of Phase I. These tests, unlike bacterial systems, reflect chromosome damage. Testing capability was established in FY 1979 with 70 chemicals scheduled for test in FY 1980.

Chemicals that are mutagenic in these assays will progress to Phase II. A certain number of chemicals giving negative results will be committed to further testing; this selection process centers mainly on known biological activity of structurally related compounds and on level of human exposure.

In Phase II, the fruit fly (*Drosophila* spp.) possesses inherent chemical metabolic activation capabilities, provides more precise information on the types and time course of the mutations induced, and demonstrates heritability of the induced mutation. Sex-linked recessive lethal mutations and heritable translocations will be measured. Testing capability was established in FY 1979; starting in FY 1980, 30 chemicals per year will be tested.

Chemicals positive in Phase II systems will be tested in whole-animal systems (Phase III) to ascertain the type mutations produced in vivo, the heritability and germ cell sensitivity of the effect, the organs involved, and dose-response information. Chemicals producing germ cell damage or mutations will be tested further using animal models to gather more information for use in risk assessment.

The potential Phase III tests are in need of validation. During FY 1980 validation efforts will commence in several laboratories using the mouse heritable translocation assay.

In conjunction with the testing of chemicals for mutagenicity, the genetic toxicology initiatives also include test system validation and new test method development for all Phases. NTP will identify not only which chemicals are mutagenic, but also which tests are most valid for determining mutagenicity. Another important aim of this activity is to foster the integration of genetic endpoints with those of other short- and long-term toxicology tests, thus allowing the same animals to be used for genetic effects and for other toxicologic endpoints.

To better compare short-term assay results with long-term bioassay data, 58 chemicals tested previously by lifetime carcinogenesis bioassays are being assayed in the *Salmonella* system. Some of these coded chemicals (listed in the NTP Annual Plan) will be tested in four laboratories to further assess interlaboratory reproducibility, while the others will be tested in a single laboratory. These studies should be completed in FY 1980.

Other assay systems being developed or validated include *Escherichia coli* WP2 uvrA, pol A+, and pol A-; and the mammalian systems L5178Y mouse lymphoma [TK+/locus] and ARL6 rat liver.

An international collaborative study evaluated a range of short-term assay systems for their ability to predict chemical carcinogenicity. Results from 30 assay systems are being analysed for 42 coded carcinogens and noncarcinogens. The chemicals tested and the assay systems used are listed in the NTP Annual Plan for FY 1980 [5,9,10]. Testing was completed in FY 1979, with decoding and combined analyses being done now; this study will be published during the latter part of 1980 [15]. A preliminary assessment of the results from this three-year study indicates:

1. Short-term tests can be used to predict carcinogenic activity, but no single assay or battery of assays was readily apparent as best suited for this purpose.
2. Reliability of data from any assay system depends on thorough understanding of the system, awareness of pitfalls and careful conduct of experiments.
3. Most assays produced false negatives and false positives; thus, to include any assay in a battery of tests requires a tradeoff between these two classes of errors.
4. Specific conclusions about test system performance and relative utility must await more detailed analysis of the data base.
5. Strong evidence for the use of a test battery was obtained, yet recommendations on test batteries must await a clear definition of their application and the relative importance of false positive and false negative results.

## General Toxicology

Before conducting and interpreting any specialized experiments in carcinogenesis, reproductive toxicology, teratology or neurobehavioral toxicology, the effect of the chemical on the general health of the test animal must be known. During FY 1980, studies will continue to develop a composite toxicologic screen that will identify vital organ damage (hepatic, renal) which results in a generalized toxicity and one that gives presumptive evidence of specific toxicities relating to fertility, reproduction, neurobehavioral toxicology and immunology. The screen should also establish the range of doses over which toxicities occur, the variability of toxicity between male and female rats and mice, and, in certain instances, the basic disposition pattern of a chemical as a function of dose and time. Then, presumptive evidence of specific organ system toxicity will be further studied using the appropriate test procedures.

NTP continues to identify and develop more sensitive methods for detection of injury to hepatic and renal function. Renal toxicity methods being reviewed and validated include kidney functions (concentrating ability and excretion rate of major nephron segments) as well as early indicators for cellular damage (presence of selected intracellular enzymes in urine).

Briefly outlined below are the major areas within the realm of general toxicology: chemical disposition, immunologic toxicology, neurobehavioral toxicology, pulmonary toxicology and reproductive and developmental toxicology.

### *Chemical Disposition*

Developing knowledge about the absorption, distribution, metabolism and excretion of chemicals selected for testing remains a major objective of NTP. Information necessary for the proper design and interpretation of toxicology and carcinogenicity studies includes knowing if a chemical accumulates in the body, causes toxic effects directly or through formation of a metabolite, and whether these events occur only at certain dose levels or if there is a species difference in pathways or rate of chemical disposition.

Resources available to NTP in FY 1979 were principally through university contracts, to be strengthened in FY 1980 by increasing the intramural component and expanding the contract capability. This will permit 12-15 chemicals to be studied in FY 1980, with a planned increase to 24 by the end of the year.

For the most efficient use of limited resources, preference in selection of work strives toward developing a core of knowledge based on chemical class characteristics that can be used to predict disposition patterns of new chemicals within that class or in chemically related classes. Studies on three major chemical classes continue: halogenated polyaromatics, benzidine-based dyes and haloalkyl phosphates.

*Halogenated Polyaromatics.* Chemicals belonging to the halogenated polyaromatics include several polychlorinated biphenyls (PCB) and octachlorodibenzodioxin, tetrachlorodibenzofuran and tetrachloroazobenzene. Disposition of selected PCB has been studied comparatively in the rat, dog and monkey; the biologic half-life of a PCB in a species depends on the capacity of that species to metabolize the PCB to an excretable polar compound. Species vary widely in ability to metabolize PCB: dog>rat≫monkey. Excretion of unmetabolized PCB is negligible in all species studied. Current work concerns identifying metabolites and establishing the disposition pattern of 3,4,3′,4′-tetrachlorobiphenyl, one of the more toxic PCB, in the rhesus monkey. These studies, to be completed in FY 1980, may advance our ability to interpret better the public health significance of PCB experimental toxicology data.

Information about the chemical disposition of chlorodibenzodioxins resides primarily on 2,3,7,8-tetrachlorodibenzo-*p*-dioxin. This knowledge base will be expanded in FY 1980 through study of octachlorodibenzodioxin, the chemically related 2,3,7,8-tetrachlordibenzofuran and the stereochemically related 3,4,3′,4′-tetrachloroazobenzene. Comparative species assessment will be done using the rat, guinea pig and monkey.

*Benzidine-Based Dyes.* The benzidine-based dye studies are designed to determine whether the biological conversion of benzidine-based dyes (as well as *o*-tolidine- and dianisidine-based dyes) to the free precursors (benzidine, *o*-tolidine and dianisidine) is a general phenomenon. A total of 13 dyes are being studied in the dog; these will be completed in early FY 1980: seven benzidine-based dyes (direct black 4, direct blue 2, direct brown 2, direct green 1, direct orange 1, direct orange 8 and direct red 28); three *o*-tolidine-based dyes (acid red 25, direct red 2 and direct red 39); and three dianisidine-based dyes (direct blue 1, direct blue 15, direct blue 218). Early results indicate that benzidine-based dyes revert to benzidine, and excretion of benzidine in urine occurs after administration or exposure to benzidine-based dyes.

*Haloalkyl Phosphates.* The haloalkyl phosphates include fire retardants and insecticides. Two of these compounds [*tris*-(1,3-dichloroisopropyl) phosphate (Fyrol FR-2) and *tris*-(2,3-dibromopropyl) phosphate (Tris)] are being studied to determine if these structurally related haloalkyl phosphates follow similar patterns of tissue distribution, metabolism, excretion and covalent binding.

A continuing priority of chemical disposition studies under NTP is the extrapolation of experimental data to humans. One way to facilitate more accurate extrapolation of chemical metabolism information from animals to humans involves developing in vitro animal and human cell cultures that proportionally reflect in vivo metabolism. The initial in vitro systems to be studied use tissues from rats, dogs and monkeys.

### *Immunologic Toxicology*

NTP is committed to studies that establish the role of immune assessment in toxicologic characterization of chemicals. Six immunologic functions were selected in FY 1979 as part of a test battery:

1. in vitro lymphocyte response to mitogens;
2. in vitro macrophage function;
3. antibody response to a T&B cell-dependent antigen;
4. delayed hypersensitivity;
5. host resistance; and
6. sensitivity to endotoxin.

In some instances, the preferred method to assess a specific immunologic function can only be determined through a comparison of methods. Research on methods selection will continue in the NTP laboratories with validation and interlaboratory comparison through contracts awarded in FY 1980. An interim immunology test battery is selectively being used in the NTP toxicology screen. Methods for in-depth characterization of immunosuppression are also being developed in the NTP laboratories, and a framework for collaborative studies has begun with selected chemicals.

### *Neurobehavioral Toxicology*

Development and validation of methods for testing neurologic and behavioral effects of chemicals continues. A test battery is being validated by investigating the effects of nine neurotoxic chemicals:

1. acrylamide,
2. *d*-amphetamine,
3. arsenic trioxide,
4. chlordecone,
5. lead acetate,
6. methylmercury,
7. PCB,
8. sodium salicylate, and
9. triethyltin.

Two objectives stand paramount: (1) determine the ability of neurobehavioral procedures to detect an *unexpected* neurotoxic effect and to ascertain the capability of each test to provide an *expected* negative result; and (2) generate a profile of effects for each substance so that tests assumed to measure the same or similar functions can be compared for relative sensitivity. The test battery includes methods that assess sensory function, motor strength and coordination, associative and cognitive factors, and emotionality.

An interim neurobehavioral test battery will also be used selectively in the NTP toxicology screen. A test capability for more extensive characterization of six chemicals per year will be developed in FY 1980. The neurobehavioral toxicity of chlordecone is being accomplished in NTP laboratories in response to public health concerns. These studies include the description and the persistence of effects in adult rats and in rats exposed during development.

*Pulmonary Toxicology*

Toxicity testing of inhaled materials rarely includes an assessment of pulmonary function. In recent years a number of techniques have been developed that measure indices of pulmonary function in rodents–static lung volumes, static and dynamic lung properties, diffusion and information about the distribution of ventilation. The applicability of these measurements in the assessment of pulmonary toxicity as well as their sensitivity compared to pathologic evaluation of lung damage remains to be demonstrated. NTP has initiated a series of studies centered around a comprehensive comparison of morphologic change vs functional change to validate the usefulness of respiratory physiology techniques. Six compounds will be evaluated using the rat and hamster at three dose levels during FY 1980 and FY 1981.

*Reproductive and Developmental Toxicology*

Fertility and reproduction are major areas that require toxicologic methods development and testing. Because these are areas in which personnel and resources available to NTP are in short supply, innovative methods development is not proposed, and efforts will be confined to general test procedures.

Teratology plans in FY 1980 represent a continuation of programs outlined in FY 1979: (1) evaluate definitive human and animal chemically associated teratology data to ensure that this information is used most effectively; (2) examine laboratory data to determine the range of doses that indicate linearity of response and permit identification of biomathematical procedures for low dose risk estimation; and (3) examine fetuses histopathologically for comparison with traditional methods to determine the adequacy of current methodology.

Testing of chemicals for teratogenic effects will continue at a rate of 10-15 per year: chemicals in progress are ethylene chlorhydrin, ethylene oxide, formaldehyde, pentachloroanisole, toluene and xylenes (*o*-, *m*-, *p*- and mixed). Results are scheduled to be reported in FY 1980. Five additional chemicals have been scheduled for testing; caffeine, dimethylaniline, ethoxy ethanol, lead monoxide and 2,3,7,8-tetrachlorodibenzofuran.

Behavioral disorders and learning deficiencies observed in children and the demonstration of behavioral dysfunctions in animals after prenatal exposure to a variety of chemicals suggest the need for behavioral evaluation of neonates in the safety assessment of new drugs and chemicals. Incorporation of behavioral evaluation into testing guidelines should be determined after reviewing data that have been produced under standardized and validated test conditions. The effects on behavior resulting from prenatal exposure to chemicals initiative (behavioral teratology) is to identify and develop screening methods which (1) yield valid and reproducible results within and among laboratories; (2) are sensitive to toxic alterations produced by a range of agents with varying toxic potential; (3) predict toxic effects in humans; and (4) are cost-efficient.

In FY 1979 a test protocol was developed and studies were initiated that will standardize these tests for the reliability and sensitivity of six behavioral methods using three chemicals known to cause behavioral teratogenic effects—*d*-amphetamine, methylmercury and vitamin A. The planned activities for FY 1980 are to conduct pilot studies, select six laboratories to conduct the studies and begin the test validation experiments.

### Carcinogenesis

During FY 1979, the National Cancer Institute/NTP tested 201 chemicals for carcinogenic potential in lifetime rodent bioassays; of these, 79 chemicals were started on bioassay in FY 1979. During the year, tests were completed and reports were issued on 95 chemicals. Under the conditions of the tests, 47 (49.5%) were considered negative, 39 (41%) positive and 9 (9.5%) equivocal carcinogens. Reports on about 30 of these chemicals are scheduled for publication in FY 1980. Depending on actual resource availability and allocation, testing of 75-100 chemicals will be initiated in FY 1980.

The NTP objective is to assure that the most important chemicals from a public health point of view are tested; that the end results are relevant to the research and regulatory agencies; and to provide better information for assessing human risks associated with those chemicals found to be carcinogenic in experimental animals.

A lifetime bioassay in rodents is the current procedure utilized to determine carcinogenic potential of a chemical. NTP does not propose alternative methods, but acknowledges a need to develop and validate less expensive and more rapid methods that may allow chemical testing priorities to be established, or in some instances to supplant the need for lifetime bioassays.

For instance, in vitro mammalian cell transformations are likely short-term assays for indicating carcinogenic potential of a chemical. Transformation assays being evaluated include BALB/c 3T3, Fischer Rat Embryo (RLV infected), hamster embryo and C3H 10T½. In FY 1979, tests on 31 chemicals were initiated in hamster embryo clonal assays and the BALB/c 3T3 focus assay. These chemicals were selected on the basis of adequate lifetime carcinogenesis bioassay results and on the mutagenicity data derived from standardized *Salmonella* assays. This validation intiative will be completed in FY 1980.

An in-progress testing program that permits comparison of standardized *Salmonella* assay results with lifetime rodent bioassays is described in the Genetic Toxicology section.

The mouse lung adenoma model is proposed as an in vivo system for determining carcinogenic potential of a chemical in a relatively short period of time. Lung adenomas are indigenous in aging strain A mice. Treating this strain with drugs and selected environmental contaminants known to be carcinogenic has shortened the period of tumor occurrence and increased the number of adenomas in a dose-related fashion. Conclusions similar to those obtained from the lifetime bioassay were obtained with this model for over 70% of a limited number of chemicals. In FY 1979 a project plan was completed that will evaluate and validate lung adenoma occurrence in the strain A mouse as a model to rapidly screen and set priorities for candidate test chemicals. Tests of 60 chemicals previously investigated in lifetime bioassays will be performed on the strain A mouse during FY 1980, and an additional 30 chemicals will be tested in FY 1981.

During FY 1980, the appearance of precursor (preneoplastic) liver lesions in hepatectomized rats treated with carcinogens will be evaluated as a potential in vivo model for predicting carcinogenesis at an earlier stage.

Carcinogenicity testing traditionally begins with young adult animals (typically six-week-old rodents). However, human chemical exposures often occur during in utero development and infancy, as well as throughout life: exposure of pregnant workers; use of drugs; accumulation, persistence and excretion via mother's milk; neighborhood contamination; and others. The adequacy of lifetime bioassay methods compared to methods that also include prenatal and neonatal exposures is being evaluated using three chemicals: a commercial polybrominated biphenyl, phenytoin (diphenylhydantoin), and ethylene thiourea.

Inhalation bioassays for carcinogenicity usually involve an arbitrarily determined duration of exposure. The required specialized facilities are expensive and commit scarce technical staff for extended periods. Ongoing studies with mice, rats and hamsters use a design which varies both the age of animals and the duration of exposure to a known carcinogen, vinyl chloride. The testing hypothesis seeks to compare tumor response among species and to analyse exposure regimens that provide a predicted carcinogenic response. These studies, projected for completion in FY 1980, may provide meaningful bioassay results using a shorter duration of exposure.

## NTP CHEMICAL TESTING

Among the eight defined areas of research and testing, NTP in FY 1979 had 397 chemicals in various stages of investigation; for FY 1980 this effort increases to 565 chemicals and expands to 678 chemicals in FY 1981.

## INFORMATION GENERATION AND DISSEMINATION

The National Toxicology Program must ascertain the toxicology of selected chemicals and assure that results will have scientific and regulatory significance. The end product is information–scientific information necessary in deciding social issues relative to public health and the environment. To provide that information, the NTP identified two important aspects: first, information must be disseminated to other scientists so that peer review and feedback assure scientific quality; second, since the scientific product helps society evaluate identified toxicological risks, information must be disseminated to not only the regulators responsible for protecting against potentially hazardous risks, but also to those exposed to the risks. Thus, the NTP will establish and use a coordinated communications network to disseminate toxicological information.

The value of information arising from NTP will depend in part on the quality and timeliness of information received into the program. The NTP will therefore actively seek information from all sources: federal, state and local governments; trade associations, industry and labor; academia; professional societies and public interest groups; the press; individuals; other countries; and all other interested parties. Information received could include nominations of chemicals to be tested; critique and questions about scientific procedures, policies, priorities and resource allocations; and any other suggestions for program improvement. To encourage multiple communication,

NTP program materials must be disseminated widely and rapidly, and questions answered in a timely manner.

### NTP Publications

In addition to the NTP technical reports, journal articles and other research documentation, the NTP makes available four publications–

1. NTP Annual Plan for Fiscal Year 1980 (NTP-79-7) [5]
2. NTP Review of Current DHEW Research Related to Toxicology (NTP-79-8) [6]
3. NTP Technical Bulletin
4. NTP First Annual Report on Carcinogens (NTP-80-50).

The 1980 NTP Annual Plan contains information on NTP research, testing and validation efforts for the coming fiscal year as well as for the previous fiscal year. This 117-page report is divided into ten sections:

1. Introduction and Executive Summary;
2. Background;
3. Participating Agencies;
4. Oversight and Review;
5. Planning Assumptions and Program Balance;
6. Organization;
7. Toxicology Research and Testing Overview;
8. Coordinative Management Activities;
9. Information Generation and Dissemination, and
10. Annual Report on Carcinogens.

The Annual Plans are published in the first quarter of the fiscal year.

A companion to the NTP Annual Plan is the 334-page NTP Review of Current DHEW Research Related to Toxicology. This compilation emphasizes three major areas: DHEW Agency Role in the Support of Toxicology Research, Testing and Method Development; Chemical Compounds Currently Being Tested by DHEW Agencies for Toxicological Properties; and Toxicology Methods Currently Being Developed by DHEW Agencies.

The NTP Technical Bulletin series serves as the NTP communication medium to keep all those interested in the NTP informed about the NTP's most current and proposed activities. The first issue (November 1979) contained key background information about the NTP, announced formation of the NTP Board of Scientific Counselors and named the eight appointees, listed the NTP Exceutive Committee members and their organizations, introduced the NTP program leaders, recorded the NTP Chemical Selection Principles. The second issue, April 1980, identified the three ad hoc subcommittees of the NTP Board of Scientific Counselors, highlighted mutagenesis activities, reported bioassay results on 12 chemicals and listed chemicals newly selected for testing. The third issue was published in September 1980.

The two-volume First NTP Annual Report on Carcinogens contains epidemiological, experimental, exposure and regulatory information on 26 chemicals evaluated by the International Agency for Research on Cancer as being associated with human cancer induction: naturally occurring chemicals (1), industrial chemicals (2), industrial processes (4), industrial by-products (1) and pharmaceuticals (8). The Second NTP Annual Report on Carcinogens will be published in September 1981.

The NTP Annual Plan for Fiscal Year 1980, the NTP Review of Current DHEW Research Related to Toxicology, the NTP Technical Bulletin and the NTP First Annual Report on Carcinogens can be obtained by writing to:

NTP Publications
National Toxicology Program
P.O. Box 12233
Research Triangle Park, NC 27709

NTP welcomes questions, comments and suggestions about the National Toxicology Program.

## ACKNOWLEDGMENTS

We thank Leslie Gardner for typing this overview and the NTP program leaders for supplying information about their projects (NTP report No. NTP-80-64).

## REFERENCES

1. Califano, J. A., Jr. "Establishment of a National Toxicology Program," *Federal Register* 43(221):53060-53061 (1978).
2. Rall, D. P. "National Toxicology Program, Meeting," *Federal Register* 44(143):43426-43435 (1979).
3. National Toxicology Program. "Annual Plan for Fiscal Year 1979 (NTP-79-1): I - Research Plan, 1-54; II - Review of Current DHEW Research Related to Toxicology, 55-361" (1979).
4. National Toxicology Program. Transcript of Proceedings, August 10, 1979, Public Meeting on the NTP Annual Plan for Fiscal Year 1979 (1979).

5. National Toxicology Program. "Annual Plan for Fiscal Year 1980 (NTP-79-7)," (1979).
6. National Toxicology Program. "Review of Current DHEW Research Related to Toxicology for Fiscal Year 1980," (NTP-79-8) (1979).
7. Huff, J. E., Ed. *NTP Technical Bulletin* 1(1):1-12 (1979).
8. Rall, D. P. "National Toxicology Program Board of Scientific Counselors: Meeting," *Federal Register* 45(8):2401 (1980).
9. Rall, D. P. "National Toxicology Program Fiscal Year 1980 Annual Plan," *Federal Register* 45(28):8888-8918 (1980).
10. Huff, J. E., Ed. NTP Technical Bulletin 1(2):1-12 (1980).
11. Walters, D. B., L. H. Keith and J. E. Harless. "Chemical Selection and Handling Aspects of the National Toxicology Program," Chapter 26, this volume.
12. National Toxicology Program. "Annual Plan for Fiscal Year 1981," NTP-80-62 (1980).
13. Rall, D. P., J. A. Moore and J. E. Huff. "National Toxicology Program," *IRPTC Bull.* 3(1) (1980).
14. Rall, D. P. "National Toxicology Program, 1-6," in *Toxic Control IV, Toxic Control in the 80's*, M. L. Miller, Ed. (Washington, DC: Government Institutes, Inc., 1980).
15. de Serres, F. J., and J. Ashby, Eds. *Short-Term Tests for Carcinogens: Report of the International Collaborative Program* (New York: Elsevier North-Holland, Inc., in press).

CHAPTER 26

# CHEMICAL SELECTION AND HANDLING ASPECTS OF THE NATIONAL TOXICOLOGY PROGRAM

**D. B. Walters**

National Toxicology Program
Public Health Service
Department of Health and Human Services
Research Triangle Park, North Carolina

**L. H. Keith and J. M. Harless**

Radian Corporation
Austin, Texas

## INTRODUCTION

Environmental health chemistry concepts are essential in the National Toxicology Program (NTP) because they are required in understanding and interrelating the various biological and toxicological aspects of this complex task. From the viewpoint of safe handling and testing of potentially hazardous chemicals, there is a need for chemistry input in the beginning information-gathering phase; through proper laboratory design, handling and management functions; for chemical monitoring, environmental control and medical surveillance; for deactivation, decontamination, spill control and emergency planning; and for final consideration of the disposal of hazardous wastes and interpretation of toxicological data based on structural considerations.

## DISCUSSION

### Chemical Nomination and Selection

The chemical selection process helps identify those compounds to which a significant number of people are exposed but which are untested, inadequately tested or raise suspicions in one or more toxicological parameters. These compounds are reviewed for human exposure and toxicologic potential and compounds which should be tested are identified. A complex toxicology testing program such as the NTP requires an orderly set of guidelines to select chemicals for testing. The chemical nomination and selection process used is diagrammed in the preceding chapter (Chapter 25, Figure 2). Nominations for a list of test chemicals are requested from each participating agency (NCI, NIEHS, NIOSH and FDA). In addition, nominations from other federal and nonfederal sources are also requested. Nominations are submitted to the chairman of the NTP Chemical Nomination Group. All nominations must be supported by the relevant information:

1. chemical identification and properties: (1) identification and chemical clarification, (2) physical and chemical properties, (3) commercial product composition, (4) exposure, production and use, (5) environmental surveillance;
2. metabolism and structure-activity: (1) pharmacokinetic data and metabolic pathways, and (2) structure-activity considerations and correlations;
3. toxicity: (1) human, (2) animal, and (3) in vitro and other short-term tests;
4. ongoing toxicological or environmental studies in the government and/or private sector;
5. rationale for choice; and
6. suggested toxicology studies to be undertaken.

Chemical information includes physicochemical properties (e.g., volatility and solubility) as well as environmental fate and stability where biological activity may effect the chemical structure and produce different products. Research may also be necessary to determine possible impurities which may be present or which may be formed during use or misuse of the chemical. Information on production, industrial uses, wastes generated and their disposal is required to determine the human exposure in the workplace and/or possible contamination of air, water, soil or food. Such knowledge is often not available or is difficult to obtain. Environmental surveillance describes the complex joint interactions of use and production patterns, health effects and exposure, environmental occurrence and regulatory status and priority.

Metabolites also contribute to the toxicological effects of a chemical.

For many chemicals metabolic alterations, storage and bioconcentration in the food chain must also be considered. Often, such information must come from structure-activity considerations and correlations.

Similarly, toxicological data are often incomplete, and the chemical must be evaluated for potential toxicological parameters on the basis of structure-activity relationships. The development and validation of short-term tests allows NTP to screen economically and rapidly many chemicals so those chemicals most likely to be toxic can be targeted for more extensive (and expensive) testing. The completed nomination package should also include a summary of ongoing relevant research, a rationale for the nomination and a listing of which toxicology studies are needed and why.

Two primary factors that suggest a chemical should be tested are its physicochemical and toxicological properties and the extent of human and environmental exposure. However, selection of chemicals is based on consideration and integration of all the abovementioned factors rather than by a sequential or categorical process. The Chemical Nomination Group (which includes four participating agencies mentioned above plus representatives from EPA, OSHA and the Consumer Product Safety Commission [CPSC]) determines if each nomination qualifies according to the principles for selection. The NTP operates under the guideline that industry will bear the burden of testing chemicals that are introduced into commerce for health and environmental effects, as intended and mandated by Congress under legislative authorities. Therefore, the NTP selects chemicals for testing using the criteria:

1. environmental chemicals;
2. substitutes;
3. structural studies;
4. validation;
5. cross-comparison of testing methods;
6. synergistic effects;
7. socially important chemicals; and
8. special chemicals.

Specifically this includes: "old chemicals" with the potential for significant human exposure which are of social importance but which generate too little revenue to support an adequate testing program. In special situations, as determined by the Executive Committee, marketed chemicals which have potential for large-scale and/or intense human exposure are considered, even if it may be possible to require industry to perform the testing. Chemicals found in the environment which are not closely associated with commercial activities are included, as well as desirable substitutes for existing chemicals, particularly therapeutic agents, that might not be developed or tested without federal involvement. Also considered are chemicals which should be tested to improve scientific understanding of structure-activity relationships and thereby assist in defining groups of commercial chemicals that should be tested by industry. Those chemicals tested by industry are included where the additional testing by the federal government is justified as a check on the validity and reliability of industry results. Previously tested chemicals are chosen for which other testing is desirable to cross-compare testing methods. And finally, there is the situation where two or more chemicals may be mixed together and combined human exposure may occur; such testing probably would not be required of industry if the products of different companies are involved.

A dossier containing additional relevant information on chemical properties, production, use, exposure, toxicity and proposed toxicologic testing needs is then compiled by the Chemical Nominations Group. The NTP Executive Committee (composed of the heads of FDA, OSHA, CPSC, EPA, NIH, NIOSH, NCI and NIEHS) receives and reviews the committee summaries and selects and prioritizes the chemicals for testing.

The selection of a chemical does not a priori commit it to testing by NTP. It does commit NTP to ascertain the specific toxicologic and regulatory concerns, i.e., to evaluate the adequacy of existing data or current efforts in government, academic or private laboratories and then to propose and conduct specific test(s) that are needed. A more complete description of the chemical nomination and selection process appears elsewhere [1].

## Chemical Repository

Chemical management aspects of the NTP begin after a chemical has been selected for inclusion in the testing program. A determination of several factors must then be made, for example, identification of the processes by which the chemical is manufactured, its intended use, grade, purity, possible impurities, additives, source, location and availability in sufficient amounts for the study. If the material is not commercially available, consideration is given to feasibility, required time, hazards and cost analysis for custom synthesis.

Contracts are awarded to provide for procurement, storage, distribution, chemical analysis, purification, synthesis and reference archiving for approximately 3000 chemicals. Capabilities are maintained for analysis of bulk chemicals, chemicals in test vehicles, samples for quality assurance, tissues, fluids, purity and stability determinations, and residual and reprocured chemicals. In addition, the purification, preparation of derivatives and routine synthesis of test chemicals are also provided.

NTP maintains the capability for sophisticated chemical analyses of the chemical and of contaminants in each chemical to be tested. In the Phase I Genetic Toxicology screening, such analyses are performed when toxicologic tests using mixtures or chemicals with impurities are positive (as well as questionable responses and selected negative response compounds), to identify the specific component(s) that may be associated with the toxic effect.

Generally, most of the analytical chemistry support for the in vivo testing aspects of NTP is currently done by Midwest Research Institute, Kansas City, MO, while most of the in vitro analytical support comes from Radian Corpoation, Austin TX. The NTP chemical repository has been established at Radian and provides for centralized management of test chemicals to characterize and assure the quality of chemicals, to minimize them as a source of variability in the testing results and to provide for maximum safety and containment. The repository is used for the receipt and transshipment of test compounds to bioassay laboratories and other programs necessary to complete the toxicological testing.

Major repository duties are:

1. open shipments received and enter into inventory system;
2. maintain a computerized inventory;
3. provide storage areas at room temperature, 5 and -20°C for 500 g each of 3000–4000 compounds;
4. eliminate or minimize possible degradation;
5. mix bulk chemicals and repack into smaller containers for storage;
6. remove aliquot for shipping;
7. package chemicals suitable for safe shipping;
8. ship chemical to testing laboratory;
9. provide two sets of documents with test materials: (1) ensure handling but maintain confidentiality, and (2) be opened only in an emergency situation;
10. perform specific requested chemical analysis and syntheses; and
11. provide quarterly summaries and annual reports.

Once a chemical has been selected for NTP genetic toxicology testing, appropriate quantities of suitably pure materials are ordered, and chemical information necessary for the bioassay laboratories is gathered. When a chemical arrives it is opened and handled only in a specially designed hazardous materials laboratory (HML) appropriate for storage, handling and analysis of carcinogens, mutagens, teratogens and highly toxic substances. A complete description of the HML is given elsewhere [2-4]. Chemicals are logged into the computerized inventory system soon after they are received. They are stored under appropriate conditions to eliminate or minimize possible degradation (e.g., heat, oxidation and ultraviolet (UV) radiation). Chemicals are homogenized to achieve uniformity and are repackaged into smaller containers to provide maximum containment and minimum contamination in the event of an accident (Figure 1). A 100-g sample of each chemical is stored for archive purposes and two 200-g aliquots are stored for bioassay, stability, chemical analysis and miscellaneous purposes. When a bioassay laboratory is scheduled to receive a chemical, a 5- to 10-g aliquot is removed from the storage container, coded to ensure a blind bioassay, and suitably packaged and shipped. All samples sent out of the repository meet and usually exceed Department of Transportation regulations. Glass hypovials with Teflon®-faced septa in steel cans, as shown in Figure 2, have been found most suitable for safe shipment of amounts under 50 g. Determination of the survivability of the primary shipping containers was performed by a destructive testing program. Sample containers were prepared with combinations of liquids and solid dyes and packaged as shown in Figure 2. Destruction was carried out by running over each container with a 3/4-ton pickup truck. One container of each type was placed end-on and one edge-on to the left front wheel (Figure 3). (Attempts to perform a top-bottom compression were unsuccessful as the cans invariably popped out from under the wheel). The calculated pressure on the body of each can was in excess of 2000 lb. All cans were badly crushed and deformed, such that they had to be opened with a band saw (Figure 4). In all instances the primary container survived intact as did the two heat-sealed plastic bags that held the primary containers.

Two sets of documents accompany all test chemicals sent to bioassay laboratories: a safety and handling document, which does not identify the material but describes types of hazards, hazard precautions, safety devices and protectors, spill and leakage information, storage precautions, disposal and waste-treatment technology and physicochemical properties, and an emergency procedures document which breaks the code number, identifies the material and provides information on synonyms, hazards, toxicology, references, personnel protection, firefighting, spills, leakage, first aid, disposal and waste-treatment technology and all other pertinent information.

These documents represent two of the many tasks performed by the repository computer system. Other computer features are:

1. computer terminal in repository area;
2. prearranged system of confidential coding to ensure blind testing;
3. inventory information (data received, lot and batch no., amount, grade, purity, source, etc.);
4. indexing by a prearranged preferred name and cross indexing;
5. physicochemical data;
6. toxicology data;
7. safety and handling information and document;
8. emergency procedures information and document; and
9. an alerting system for reordering.

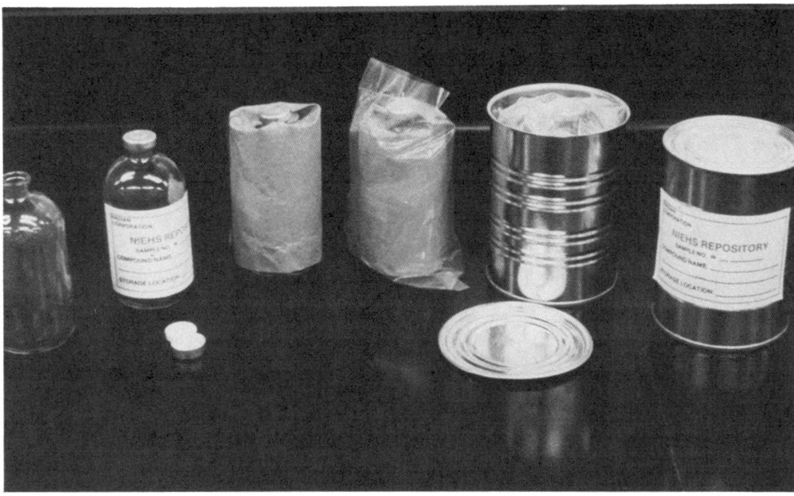


**Figure 1.** Preparation of sample for storage in NTP repository.

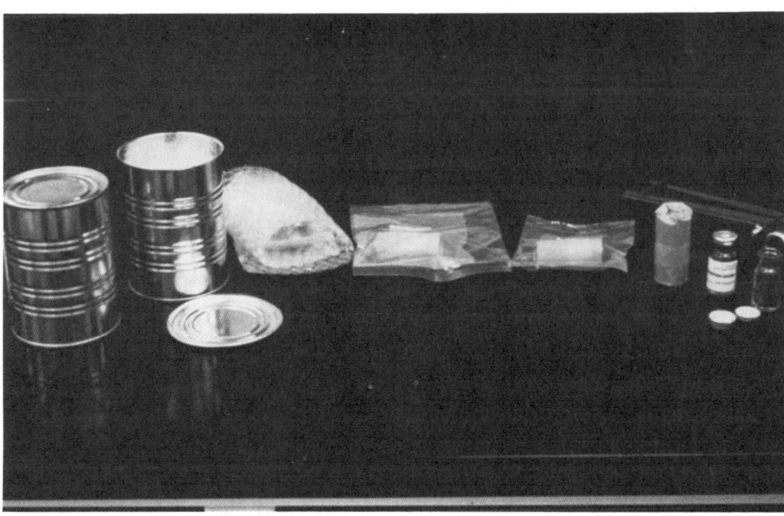

**Figure 2.** Preparation of aliquot for shipment from NTP repository.

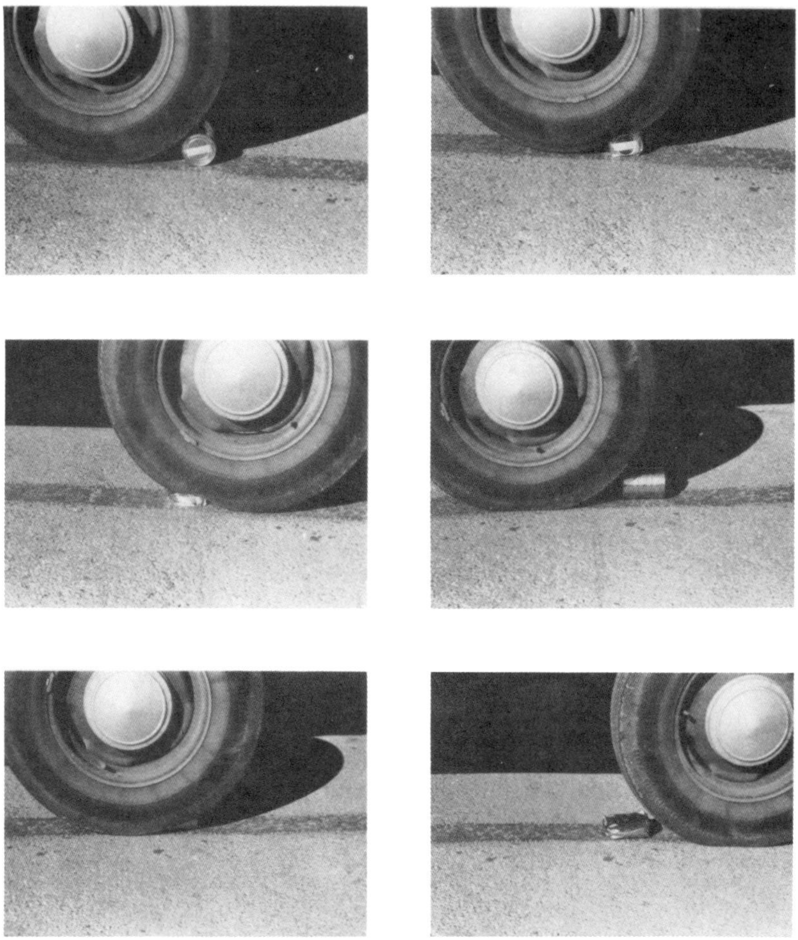

**Figure 3.** Durability test of hazardous materials shipping container.

A computer terminal containing a keyboard, CRT display and line printer is located inside the repository's HML. In addition, a desk for records preparation and maintenance is provided. The terminal is connected to the repository's central computer system where all inventory, safety and transaction information for chemicals stored in the HML is maintained. The incorporation of a computer terminal in the HML allows Radian to successfully manage repository operations for the NTP where hundreds of compounds are stored and cataloged, and where aliquots are removed and shipped to various laboratories around the world. As many as possible of the repository's tasks are

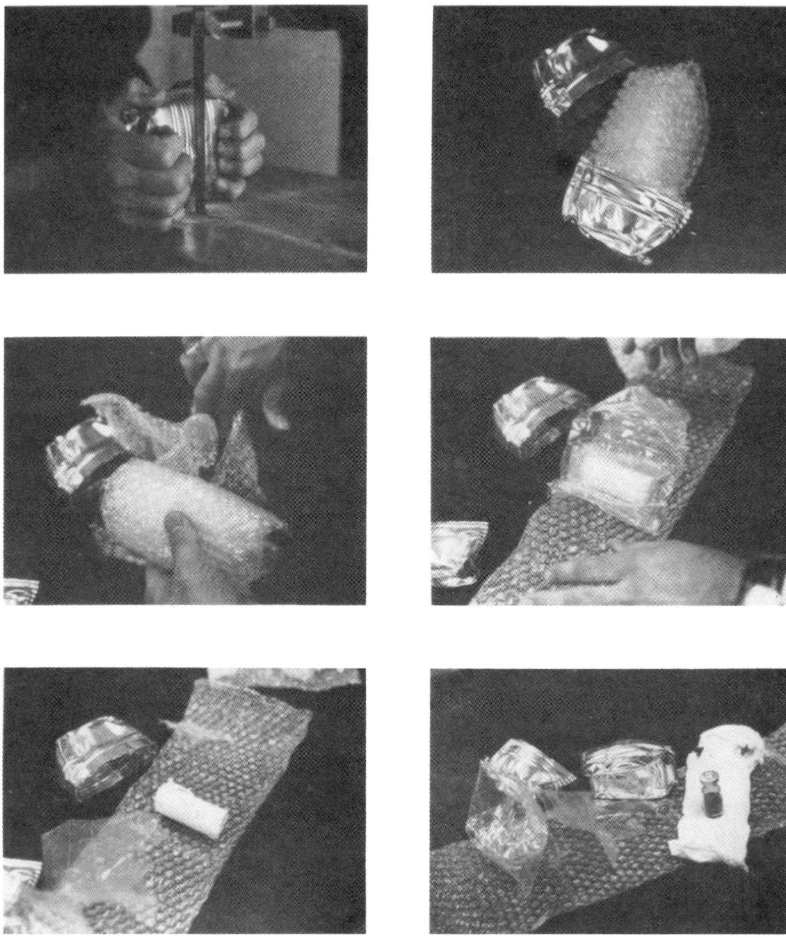

**Figure 4.** Contents of crushed hazardous materials shipping container after opening.

computerized to provide efficient and effective use of information for interface with the diverse NTP areas.

Table I lists the items for which information is sought on each chemical. Several of these items are composed of subsections, into which the data are categorized: For example, Item 11 (solubility) is subcategorized into solubilities in water, ethyl alcohol, diethyl ether, acetone, benzene, chloroform, DMSO and selected other solvents. Solubility categories also have been defined:

**Table I. Subject Categories Searched for Each Chemical**

| | |
|---|---|
| 1. Secondary ID No. | 23. Carcinogenicity |
| 2. Primary Name | 24. Mutagenicity |
| 3. CAS No. | 25. Teratogenicity |
| 4. WLN | 26. Other Comments |
| 5. Formula | 27. Sources |
| 6. Synonyms | 28. Types of Hazard |
| 7. Molecular Weight | 29. Hazard Precautions |
| 8. Density | 30. Safety Devices and Protectors |
| 9. Melting Point, °C | 31. Storage Precautions |
| 10. Boiling Point, °C | 32. Physical Description |
| 11. Solubility | 33. Toxicity |
| 12. Flammability | 34. Volatility |
| 13. Reactivity | 35. Other Instructions |
| 14. Stability | 36. Personal Protection |
| 15. NIOSH Registry No. | 37. Fire Fighting |
| 16. Toxicity | 38. First Aid |
| 17. AQTX/TLM96 | 39. Spills and Leakage |
| 18. SAX Toxicity Evaluation | 40. Disposal and Waste Treatment |
| 19. Acute Local | 41. Hazards |
| 20. Acute Systemic | 42. Toxicology |
| 21. Chronic Local | 43. Citations |
| 22. Chronic Systemic | |

1. insoluble–less than 0.1 g/100 ml solvent
2. slightly soluble–0.1-1.0 g/100 ml solvent
3. soluble–1-10 g/100 ml solvent
4. very soluble–greater than 10 g/100 ml solvent

This information is then composed into several formats when retrieved from the computer. The emergency procedures information discussed previously is just one of many useful listings available.

The general categories of analytical duties required of the repository are:

1. purity and stability analyses;
2. separation and isolation of complex mixtures;
3. qualitative and quantitative analysis and identification of mixtures;
4. analysis and purification of compounds synthesized onsite for NTP; and
5. monitoring of repository laboratory.

Procedures for chemical analysis may be developed for analysis of materials before, during or after toxicological testing. These analyses include purity determination and stability and storage analysis at the percent level. Often required is the application of separation and isolation techniques to complex mixtures to analyze qualitatively and quantitatively trace impurities at ppm or ppb levels. (Level of detection is determined on a case-by-case basis.) It is not uncommon to request that the repository derivatize existing compounds to obtain materials more amenable with bioassay testing requirements or to synthesize chemicals which are not commercially available or are not available in sufficient purity. In all cases the final products are subjected to the necessary cleanup procedures and are then chemically analyzed. In addition, the HML area is periodically subjected to chemical monitoring for detection of hazardous materials. The presence of such materials is often the first indication of either a malfunction of engineering controls designed to provide containment or improper personnel operational procedures. In either case, repository work stops until the cause of the contamination is ascertained and the problem is corrected. These efforts are coordinated with appropriate medical, safety, industrial hygiene, engineering and chemistry staff. It should be noted that all repository personnel receive baseline medical exams before starting work in the area as well as periodic medical surveillance exams.

Operation and safety concerns of the repository's HML are facilitated by use of the specially prepared documents listed below:

1. Design and Operation of a Hazardous Materials Laboratory Manual;
2. Safety Manual;
3. Operational Procedures Manual;
4. Manual on Analysis and Storage of Hazardous Chemicals;
5. Inventory and Systems Design Document;
6. Manual on Shipment of Hazardous Chemicals; and
7. Information and Procedures Manual for Bioassay Testing Laboratories.

The establishment of a sound NTP safety program is based on the application of the principles of industrial hygiene, chemistry, toxicology and engineering control. The basis of the safety program is reliance on containment and engineering controls rather than on personnel protection. Common throughout the NTP is the fact that all substances under study in the program are chemicals which behave according to their physicochemical properties. These properties are considered along with the known biological properties of these substances. The HML of the NTP repository was designed to meet these needs. Some of the HML special design features are:

1. isolated building;
2. dressing/shower area;
3. subatmospheric pressure;
4. filtered exhaust air;
5. treated wastewater;
6. external utilities;
7. emergency power;
8. computer terminal;
9. intercom system;
10. three repository rooms;

11. air lock for receiving and exiting equipment and chemicals;
12. isolated chemical manipulation rooms;
13. alarm systems for temperature failure, atmospheric pressure failure, electrical failure, wastewater treatment failure, and accidents and spills;
14. seamless vinyl coved flooring; and
15. visual access to all working areas.

As stated above, a complete description of many of these features including design, engineering controls, monitoring, operation procedures and functional capabilities are given in the next chapter and elsewhere [2,4]. This section will highlight those aspects of the repository.

Entrance to the HML is achieved from the viewing hall (Figure 5) through a dressing area. The viewing hall is an important safety feature of the laboratory because it allows external visual monitoring of personnel working in the facility and of the safety shower area. In case of an accident inside the laboratory, personnel outside the facility can assess the situation and determine appropriate responses from a safe vantage point. Intercom communications is also provided between the viewing area and the main laboratory area.

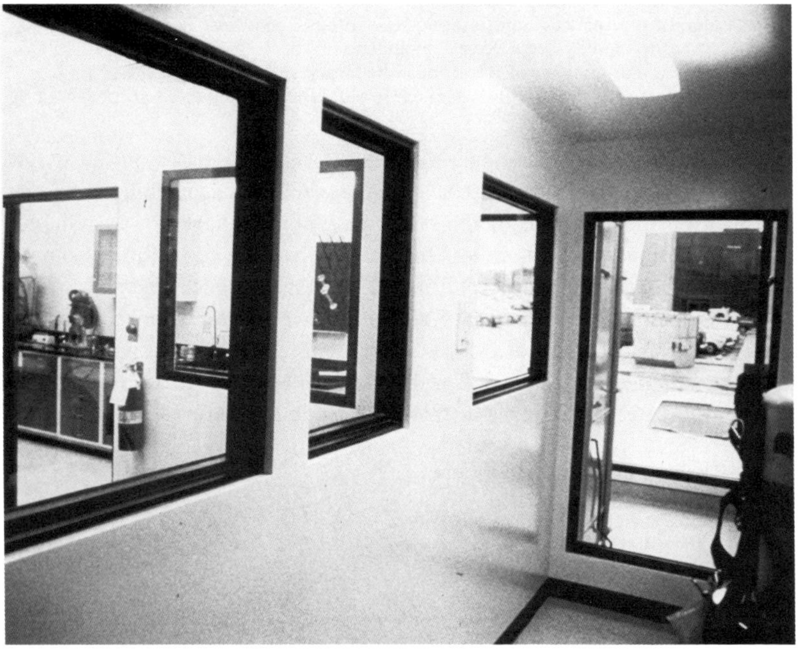

**Figure 5.** View of the HML from the viewing hall.

The laboratory workspace of the repository is shown in Figure 6 (a photograph taken from one of the viewing windows). Visible features are: the main preparative workspace area, the glove box, two subambient storage areas and the two chemical manipulation rooms.

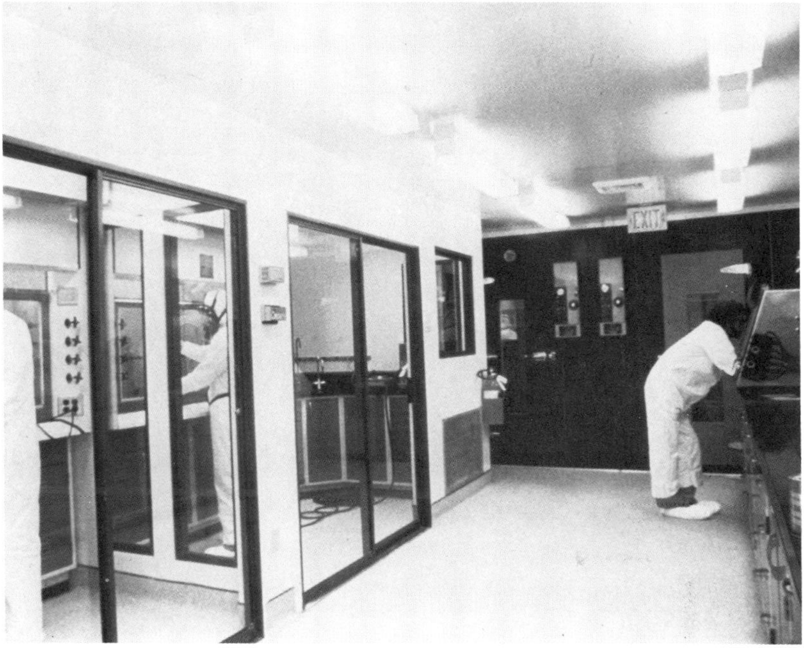


**Figure 6.** Interior of the HML.

The main laboratory area is designed as a general-purpose workspace, although it is not used for handling chemicals. Approximately 20 feet of benchtop work area and undercounter storage are provided. This space is occupied by a controlled-atmosphere glove box (Figure 7), general workspace and a large glassware-cleaning area. The glove box is the only place in this area where chemicals can be handled, and it is usually used for chemicals too hazardous or unstable to be manipulated in a fume hood. Utilities provided in this area include breathing air, compressed air, argon, nitrogen, natural gas, vacuum, and hot, cold, and deionized water.

A 16-sprayhead safety shower and eyewash station is also located in the main laboratory area. An emergency alarm button is provided adjacent to the shower for easy access in case of personnel injury or contamination.

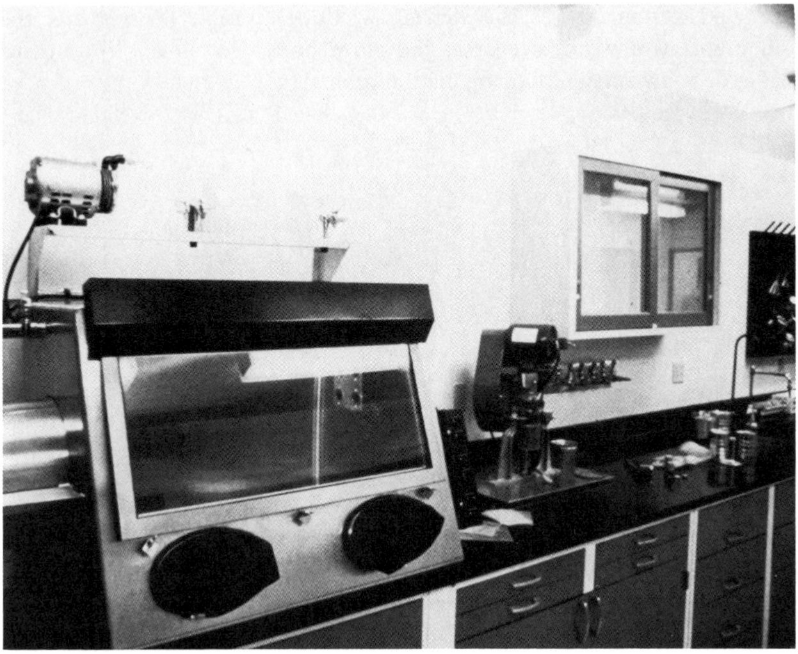

**Figure 7.** Glove box and canner in main laboratory area.

Once activated, the alarm system sounds throughout the Radian office/laboratory complex.

The chemical manipulation rooms (Figure 8) were designed to house the majority of operations conducted in the HML. Each room is isolated and operated at a negative pressure with respect to the remainder of the laboratory; therefore, any chemical released in these rooms is isolated. Each room is equipped with a six-foot stainless steel fume hood and approximately ten feet of benchtop workspace and undercounter storage. The fume hoods selected for this facility were Kewaunee "Solvent Sweep" auxiliary air hoods. These hoods are especially versatile because they are designed to provide approximately four feet of interior vertical clearance, enough to allow the use of tall reflux and distillation columns commonly required for chemical synthesis. A minimum face velocity of 150 feet per minute is maintained across the face of each hood with the sash in the fully open position. Utilities supplied to each room include breathing air, vacuum, compressed air, argon, nitrogen, natural gas, and hot, cold and deionized water. An emergency alarm button is located inside each manipulation room for use in personal injury or contamination situations. The various kinds of protective clothing and equipment used in the HML are also illustrated in Figure 8.

The large storage facilities (Figure 9) incorporated into the area are necessary for maintaining chemical repository services. Commercial, walk-in, refrigerated chambers are used to maintain chemicals at 5 and -20°C, and a third area is used to store materials at ambient temperatures. Five to six

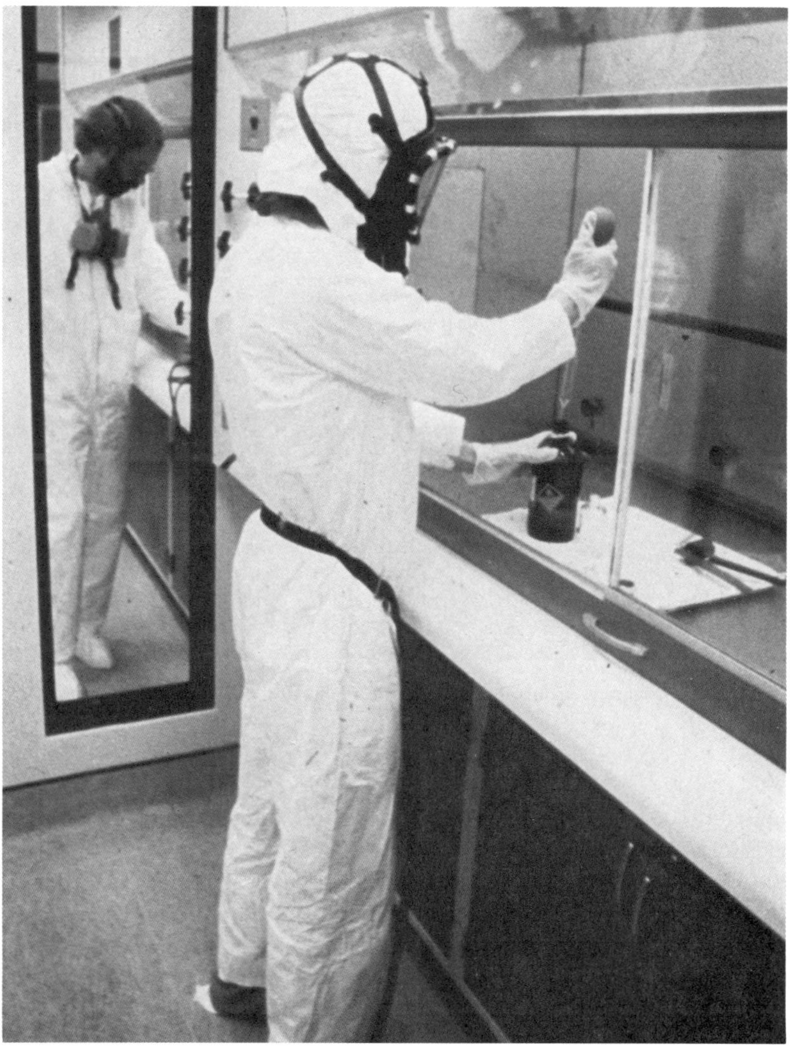

**Figure 8.** Chemical manipulation rooms.

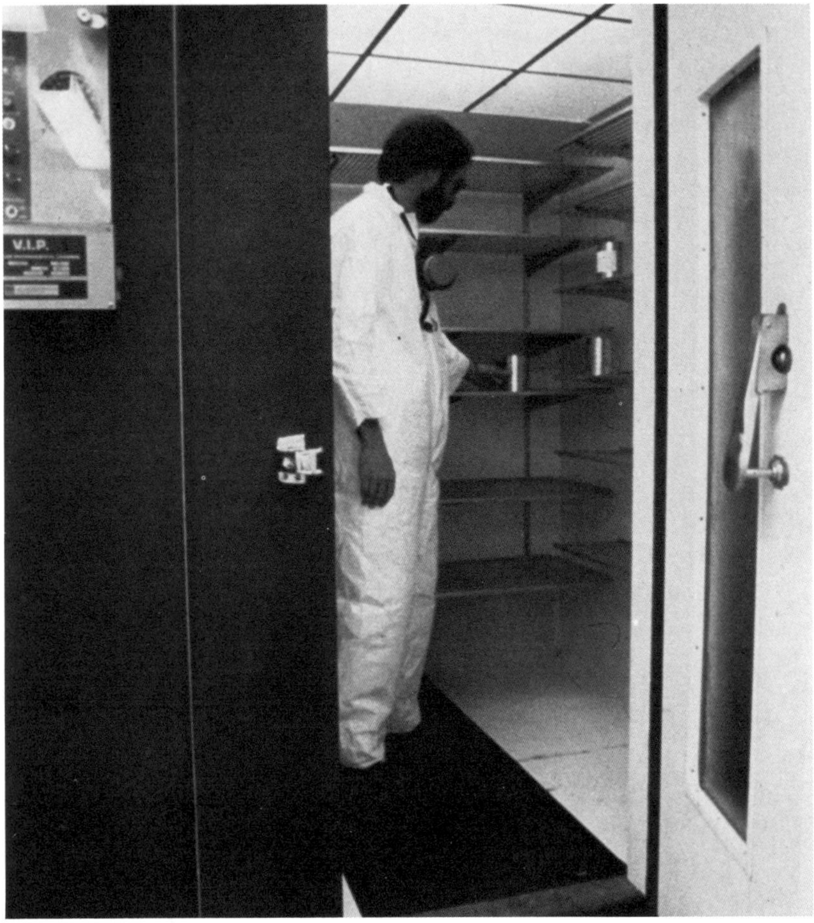

**Figure 9.** Controlled-temperature repository storage area.

thousand 100-gram lots of chemicals can be stored in the present HML repository area (which is currently being expanded to an area about three times its present size). The storage areas are an integral part of the laboratory and are therefore isolated from the surrounding environment. The refrigeration units for the subambient storage areas are located in the overhead chase space for ease of maintenance. The temperature of each refrigerated area is constantly monitored, and an alarm is activated inside the HML, on the master control panel and in the Radian offices if the temperature rises above the normal operating range.

## CONCLUSIONS

Selection and control of potential carcinogenic, mutagenic, teratogenic and highly toxic chemicals in a multifaceted organization such as NTP presents special problems of management and program implementation. Critical to the effective long-term operation of NTP is the chemical nomination and selection process. This process has recently been reviewed, and NTP has initiated a "Testing Needs Study." The purpose of this is to estimate the number of compounds to which a significant number of people are exposed but which are untested, inadequately tested or raise suspicions in one or more toxicological parameters. With this information, better projections can be made about chemicals that need testing over the next several years. During this study, a large number of compounds will be reviewed for both human exposure and toxicologic potential, and this review will identify compounds that should be tested. Although this study will take at least two years to complete, useful information will be produced as the study progresses.

The two primary areas on which decisions are based for safe handling of a chemical are the physicochemical and toxicological properties of the chemical. Unfortunately, for too many chemicals, little is known about either of these areas. In these situations the chemical must be assessed for safe handling and use on the basis of its structure and relationship to other chemicals of similar structure for which data are already available. The groups of chemicals to which the one under consideration is compared must be close relatives, and careful comparisons are imperative. Implementation of control procedures is best accomplished by close interdisciplinary cooperation with a firm chemical-safety basis. In this manner a suitable safety program can be devised which is applicable to research settings and which has a sound chemistry foundation. Such a safety program should include appropriate safety manuals, hazardous agent use protocols [5] and an effective protocol review system.

The designs and procedures presented in this chapter are not necessarily the final answers to the problems associated with chemical operations with hazardous compounds, but they are at the forefront of current technology. Hopefully they will serve as catalysts in the evolutionary development of better laboratory designs and procedures.

## REFERENCES

1. National Toxicology Program. "Annual Plan, Part 1, Fiscal Year 1980," U.S. Department of Health, Education and Welfare.
2. Harless, J., K. E. Baxter, L. H. Keith and D. B. Walters. "Design and

Operation of a Hazardous Materials Laboratory," in *Safe Handling of Chemical Carcinogens, Mutagens, Teratogens and Highly Toxic Substances, Vol. 1,* D. B. Walters, Ed. (Ann Arbor, MI Ann Arbor Science Publishers, Inc., 1980).

3. Ward, J. T., C. H. Williams, Jr., C. D. Wolbach, L. H. Keith and D. B. Walters. "Transportation of Materials from Radian Corporation's Hazardous Materials Laboratory," in *Safe Handling of Chemical Carcinogens, Mutagens, Teratogens and Highly Toxic Substances, Vol. 1,* D. B. Walters, Ed. (Ann Arbor, MI: Ann Arbor Science Publishers, Inc., 1980).
4. Keith, L. H., J. M. Harless and D. B. Walters. "Analysis and Storage of Hazardous Environmental Chemicals for Toxicological Testing," Chapter 27, this volume.
5. Walters, D. B., J. D. McKinney, A. Norstrom and N. DeWitt. "Control of Potential Carcinogenic, Mutagenic and Toxic Chemicals via a Protocol Review Concept and a Chemistry Containment Laboratory," in *Safe Handling of Chemical Carcinogens, Mutagens, Teratogens and Highly Toxic Substances, Vol. 1,* D. B. Walters, Ed. (Ann Arbor, MI: Ann Arbor Science Publishers, Inc., 1980).

# CHAPTER 27

# ANALYSIS AND STORAGE OF HAZARDOUS ENVIRONMENTAL CHEMICALS FOR TOXICOLOGICAL TESTING

**Lawrence H. Keith and James M. Harless**

Radian Corporation
Austin, Texas

**Douglas B. Walters**

Environmental Chemistry Branch
National Institute of Environmental Health Sciences
Research Triangle Park, North Carolina

## INTRODUCTION

As a result of new tests to determine mutagenic activity of chemicals, the National Institute of Environmental Health Sciences (NIEHS) through the National Toxicology Program (NTP), has begun large-scale screening of environmental chemicals that are potentially hazardous to public health. These chemicals are stored and dispensed as blind samples for mutagenic testing.

Radian Corporation, as a contract laboratory to NTP, obtains sources of the desired chemicals, orders them, places them in inventory when they arrive, and gathers and computerizes information on their chemical, physical and toxicological properties. Aliquots of the chemicals are sent to other contract laboratories which subject these materials to blind mutagenic testing. Compounds that exhibit positive mutagenic response (as well as questionable response and selected negative compounds) are then subjected to chemical fractionation, analysis and further testing to learn whether the parent compound or an impurity is responsible for the mutagenic activity.

To successfully carry out such a program, four requirements are necessary: (1) adequate storage and handling facilities; (2) a comprehensive safety program; (3) a modern analytical laboratory with state-of-the-art equipment; and (4) chemists experienced in working with hazardous materials and analyzing for trace organic and inorganic constituents. In addition, it is useful to have computer hardware and software capable of storing and processing the mass of chemical, physical and toxicological data associated with the handling of large numbers of bulk chemicals and their aliquots.

The following sections describe Radian's approach to implementing these four requirements into a cohesive program that safely and efficiently handles the procurement, storage, handling and analysis of hundreds of hazardous environmental chemicals each year.

## STORAGE AND HANDLING FACILITIES

Radian's hazardous materials laboratory (HML) was designed and built for safe handling of toxic and mutagenic materials. In addition to serving as a chemical repository of hazardous materials from three government agencies [NIEHS, National Cancer Institute (NCI) and the U.S. Environmental Protection Agency (EPA)] , it is used for many other chemical activities that are specially designed facilities for manipulating these chemicals.

The initial commitment to build the HML was made because Radian chemists were increasingly being exposed to potentially hazardous chemicals that were constituents of environmentally derived samples. For example, samples from landfills used to store chemical waste can contain significant amounts of toxic chemicals. Samples from energy related wastes can contain cyanides, polynuclear aromatic hydrocarbons (PAH), and noxious sulfur and nitrogen gases. Samples from industrial wastes can contain all of the above plus heavy metals and a large variety of organic chemicals, the hazards of which are not yet defined. Currently, all environmental samples suspected of containing hazardous materials are prepared for analysis in the HML.

Another use of the HML is for the separation, purification and synthesis of large quantities of hazardous chemicals such as many of EPA's priority pollutants. After synthesis, distillation and recrystallization of large amounts of these compounds are carried out entirely within the confines of this laboratory.

Finally, the HML is also used to prepare and store standard solutions of hazardous environmental chemicals such as 2,3,7,8-tetrachlorodibenzo-*p*-

dioxin (TCDD), nitrosamines and pesticides. These compounds are often needed in dilute solutions for qualitative and quantitative reference standards. They may be needed for an identity confirmation or for a standard against which an identified compound is referenced for quantification. However, for whatever purpose they are required, all of these procedures with the concentrated or pure compounds are carried out in the HML.

## Design of the Radian HML

The principal design philosophy behind the Radian HML was to create a highly versatile facility while ensuring maximum protection against the uncontained exit of contaminating chemicals. This philosophy was translated into a controlled-access structure containing workspaces and equipment capable of supporting a full range of chemical operations. The laboratory building and its utilities/mechanical support system, air handling system and wastewater purification system were all designed to assure operational safety and containment of hazardous materials.

### *Structural and Floor Plan Design*

The Radian HML was constructed as a new facility rather than as a remodeled existing facility. By using this approach, all of the interrelated systems and the desired versatility could be designed without prior constraints imposed by an existing structure. A floor plan of the Radian HML is shown in Figure 1. Although it was built adjacent to an existing building, none of the actual laboratory walls are common to any existing walls; the actual laboratory space and the existing building are separated by utility areas (G and H in Figure 1) and walkways. This arrangement provides a buffer zone between the HML and surrounding structures in case there is an escape of contaminating materials.

The building was designed to easily connect with future additions through existing window openings in the north exterior wall in both the laboratory and dressing areas (C and B, respectively, in Figure 1). It is 1.5 stories high. The main floor of the building houses the showers, dressing rooms and laboratory facilities, and the upper half-floor contains most of the utilities and mechanical equipment serving the laboratory. Interior walls are gypsum wallboard covered with three coats of epoxy polymer based paint. Floors are covered with vinyl sheet flooring, and all seams are sealed by thermal welding. The flooring is coved 6 inches onto all wall surfaces in the laboratory portions of the building. These special coatings, seams, etc., are necessary to reduce leakage, facilitate cleanup, and contain and control contamination.

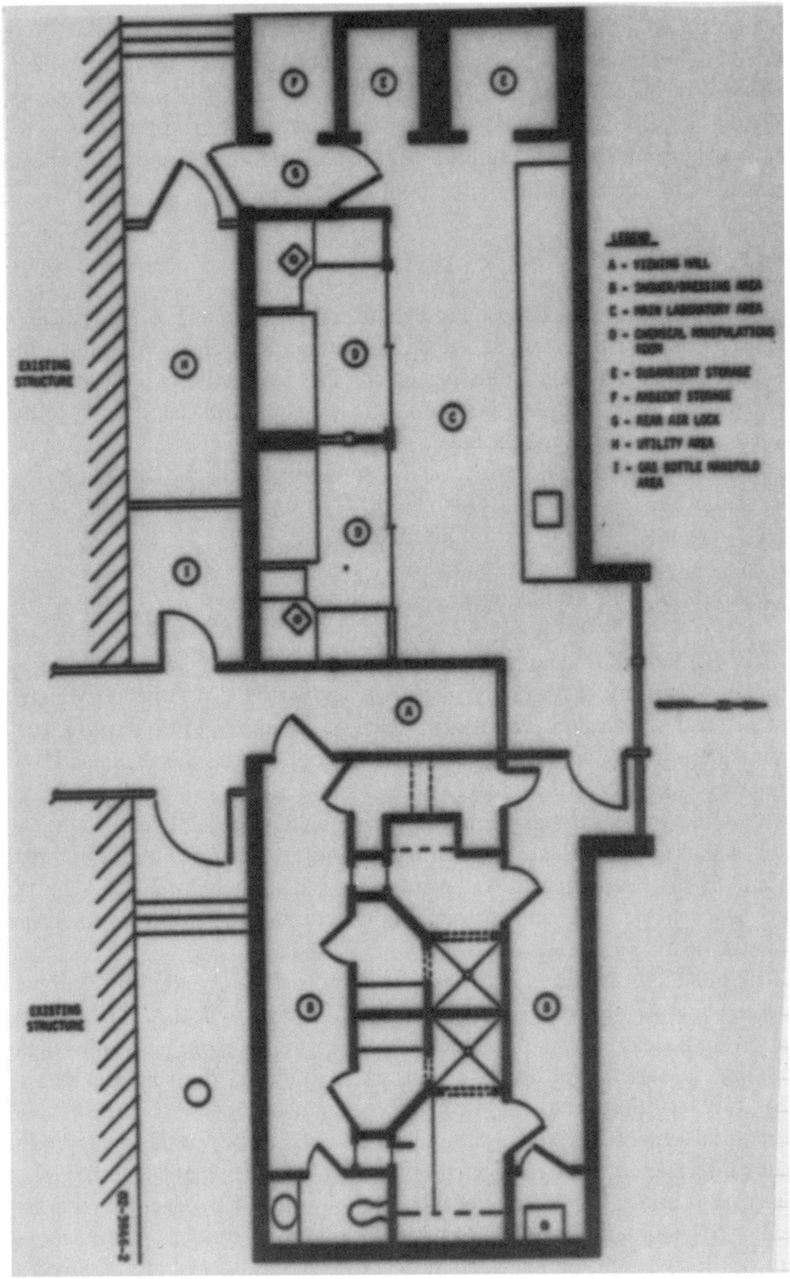

Figure 1. Floor plan of Radian's HML.

Visual observation of virtually all laboratory workspaces is provided by the viewing hall (Area A in Figure 1). A clear view of the fume hood workrooms (D), main laboratory room (C), subambient storage area (E) and safety shower is available in the Radian HML from this hallway. Also located in this hallway is the master control and monitoring panel for the laboratory mechanical support functions. Control switches, operating monitors, and malfunction alarms for the fume hood exhaust and auxiliary air blowers, exhaust air filtering systems, laboratory air conditioning system, lighting and subambient storage areas are located on this panel. By arranging the layout of equipment in this way, visual checks of personnel who are manipulating toxic chemicals, and maintenance of major pieces of equipment can be made without the need to enter the room itself.

The shower and dressing area of the HML (Area B in Figure 1) provides personnel access to the laboratory. Facilities are provided for removal and storage of street clothes, dressing into laboratory clothing and showering. Laboratory clothing and respirators are stored in the inner dressing area and in the inner hallway. Hampers for containment of used, washable materials are provided; these are emptied from the exterior hallway. Passage between the dressing areas is accomplished by going through the shower area, although a shower is required only when leaving the facility at the end of a work period. Restroom facilities are provided in the external area of the dressing area to ensure that the laboratory personnel go through the proper decontamination procedures before using these facilities.

The main laboratory (Area C in Figure 1) contains general workspaces and storage areas. This area is always operated at a negative pressure with respect to both the dressing area and the outside atmosphere. This is to prevent the escape of any chemical material that might be present in the laboratory atmosphere.

The chemical handling rooms (Area D in Figure 1) are isolated from the main laboratory area by glass walls and sliding glass doors, and are operated at a negative pressure with respect to the main laboratory area. All hazardous materials are handled in these rooms unless a glove box is required. The handling rooms are equipped with stainless steel fume hoods and epoxy-topped laboratory benches. All air leaving the facility is exhausted through the fume hoods in these rooms and is filtered and decontaminated before release to the atmosphere.

Chemical storage areas are located at the west end of the main laboratory (Areas E and F in Figure 1). Two subambient storage areas (E), one at 5°C and the other at 20°C, and an ambient temperature storage area (F) are available.

The airlock (Area G in Figure 1) for receiving and exiting of chemicals and equipment is located at the rear of the facility. This area was incorporated into the building design so that materials could be transferred into and out of the laboratory without allowing direct contact between the outside environment and the laboratory atmosphere. The airlock is operated so that both doors cannot be opened at the same time.

The electrical control panels, hot water heater, vacuum pump and laundry facilities are located in the utility area (H). Access to mechanical services located in the chase area above the laboratory and on the roof is provided through this room. Compressed air, argon and nitrogen are supplied to the laboratory from gas bottle manifolds (Area I in Figure 1).

Several areas of the HML are not shown in Figure 1. The wastewater treatment area and the emergency auxiliary generator are located outside the west end of the building. A five-foot high space over the entire structure provides access to all plumbing, electrical conduits and relays, refrigeration equipment for the subambient storage rooms, and some of the air handling equipment. Supply and exhaust blowers for the fume hoods, the exhaust air purification system and cooling equipment are located on the roof of the laboratory building.

*Mechanical/Utilities Design*

In the layout for the building, all pipes and conduits carrying utility services were located in the overhead space above the laboratory whenever possible, and entrance into the laboratory facility was accomplished through the ceiling or walls as required. Whenever a hole had to be cut in the wall, the area around the incoming pipe or conduit was completely sealed, first by polyurethane foam and then by a silicone polymer sealant. This was done to assure minimal release of air contaminants to the atmosphere except by passage through air pollution control equipment.

Hot, cold and deionized water are all supplied to the laboratory from pre-existing facilities. All water outlets in the HML are fitted with vacuum-breakers to prevent backflow of water into the service lines.

Electricity is normally supplied to the HML through electrical circuit panels in Utility Room H (Figure 1). However, because hazardous materials are stored at subambient temperatures in the HML and the isolation of the facility depends on the maintenance of negative pressure inside, the HML electrical system is equipped with an auxiliary generator. This natural gas-fired, 30-kW generator is designed to automatically begin operation and supply enough power to support critical laboratory functions in the event of a power failure. The fume hood exhaust blowers, the air conditioner fans, the subambient storage refrigeration units and approximately half of the laboratory lighting are supplied electricity from the auxiliary generator. After restoration of normal electrical power, the generator turns off, and full operation of all electrical equipment is restored.

The design of the air handling and purification system was the most complex part of Radian's HML development. A schematic of the air movement system in the HML is shown in Figure 2. The system consists basically of three parts: one exhaust section consisting of the two fume hood exhaust blowers, and two air supply sections, one of which is the air conditioning system which supplies heated or cooled air to the working portions of the laboratory, and the other is the fume hoods' auxiliary air blowers, which supply makeup ambient air for the hood exhausts. The total exhausted air is balanced against the total supplied air so as to create a negative pressure inside the HML dressing area (-0.03 in. wp static pressure) and main laboratory area (-0.006 in. wp static pressure) with respect to atmospheric pressure. Negative pressure (-0.1 in. wp static pressure) is also maintained in the chemical manipulation rooms relative to the main laboratory room.

The airflows inside the laboratory are governed by the amount of air exhausted through the fume hoods. These exhausts are set to establish a 125-ft/min or greater face velocity across the hood openings with the sashes in the fully opened position. Approximately 60% of this exhausted air is supplied by the auxiliary air blowers associated with each hood, and 40% is supplied by the air conditioning system.

Air passes continuously into the laboratory area from the dressing/shower area at a rate of 100 $ft^3$/min through a bypass vent located above the entrance door. When the door is opened, the vent closes, and the air is swept through the door opening. This prevents any air inside the laboratory from escaping into the outer areas. A similar flow pattern is established at the entrance to the chemical manipulation rooms. An airflow of 450 $ft^3$/min is maintained through bypass vents until the doors are opened. The air is then drawn through the door opening to prevent escape of air from the rooms into the main laboratory area.

All of the air exhausted from each fume hood is drawn through a filtration/purification unit before discharge into the atmosphere (see Figure 2). One Flanders Model E2 bag-out filtration unit is used for each hood exhaust system and is located just upstream of the exhaust blowers. This system employs a 24- x 24-in. HEPA 0.5-$\mu$ prefilter for collecting dusts and mists, a 24- x 144- x 2-in. charcoal adsorbent bed for trapping organic vapors, followed by a second 24- x 24-in. HEPA filter to trap any contaminated carbon dust that might be released from the carbon filter. This system is adequate for the ~1200-$ft^3$/min exhaust flow from each hood. The status of each HEPA filter is continuously monitored on magnehelic gauges located in the main control panel (Area A, Figure 1). They indicate the pressure drop ($\Delta$P) across each HEPA filter, and when the $\Delta$P across a filter reaches a value approximately three times that registered when the filter is new, the filter is changed. A system for monitoring the activity of the carbon adsorbent for the wide range of compounds stored and used in the repository has not yet been

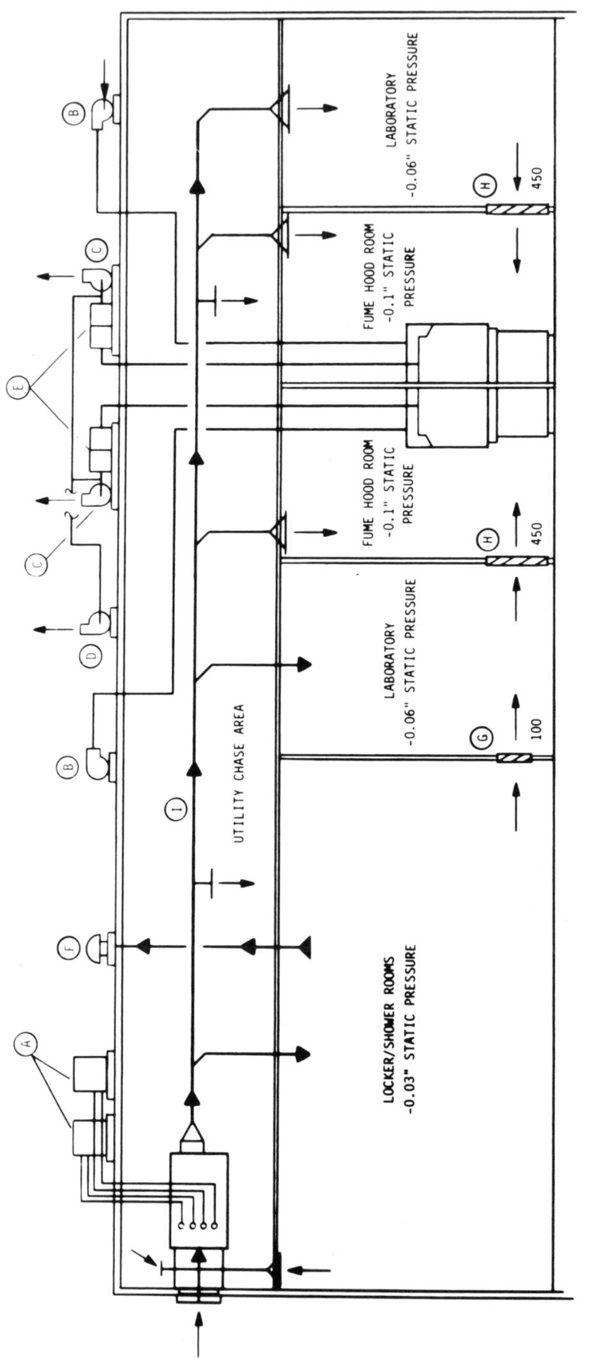


**Figure 2.** Schematic of the Radian HML air handling system.

devised; that filter is routinely changed every 6–12 months depending on the number of hours the fume hoods are in use and the types of operations performed in them.

Filter changing is performed using the Flanders bag-out system. When the filters are installed, large plastic bags are attached around the filter access opening. When a filter is changed, it is disconnected and pulled into the bag with the bag serving as a barrier between the person changing the filter and the contaminated filter. After removal, the filter is sealed in the bag, and the whole unit is incinerated at temperatures exceeding 2000°F.

As shown in Figure 2, an auxiliary exhaust blower was designed into the fume hood exhaust system. Under normal operating conditions, the two main exhaust blowers are used, one for each fume hood. An auxiliary blower is inoperative and isolated from the exhaust ducts by dampers. If a main exhaust blower fails for any reason, pressure sensors in the duct sense the resulting pressure change and automatically activate the auxiliary exhaust blower. The appropriate dampers are also actuated to isolate the malfunctioning blower and open the exhaust duct to the auxiliary blower. Simultaneously with the above activity, the pressure sensors also activate the main alarm system in the control panel. A second alarm sounds if the auxiliary blower has not returned the exhaust system to normal operation within 2-3 min after failure of the main exhaust blower. Once the main blower is placed back in full operation, the auxiliary blower stops operation, and the dampers return to their normal positions.

The design of the wastewater treatment system for Radian's HML is based on a system reported by Nony et al. [1]. The design is based on application of physical separation processes involving solid-liquid contacting equipment. The system, shown schematically in Figure 3, consists of a holding tank, pump, solid particulate filters and activated carbon and nonionic polymeric resin adsorbents arranged in series. The Radian system uses a 500-gal holding tank to receive all the waste water from the main laboratory and chemical manipulations areas of the HML. As the tank fills, a level sensor activates the pump which draws water from the tank and forces it through the filtering and adsorbing system and then into the city sanitary sewer network. The water flows sequentially through 40-, 25- and 5-$\mu$ particulate filters, ~0.75 ft$^3$ of activated charcoal and ~0.75 ft$^3$ of Amberlite XAD-2 resin. The system is constructed using two parallel filtering/adsorbing trains so that one train is available for use while the other is being replaced. The particulate filters and adsorbents are replaced twice yearly unless routine analysis of the effluent reveals that organic materials from the laboratory are present.

The operation of the wastewater purification system is continually monitored by a level sensing switch located inside the tank. The switch is con-

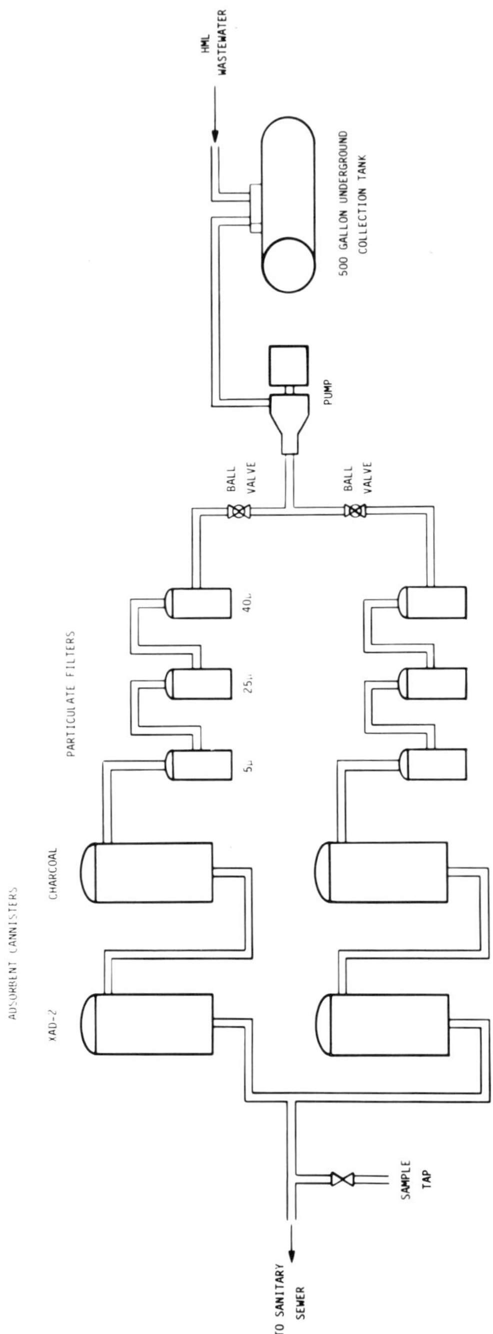


**Figure 3.** Schematic of the Radian HML wastewater treatment system.

nected to a time delay relay so that if the pump does not reduce the water level in the tank within 3 min after it is turned on, an alarm is activated on the main control panel.

## COMPREHENSIVE SAFETY PROGRAM

Safety in the HML is even more important than it is in Radian's other laboratories because of the higher risk factor associated with exposure to hazardous chemicals. In addition to a comprehensive safety and operations manual that everyone working in the HML is required to read and abide by, HML personnel are trained in location and operation of all the emergency equipment, firefighting, decontamination procedures and first aid.

Safety is also integrated into all the operating procedures of the HML. These procedures cover the four primary areas involved in daily laboratory operation: personnel protection, materials handling, waste disposal and decontamination.

It should be emphasized that the first line of defense in handling hazardous materials must always be institution of containment principles and proper engineering controls. Employees need to exercise caution and not become overly reliant on personnel protective devices. A false sense of security can develop which can lead to poor work practices and a resulting covert exposure to hazardous chemicals.

Personnel protection must be designed to provide maximum protection for personnel working in the facility, and they must minimize the risk of accidental contamination of outside areas by laboratory personnel. The principal personnel protection procedures for the Radian HML include procedures for entrance into the laboratory, protection during normal operations and exit from the laboratory.

Personnel entering the HML first remove all street clothing in the exterior dressing room. After passing through the shower area and into the interior dressing room, they don washable, two piece laboratory scrub suits and tennis shoes. Disposable coveralls and shoe covers made of Tyvek® (DuPont Corporation, 100% high density polyethylene fibers) are then put on over the washable undersuits; Tyvek head covers are also used when working with highly hazardous materials. The Tyvek lab wear is impervious to most chemicals and affords good protection from spilled materials. The outer Tyvek clothing is discarded and the scrub suits and shoes are laundered in the HML laundry facility. Before entering the laboratory, personnel put on two pair of gloves to prevent contamination of the hands. The first pair are latex surgeon's gloves and the outer pair are vinyl plastic or other suitable material. Gloves of different materials, hence different permeabilities for chemicals encountered, are used to decrease the chances of a chemical permeating through the gloves to the skin.

Personnel in Radian's HML are required to wear some type of respiration device whenever they are working with open chemicals (except in the glove box) and when they enter any of the three chemical storage areas. Half-face and full-face respirators (equipped with both particulate and organic vapor cartridges), and airline respirators are provided. Cartridge respirators are used when compounds of low to moderate hazard are being manipulated, and airline respirators are used when working with highly hazardous compounds such as known carcinogens and toxins.

The second area of procedures design involving personnel protection is work area selection. In Radian's HML, the two work areas for handling chemicals are the fume hoods and the glove box. Compounds determined to be highly hazardous or air-sensitive are handled in the glove box, and all others are handled in the fume hoods.

Procedures for exiting the HML have been developed for two situations: (1) leaving the laboratory during regular work periods but remaining inside the Radian complex, and (2) leaving the Radian premises. When leaving for short periods of time, the HML personnel are required to remove all Tyvek protective clothing, shoe covers, respirators and gloves, and wash all exposed skin surfaces (face, neck, arms and hands) with soap and water. They may then exit wearing their scrub suits and tennis shoes. Full showers are not required for exit under these circumstances. When personnel exit the laboratory to leave the Radian complex, they remove and discard the Tyvek clothing and remove and store all other laboratory apparel. Filter cartridges are removed from respirators, and the respirators are washed with soap and water. Washings are processed through the Radian wastewater treatment system shown in Figure 3. After they shower, they can then leave the facility.

## Materials Handling Procedures

The three material handling operations normally conducted in the HML are chemicals storage, chemicals manipulation and transfer of materials out of the laboratory. Chemicals stored in the HML are packaged in hypovials or in screw-cap glass bottles and steel cans.

All chemical manipulations are performed on plastic trays covered with abosrbent paper to provide initial containment of any spills. Packages of materials received from outside sources are placed on trays and opened in a fume hood. The fume hood sash is closed to a position to assure an air velocity of greater than 150 ft/min across the opening before the packages are opened. Tests have shown that dusts arising from packing materials are swept into the hood exhaust under these conditions.

Hazardous materials transported within the Radian facilities are crimp-sealed in hypovials fitted with Teflon®-face septa, the vials are decontaminated by washing with one or more appropriate solvents, and the washings are treated as described above.

*Waste Disposal Procedures*

The major nonaqueous wastes generated from the Radian HML are the discarded expendable laboratory materials and waste chemicals. These wastes are divided into burnable and non-burnable materials inside the laboratory and are disposed of accordingly. Burnable materials, including most chemicals, laboratory clothing and packaging materials, are incinerated at greater than 2000°F in a commercial natural gas-fired incinerator. Noncombustible packing materials such as vermiculite are buried at a commercial chemical disposal site. All waste materials leaving the HML are double-bagged in heavy polyethylene bags and labeled as biohazard materials.

*Contamination Monitoring and Decontamination Procedures*

The Radian HML is periodically monitored for build-up of chemical contamination both in the air and on laboratory surfaces. Routine decontamination of the laboratory work surfaces are performed weekly, and when indicated by monitoring procedures or a chemical spill, additional decontamination procedures are initiated.

Routine air monitoring in the HML is performed at least quarterly using the NIOSH charcoal tube sampling procedure. Laboratory air is drawn through the tube for an 8-hr period, and the charcoal adsorbent is extracted with carbon disulfide or other suitable solvent. The extract is analyzed by gas chromatography using flame ionization and electron capture detectors, and chromatograms from each sample are compared to those from blank samples collected before initiation of HML operation. The presence of new compounds or higher concentrations of preexisting compounds indicates that a contamination problem exists.

Laboratory surface samples are also collected and analyzed at least quarterly to monitor contamination levels. Cotton swabs saturated with hexane and methylene chloride are used to collect samples from six 100-$cm^2$ surface areas in the laboratory. These areas are on walls in the main laboratory area, each manipulation room and each storage area. The swabs are extracted with acetone and analyzed by hexane and methylene chloride methods analogous to the charcoal extracts above.

Figure 4 shows a gas chromatogram of one of the background wall swipes taken before the HML was placed into operation. Superimposed above it is the chromatogram of a wall swipe taken three months later and analyzed under identical conditions. One large peak is seen to have built up during this time. Figure 5 shows the total ion chromatogram and the mass spectrum of the compound that comprised that peak. Analysis of the data reveals that the new peak is caused by *bis*(2-ethylhexyl) phthalate, a common and ubiquitous contaminant. Although no hazardous compounds have yet been

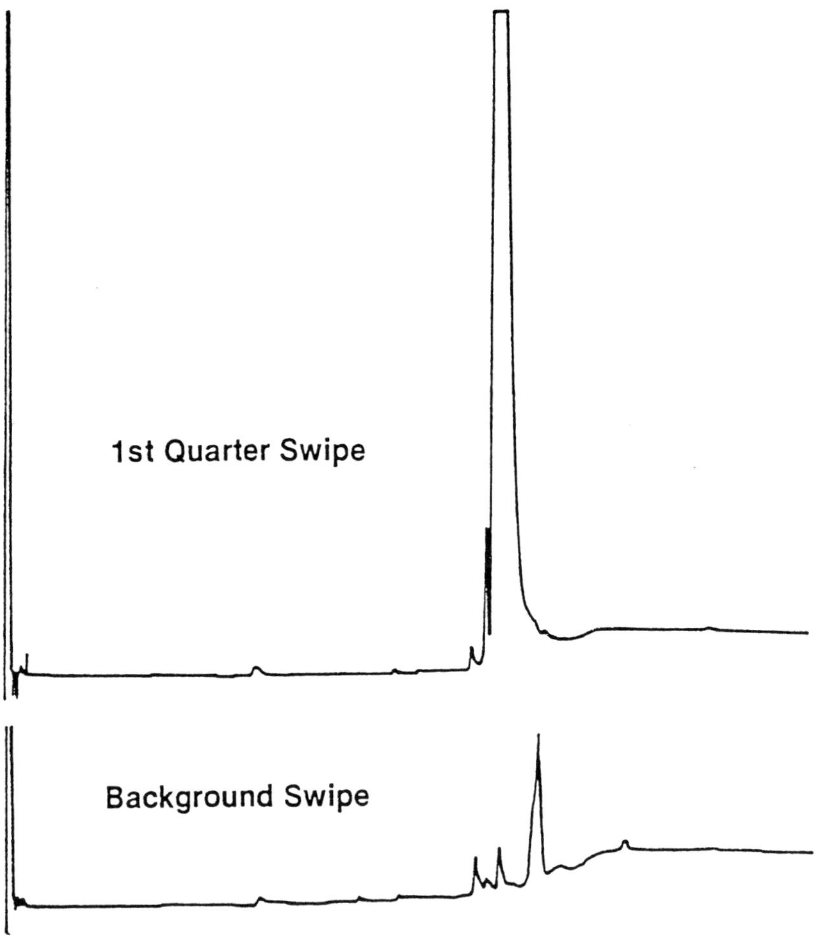


**Figure 4.** Gas chromatogram using $^{63}Ni$ electron capture detector of HML wall swipes.

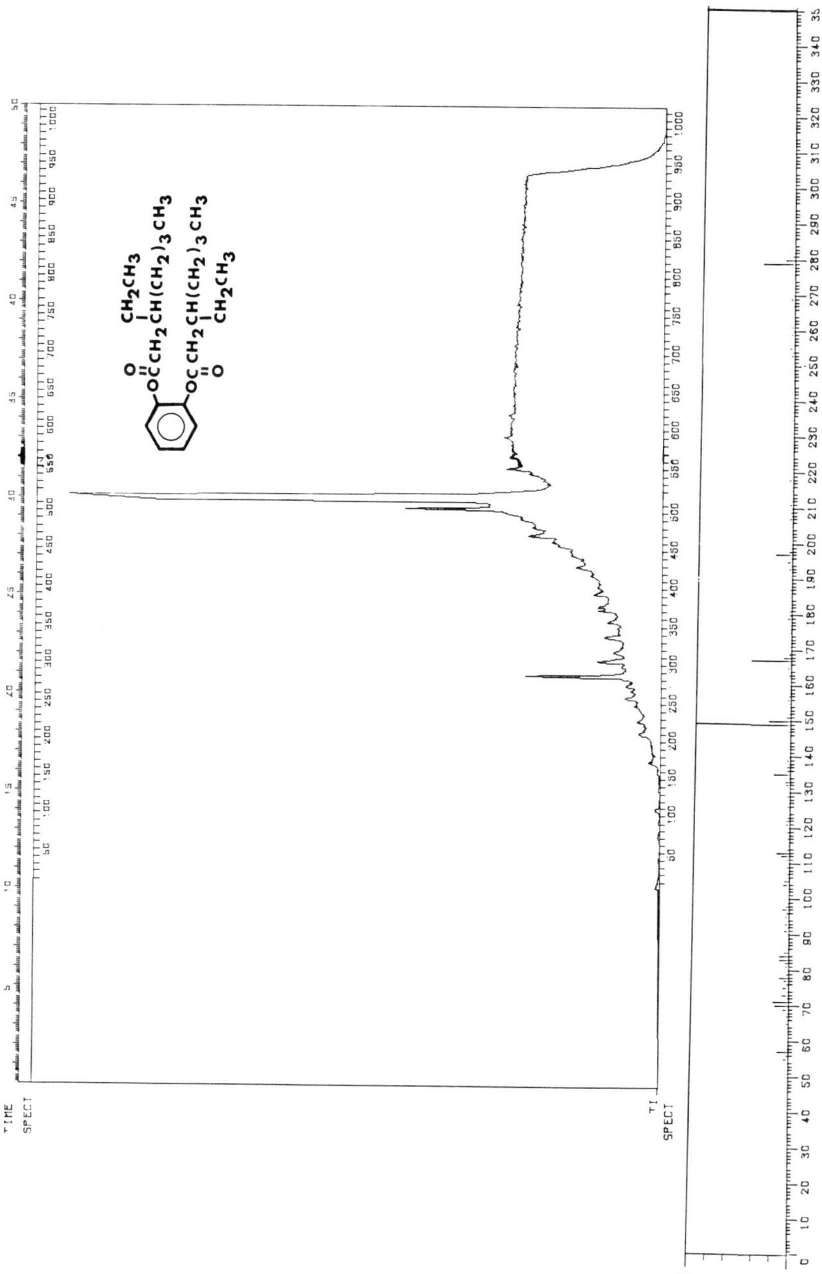

**Figure 5.** Total ion chromatogram and mass spectrum of contaminant *bis* (2-ethylhexyl) phthalate.

found to be building up in the HML, the monitoring techniques employed should provide an indication if this occurs. Compounds that are not sensitive to the electron capture detector (and the majority of the hazardous chemicals are) will be sensitive to the general purpose flame ionization detector.

Routine decontamination of the HML consists of weekly washings of the floor and all horizontal surfaces where chemical deposits might build up. Decontamination is done using strong detergent solutions with all washings treated by the system shown in Figure 3. If air or swab samples indicate that a contamination problem exists, the entire laboratory area will be thoroughly washed with a strong detergent solution. Solvent washes will be used if the contamination persists. Sponges and mops used for laboratory cleaning are discarded after each use.

Decontamination procedures used for chemical spills are divided into two methods, one for liquids and one for solids. Liquid spills are generally handled by collecting the material onto absorbent paper followed by washing the area with strong detergent. Absorbent paper saturated with an appropriate solvent is then used for a final wash of the area. Solids spilled in the laboratory are collected on dampened absorbent paper, and the area is cleaned as above. All laboratory clothing worn during decontamination procedures is immediately removed and replaced with new clothing. All contaminated materials are double-bagged in polyethylene bags and incincerated. Self-contained, acid-resistant suits are used to remove spills of highly hazardous materials which would pose a threat to personnel in normal laboratory attire. These suits are located outside of the HML to prevent them from being contaminated and to prevent decontamination teams from being exposed to hazardous chemicals before they are fully protected. Spill cleanup procedures are the same as described earlier.

## COMPUTERIZED INVENTORY

The large number of compounds being handled and the mass of data associated with each one can be handled reasonably only by a computer. A software program was written by Radian computer personnel especially for managing these data. It is designed so that chemists and technicians with no previous computer experience can use it after receiving rudimentary instruction.

The computerized data fall into three main categories: inventory information (e.g., quantity, purity and date of receipt), aliquot information (e.g., where and when the chemical was shipped and how much was sent) and catalog information (e.g., chemical, physical and toxicological properties, and safety procedures). Data forms are provided with spaces for all the required information for all three types of data. These are filled out and filed to provide a permanent original copy of all computerized data. Generally, standard references [2-14] are consulted for the relevant information. If insufficient data are located, selected special sources are searched and these are chosen individually as the situation requires.

The information is entered into a Data General M-600 Eclipse computer using one of two Radian/Unitech terminals equipped with cathode ray tubes (CRT) and dual floppy discs. The software program is interactive, providing a dialog between the computer and the chemical technician.

Figure 6 lists the 16 interactive options that are used to enter or to retrieve data. The first option (0) provides one of the unique safety features of Radian's HML. By typing "0" plus any "key identifier," emergency information is called up and immediately displayed on the CRT for the compound of concern.

**Enter the Number of One of These Items:**

0. Emergency treatment and measures
1. Add data about a new chemical to the catalog
2. Delete a catalog entry
3. Log in a new sample (inventory information only)
4. Log out an aliquot
5. Log an unused aliquot back into the repository
6. Change catalog or inventory data
7. Get catalog data about a chemical
8. Print catalog summary table
9. Get inventory status information for a sample
10. Get inventory alert information
11. Get data about an aliquot
12. Get aliquot shipping information
13. Print safety/emergency documentation
14. Get catalog data for all chemicals
15. Log out of the system
16. Help

**Figure 6.** Software options.

"Key identifers" include the primary name under which the compound is cataloged, synonyms, the Radian HML repository number, a secondary identification number or the Chemical Abstracts Service (CAS) number. Figure 7 illustrates the type of information that is available from the emergency data output. Because one of the two Radian/Unitech terminals is located in the main laboratory area of the HML, access to this information is immediate by the personnel working with the hazardous compounds.

## NIEHS REPOSITORY
## 1,1-DICHLOROETHYLENE

## EMERGENCY TREATMENT AND MEASURES

**PERSONAL PROTECTION:**

In an emergency situation involving this chemical, all personnel must be protected from any exposure or contact with the chemical, its vapor or decomposition products.

Choose from among the following personal protection devices on the basis of their availability, the hazards of the chemical compound and the degree of risk in the emergency situation:

* An impervious full-body suit equipped with an air line respirator or a self-contained breathing apparatus, e.g. an MSA neoprene acid suit.

or

* A full-body impervious jump suit (e.g. of Tyvek [TM]), one or two pairs of gloves of neoprene, nitrile or latex rubber taped to form a seal with the jump suit, rubber boots or impervious shoe covers, an impervious hood, and most importantly, a full-face airline respirator. A full-faced or half-face (plus goggles) cartridge respirator can also be used if equipped with an organic vapor or combination organic vapor + particulate cartridge.

  Refer to other instructions for special precautions or safety devices for this chemical.

**FIRE FIGHTING:**

The inhalation of smoke from a fire involving this chemical is dangerous and potentially fatal. Firefighters should wear an impervious full-body suit with an air line or self-contained breathing apparatus. Extinguish fires with a dry chemical, carbon dioxide, foam or halon extinguisher. A water spray can also be used.

**FIRST AID:**

Skin contact - Flood skin with water from a safety shower or faucet. Remove any contaminated clothing. Wash affected skin area thoroughly with soap and water.

Eye contact - Flush eyes immediately with water from any source for 15 minutes. Remove contact lenses at once. Do not use oil or ointment in the eyes. If eyes become light sensitive, cover with a loose dressing.

Inhalation - Remove personnel to open air. Administer oxygen or artificial respiration as required.

Ingestion - If victim is convulsing or unconscious, do not attempt first aid, but transport immediately to hospital emergency room or poison control center. If victim is conscious, do not induce vomiting. Have the patient drink up to one quart of one of the following to dilute the poison and slow absorption: milk, beaten eggs or activated charcoal in water (1 gram charcoal/100 mg poison ingested). Transport immediately to medical facility for gastric lavage (stomach pumping) or emesis (induced vomiting).

Important! With any exposure and after any initial treatment, victim should be transported promptly for medical examination. Report the incident to a supervisor or company official.

**SPILLS AND LEAKAGE:**

Use absorbent paper to pick up small quantities of spilled material: dry paper for liquids, moistened paper for solids. Observe all measures of personal exposure protection listed above in cleaning up spilled chemical. Contaminated clothing and absorbent paper should be sealed inside vapor-tight, double-sealed plastic bags for eventual high temperature incineration. Wash contaminated surface areas with strong detergent and water or with the solvent listed in the safety and handling document.

**DISPOSAL AND WASTE TREATMENT:**

Destroy all waste and contaminated materials in a special, high temperature (>2000 degrees F) chemical incinerator facility.

**Figure 7.** Emergency treatment data output.

The Catalog Summary Table (Option No. 8 in Figure 6) lists each compound in inventory and provides its Radian HML repository number, any secondary identification number assigned and its CAS number. Another option used is the request for information on a certain chemical in the Repository. The format and type of information obtainable for each compound is listed in Figure 8. A variation on this format is provided by Option No. 9 in Figure 6. Inventory status information consists of the primary chemical name, the amount present in inventory and the "status" of the inventory. The latter refers to a predetermined amount of each chemical below which the inventory is not wished to drop. If the amount in inventory is below the "alert status" quantity, an asterisk is printed in the "status" column. This serves to notify HML personnel that additional material should be ordered. Generally, the alert status is 10–25 g, unless a particular compound is very expensive and not obtainable in 100-g quantities. Originally, 100-g amounts of each chemical were inventoried but this quantity has now been increased to 500-g amounts when practical. Figure 9 shows an example of the option that details all of the inventory information concerning a particular compound. It not only keeps a running account of the inventory supply but also lists where the compound was purchased, how much was received, when it was received, the alert (minimum) amount to be kept in inventory and other pertinent comments.

All of the catalog information about a chemical can be retrieved using Option No. 7 in Figure 6. This information is divided into four categories: identifiers, physical data, toxicity data and emergency treatment and measures. An example of the type of physical and toxicity data available from this output is shown in Figure 10.

Aliquot information is also stored in the data base and is available on demand. Aliquots are shipped as unknown samples to various laboratories for mutagenic testing. Blind samples are necessary to ensure the validity of the data since known mutagens and known nonmutagens are interspersed with test samples. A random six digit number is generated by the computer for

| Sample | Amount | Location | Status |
|---|---|---|---|
| Benzo(a)pyrene | 14.7 | A1L | |
| Dimethylnitrosamine | 94 | C1L | |
| Hexachloroethane | 298.5 | C1L | |
| Calcium Chromate (1:1) Anhydrous | 94.7 | A1L | |
| Potassium Chloride | 88.9 | A1L | |
| Choline Chloride | 219.9 | C1L | |
| Glycine | 131.3 | A1LP | |
| Glycerol | 229.65 | A1L | |
| 2,3-Dichlorophenol | 93.8 | C2L | |
| 1,4-Dichlorobenzene | 91.52 | C2L | |
| 3,4-Dichloronitrobenzene | 94.9 | C2L | |
| 2,4-Dichlorophenol | 83.79 | | |
| 2,3-Dichloronitrobenzene | 93.4 | C2L | |
| Pentachlorobenzene | 89.5 | C3L | |
| 2,4-Dichloronitrobenzene | 102.67 | C3L | |
| Dimethylcarbamyl Chloride | 108.3 | C1L | |
| Streptomycin Sulfate (2:3) (Salt) | 93.48 | C1L | |
| 2′-Methyl-4-(Dimethylamino)azobenzene | 9.4 | C1L | |
| 4-Aminobiphenyl | 90.3 | C1L | |
| Sodium Azide | 96.4 | A1L | |
| 1,2-Dichlorobenzene | 198.38 | A2L | |
| 1,2-Propylene Glycol | 203 | A2L | |
| Beta-Picoline | 135.72 | C2L | |
| Thioglycolic Acid, Sodium Salt | 107.6 | A2L | |
| Tetrachlorophthalic Anhydride | 302.8 | C2L | |
| Carbon Disulfide | 393.3 | C2L | |
| Meta-Cresol | 0 | | |
| Para-Cresol | 466.05 | | |
| Morpholine | 182.28 | B1L | |
| 4-Chloronitrobenzene | 263.63 | C2L | |
| 2-Chloronitrobenzene | 210.63 | C1L | |
| Ethylenediamine | 140.26 | C3L | |

**Figure 8.** Current inventory status output.

each aliquot that is shipped under the NTP. This ensures a number is impossible to decode. It is kept secret and requires a secret access password to be obtained from the computer. Figure 11 is an output from a dummy aliquot file used to show this information that is available and its format.

Two types of computer-generated documents are sent with every aliquot shipped to a testing laboratory: a Safety and Handling Document (SHD) and an Emergency Procedures Document (EPD). The SHD provides all the information necessary to safely work with that chemical without divulging its identity. In addition, a physical description of the chemical is provided so that the receiving laboratory can verify that the compound has

**INVENTORY STATUS INFORMATION**

**TRANS-1,2-DICHLOROETHYLENE**

**RADIAN ID #N-000138** **SECONDARY ID #79-072**

| | |
|---|---|
| STORAGE LOCATION: | BIL |
| SUPPLIER: | ALDRICH |
| SUPPLIER'S CATALOG #: | D6,220-9 |
| LOT/BATCH #: | MC 092887 |
| CONDITION RECEIVED: | OK |
| QUANTITY RECEIVED (GM): | 100 |
| DATE OF RECEIPT: | 09/04/79 |
| AMOUNT INVENTORIED (GM): | 96.12 |
| DATE OF INVENTORY: | 10/05/79 |
| INVENTORIED BY: | HRP |
| ALERT AMOUNT (GM): | 15 |
| GRADE: | 98 PER CENT |
| COMMENTS (ANALYSIS): | NOT SPECIFIED |
| CURRENT AMOUNT (GM): | 96.12 |
| ALERT STATUS: | 0 |
| DATE ENTERED: | THU 16 AUG 79 |
| DATA ENTERED BY: | HRP |

**Figure 9.** Variation available in inventory status information.

not changed composition during the shipment. For example, if the physical description accompanying an aliquot was "colorless liquid" and the compound received was amber in color an immediate problem would be identified. An example of an SHD is shown in Figure 12.

The EPD accompanies the SHD but is in a separate, sealed colored envelope. The seal is such that it cannot be tampered with without evidence of the tampering being obvious. At the same time the envelope is easily opened in an emergency, such as a spillage. The EPD identifies the material and contains all relevant safety and emergency information that Radian chemists have been able to find on it. An example of an EPD is shown in Figure 13.

## ANALYTICAL REQUIREMENTS

Two general types of analyses are required when working with hazardous materials that are being tested for biological activity. The first type is a chemical assay. The assay simply determines or verifies the purity of the chemical(s) to be tested. If there are major impurities (greater than 1%) in the sample these are usually identified and quantified. The importance of con-

## NIEHS REPOSITORY
## TRANS-1,2-DICHLOROETHYLENE

### PHYSICAL DATA

**MOLECULAR WEIGHT:** 96.94

**DENSITY:** 1.2743 @ 25/4

**MP(DEG C):** -49.4

**BP(DEG C):** 47.2 @ /745

**SOLUBILITY:**

Water: Slightly (0.1-1g/100 ml)
Alcohol: Very (> 10g/100 ml)
Ether: Very (> 10g/100 ml)
Acetone: Very (> 10g/100 ml)
Benzene: Very (> 10g/100 ml)
Chloroform: Very (> 10g/100 ml)

**FLAMMABILITY:** 3
Material can be ignited under most ambient conditions.

**REACTIVITY:** 2
May release explosive chloroacetylene on contact with copper and alloys.

**STABILITY:** Not specified

### TOXICITY

**NIOSH REGISTRY NUMBER:** KV94000

**TOXICITY:**

| TYP. Dose | Mode | Specie | Amount | Unit | |
|---|---|---|---|---|---|
| TCLO | IHL | HMN | 4800 | MG/M3/10M | TFX:CNS |
| LCLO | IHL | MUS | 75000 | MG/M3/2H | |
| LD50 | ORL | RAT | 770 | MG/KG | |

**AQTX/TLM96:** Not specified

**SAX TOXICITY EVALUATION:** Not specified

Acute Local: Inhalation 1
Acute Systemic: Ingestion 2; Inhalation 2; Skin Absorption 2
Chronic Local: Irritant 1
Chronic Systemic: Unknown

**CARCINOGENICITY:**
NIO, VOL. 1, CH.2
OSHA: Not listed

**MUTAGENICITY:**
NIO, VOL. 1, CH. 4 – Not listed

**TERATOGENICITY:**
NIO, VOL. 1, CH. 3 – Not listed
NIO, VOL. 1, CH. 5

**OTHER COMMENT:** Flash Point . . . 43 F.
TLV . . . 200 ppm.
Shipping Regulation: (Rail) Red Label
(Air) Flammable Liquid Label

**SOURCES:**
NIOSH Registry of Toxic Effects (1977): Listed
CRC Handbook of Chemistry (56th): Pg. C-292
The Merck Index (9th): Pg. 12
Dangerous Properties of Industrial Materials (4th): Pg. 629
Toxic and Hazardous Industrial Chemicals Safety Manual (1978): Pg. 165
Condensed Chemical Dictionary (9th): Pg. 279
Aldrich Catalog Handbook of Fine Chemicals (1979-1980): Pg. 293
Chemical Hazards of the Workplace (1978): Not listed
Toxic Substances Control Act Chemical Substances Inventory (1979): Listed
CRC Handbook of Lab Safety (1976): Pg. 754

**Figure 10.** Chemical, physical and toxicity data available.

**ALIQUOT STATUS INFORMATION**

**TRANS-1,2-DICHLOROETHYLENE**

**RADIAN ID #N-000138** **SECONDARY ID #79-072**

ALIQUOT CODE: 785794
ALIQUOT SIZE (GMS): 0
ALIQUOTTED BY: HRP
SHIPPED TO: 1
DATE SHIPPED: 00/00/00
SHIPMENT CARRIER: AIR FREIGHT
BILL OF LADING #: 1111111
RECEIPT CONFIRMATION DATE: 00/00/00
COMMENT: SHIPPED UNDER DRY ICE.
DATE ENTERED: THU 16 AUG 79
DATA ENTERED BY: HRP

**Figure 11.** Output from aliquot file used for shipping samples.

## NIEHS REPOSITORY FOR MUTAGENIC TESTING

## SAFETY AND HANDLING DOCUMENT

## ALIQUOT NUMBER 785794

### TYPES OF HAZARD

Toxic. Irritant. Flammable.

### HAZARD PRECAUTIONS

Handle unknown chemicals with extreme care. Avoid all skin contact, inhalation or ingestion of this chemical or its vapor, solutions or decomposition products, such as smoke or fume. Protect from high temperatures and ignition sources, such as flames or sparks. Personnel handling this chemical should be experienced, aware of its hazards and protected by a complete set of personal protection devices (described below). Report any spill, leakage or personnel exposure to a supervisor or laboratory official. Refer to other instructions below for any special precautions or protective devices for this chemical.

Important! In case of an emergency, open the accompanying sealed emergency procedure document with the same aliquot number. This sealed document will identify the test chemical and give specific first aid instructions. Exposed personnel must receive medical evaluation as soon as possible.

### SAFETY DEVICES AND PROTECTORS

Handle only in an approved fume hood with auxiliary personal protection devices including rubber gloves, impervious disposable lab coat, goggles and a half-face respirator with a combination particulate-organic vapor cartridge. Handle on a tray covered with absorbent paper to contain any spill or leakage.

Firefighters must wear an impervious full-body protection with a self-contained breathing apparatus or air line. One or more of the following types of fire extinguishers must be immediately available: dry chemical, carbon dioxide, foam or halon.

Personnel handling the test chemicals must be trained in and thoroughly familiar with the use of the personal protection devices listed above.

### SPILLS AND LEAKAGE

Use absorbent paper to pick up small quantities of spilled material: dry paper for liquids, moistened paper for solids. Observe all measures of personal exposure protection listed above in cleaning up spilled chemical. Contaminated clothing and absorbent paper should be sealed inside vapor-tight, double-sealed plastic bags for eventual high temperature incineration. Wash contaminated surface areas with strong detergent and water or with the solvent listed in the safety and handling document.

### STORAGE PRECAUTIONS

Protect the glass vial from physical damage. Reseal the crimp top vial using only unperforated teflon-faced septa. Store in an explosion-proof refrigerator (5 degrees C) or freezer (-20 degrees C).

### DISPOSAL AND WASTE TREATMENT

Destroy all waste and contaminated materials in a special, high temperature (>2000 degrees F) chemical incinerator facility.

Physical Description: Colorless liquid.
Solubility: Slightly soluble in water. Very soluble in acetone.
Toxicity: Moderate.
Flammability: High . . . flash point $<$50 F.
Volatility: High . . . boiling point $<$100 C.
Stability: Unknown.

**OTHER INSTRUCTIONS**

Not specified

**Figure 12.** Safety and handling document.

**NIEHS REPOSITORY FOR MUTAGENIC TESTING**

**EMERGENCY PROCEDURES DOCUMENT**

**ALIQUOT NUMBER 785794**

**PRIMARY NAME** Trans-1,2-Dichloroethylene

**RADIAN ID** #N-000138 **CAS** #000540590 **NIOSH REGISTRY** #KV94000

**SYNONYMS**

Trans-acetylene Dichloride
NCI-C54591

**HAZARDS**

Toxic. Irritant. Suspect Carcinogen. Flammable.

**TOXICOLOGY**

Acute Toxicity: Lethal Dose in Rats (LD50 ORL-Rat). . . .770 mg/kg.

Toxic Exposure Routes: Ingestion, Inhalation, Skin Absorption.

Acute Response: Narcotic in High Concentrations, Nausea, Vomiting, Weakness, Tremor and Cramps, Dermatitis.

**CITATIONS**

SAX 4th ed., pg. 629
Merck 9th ed., no. 85
NIOSH: Suspect Carcinogen.

**PERSONAL PROTECTION**

In an emergency situation involving this chemical, all personnel must be protected from any exposure or contact with the chemical, its vapor or decomposition products.

Choose from among the following personal protection devices on the basis of their availability, the hazards of the chemical compound and the degree of risk in the emergency situation:

* An impervious full-body suit equipped with an air line respirator or a self-contained breathing apparatus, e.g. an MSA neoprene acid suit.

or

* A full-body impervious jump suit (e.g. of Tyvek [TM]), one or two pairs of gloves of neoprene, nitrile or latex rubber taped to form a seal with the jump suit, rubber boots or impervious shoe covers, an impervious hood, and most importantly, a full-face airline respirator. A full-faced or half-face (plus goggles) cartridge respirator can also be used if equipped with an organic vapor or combination organic vapor + particulate cartridge.

Refer to other instructions for special precautions or safety devices for this chemical.

**FIRE FIGHTING**

The inhalation of smoke from a fire involving this chemical is dangerous and potentially fatal. Firefighters should wear an impervious full-body suit with an air line or self-contained breathing apparatus. Extinguish fires with a dry chemical, carbon dioxide, foam or halon extinguisher. A water spray can also be used.

**SPILLS AND LEAKAGE**

Use absorbent paper to pick up small quantities of spilled material: dry paper for liquids, moistened paper for solids. Observe all measures of personal exposure protection listed above in cleaning up spilled chemical. Contaminated clothing and absorbent paper should be sealed inside vapor-tight, double-sealed plastic bags for eventual high temperature incineration. Wash contaminated surface areas with strong detergent and water or with the solvent listed in the safety and handling document.

**FIRST AID**

Skin contact - Flood skin with water from a safety shower or faucet. Remove any contaminated clothing. Wash affected skin area thoroughly with soap and water.

Eye contact - Flush eyes immediately with water from any source for 15 minutes. Remove contact lenses at once. Do not use oil or ointment in the eyes. If eyes become light sensitive, cover with a loose dressing.

Inhalation - Remove personnel to open air. Administer oxygen or artificial respiration as required.

Ingestion - If victim is convulsing or unconscious, do not attempt first aid, but transport immediately to hospital emergency room or poison control center. If victim is conscious, do not induce vomiting. Have the patient drink up to one quart of one of the following to dilute the poison and slow absorption: milk, beaten eggs or activated charcoal in water (1 gram charcoal/100 mg poison ingested). Transport immediately to medical facility for gastric lavage (stomach pumping) or emesis (induced vomiting).

Important! With any exposure and after any initial treatment, victim should be transported promptly for medical examination. Report the incident to a supervisor or company official.

**DISPOSAL AND WASTE TREATMENT**

Destroy all waste and contaminated materials in a special, high temperature (>2000 degrees F) chemical incinerator facility.

**OTHER INSTRUCTIONS**

Not Specified

**Figure 13.** Emergency procedures document.

ducting a chemical assay to verify the integrity of the material to be tested cannot be overemphasized. It is common to find that a given material does not meet the specified purity requirements or that it contains toxic or mutagenic impurities in large enough amounts to influence the test results.

The second type of analysis is "comprehensive chemical analysis." In a comprehensive analysis, all possible chemical components of a mixture are identified and quantified. This includes trace impurities which may be at parts-per-thousand or even parts-per-million levels in the test material. This is necessary because sometimes small amounts of a strongly mutagenic impurity in the chemical being tested can significantly influence the test results. A classic example is the presence of trace amounts of TCDD in the herbicide 2,4,5-T.

In the NTP, selected materials that give strongly positive mutagenic tests as well as questionable response and selected negative compounds will undergo comprehensive analyses to determine if any of the impurities may be responsible for the positive tests. If the material is a mixture, separation of the components will be attempted, and each of these then retested to determine the source of the mutagenicity. The separation techniques that are chosen must:

1. not alter the composition of the mutagenic compounds;
2. maximize conservation of all chemical components;
3. maximize separation of individual chemical components; and
4. minimize introduction of impurities.

Even if all of these objectives are met, the situation of testing synergists or cocarcinogens that are separated and therefore provide negative mutagenic tests may present itself. A program involving selected mixing and restesting would then be necessary.

Typical separation techniques commonly used at Radian include:

1. solvent extractions at one or more pH;
2. column chromatography on alumina, silica gel or Florisil;
3. thin-layer chromatography using alumina or silica gel;
4. high performance liquid chromatography;
5. gel permation chromatography;
6. ion chromatography of inorganic species;
7. gas chromatography using packed, support coated open tubular or glass capillary columns and a variety of detectors;
8. spinning band distillations; and
9. recrystallization techniques.

Usually, success in separating components of a mixture can be gained through combinations of several of the above techniques if any of them proves insufficient.

Once the components of a mixture are separated from one another, identification and quantification becomes feasible. Analytical techniques commonly used are:

1. mass spectrometry (both electron impact and chemical ionization);
2. nuclear magnetic resonance spectroscopy;
3. infrared spectrophotometry;
4. ultraviolet spectrophotometry;
5. fluorescence spectrophotometry;
6. gas chromatography with selective detectors (flame photometric, thermionic, Hall electrolytic conductivity, photoionization, thermal conductivity or mass spectrometer) and with general purpose flame ionization detectors;
7. atomic absorption spectroscopy; and
8. inductively coupled plasma emission spectroscopy.

The cornerstone of organic analyses is mass spectrometry. Likewise, the principal method of elemental analyses is ICPES. Both methods utilize computer-controlled instruments and computer-assisted analysis of the data. Although the capital investment in each instrument is extremely large, the analyses themselves are cost-effective if sufficient samples are available to utilize the instruments constantly.

## CONCLUSION

The decision to become involved with the storage and analysis of hazardous chemicals is not one to be taken lightly. The capital costs are very large, the personnel must be highly trained and the analytical challenges are great. The alternatives, to take shortcuts or use inferior facilities can be disastrous. On the positive side, however, there is a need for this kind of work to be performed. We are in the beginning phases of learning which of the thousands of chemicals we are exposed to in our highly industrialized environment are hazardous and why.

## REFERENCES

1. Nony, C. R., E. J. Treglown and M. C. Bowman. *Sci. Total Environ.* 4:155 (1975).
2. *NIOSH Registry of Toxic Effects of Chemical Substances, Volume II,* (1977). Edition.
3. *Handbook of Chemistry and Physics* 56th ed. (Cleveland OH:CRC Press, Inc., 1975-1976).
4. *The Merck Index*, 9th ed. (Rahway, NJ: Merck and Company, Inc., 1976).

5. *Dangerous Properties of Industrial Materials*, 4th ed. (New York: D. Van Nostrand Reinhold Company, 1975).
6. *Toxic and Hazardous Industrial Chemicals Safety Manual*, (Tokyo: International Technical Information Institute, 1978).
7. *The Condensed Chemical Dictionary*, 9th ed. (New York: D. Van Nostrand Reinhold Company, 1977).
8. *Aldrich Catalog Handbook of Fine Chemicals, 1979-1980, Catalog 19,* (Milwaukee, WI: Aldrich Chemical Company, 1979).
9. *Chemical Hazards of the Workplace.* (New York: J. B. Lippincott Company, 1978).
10. *Toxic Substances Control Act Chemical Substances Inventory,* U.S. Environmental Protection Agency (1979).
11. *CRC Handbook of Laboratory Safety,* 2nd ed. (Cleveland, OH: CRC Press, Inc., 1978).
12. "OSHA Carcinogen Listing" (Tentative List) Occupational Safety and Health Administration (July 1978).
13. "Environmental Mutagenic Information Center" (Toxline Subfile) (1960-Present).
14. "Environmental Teratogenic Information Center" (Toxline Subfile) (1975-Present).

# CHAPTER 28

# THE DEVELOPING ROLE OF CHEMISTRY IN TOXICOLOGY: ASPECTS OF TEST MATERIAL DEFINITION AND MECHANISM OF ACTION

**Thomas Cairns**

Food and Drug Administration
National Center for Toxicological Research
Jefferson, Arkansas

## INTRODUCTION

With the growing importance of toxicology and its implications to modern society, the basic disciplines, in combination, embrace this new interdisciplinary science and have their own importance in the reinforcement of their respective participations. Of fundamental and paramount interest is the key role that chemistry can and must play to ensure a productive subordinate or surrogate partnership. Like most interdisciplinary marriages, the strength of that new science depends wholly on the individual successes of the component disciplines.

In the last decade, the principal role played by chemistry has gained much momentum and respect, probably through quantum leaps in analytical technologies and increased awareness of precision and accuracy–terminologies that have been commonplace to analytical chemistry for a long time. It is the successful application of these advancements and principles that have permitted chemistry to develop an increased role in the arena of modern toxicology. The matrix that perhaps best defines the science of toxicology is the planning tree (Figure 1) developed at the National Center for Toxicological Research (NCTR). Such a planning tree or decision chart gives a

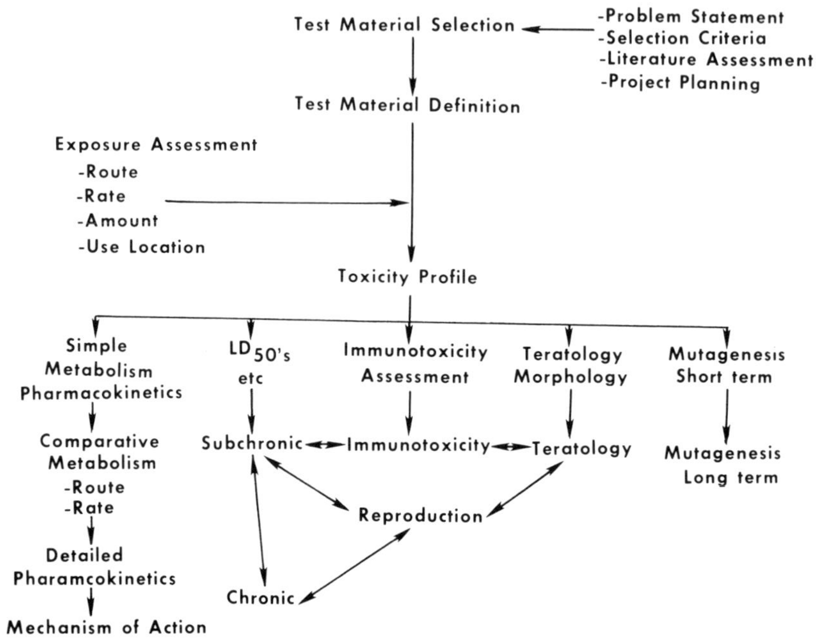


**Figure 1.** Schematic layout of toxicology planning tree.

strong indication of the complexity of the science and its implementation. Two distinct areas have been selected from this conceptual effort to illustrate the present and future roles that chemistry can and will play to provide answers and resolutions.

## TEST MATERIAL DEFINITION

Synonymous with current concepts of good laboratory practices (GLP) [1] for nonclinical studies, implications on the chemistry of the test material definition can be summarized in six important areas.

### Identity, Purity, Chemical Properties and Stability of the Test Substance

The compound 2-acetylaminofluorene (2-AAF) was a known model carcinogen selected for a 33-month study at NCTR involving 24,192 female

BALB/c mice fed 30, 35, 45, 60, 75, 100 and 150 ppm plus a control [2]. The initial 10-kg batch of 2-AAF acquired was found to be 85-90% pure. However, the impurities were volatile enough to ensure a 99.6% purity after oven-drying. This level of purity was deemed adequate for the study. During the actual 33-month study it became apparent that the initial supply of 2-AAF was inadequate for continued testing, and an additional supply had to be purchased. This new shipment of 2-AAF assayed 16.2% pure, and had this single fact gone undetected, the entire investment in the long-term study might have been lost or, even worse, erroneous data may have been reported. Subsequently, additional supplies were obtained from another source which assayed out to be 99.4% pure and hence satisfied the purity criterion.

## Handling and Storage of the Test Substance

With reference to safe handling and storage of test compounds, particularly suspected carcinogens, they are treated as if they were radioisotopes. All suspected carcinogens are handled in a glove box equipped with a HEPA filter (retains 99.1% of particles of 0.3 $\mu$m diameter or larger) and kept under reduced pressure (0.5 in. water) during operation. Only very dilute preparations of the test substances are removed from the box, as suggested by OSHA guidelines.

## Analysis of the Bioassay Supplies for Essential and/or Deleterious Ingredients

During a long-term animal experiment the integrity of the concurrent bioassay systems (diet) necessarily must conform to certain well-defined standards, both essential (Table I) and deleterious (Table II). Such analysis can also be extended to include besides the diet or chow, cardboard feeder boxes, bedding and drinking water.

**Table I. Analysis of the Bioassay Supplies: Specifications for Essential Nutrients**

| Substance | Specifications |
|---|---|
| Calcium | 0.75% min |
| Copper | 8.0 ppm min |
| Selenium | 0.05 ppm min; 0.65 ppm max |
| Zinc | 75 ppm min |
| Vitamin $B_1$ | 0.075 mg/g min; 0.125 mg/g max |
| Vitamin A | 15 IU/g min; 75 IU/g max |
| Total Fat | 4.3% min; 6.7% max |
| Total Protein | 21.0% min 28.0% max |

**Table II. Analysis of Bioassay Supplies: Acceptable Contamination Levels**

| Substance | Specifications |
|---|---|
| Aflatoxins ($B_1$, $B_2$, $G_1$, $G_2$) | 5 ppb max |
| Estrogenic Activity | 5 ppb equivalents of DES max |
| Arsenic | 1.0 ppm max |
| Cadmium | 250 ppb max |
| Lead | 1.5 ppm max |
| Mercury | 200 ppb max |
| Dieldrin | 20 ppb max |
| Heptachlorepoxide | 20 ppb max |
| Lindane | 100 ppb max |
| Malathion | 5 ppm max |
| Polychlorinated Biphenyls | 50 ppb max |
| Total DDT-Related Substances | 100 ppb max |

## Homogeneity, Stability and Proper Concentration of the Test Substance in the Dosage Form

The test substance is normally administered to the animals in either the diet or drinking water. If the compound is sufficiently soluble and stable, drinking water is the preferred route of exposure. In the case of benzidine dihydrochloride, between 50 and 500 ppm, the acidity should be maintained at pH 2 to ensure stability and thus allow ease of quantification (i.e., reduce manpower) via spectrophotofluorescence to levels of 10 mg/ml [3]. Very often, a judicious choice of matrix and method of analysis can be a cost-effective exercise.

## Safety Surveillance of Personnel and Work Areas

In studies conducted at NCTR, such as the benzidine series [3], routine monitoring of air, work areas and human urine are performed to detect any possible accidental exposure to personnel.

## Safe Disposal of the Chemical and Contaminated Experimental Material

Obviously, during normal operations of conducting nonclinical studies using mice, rats, monkeys, etc., a tremendous amount of contaminated experimental material is accumulated. To decontaminate animal cages, for example, large volumes of water are used, and the resultant waste water contains traces of all test substances currently under study. At NCTR, an adsorption system was developed to remove trace quantities of chemical carcinogens [4] from such industrial waste water. Basically, the system involved a tandem arrangement of filters, activated carbon and nonionic polymeric resin (XAD-2). It provided a highly efficient, low-cost, minimal-operation technology. The success of this pilot study has resulted in the construction of a wastewater treatment system at NCTR capable of handling 100,000 gal/day (Figure 2). Chemical surveillance has been developed [3] to ensure that no detectable levels pass through the system (i.e., sub-ppb). All contaminated solid waste, such as the spent carbon adsorbers, bedding, carcasses, diet, cardboard feeder boxes, clothing and apparatus, is burned at 900°C in a two-chamber incinerator for disposal.

As illustrated above, the implications of defining the test substance are a mammoth task involving all facets of analytical chemistry and trace analysis. It should be stressed, however, that such rationalizations ensure the integrity of the study in a serious attempt to prevent erroneous data and subsequent misinterpretation of the results.

## MECHANISM OF ACTION

The lay public and fellow scientists have long been bitter critics of the currently accepted dose level studies for in vivo carcinogenicity testing. Extrapolation of test results of high-dose (MTD) to low-dose levels and to the genetically diverse human population is an accepted regulatory posture [5]. In an attempt to explore the shape of the dose-response curve one order of magnitude lower than that previously monitored NCTR conducted the so-called ED01 study to determine the dosage necessary to produce a 1.0% tumor rate [2], as compared to current NCI bioassay screening procedures or ED10 (Table III). This exploration of one order of magnitude difference resulted in a much larger number of animals and hence resultant costs. An ED10 study (Figure III) has a price tag between $300,000 and $500,000. This dilemma has resulted in extensive research into biochemical indicators of carcinogenicity at extremely low doses, rather than conventional pathological indicators (e.g., bladder tumors). In very simple terms, via metabolic activation, certain compounds have the ability to become electrophilic or electrodeficient entities and then bind covalently to informational macromolecules (e.g., DNA, RNA, and proteins). Residues, once covalently bound, may lead to carcinogenesis and tumor formation (pathological endpoint). Such events are at the molecular level, and analytical techniques are now

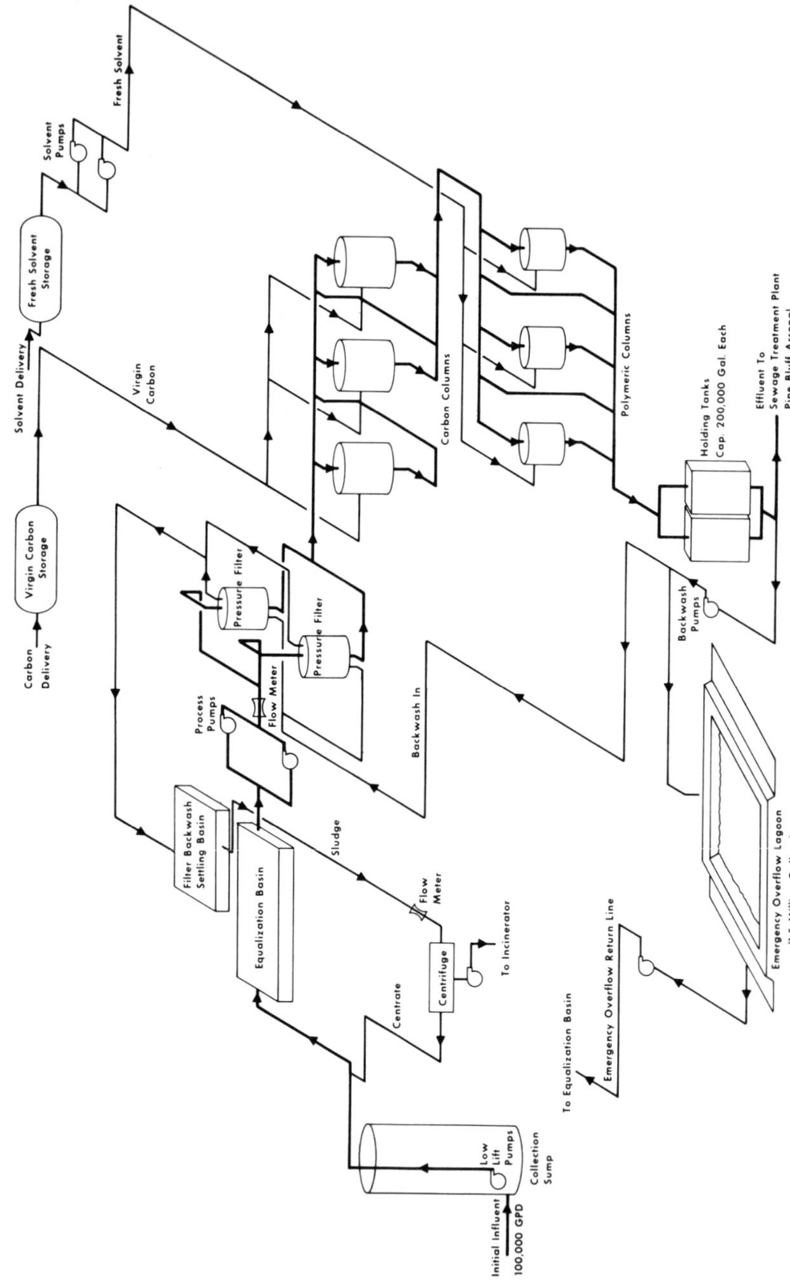


**Figure 2.** Schematic of wastewater treatment facility currently under construction.

Table III. Approximate Number of Animals Required for 95% Confidence Interval Equal to Size of the Effect (Spontaneous Background Rate = 0.01)

| | Proportion of Animals with Tumors | | | Confidence Interval (95%) | Approximate Sample Size (each) |
|---|---|---|---|---|---|
| CASE | Treated | Control | Excess | | |
| ED001 | 0.011 | 0.01 | 0.001 | ±0.001 | 80,000 |
| ED01 | 0.02 | 0.01 | 0.01 | ±0.01 | 1,100 |
| ED10 | 0.11 | 0.01 | 0.10 | ±0.10 | 40 |

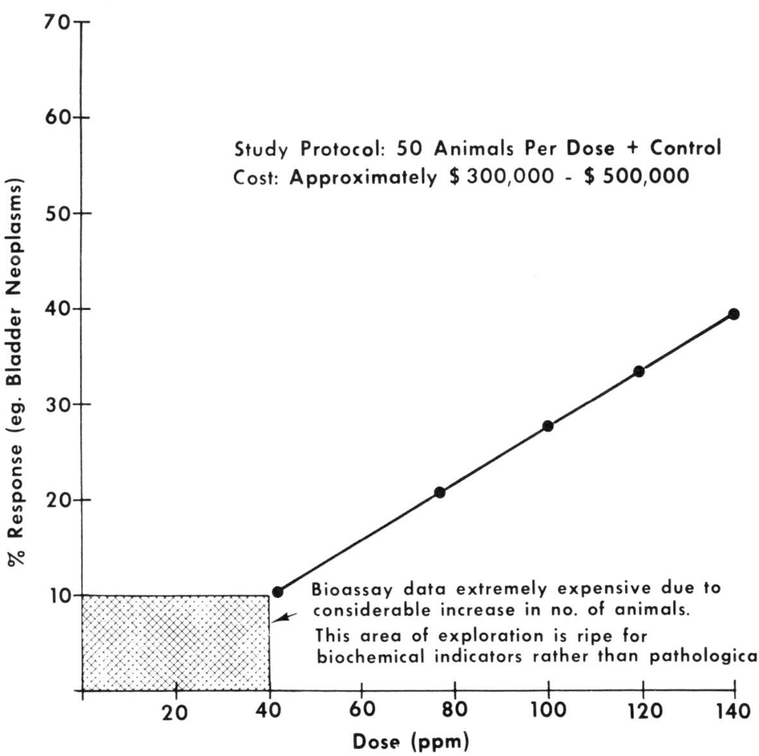


Figure 3. Typical dose-response curve from long-term bioassay protocol.

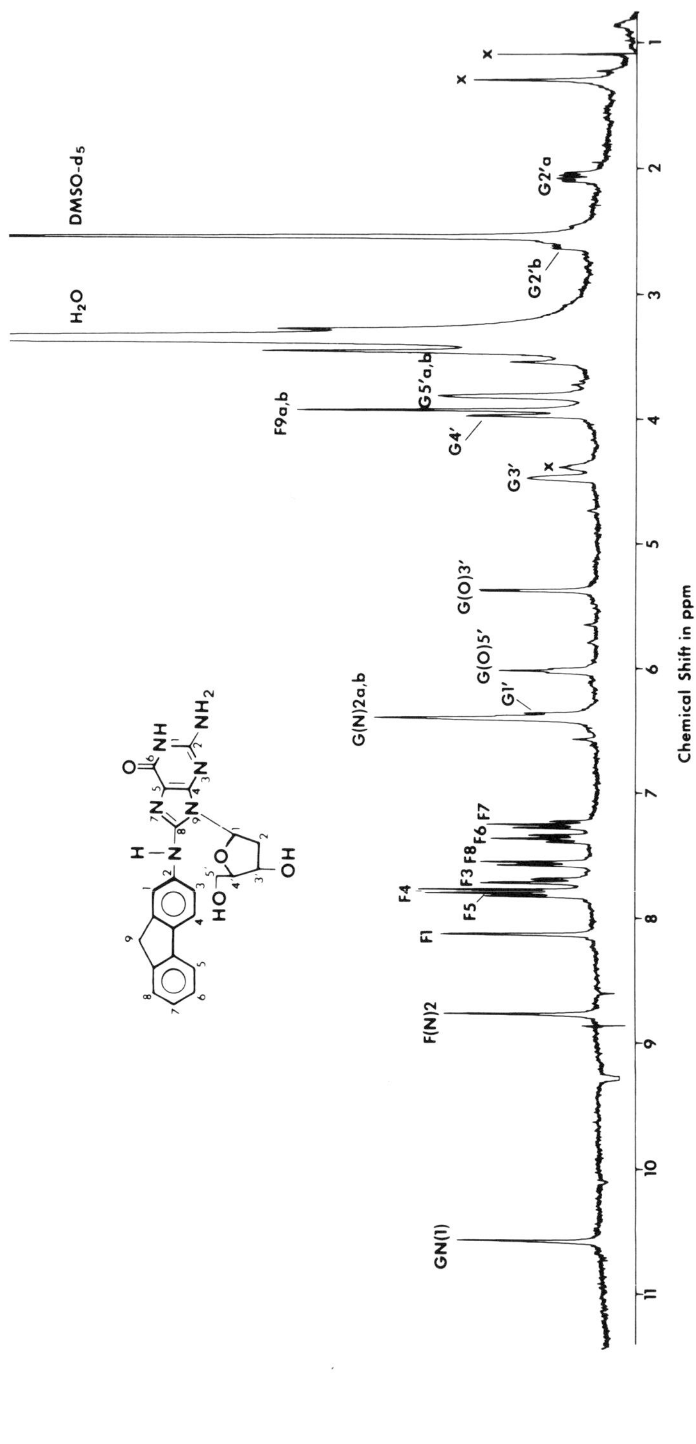


**Figure 4.** 270 MHz proton NMR spectrum of N-(deoxyguanosin-8-yl)-2-aminofluorene.

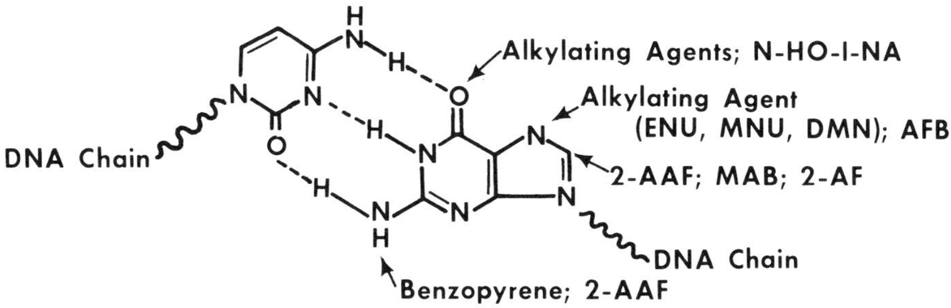


Cytosine - Guanine

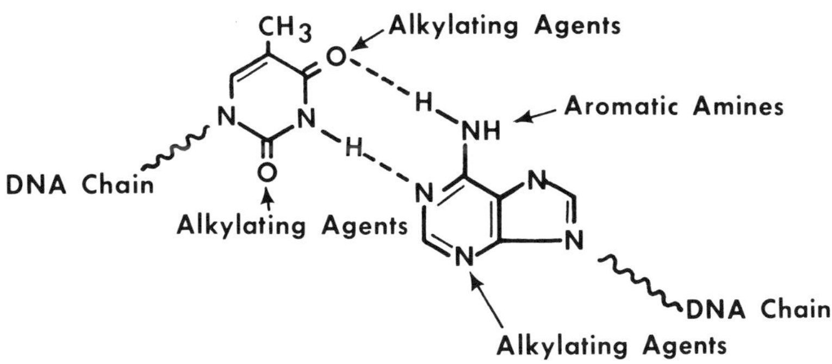


Thymine - Adenine

**Figure 5.** Sites of interaction of chemical carcinogen with DNA in vivo.

available to identify these adducts and their sites of formation. With the availability of high-resolution nuclear magnetic resonance (NMR), the site of interaction can be determined (Figure 4). Extensive studies at NCTR have resulted in a data base compiling the various possible sites of interaction [6] on the base-pairs of DNA (Figure 5). Through basic mechanism studies of this type there is hope to replace someday the expensive, time-consuming bioassay procedure with molecular event chemistry. However, it is optimistic to predict such a breakthrough in the near future. Nevertheless, it is also optimistic to continue basic biochemical studies of adduct formation in the hope of gaining insight, however slight, into the possible mode of action of carcinogens.

## CONCLUSIONS

With increased emphasis on modern toxicology, the demands on the component disciplines such as chemistry must also inevitably increase. Explorations in analytical technologies have allowed the developing role of chemistry to become extremely important in the hierarchy of toxicology and to play an ever-increasing part in the scheme of design, conduct and basic research relevant to all ramifications of the toxicology knowledge tree.

Hopefully, chemistry will continue to provide the necessary support to establish the integrity of animal studies and allow cost-effective managment of resources to achieve objectives without sacrificing the prerequisite controls.

## REFERENCES

1. "Non Clinical Laboratories Studies," *Federal Register* December 22, 1978.
2. Cairns, T. "The $ED_{01}$ Study: Introduction, Objectives and Experimental Deisgn," *J. Environ. Pathol. Toxicol.* 3(3):1-7 (1979).
3. Bowman, M. C. "Trace Analysis: A Requirement for Toxicological Research with Carcinogens and Hazardous Substances," *J. Assoc. Off. Anal. Chem.* 61(5):1253-1262 (1978).
4. Nony, C. R., E. J. Treglown and M. C. Bowman, "Removal of Trace Levels of 2-Acetylaminofluorene (2-AAF) from Wastewater," *Sci. Total Environ.* 4:155-163 (1975).
5. "Scientific Basis for Identification of Potential Carcinogens and Estimation of Risk," *J. Nat. Cancer Inst.* 63(1):245-268 (1979).
6. Kadlubar, F. F. et al. "Formation of DNA Adducts by the Carcinogen N-Hydroxy-2-Napthylamine," *J. Nat. Cancer Inst.* (in press).

# CHAPTER 29

# STRUCTURAL CORRELATES OF CARCINOGENICITY AND MUTAGENICITY AND POTENTIAL REGULATORY APPLICATIONS

**I. M. Asher and C. Zervos**

Scientific Liaison and Intelligence Staff
U. S. Food and Drug Administration
Rockville, Maryland

## INTRODUCTION

Some 25,000 chemicals are currently produced in bulk in the United States. It is the thankless, almost hopeless and nonetheless vital task of U. S. regulatory agencies such as the Food and Drug Administration (FDA), Environmental Protection Agency (EPA), and Occupational Safety and Health Administration (OSHA) to protect the public from the potential hazards of such materials. The standard methods for risk analysis place heavy reliance on data from animal models. Despite the difficulty of extrapolating from animals to humans, in vivo animal testing is still generally regarded as one of the most precise tools available for carcinogen screening, and as such forms much of the basis for FDA regulatory action.

Such bioassays are complex, lengthy, and extremely expensive. Practical limitations on facilities, funds and trained personnel clearly prohibit the full in vivo testing of all chemicals to which the public–deliberately or inadvertently–is exposed. Clearly, a way to assign testing priorities to the most critical materials is needed. The numerous factors that do–or should–impinge on such decisions, the need to quantify and assign relative weights to them, and the complexities of their interaction (Figure 1 shows only one

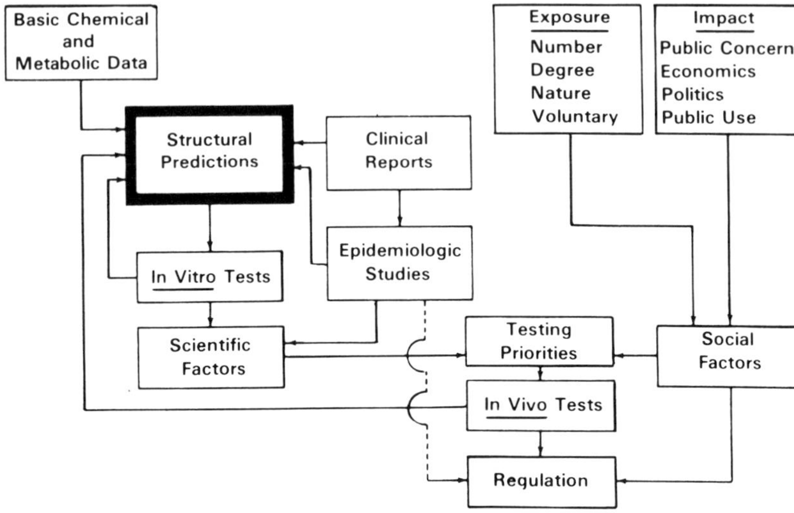


**Figure 1.** Numerous scientific and social factors impinge on the setting of testing priorities; one possible scheme is presented in this figure.

of many possible schemes) make this a difficult task. Scientific factors include the results of chemical studies, epidemiological studies and in vitro tests. Social considerations include the amount of the chemical produced, the risk of public exposure, the size and age of the exposed populations, economic impact, and the voluntary or involuntary nature of the exposure.

Recent advances in correlation analysis and pattern recognition computer programs, large accumulations of in vivo and in vitro test data and advances in understanding some of the chemical events and properties associated with carcinogenesis suggest that quantitative structure-activity relationships (QSAR) may be of significant help in this effort.

This possibility was discussed intensively at a recent FDA Science Symposium [1]. The symposium sought to clarify the state-of-the-art in QSAR and its potential usefulness as a guide to carcinogen testing priorities. Much time was also devoted to examining empirical correlations already uncovered by standard toxicological methods. It is now known, for example, that many carcinogens are highly reactive electrophiles, although many such ultimate carcinogens are the metabolic products of at-first-glance innocuous precarcinogens in the environment (liver enzymes seem particularly good at such activation). Thus, chemical features facilitating activation, transport to target sites and interaction with DNA can all be expected to be significant (Figure 2). Other important metabolic considerations involve the possible saturation of detoxification pathways—or, conversely, the triggering of defense mech-

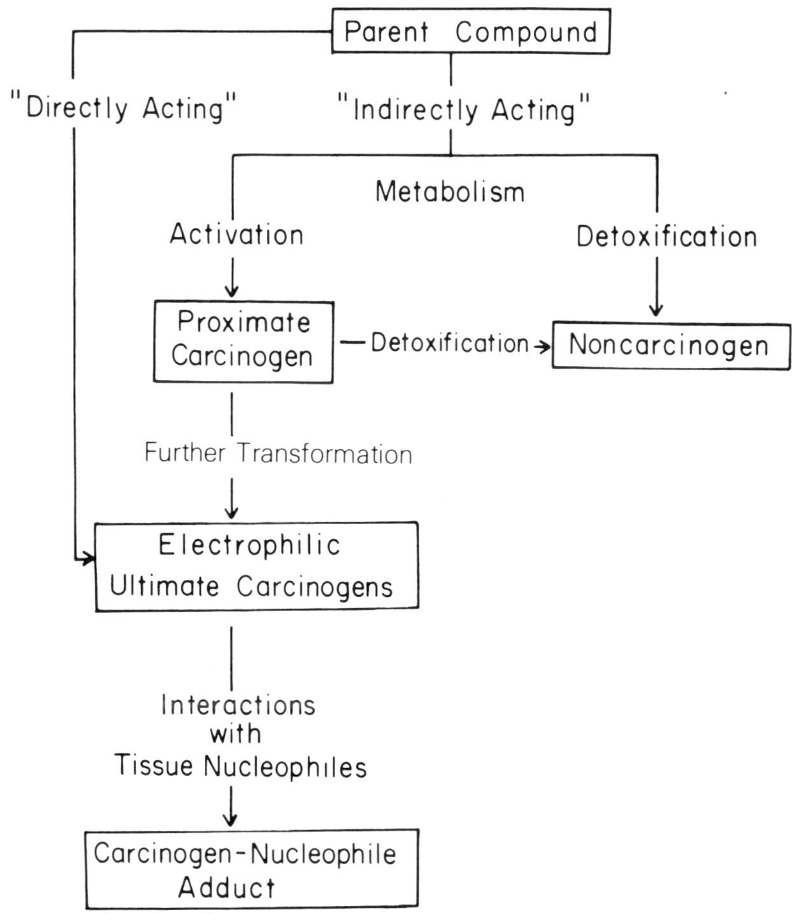


**Figure 2.** Examples of the electrophilic activation of several major classes of carcinogens.

anisms—at the high dosage levels used in animal experiments, but not at the lower levels typical of normal human exposure. From the very outset, however, one must recognize current limitations of a priori knowledge of the basic chemical events underlying carcinogenesis and the equally important limitations on the accuracy and relevance of the toxicological data available for correlation.

Of the 35 invited speakers, 11 reviewed current knowledge of the effects of chemical structure on carcinogenicity for epoxides, haloethers, polynuclear aromatic hydrocarbons (PAH), aromatic amines, nitrosamines, halogenated saturated and unsaturated hydrocarbons, hydrazines, esters, benzylic alcohols, and natural products. Space limitations prevent summarizing their informative presentations here. The remainder of this chapter will, instead, concentrate on the wide variety of mathematical approaches to correlating chemical structure and carcinogenicity. The 11 speakers in those areas emphasized Hansch, Free-Wilson and pattern-recognition techniques.

## MATHEMATICAL METHODS

### Hansch Analysis

The "Hansch" approach uses multiple regression techniques to identify a small number of appropriate empirical parameters (e.g., octanol-water partition coefficients) for use in QSAR calculations. These are simple extensions of the linear-free energy relationships (LFER) used in classical chemistry, and the required parameters can usually be calculated to the necessary accuracy using data on structural fragments. However, there are theoretical problems (Figure 3) in the wholesale extrapolation of such equilibrium-based equations as the Hammet equation:

$$\log K_i = \sigma_i + \log K_o \tag{1}$$

which describes the ionization constant of substituted benzoic acids ($K_i$) in terms of benzoic acid ($K_o$) and an appropriate substituent constant $\sigma_i$, to biological reactivity (BR) equations such as:

$$\log (BR) = \log (1/C) = a\sigma + b\,\pi + cE_s + d \tag{2}$$

based on electronic ($\sigma$), hydrophobicity ($\pi$) and Taft steric parameters ($E_s$). The reactivity is usually measured in terms of the concentration (C) of agent required to produce the desired effect (e.g., drug action, acute toxicity or carcinogenicity).

Closely related to entry and bioaccumulation mechanisms, the $\pi$-parameter has been found to be of great importance in empirical studies of drug action. It is related to the relative octanol-water partition coefficients of substituted ($P_i$) and unsubstituted ($P_o$) compounds by $\pi = \log (P_i/P_o)$. Although chosen for historical reasons, octanol-water P values are as good or better than those utilizing other solvents for most biological endpoints and test solvents examined to date. Perhaps octanol—unlike nonpolar lipids or $CHCl_3$—is a good model compound for natural lipid bilayers and carrier proteins which have both polar and nonpolar regions.

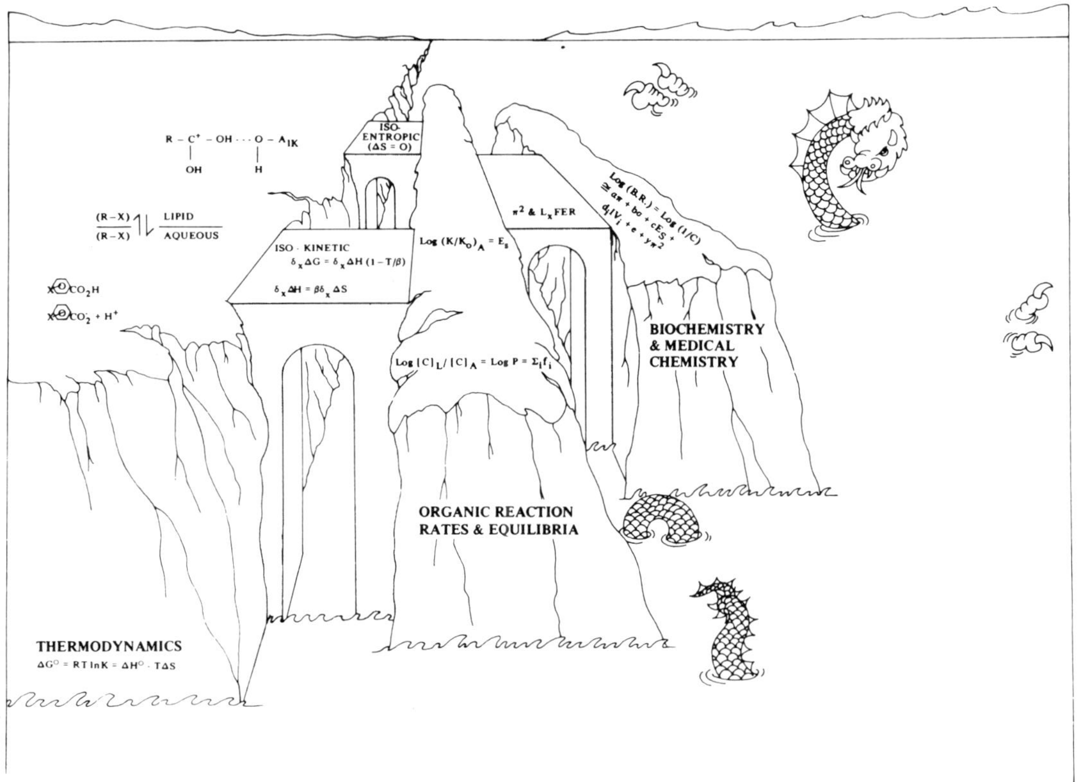


**Figure 3.** The extension of thermodynamic concepts and equations to biochemical and medical problems is not without its pitfalls.

Although sufficient for some simple cases, Equation 2, which is linear in $\pi$, cannot account for the fact that in some transport phenomena an optimal hydrophobicity is apparent. Hansch and others explained such non-linear phenomena using a kinetic model in which a series of lipid/aqueous compartments had to be traversed by the drug with partitioning occurring between each phase boundary. This can give such parabolic equations as:

$$\log (1/C) = a\sigma + b\pi + cE_s - d\pi^2 + e \qquad (3)$$

However, statistical considerations will require *over* four examples for every independent variable; thus, for Equation 3 some 20 (preferably 30) or so test compounds and their activities (expressed as C) would be required as initial input to fix a, b, c, d and e for subsequent predictions.

The initial test compounds ("input") must be chosen with care. For example, Craig reported an analysis of antimalarial phenanthrenes (Figure 4). Some 244,800 compounds were initially considered; these were later reduced to 18,000–each of which would require \$3000–4000 to test. Using 40 analogs, a simple equation based only on substituent $\pi$ and $\sigma$ values was developed. The ED50 was calculated for the two compounds of Figure 4b,c which were then synthesized and assayed. The predictions, accurate for compound 4c, were off by a factor of four for compound 4b. The problem was that the 40 analogs on which the original equation was based contained only halogen, trifluoromethyl and methoxy substituents. They did not span the parameter space, i.e., they were roughly colinear in the $\pi$, $\sigma$ plane (Figure 5). A more complete Hansch analysis utilizing 102 test compounds–some of which were in the $(+\pi, -\sigma)$ and $(-\pi, +\sigma)$ quadrants, and differentiating between substituents on the central and outside rings–has given excellent predictions for the over 200 analogs prepared and tested to date.

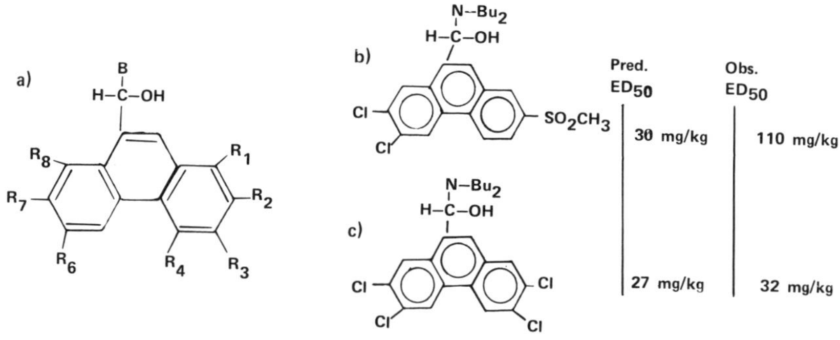


**Figure 4.** Substitutions give a large number of phenanthrenes to test for antimalarial activity. Of two phenanthrenes predicted to be active on structural grounds (Hansch analysis), the second has, in fact, only 25% the predicted activity.

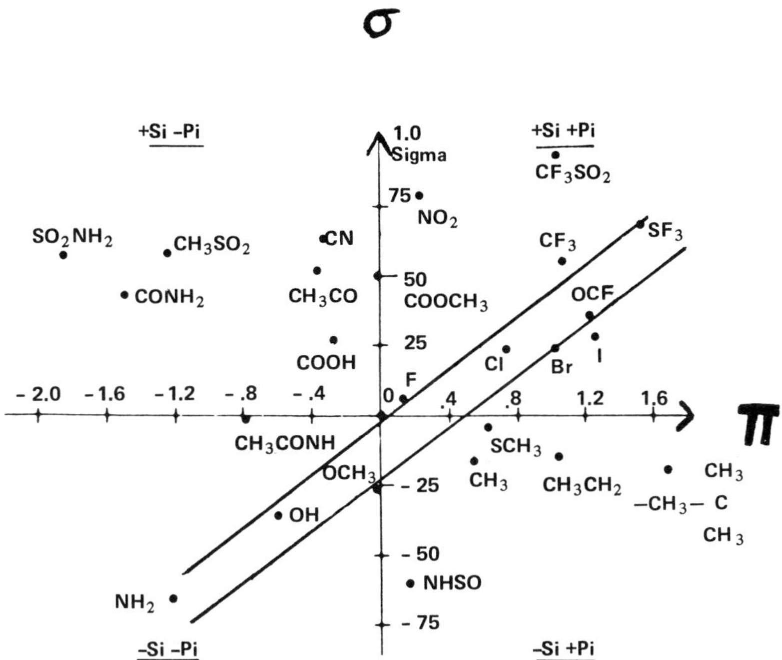


Figure 5. Two-dimensional plot of pi vs sigma constants for aromatic substituents. The constants for the particular groups used in the Hansch analysis calculation of Figure 4, lie essentially on a straight line (reproduced with permission).

## Free-Wilson Analysis

"Free-Wilson" methods assume that a substituent group makes a roughly constant contribution to biological activity every time it appears in the same substituent position. There is no assumption that any particular set of physical parameters ($\pi$, $\sigma$, etc.) are of interest. The only inputs are the biological activities of a set of N related test compounds and their chemical structure; each substituent at each available position is, in effect, an independent variable. Three or more examples are desirable for each substituent group. The N resulting equations are solved by high-speed computer to yield the substituent constants. Table I gives the results for the same set of phenanthrenes (Figure 4) examined by Hansch procedures above. Such analyses are very helpful to drug design; for example, replacing $OCH_3$ with $CF_3$ at position 6 results in a tenfold change in activity.

The Hansch and Free-Wilson approaches yield roughly equivalent results, and structural fragments arranged in the order of their substituent constants

**Table I. Results of a Free-Wilson Analysis of the Antimalarial Phenanthrenes of Figure 4[a]**

| Position | Group | No. of Examples | Substituent Constant | Range |
|---|---|---|---|---|
| $R_1$ | Cl | 3 | 0.130 | |
| | H | 39 | -0.001 | |
| | Br | 1 | -0.338 | 0.468 |
| $R_2$ | Cl | 7 | 0.301 | |
| | $CF_3$ | 1 | 0.292 | |
| | H | 35 | -0.069 | 0.370 |
| $R_3$ | $CF_3$ | 7 | 0.384 | |
| | Br | 1 | 0.296 | |
| | Cl | 10 | 0.155 | |
| | I | 1 | 0.129 | |
| | F | 2 | -01.93 | |
| | H | 22 | -0.194 | 0.578 |
| $R_4$ | Cl | 1 | 0.273 | |
| | $CF_3$ | 1 | 0.043 | |
| | H | 41 | -0.008 | 0.280 |
| $R_6$ | $CF_3$ | 18 | 0.451 | |
| | Br | 2 | 0.363 | |
| | Cl | 6 | -0.187 | |
| | F | 2 | -0.196 | |
| | H | 13 | -0.477 | |
| | $OCH_3$ | 2 | -0.570 | 1.021 |
| B | 2-Piperidyl | 13 | 0.037 | |
| | N-$Bu_2$ | 13 | 0.0142 | |
| | N-$Hept_2$ | 17 | -0.056 | 0.093 |

[a] For the overall regression, $R^2 = 0.853$, $s = 0.274$, $F = 7.83$ ($F_{24,18} = 2.7$ for 1%).

also tend to be in order relative to their $\pi$, $\sigma$ values (Table II). Combined methods, such as the Fujita-Ban method, are also becoming increasingly popular. At present, such techniques are being used successfully to predict drug activity; application to acute toxicity prediction has been more difficult, but is progressing. Can such QSAR methods be used to predict carcinogenic potential with at least sufficient accuracy to enrich significantly the positives among the chemicals selected for testing? Work is just beginning in this area. One problem is the difficulty of quantifying the results of carcinogenicity assays, as is done for acute toxicological endpoints.

**Table II. A Comparison of Hansch and Free-Wilson Results for the Phenanthrene Example**

| Group | $R_8$[a] s.c. | $\pi$ | $\sigma$ (para) | $R_6$[b] s.c. |
|---|---|---|---|---|
| $CF_3$ | 0.332 | 1.16 | 0.54 | 0.476 |
| Br | 0.223 | 0.86 | 0.23 | 0.388 |
| Cl | 0.688 | 0.71 | 0.23 | -0.118 |
| H | -0.257 | 0 | 0 | -0.431 |
| F | -0.265 | 0.14 | 0.06 | -0.159 |
| $OCH_3$ | | -0.02 | -0.27 | -0.510 |

[a] Range = 0.60.
[b] Range = 0.98.

## Pattern Recognition Methods

In many simple Hansch analyses substituent chemical groups can be characterized by their $\pi$, $\sigma$ values, and represented as a point in the $\pi$, $\sigma$ plane (Figure 5), a two-dimensional variable space. In Free-Wilson analyses, the biological activity of a compound is estimated from the sum of the activities of its chemical fragments and other structural features. Pattern recognition methods utilized multidimensional spaces defined by *large* numbers—often hundreds—of variables, each of which represents a molecular parameter (e.g., molecular weight) or the absence or presence of a given structural fragment (e.g., a 5-carbon ring). One tries to identify transformations of the space (e.g., nonlinear, eigenvector plane or discriminate plane mapping) which maximize the clustering of "toxic" and "nontoxic" compounds, and their "separation" from each other. The variables most useful for this separation can thus be identified and used for making "decisions" on the toxicity of new compounds. No a priori identification of such variables is required. All these procedures are in essence "learning" systems, in that they require the initial input of considerable numbers of compounds, of known structure and toxicity, spanning the chemical classes of interest. Such data—especially if in vitro assays are included—are becoming increasingly available.

Several different algorithms have been developed. Nonlinear mapping projects the points (chemicals) onto a plane while attempting to preserve distances, i.e., if two points are "close" to each other in the original N-dimensional space, they should remain close on some optimal two-dimensional plane. Eigenvector mapping locates the plane in N-dimensional space that minimizes the sum of all the squared distances from the points to the plane;

this requires finding the eigenvectors of the data covariance matrix. The two axes of the plane are the eigenvectors corresponding to the two largest eigenvalues. Discriminant plane mapping projects the points on a plane which enhances separation into and discrimination between two distinct data classes (e.g., "toxic" and "nontoxic" chemicals). New points falling into a given class are then assumed to share the properties of that class (Figure 6). Discrimination techniques have been expanded, using ISODATA, a clustering algorithm, which can partition the variable space into any number of disjoint subsets. After an initial partition around arbitrary "seed points," the partitioning is refined to optimize the similarities between the points in each cluster. ISODATA then gives the location, size and membership of each cluster as well as measures of the "distance" in variable space between clusters. The system can use either atom-centered fragments (as used by Chemical Abstract retrieval services) or CIDS (Chemical Informations Data System) to describe the molecular structures provided as input. A simpler pseudo-clustering algorithm SIMP is also in use, both to estimate control parameters for ISODATA or to yield limited structure-activity information. SIMP can identify all points (compounds) within any specified "distance" of any given point (compound).

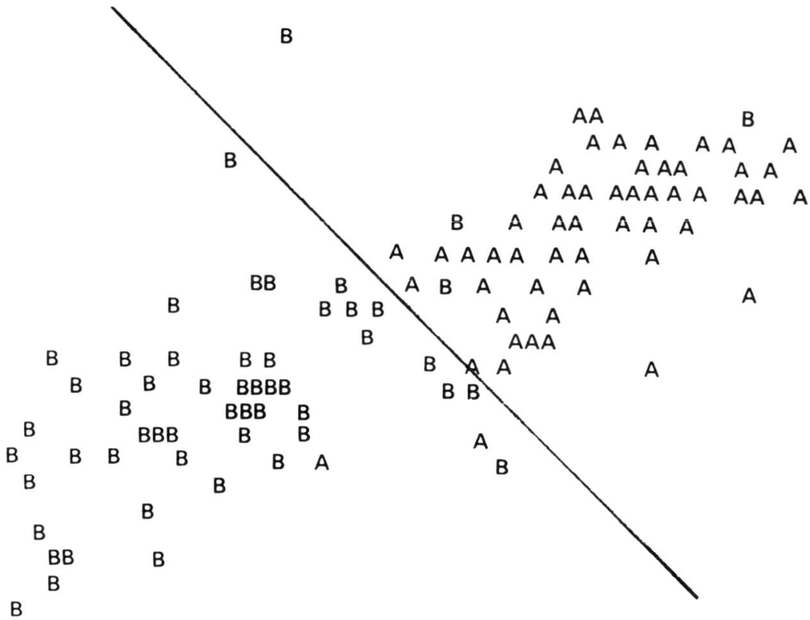

**Figure 6.** Discriminant planning mapping seeks to maximize the separability of two classes of "points" (compounds).

Using appropriate decision rules, computerized discrimination and clustering methods have provided 80-90% accuracy in discriminating "toxic" from "nontoxic" carbamates and organophosphates, and high- from low-therapeutic ratio glycolates. In one study of drug mixtures with one component from each of three different classes of drugs, ISODATA clustering led to the selection of 21 prototype mixtures that spanned the variable space. Seven of the ten most efficacious mixtures (as determined by animal tests of 168 prime candidates selected by experts) were 150 DATA prototypes. Since $(7/21) \gg (10/168) \gg (10/\text{total number of candidate mixtures})$, use of ISODATA would have considerably enriched the fraction to be tested. Can such increased testing efficiency be achieved for carcinogenesis? Again, the answer depends on the availability of appropriate data sets, and–if physicochemical as well as structural parameters are to be included–increased knowledge of chemical mechanisms relevant to carcinogenesis.

## CONCLUSIONS

There was considerable spirited discussion during and between the presentations and at special full-evening open discussion sessions [1]. Numerous examples of the application of QSAR methods to the prediction of acute toxicity and carcinogenicity were presented. The merits and limitations of each approach, their potential usefulness relative to other decision-making tools (e.g., short-term in vitro assays) and to each other, and alternative directions for further growth were energetically discussed. Some felt that current procedures are still too tightly limited to homologous series which present less of a regulatory decision-making problem than totally new or untested series of compounds: the amount of input data required leads to overreliance on in vitro data (which present several unresolved problems); and these methods are more appropriate to areas of toxicity other than carcinogenesis. Others disputed each of these points, and pointed to the considerable progress already made. Furthermore, such "QSAR-type" arguments are already being made in practice, and used by individuals disguised as "experience" or "intuition." The current availability of powerful off-the-shelf programs and the small (compared to bioassay) costs involved were also stressed. Although no agreement on technical details was reached, all agreed that this area will be undergoing rapid growth, and assuming an enhanced regulatory significance, in the years ahead.

## REFERENCES

1. Proceedings of Symposium on "Structural Correlates of Carcinogenesis and Mutagenesis. A Guide to Testing Priorities," A. M. Asher and C. Zervos, Eds., Office of Science, FDA, HEW Publication No. 78-1046 (1977).

# INDEX